Vascular Smooth Muscle in Culture

Volume II

Editors

Julie H. Campbell, Ph.D.
Head
Cell Biology Laboratory
Baker Medical Research Institute
Senior Research Fellow
National Health and Medical
Research Council of Australia
Melbourne, Victoria, Australia

Gordon R. Campbell, Ph.D.
Reader in Anatomy
Head
Cardiovascular Research Unit
Department of Anatomy
University of Melbourne
Melbourne, Victoria, Australia

CRC

CRC Press, Inc.
Boca Raton, Florida

Library of Congress Cataloging-in-Publication Data

Vascular smooth muscle in culture.

Includes bibliographies and index.
1. Vascular smooth muscle. 2. Tissue culture.
I. Campbell, Julie H. II. Campbell, Gordon R.
[DNLM: 1. Muscle, Smooth, Vascular--cytology. 2. Tissue Culture. WE 500 V3308]
QP110.V37V358 1987 591.1′16 86-30953
ISBN 0-8493-4325-9 (set)
ISBN 0-8493-4326-7 (v. 1)
ISBN 0-8493-4327-5 (v. 2)

This book represents information obtained from authentic and highly regarded sources. Reprinted material is quoted with permission, and sources are indicated. A wide variety of references are listed. Every reasonable effort has been made to give reliable data and information, but the author and the publisher cannot assume responsibility for the validity of all materials or for the consequences of their use.

Direct all inquiries to CRC Press, Inc., 2000 Corporate Blvd., N.W., Boca Raton, Florida, 33431.

International Standard Book Number 0-8493-4325-9 (Set)
International Standard Book Number 0-8493-4326-7 (Volume I)
International Standard Book Number 0-8493-4327-5 (Volume II)

Library of Congress Card Number 86-30953
Printed in the United States

PREFACE

Smooth muscle was first grown in culture in 1913/1914 by Champy,[1] Laquer[2] and Lewis and Lewis.[3] For the next 55 years, most of the reports were descriptive. However, from the late 1960s onwards, there has been an ever-increasing interest and volume of papers on cultured smooth muscle, many concerned with the vascular smooth muscle cell and its role in arterial disease. For example, in 1966, 135 papers were published on smooth muscle in culture, while in 1984, there were 847, of which 416 were specifically on vascular smooth muscle.

For these volumes we invited contributions from several of the major laboratories in the world which use cell culture as a tool to study the biology of vascular smooth muscle. These contributions cover methodology, structural and functional modulation, alterations in contractile and cytoskeletal proteins, differentiation, growth factors, growth inhibitors, collagen, glycosaminoglycan and elastin synthesis and degradation, production of prostaglandins, lipoprotein metabolism, endothelial-smooth muscle interactions, vasoactive hormone receptor expression and regulation, hypertrophy, hyperploidy, and innervation. The books thus provide a near-complete dossier of what is currently known about the vascular smooth muscle cell in culture.

Julie H. Campbell
Gordon R. Campbell
Melbourne, 1985

REFERENCES

1. **Champy, C.,** Quelques resultats de la methode de culture des tissus. I. Generalities. II. Le muscle lisse (note preliminaire), *Arch. Zool. Exp. Gen.*, 53, 42, 1913/1914.
2. **Laqueur, E.,** Zur Uberlebensdauer von Saugetierorganen mit Automatie, *Zentralbl. Physiol.*, 28, 728, 1914.
3. **Lewis, M. R. and Lewis, W. H.,** Mitochondria in tissue culture, *Science,* 39, 330, 1914.

THE EDITORS

Julie H. Campbell, Ph.D., is a Senior Research Fellow with the National Health and Medical Research Council of Australia and Head of the Cell Biology Laboratory, Baker Medical Research Institute, Prahran, Victoria, Australia.

Dr. Campbell received her B.Sc. (Hons) degree from the University of New South Wales, Sydney, Australia in 1968, and her Ph.D. degree in 1973 from the University of Melbourne, Australia. After two postdoctoral fellowships at the University of Melbourne, she was awarded the John H. Halliday Travelling Fellowship of the Life Insurance Medical Research Fund of Australia and New Zealand and further studied at University College, London, England, the University of Iowa, Iowa City and the University of Washington, Seattle, during 1976-1977. In 1978, she assumed her present position at the Baker Medical Research Institute in Melbourne, Australia.

Dr. Campbell is a member of the Australian and New Zealand Society for Cell Biology, and the Australian Society for Experimental Pathology. During 1985, she was Chairman of the Australian Atherosclerosis Group, a Committee Member for the 7th International Conference on Atherosclerosis, in Melbourne, and co-organizer for its satellite symposium "Cell Biology of the Artery Wall" held at Hamilton Island, Australia.

Dr. Campbell is the author of more than 80 papers and is coauthor of a book on cardiac muscle. Her current major research interests relate to the role of smooth muscle cells in the etiology of atherosclerosis.

Gordon R. Campbell, Ph.D., is Reader in Anatomy in the School of Medicine at the University of Melbourne, Australia. He is also Head of the Cardiovascular Research Unit within the Department of Anatomy.

Dr. Campbell received his B.Sc. (Hons) and Ph.D. degrees at the University of Melbourne in 1969 and 1974, respectively. After gaining postdoctoral experience at the University of Melbourne, University College, London, England, the University of Iowa, Iowa City and the University of Washington, Seattle, he was appointed Head, Morphology and Cell Biology Laboratory at the Baker Medical Research Institute, Prahran, Victoria, Australia in 1978. In 1980, he was appointed Senior Lecturer in the Department of Anatomy, University of Melbourne, and Reader in the same department in 1984.

Dr. Campbell is a Fellow of the Royal Society of Medicine, London, England and a member of the American Society for Cell Biology. He is also a member of the Australian and New Zealand Society for Cell Biology, the Australian Atherosclerosis Society, the Australian Society for Experimental Pathology and the Anatomical Society of Australia and New Zealand. In October 1985 he was co-organizer of an international symposium "Cell Biology of the Artery Wall" held at Hamilton Island, Australia.

Dr. Campbell is the author of more than 80 papers and the coauthor of two books on muscle structure and function. His current major research interests relate to the role of smooth muscle cells in the etiology of arteriosclerosis.

CONTRIBUTORS

R. Wayne Alexander, Ph.D., M.D.
Associate Professor of Medicine
Harvard Medical School
Cardiologist
Division of Cardiovascular Medicine
Brigham and Women's Hospital
Boston, Massachusetts

Edwin L. Bierman, M.D.
Professor of Medicine
Department of Medicine
University of Washington
Seattle, Washington

Alex Bobik, Ph.D.
Associate Director
Biochemical Pharmacology Laboratory
Alfred Hospital and Baker Medical Research Institute
Prahran, Victoria, Australia

Jacques Bonnet, M.D.
Chef de Clinique — Assistant
Department of Cardiology
Groupe Hospitalier Haut-Levêque-Xavier Arnozan
Pessac, France

Paul Bornstein, M.D.
Professor of Biochemistry and Medicine
Department of Biochemistry
University of Washington
Seattle, Washington

Daniel Bowen-Pope, Ph.D.
Research Assistant Professor
Department of Pathology
University of Washington
Seattle, Washington

H. Bricaud, M.D.
Professor of Cardiology
Chief
Department of Cardiology
Groupe Hospitalier Haut-Leveque-Xavier Arnozan
Pessac, France

John J. Castellot, Jr., Ph.D.
Assistant Professor
Department of Pathology
Harvard Medical School
Boston, Massachusetts

Alan Chait, M.D.
Professor of Medicine
Department of Medicine
University of Washington
Seattle, Washington

Peter F. Davies, Ph.D.
Associate Professor of Pathology
Department of Pathology
Brigham and Women's Hospital
Harvard Medical School
Boston, Massachusetts

B. Dorian, Ph.D.
Assistant
Unité de Recherches de Cardiologie
INSERM U8
Pessac, France

Michael A. Gimbrone, Jr., M.D.
Professor of Pathology
Brigham and Women's Hospital
Harvard Medical School
Boston, Massachusetts

David Gordon
Department of Pathology
University of Washington
Seattle, Washington

M. Daria Haust
Professor
Department of Pathology
University of Western Ontario
London, Ontario, Canada

William Hornebeck, Ph.D.
Laboratoire de Biochemie du Tissu Conjonctif
Faculte de Medicine
Universite Paris val de Marne
Creteil, France

Olli Jaakkola, M.Sc.
Assistant
Department of Biomedical Sciences
University of Tampere
Tampere, Finland

Olli-Pekka Kallioniemi, M.D.
Department of Biomedical Sciences
University of Tampere
Tampere, Finland

Morris J. Karnovsky
Professor
Department of Pathology
Harvard Medical School
Boston, Massachusetts

J. Larrue, Ph.D.
Directeur de Recherche
Unité de Recherches de Cardiologie
INSERM U8
Pessac, France

James R. A. Leushner
Department of Pathology
University of Western Ontario
London, Ontario, Canada

Richard A. Majack, Ph.D.
Research Scientist
Atherosclerosis and Thrombosis Research
The Upjohn Company
Kalamazoo, Michigan

Mark W. Majesky, Ph.D.
Postdoctoral Fellow
Department of Pathology
School of Medicine
University of Washington
Seattle, Washington

M. J. Merrilees, Ph.D.
Senior Lecturer
Department of Anatomy
University of Auckland
Auckland, New Zealand

Richard A. Murphy, Ph.D.
Professor of Physiology
Department of Physiology
University of Virginia School of Medicine
Charlottesville, Virginia

Seppo Nikkari, M.D.
Department of Biomedical Sciences
University of Tampere
Tampere, Finland

Tapio Nikkari, M.D.
Professor
Department of Biomedical Sciences
University of Tampere
Tampere, Finland

Susan E. O'Connor
Department of Pathology
Brigham and Women's Hospital
Harvard Medical School
Boston, Massachusetts

John F. Oram, Ph.D.
Research Assistant Professor
Department of Medicine
University of Washington
Seattle, Washington

Gary K. Owens, Ph.D.
Assistant Professor
Department of Physiology
University of Virginia School of Medicine
Charlottesville, Virginia

Kari Pietilä, M.D.
Special Lecturer
Department of Biomedical Science
University of Tampere
Tampere, Finland

Leslie Robert, M.D., Ph.D.
Director of Research
Laboratoire de Biochimie du Tissu Conjonctif
Faculte de Medicine
Universite Paris val de Marne
Creteil, France

Russell Ross, Ph.D.
Professor and Chairman
Department of Pathology
University of Washington
Seattle, Washington

Arthur S. Rovner, Ph.D.
Postdoctoral Fellow
Department of Physiology
University of Virginia School of Medicine
Charlottesville, Virginia

Stephen M. Schwartz, Ph.D.
Associate Professor
Department of Pathology
University of Washington
Seattle, Washington

George A. Truskey, Ph.D.
Assistant Professor of Chemical Engineering
Department of Chemical Engineering
Tufts University
Medford, Massachusetts

TABLE OF CONTENTS

Volume I

Volume II

Chapter 11

BIOSYNTHESIS AND DEGRADATION OF ELASTIN

W. Hornebeck and L. Robert

TABLE OF CONTENTS

I. INTRODUCTION

The extracellular matrix (EM) comprises macromolecules belonging essentially to four different families: collagens, elastin(s), proteoglycans, and structural glycoproteins. Phylogenetically speaking, elastin is the "youngest" of these macromolecules. Collagen, as well as certain structural glycoproteins, appears from the very first metazoans, the sponges;[1,2] proteoglycans are found in invertebrates,[3] but elastin appears only from the vertebrates such as fishes.[4]

The connective tissue protein elastin is mainly responsible for maintaining the elasticity of major blood vessels, lung tissue, and the dermis; indeed, the elastic fiber can be extensively deformed and yet return to its original conformational state.[5] Although the soluble precursor of elastin(s) is very susceptible to degradation by many proteinases,[6] mature elastin possesses a low turnover rate. Some physiological events, such as growth and pregnancy, are accompanied by elastic fiber lysis. However, the rate of elastin degradation is considerably accelerated under a variety of pathological conditions, such as emphysema and atheroarteriosclerosis.[7,8] Obviously, agents which are implicated in these destructive changes will play a major role in the pathogenesis of these diseases.[8,9]

Elastin was first isolated at the end of the 19th century through its very strong resistance to physical and chemical aggressions. Still today, the easiest method for purifying elastin consists of boiling the defatted and salt-extracted tissues in 0.1 *M* NaOH for 45 min.[10,11] The residual material obtained by this treatment is composed essentially of a fibrous mass that is designated as "elastin" but still contains some associated glycoprotidic and lipidic substances.[12,13]

The richest source of elastin is bovine ligamentum nuchae (~80%), but other tissues such as aorta, lung, skin, and elastic cartilage also contain appreciable amounts of this macromolecule. The amino acid composition of elastins purified by the above procedure or by milder treatments are shown in Table 1. They consist essentially of aliphatic, hydrophobic amino acids and only a small proportion of polar amino acids.

Most of the dicarboxylic amino acids are found in the amidated form in purified elastin,[14] and a large proportion of the lysine residues are engaged in cross-links as lysinonorleucine[15] and desmosines, first discovered by Thomas et al.[16] Together with these crosslinks, the hydrophobic interactions could be considered as the main stabilizing forces of elastic fibers, conferring on them their great resistance to physical and chemical agents. We originally demonstrated in the early 1960s that this great resistance to the degradation by alkali ions is dramatically decreased in the presence of organic solvents.[17,18] The resulting soluble elastin peptides (κ-elastin) can be easily analyzed and provide a useful tool for studying the properties and structure of elastin.[8,19] Another method for "solubilizing" elastin was designed by Partridge et al.[20] It consists of boiling fibrous elastin in 0.25 *M* oxalic acid until solubilization. This solution was designated as α-elastin and the lower-molecular-weight fractions as β-elastin.

However, the isolation of a soluble precursor form of elastin (e.g., tropoelastin from animals such as pigs and calves maintained on a copper-deficient diet) was a major breakthrough in elastin research as it provided a way to understanding the biosynthesis and structure of the precursor of elastin.[21] Tropoelastin(s) is a single polypeptide chain of about 800 amino acid residues (68 to 70 kdaltons).[22]

II. BIOSYNTHESIS OF ELASTIN

A. General Considerations

A sheep elastin cDNA clone was recently isolated and characterized.[23] It was found to hybridize to a single 3.5 kb mRNA species upon blot hybridization. Similar-sized

Table 1
AMINO ACID ANALYSIS OF SEVERAL ELASTIN SAMPLES PURIFIED FROM VARIOUS TISSUES (EXPRESSED AS RESIDUES PER 1,000)

Amino acid	Bovine ligamentum nuchae	Human aorta: Nonpathological state	Human aorta: Marfan syndrome	Human breast cancer
Hydroxyproline	8.1	10	35	12
Aspartic acid	5.8	8	30	25
Threonine	9.3	7	23	18
Serine	8.7	9	23	8
Glutamic acid	15.4	17	59	43
Proline	115.5	104	113	118
Glycine	238.1	324	304	307
Alanine	227.0	224	165	219
Valine	131.6	143	70	103
Half cysteine	0.0	0.0	0.0	0.0
Methionine	0.0	0.0	10	2.0
Isoleucine	23.9	27	23	25
Leucine	59.4	65	50	54
Tyrosine	5.9	9	12	3
Phenylalanine	29.3	26	25	22
Hydroxylysine	0.0	0.0	0.0	0.0
Lysine	3.3	5	22	25
Histidine	0.5	1.0	8.0	1.0
Arginine	5.8	5.0	3.0	9.0
Amide	16.6	ND	ND	ND
Aldol condensation products	4.3	ND	ND	ND
Dehydrolysinonorleucine	0.0	ND	ND	ND
Lysinonorleucine	2.2	ND	ND	ND
Dehydromerodesmosine	0.2	ND	ND	ND
Merodesmosine	0.5	ND	ND	ND
Isodesmosine[a]	5.4	4	3	2.5
Desmosine[a]	10.1	18	5	3.0

Note: ND, not determined.

[a] Expressed as lysine equivalents.

From Jacob, M. P. and Hornebeck, W., *Frontiers of Matrix Biology,* Vol. 10, S. Karger, Basel, 1985, 92. With permission.

mRNAs were also identified from chick aorta mRNA preparations.[24] It is now generally assumed that tropoelastin polypeptides are synthesized on membrane-bound polyribosomes and discharged into the lumen of the endoplasmic reticulum by the cotranslational removal of a signal peptide.[22,25,26] The primary sequence of the leader peptides have been completed in the chick and in the sheep;[22] double residues were found at a few locations in the sheep leader peptide sequence, suggesting that two types of elastin may exist. Indeed, Karr and Foster[27] identified two tropoelastin chains designated as "a" (molecular weight = 73 kdaltons) and "b" (molecular weight = 70 kdaltons), which could be differentiated by immunological techniques using monoclonal antibodies as probes.[27]

These elastin types may be somehow associated with the developmental maturation of the animals. Also, it was found that aortic tissue contains a high proportion of tropoelastin b, whereas lung tissue possesses approximately equal amounts of the two forms. In the two tissues, elastin mRNAs coding for both tropoelastin a and b were found. However, the presence of two elastin genes remains controversial. Another hypothesis (still to be verified) is that alternative splicing of the primary transcript of one single and complicated gene could result in several mRNAs and translation products, as was demonstrated for the fibronectin gene.[30] Since the amino acid composition of elastin is rather peculiar, as far as it is poor in polar amino acids, such small differences at critical sites in the peptide chain could not be easily detected. This hypothesis remains compatible with the progressive increase in the "polar" components of the elastic fibers of human aorta with age and atherosclerosis.[31] The compositional changes during maturation and aging could be explained by an increasing ratio of microfibrils being crosslinked, e.g., through free radical mediated processes to the elastic fibers consisting of tropoelastin polymers. This hypothesis will need experimental confirmation.

The hydroxylation of proline residues (at the fourth position) and the oxidative deamination of lysine residues are the two main posttranslational events of the biosynthesis of elastin. These reactions are catalyzed by the enzymes prolyl hydroxylase and lysyl oxidase.[32-35]

In contrast with collagen biosynthesis, the hydroxylation of proline residues in tropoelastin molecules is not a prerequisite of the secretion of the precursor form of elastin.[36] Also, it does not play a crucial role in stabilizing the elastin structure. In contrast, it was demonstrated that the overhydroxylation of synthetic model peptides of elastin results in an increase of the coacervation temperature.[37] We also showed conclusively that over-proline hydroxylated elastin samples purified from pathological aortas (Marfan syndrome, aneurysms) presents a higher sensitivity to hydrolysis catalyzed by porcine pancreatic elastase.[38] These results point towards a destabilizing effect of the hydroxylation of certain proline residues in the elastin structure.

B. Role of Microfibrils

As a result of detailed electronmicroscopical studies,[12,39-42] it became apparent from the mid-1960s that elastic fiber formation occurs on a microfibrillar scaffolding. The microfibrillar component can be visualized by contrasting procedures (Figure 1) whereby the depositing elastic material appears translucent to electrons. It was also shown by Ross and Bornstein[41] and Robert and co-workers[12] that with maturation and aging the microfibrillar components of elastic fibers decrease and the amorphous component, consisting apparently of crosslinked elastin, increases. These microfibrils, however, never completely disappear, and even the roughest treatment such as boiling in 0.1 *M* sodium hydroxide cannot eliminate them completely.[10,11]

We postulated several years ago that the microfibrillar material deposited by the mesenchymal cells engaged in elastin biosynthesis serves for the guidance of the ordered ("vectorial") deposition of tropoelastin molecules.[8,12] Figure 2 depicts the hypothesis that electrostatic forces between the negatively charged glycoprotein microfibrils and the positively charged tropoelastin(s) (containing about 47 lysine residues per thousand residues) would be sufficient to ensure the interaction between the two EM components and that the properly orientated tropoelastin is extensively crosslinked (see later). It must be mentioned, however, that similar or identical microfibrillar material has been identified in many different connective tissues[13,43] and is not always accompanied by the deposition of elastin.

The oxytalan fibers originally described by Fullmer and Lilly[44] and recently quantitatively studied in many tissues in our laboratory using morphometric procedures also correspond to such microfibrillar components of elastin-rich tissues. It must be pointed out, however, that they are also present in most other connective tissues such as ten-

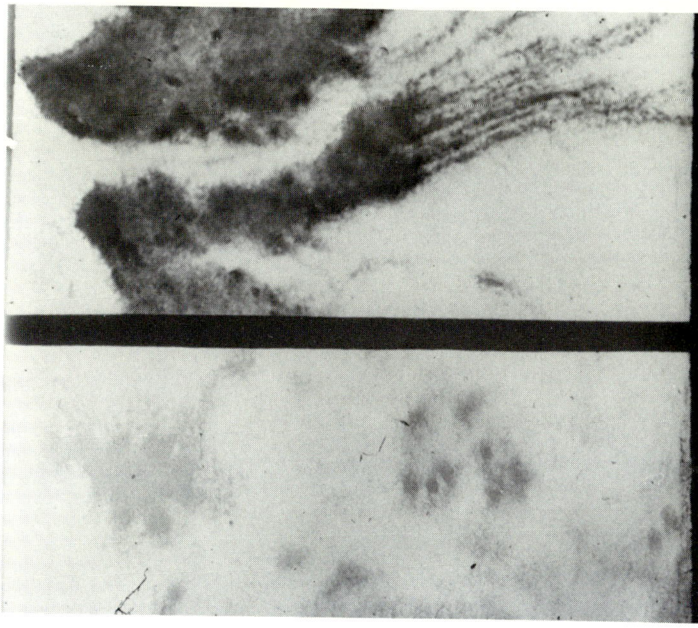

FIGURE 1. Structural relationship between the microfibrils (mf) and the amorphous elastin (E). Uranyl acetate + Pb. (Magnification × 31,000.) (From Kadar, A., *Frontiers of Matrix Biology: Biology and Pathology of Elastic Tissues*, Vol. 8, Robert, A. M. and Robert, L., Eds., S. Karger, Basel, 1980, 54. With permission.)

don, ligament, fascia, gingiva, etc.,[45,46] suggesting, therefore, that elastogenesis may not always proceed to completion.

Lysyl oxidase plays a crucial role in elastin biosynthesis by oxidizing peptidyl lysine in tropoelastin(s) to peptidyl ε-aminoadipic δ-semi aldehyde, the reactive precursor to the covalent crosslinkages of the EM component. This enzyme contains copper in its active site and requires also molecular oxygen and pyridoxal phosphate as cofactors. It was recently purified and characterized by Kagan et al.[34] and Harris et al.,[35] and its composition appears to be quite similar to that of the structural glycoprotein microfibrils (sgpmf) associated with elastin. It is not unreasonable to assume that it may well be part of (or strongly associated with) the microfibrillar assembly, and also that its action can be strictly localized in space on selective lysine residues as represented in Figure 2, resulting in a unidimensional crosslinking of tropoelastin subunits.[8]

It was also shown that the interaction between tropoelastin and lysyl oxidase is markedly influenced by amphiphilic substances known to bind strongly to elastin.[34] As an example, fatty acids and bile salts can completely inhibit the oxidation of lysine in elastin catalyzed by lysyl oxidase. It has to be pointed out that identical anionic amphiphilic ligands have an opposite effect on the degradation of elastin by elastase-type proteases.

Careful electron microscopic investigations by Gotte et al.[47] and physicochemical studies by Urry[48] strongly support a fibrillar structure for elastin obtained through the unidimensional cross-linking of vicinal tropoelastin molecules. Part of the sequence of tropoelastin from porcine aorta was established by Sandberg and co-workers[49] and was shown to contain two families of repeating units: the family of the tetra-, penta-, or hexapeptides, which contain exclusively glycine, proline, and valine as amino acids, as well as the polyalanine family (Figure 3). Synthetic high-molecular-weight elastin

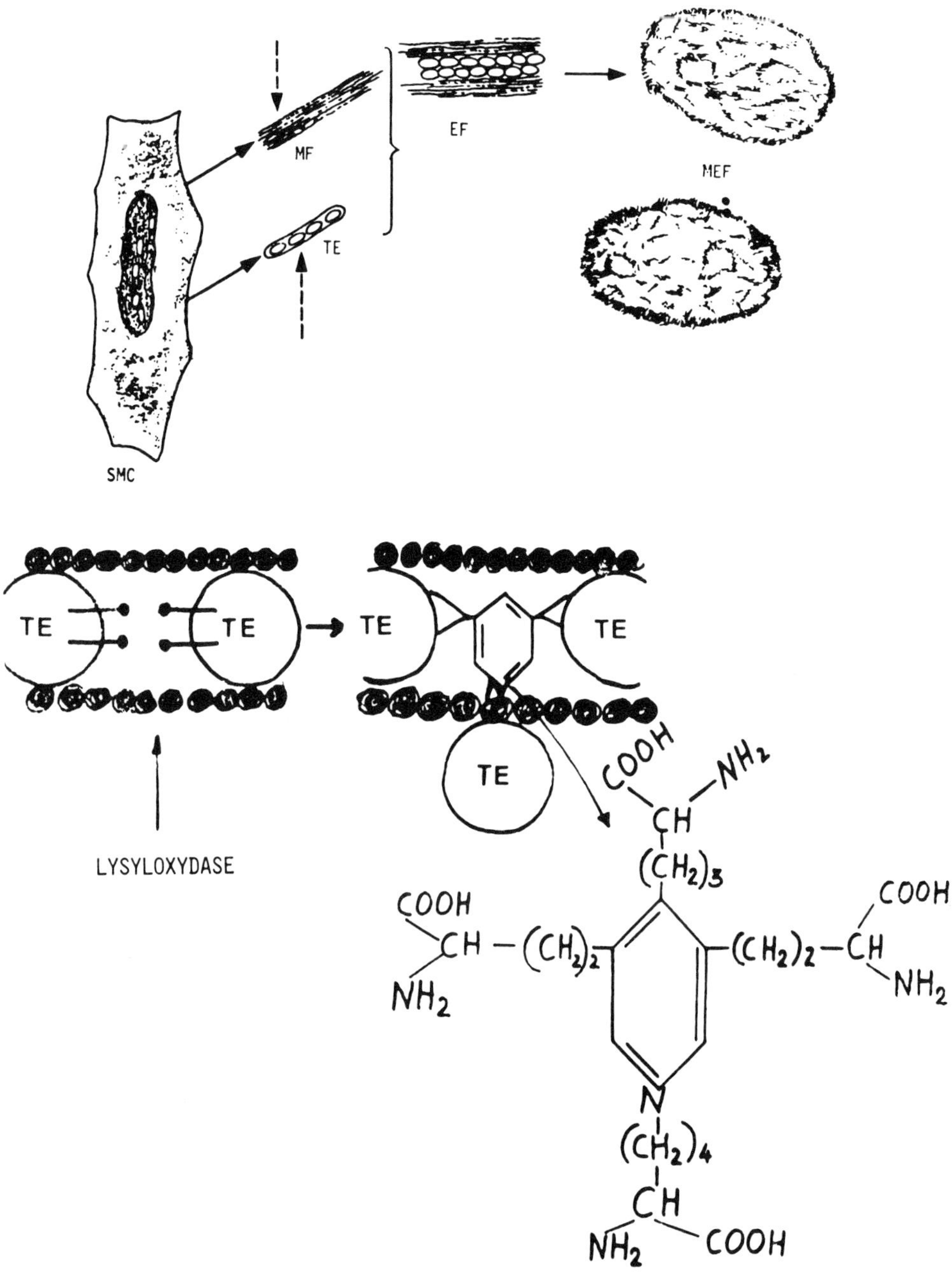

FIGURE 2. Schematic representation of elastogenesis. SMC synthesizes structural glycoprotein-microfibrils (sgp-mf) (a) and also tropoelastin. These two types of molecules interact to form first the young elastic fiber, which then become mature elastic fibers.

models obtained by the polymerization of the penta- or hexapeptide subunits result in a fibrous material with similar hydrophobic elastic properties such as native elastin. Fibrillogenesis can also be obtained from such synthetic peptides and also from peptides derived from alkaline and/or acid hydrolysis of insoluble elastin.[50] These investigations, which are described in detail elsewhere, led to the proposition by Gotte et al.[47] and Urry[48] of an essentially fibrous structure for elastin consisting mainly of β-

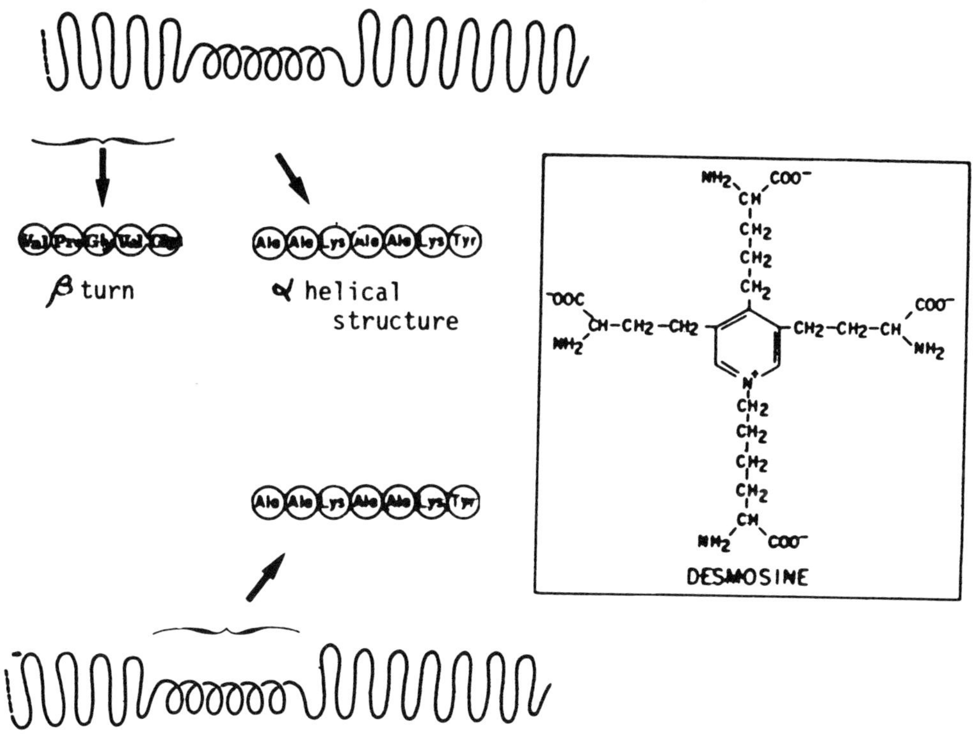

FIGURE 3. Proposed model of elastin structure. Elastin is composed of two parts: a β-turn region enriched in apolar residues and α-helical area which contains polyalanine-lysine sequences. These α-helical structures are the site of crosslinks (desmosine and isodesmosine) formation.

turns and interspaced α-helical sequences. The α-helical sequence enriched in alanine and lysine residues is involved in the crosslinking process; the β-turn containing sequences play an important role in the hydrophobic elasticity of elastin.[51]

C. Biosynthesis of Elastin by Smooth Muscle Cells

As the major arteries such as aorta are the richest tissues in elastin in the organism, and as the major constituents of the media of the aorta are smooth muscle cells (SMC), it is logical to assume that these cells are actively engaged in elastin biosynthesis. This was conclusively demonstrated by several investigators when in vitro culture systems for SMC were developed. Cultured SMC synthesize appreciable amounts of extracellular matrix, which contains elastic fibers with the typical ultrastructural and morphological appearance. Biosynthetic experiments have also been carried out using radioactive precursors that become incorporated into elastin synthesized by SMC.

Early studies were performed using aorta explants in organ culture whereby the media of newborn, young, and adult rabbits were dissected under sterile conditions, eliminating the endothelium and the adventitia. The media was cut into 1 mm^3 fragments and incubated in Eagle's minimum essential medium for 4 to 24 hr at 37°C in the presence of radioactive precursors such as ^{14}C lysine or ^{3}H glucosamine.[52] After sequential extraction of the macromolecules of the thoroughly washed explants, elastin could be isolated that contained radioactive desmosine derived from ^{14}C lysine added to the medium. It is interesting to notice in these experiments that the highest specific activity of desmosine was found in a fraction of elastin which could be solubilized by 4 *M* guanidinium. This finding is in favor of the contention that crosslinking of elastin occurs progressively on tropoelastin molecules aligned on a microfibrillar scaffolding.

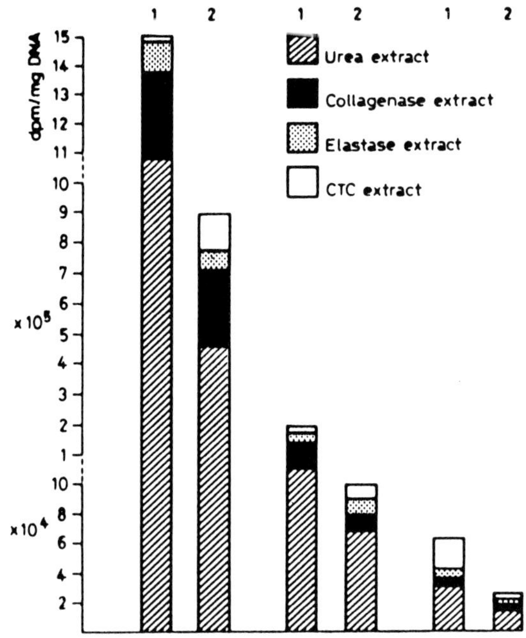

FIGURE 4. Incorporation of ^{14}C lysine (1) and ^{3}H glucosamine (2) in rabbit aorta kept in organ culture. Newborn (a), young 400-g rabbit (b), adult rabbit (2.5 to 3.5 kg) (c), 3 days incorporation in organ culture conditions. The radioactivity in the extracts is expressed as dpm/mg DNA. The calcium chloride extract contains diffusible macromolecules. The 6 *M* urea-0.1 *M* mercaptoethanol extract contains the structural glycoproteins, proteoglycans, and some collagen and elastin oligomers. The collagenase extract contains most of the polymeric collagen, and the elastase extract contains the polymeric elastin. (From Moczar, M., Ouzilou, J., Courtois, Y., and Robert, L., *Gerontology,* 22, 461, 1976. With permission.)

Under these conditions, one should observe partially crosslinked tropoelastin subunits. Such tropoelastin oligomers could have been extracted with the guanidinium solvent, and could explain the high specific activity of this guanidinium-extractable desmosine. The guanidinium insoluble elastin fraction also contained radioactive desmosine at a lower specific activity, which can be attributed to the fact that the freshly synthesized crosslinked tropoelastin oligomers are progressively incorporated in the strongly crosslinked fibrillar elastin that resists extraction with 4 *M* guanidinium.

Figure 4 shows one essential finding made during these studies: i.e., the strong decrease in the incorporation of lysine and glucosamine into matrix macromolecules of rabbit aorta with the age of the animal. As the results are expressed as dpm/mg DNA, these experiments suggest a decreasing biosynthetic activity of aorta SMC after the completion of the ontogenetic process in the rabbit aorta.

Nevertheless, even in the adult animal, a measurable incorporation of lysine into desmosines could be demonstrated. Similar results were obtained with the incorporation of glucosamine into glycosaminoglycans and glycoproteins. The figure shows also that the highest incorporation both of lysine and glucosamine in the newborn rabbit aorta explants was obtained in a 1 *M,* $CaCl_2$-soluble glycosaminoglycan and glycoprotein-rich extract. It appears, therefore, that the major biosynthetic activity of the young, developing aorta SMC concerns glycoproteins and glycosaminoglycans. A small fraction of this incorporation is directed towards polymeric collagen and elastin. This fraction increases somewhat in the young, growing animals and becomes even more important in adults, although the total biosynthetic activity decreases.

In these same experiments, SMC were cultured from explants of newborn and adult rabbits and the incorporation of lysine and glucosamine studied in the fourth serial subculture. No decrease of the total incorporation into matrix macromolecules recovered from the medium or cell layer could be demonstrated, although qualitative differences affecting mainly structural glycoproteins were observed.

This difference between the explant culture experiments and the cell culture experiments clearly shows the importance of cell-matrix interactions in the regulation of biosynthetic activity of SMC. It also suggests that SMC derived from explants may not be representative in some respects to the biosynthetic activity of whole aorta.

The biosynthesis of elastin by SMC was also extensively studied by Franzblau and Faris,[53] who demonstrated that long-term cultures of rabbit aortic SMC at the second passage continue to accumulate elastin over a period of several weeks. They also pointed out the low content of desmosine and isodesmosine in aortic SMC cultures and suggested that an additional enzymatic oxidation, not functional in cell cultures, was necessary to achieve the complete crosslinking of elastin.

Also reported in the literature were many experiments with different cell types or with embryos. For these reasons, we will briefly mention only some of them. Of significance, for example, Shibahara et al.[54] reported that the elastin production in developing fetal lung is partly modulated by the quantity of available translatable elastin mRNA present in the tissue.

It was conclusively shown by Lenny et al.[55] that SMC grown on elastic fibers are induced to secrete more EM components when these fibers are subjected to continuous stretch and relaxation. The recent studies of Gardner et al.[56] confirm that blood pressure strongly influences the rate of elastin biosynthesis. They studied the net accumulation of aorta elastin in the chick from day 1 to 14 posthatching and found that deoxycortisone acetate plus dietary NaCl causes a significant increase in protein synthesis in the aorta. In contrast, the administration of a sympathetic nerve poison, 6-hydroxydopamine, known to decrease the blood pressure and depress heart rate, causes a marked reduction in elastin accumulation.

Other significant experiments by Mecham and co-workers[57,58] showed that undifferentiated (nonelastin-producing) bovine ligament fibroblasts from early gestation animals initiate elastin synthesis when grown on EM substratum prepared from late gestation ligamentum nuchae rich in elastin. From these experiments, it appears that cell matrix interactions play a crucial role in the process of differentiation and probably even more in the maintenance of a differentiated phenotype for elastin synthesizing cells. In this respect, Frish and Werb[59] have recently observed that changes in cell shape may regulate elastin gene expression in rat aortic SMC. In elastic tissues such as blood vessels which are comprised of different cell types, the various EM components could interact to play a regulatory role in directing differentiation.[60]

III. DEGRADATION OF ELASTIN BY ELASTASES

The degradation of elastin can be observed with aging and is strongly accelerated during the atherosclerotic process in the arterial wall and during the development of emphysema in lung alveoli.[7,8] Several skin diseases are also accompanied by a strong local elastolysis.[61] Degradation seems to be accelerated by the interaction of elastin with lipids, mainly fatty acids and cholesterol esters.[8] It was shown by in vitro and in vivo experiments that such lipids have a high affinity for mature elastic fibers[62] (Table 2). It was also shown that calcium salts interact strongly with elastin; according to

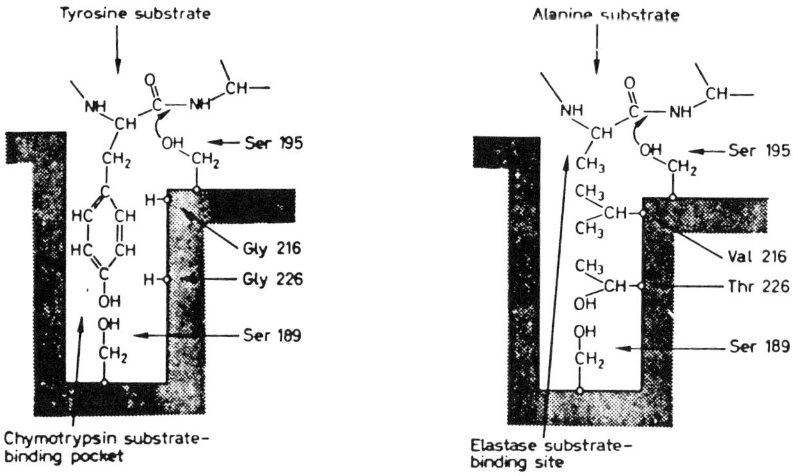

FIGURE 5. Cholesterol bound by insoluble elastin (a) and by soluble elastin peptides (b) as a function of cholesterol concentrations. (a) Insoluble elastin: in presence of sodium ions (0.18 *M)* at 37°C during 72 hr, in presence of calcium ions (0.06 *M)* at 37°C during 72 hr, in presence of sodium ions (0.18 *M)* at 65°C during 72 hr, in presence of calcium ions (0.06 *M)* at 65°C during 72 hr; (b) soluble κ-elastin: in presence of sodium ions (0.18 *M)* at 37°C during 72 hr (the solutions are then allowed to coacervate at 65°C), in presence of calcium ions (0.06 *M)* at 37°C during 72 hr (the solutions are then allowed to coacervate at 65°C). (From Jacob, M. P., Hornebeck, W., and Robert, L., *Int. J. Biol. Macromol.*, 5, 275, 1983. With permission.)

Urry,[48] this could be due to the fact that the β-turns of elastin represent natural chelating sites for calcium ions. It was further demonstrated that the interaction between elastin and lipids is potentiated by the presence of calcium ions.[63,64]

Figure 5 shows the results of an experiment in which the transfer of ^{14}C cholesterol from taurodeoxycholate micelles to fibrous and kappa-elastin was studied. The uptake of ^{14}C choleterol by fibrous elastin was quantitated by centrifugation and washing of the fibers and measuring the associated radioactivity after elastase digestion. With kappa-elastin, coacervation was induced by heating to 65°C followed by centrifugation to separate the coacervated phase in which the trapped radioactivity could be determined.

When sodium ions containing buffers are used during this interaction procedure, saturation curves can be obtained for the accumulation of radioactive cholesterol in fibrous or kappa-elastin. When calcium ions are replacing sodium ions, much higher cholesterol uptake by both forms of elastins can be seen. In the range of cholesterol concentrations used, no saturation effect is obtained. Lipid-saturated elastin loses its elasticity, and its rate of degradation by elastases is increased. This is especially significant when fatty acids are taken up by fibrous elastin, as also shown by Jordan et al.[65]

This finding has biological importance since fatty acids strongly increase in vivo in human aorta with age and atherosclerosis.[8] Table 2 shows the result of our determinations on post-mortem aorta samples after the isolation and purification of elastin by a sequential extraction procedure.[62] A strong increase of the lipid content of this elastin could be demonstrated, which is particularly evident when the fatty acids are analyzed. There is a strong increase in the long chain and odd chain fatty acids with the degree of atherosclerosis.[62] This could explain the loss of elasticity and the increased rate of degradation of elastic fibers in these pathological conditions.

Table 2A
FATTY ACID COMPOSITION OF THE NEUTRAL LIPIDIC FRACTION OF THE UREA - EXTRACT OF HUMAN AORTAS (THIRD LIPID EXTRACT, SEE REFERENCE 62)

Results are Given in Microgram Fatty Acid per Gram Fresh Tissue

	Cholesterol esters		Triglycerides		Free fatty acids		TOTAL	
Fatty acid	Group 1	Group 2	Group 1	Group 2	Group 1	Group 2	Group 1	Group 2
13:1[a]			2.17	3.56			2.17	3.56
14:0				0.64	0.88		0.88	0.64
16:0	1.48	2.38	3.05	4.15	6.67	9.02	11.2	15.55
16:1	0.99	1.51	0.93	1.23	1.17	2.26	3.09	5.00
18:0	0.62	0.38	1.07	1.49	4.45	6.28	6.14	8.15
18:1	2.07	3.67	5.00	6.51	3.64	9.54	10.71	19.72
18:2	0.83	2.02	0.93	0.90	1.64	1.38	3.4	4.3
18:3				0.26				0.26
19:1[a]	0.26	0.72	1.52	0.69			1.78	1.41
TOTAL	6.25	10.68	14.67	19.43	18.45	28.48	39.37	58.59

Note: Group 1, normal or slightly pathological aortas; Group 2, strongly atherosclerotic aortas. For details, see Reference 62.

[a] Calculated identification.

Table 2B
FATTY ACID COMPOSITION OF NEUTRAL LIPIDIC FRACTION OF THE FOURTH LIPIDIC EXTRACT (LIPIDS ASSOCIATED WITH ELASTIN)

Results are Given in Microgram Fatty Acid per Gram Fresh Tissue

	Cholesterol esters		Triglycerides		Free fatty acids		TOTAL	
Fatty acid	Group 1	Group 2	Group 1	Group 2	Group 1	Group 2	Group 1	Group 2
11:?	0.05	0.06	0.04	0.09	0.08	0.12	0.17	0.27
12:0	0.07	0.31	0.21	0.17	0.41	1.01	0.79	1.49
3:1[a]	0.07	0.31	0.21	0.17	0.51	1.01	0.79	1.49
14:0	0.09	0.08	0.46	0.40	0.38	0.95	0.93	1.43
15:0			0.20	0.16	0.21	0.49	0.41	0.65
15:1[a]	0.30	0.37					0.30	0.37
16:0	0.37	0.36	2.00	1.16	2.84	5.84	5.21	7.36
16:1	0.70	0.69	0.79	0.53	0.54	1.27	2.03	2.49
17:1[a]	0.33	0.44	0.11	0.11	0.13	0.37	0.57	0.92
18:0	0.23	0.15	0.45	0.30	1.46	2.93	2.14	3.38
18:1	0.51	0.69	1.86	0.95	1.60	5.10	3.97	6.74
18:2			0.72	0.30	0.15	0.26	0.87	0.56
19:1[a]	0.19	0.51	0.13	0.32	0.29	0.20	0.61	1.03
19:2[a]	0.06	0.23	0.11	0.52			0.16	0.75
20:1	0.07	0.23			0.43	0.39	0.50	0.62
21:1[a]		0.11		1.06	0.54	0.39	0.54	1.56
22:1					0.55	0.35	0.55	0.35
TOTAL	3.01	4.26	7.15	6.15	9.82	19.94	19.97	30.35

Note: Group 1, normal or slightly pathological aortas; Group 2, strongly atherosclerotic aortas.

[a] Calculated identification.

As far as recognizing the enzymes responsible for this degradation are concerned, a great deal of progress was made during the last decade. The first enzyme shown to be able to degrade elastin was the pancreatic elastase first identified by Banga and Balo.[66] This enzyme has a very similar structure to the other pancreatic proteases such as trypsin and chymotrypsin, but there is a significant difference at the level of the active site of the enzyme, as shown in Figure 6. In this active site, the intrusion of an aliphatic aminoacid side chain renders impossible the acceptance of relatively large aminoacid residues. Therefore, only relatively short chain aliphatic aminoacid residues can be introduced in this cleft, resulting in a relative specificity of this enzyme for peptides rich in aliphatic aminoacids such as elastin. However, this protease is able to act on other proteins, and it cannot be considered as specific for elastin.[67] This is the case for all the other enzymes which were later characterized and shown to be able to degrade elastin.

Another important physicochemical feature of elastase action on elastin can be demonstrated, which probably accounts for the relative specificity of pancreatic elastase for elastic fibers: purified elastic fibers exhibit a very high affinity for this enzyme, which can be adsorbed from dilute solutions to the fibers and then resists washing.[68] Adsorption isotherms can thus be obtained, showing that there is a limited number of sites on elastic fibers capable of interacting and adsorbing strongly pancreatic elastase.

Figure 7 shows such an adsorption isotherm. This was obtained by mixing increasing amounts of elastase with highly purified fibrous elastin. After washing, these elastic fibers were put in a pH 8.6 buffer, and the rate of elastolysis measured. The adsorption itself is carried out at pH 4.5 in acetate buffer where elastolysis does not progress or is negligible. This strong adsorption of elastase on elastic fibers is probably the main factor responsible for the higher rate of its action on elastic fibers than on soluble proteins. When elastin-derived peptides (kappa-elastin) are separated by gel permeation chromatography, their rate of elastolysis as recorded by Titrigraphic measurements is directly related to their apparent molecular weight[11] (Figure 8).

Another important finding contributing to the high affinity and rate of attack of pancreatic elastase on insoluble elastic fibers is that the desorption of elastase can be obtained only after a certain amount of peptide linkages are cleaved. This was shown by adsorbing pancreatic elastase onto elastic fibers labeled with ^{125}iodine and washing and mixing these fibers with another batch of elastic fibers labeled with ^{131}iodine.

Figure 9 shows the rate of elastolysis of both elastases as determined by the selective counting of the two iodine isotopes. It can be seen that the ^{131}I-labeled elastin is much more slowly hydrolyzed than the ^{125}I-labeled elastin onto which elastase was adsorbed. The two hydrolysis curves approach each other only after a certain fraction of the total peptide linkages are cleaved.

This high affinity of pancreatic elastase for elastic fibers also explains the partial inhibition which can be obtained even with the most potent elastase inhibitors such as α_1-proteinase inhibitor and α_2-macroglobulin when added to the enzyme previously mixed with the elastic fibers.[7,69]

Figure 10 shows such an experiment, whereby adding the inhibitor to elastase before the elastic fibers are added to the medium completely inhibits the action of elastase on elastic fibers. When, however, this same inhibitor is added after mixing elastase and elastic fibers, only about 40 to 50% inhibition is obtained.

This finding is probably of physiopathological significance and may explain the fact that when elastase is injected into the bloodstream, even in quantities inferior to the amount which can be neutralized by circulating α_1-antiprotease, the elastic fibers of the aorta and the lung are attacked.[70] It also can explain that in the large majority of emphysematous patients, no deficiency of α_1-antiprotease can be demonstrated, and yet an active elastolytic process seems to be involved in the progressive destruction of the alveolar wall elastic fibers.

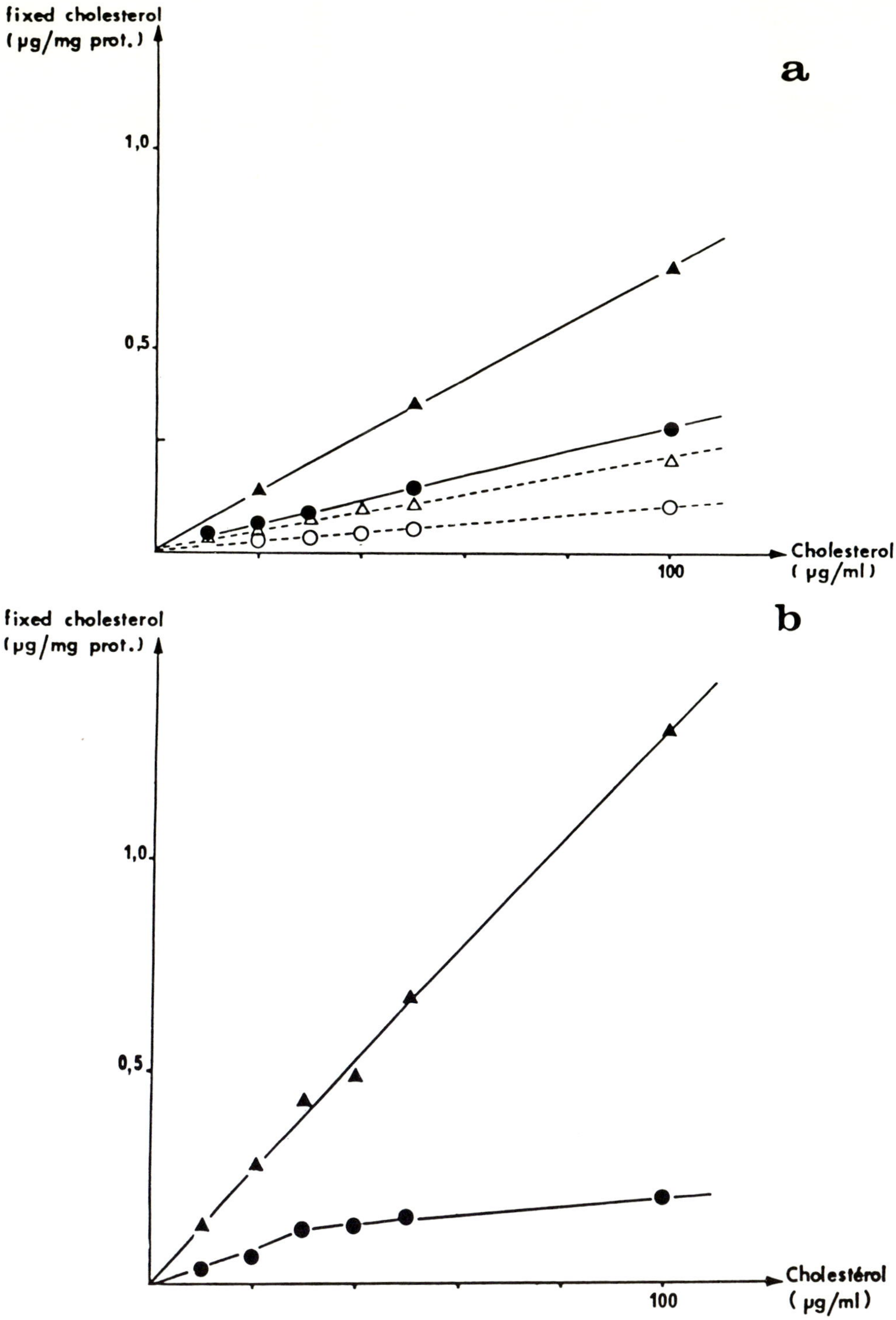

FIGURE 6. Comparison between the binding site of porcine pancreatic chymotrypsin and elastase. (From Bieth, J., *Frontiers of Matrix Biology*, Vol. 6, S. Karger, Basel, 1978, 1. With permission.)

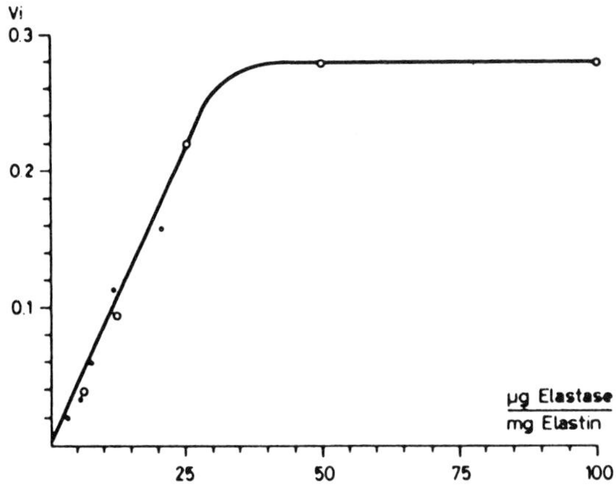

FIGURE 7. Adsorption isotherm of porcine pancreatic elastase on elastin. Increasing amounts of elastase were preadsorbed at pH 4.5 on fibrous elastin and after washing put in pH 8.6 buffer at 37°C, and the speed of elastolysis was recorded. O and • represent the results of two independent experiments. Abscissa: microgram of pancreatic elastase preadsorbed per milligram elastin Ordinate: Initial rate of hydrolysis (milligram elastin solubilized per minute). (From Robert, B., Hornebeck, W., and Robert, L., *Biochimie*, 56, 239, 1974. With permission.)

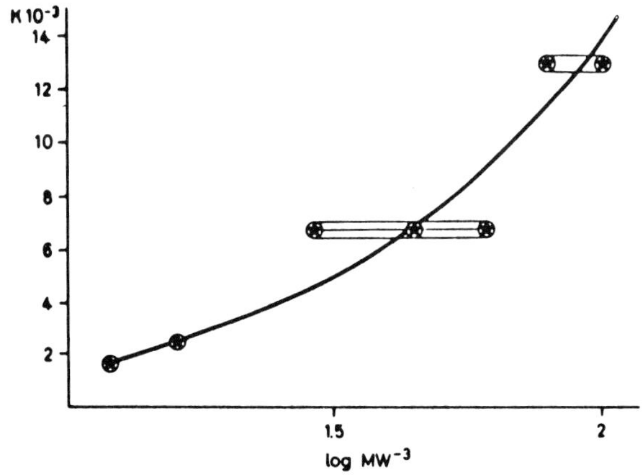

FIGURE 8. Rate constant of elastolysis of elastin peptides (kappa-elastin) determined by titrigraphy as a function of the size of the elastin peptides. Abscissa: log MW^{-3}. Ordinates: Rate of release of protons per minute 10^{-3}. Horizontal bars indicate rates determined on partially purified peptides having the indicated apparent molecular weight. (From Robert, L. and Robert, A. M., *Frontiers of Matrix Biology: Biology and Pathology of Elastic Tissues*, Vol. 8, Robert, A. M. and Robert, L., Eds., S. Karger, Basel, 1980, 130. With permission.)

The second elastase-type protease isolated was from polymorphonuclear leukocytes.[71,72] This enzyme is also a serine protease and occurs in humans as three isoforms. It is a glycoprotein, but the glycane part is not essential for its enzymatic action. Although its action on fibrous elastin is slower than that of pancreatic elastase, it is still

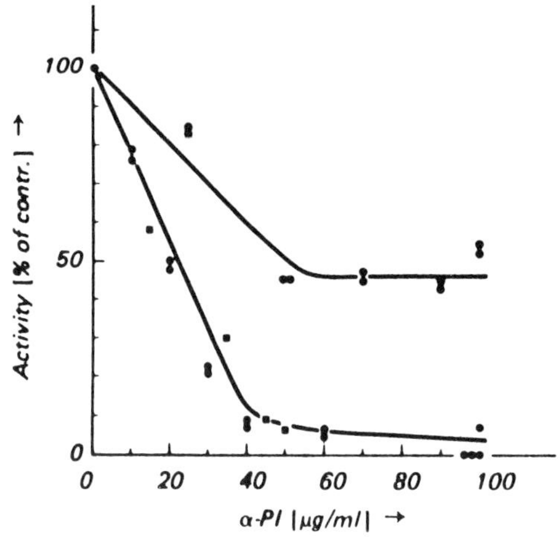

FIGURE 9. Substrate competition in pancreatic elastase catalyzed elastolysis. (a) pancreatic elastase was preadsorbed on elastin labeled with ^{125}I. After washing, elastin labeled with ^{131}I was added, and solubilization of peptides was determined in a scintillation spectrometer. The curves represent the rates of liberation of peptides from the two different labeled elastins. (Robert, B., Hornebeck, W., and Robert, L., *Biochimie*, 56, 239, 1974. With permission.)

an enzyme which can relatively rapidly hydrolyze ("solubilize") fibrous elastin. This enzyme is present in the granules (lysosomes) of polymorphonuclear leukocytes and is liberated during degranulation after phagocytosis or contact with other foreign bodies or cell surfaces. It is supposed to be an important enzyme in the development of the emphysematous lesion, and as a serine protease, it can be inhibited by α_1-antiprotease and also α_2-macroglobulin.[72] The same limitations for the biological role of these inhibitors as protectors against elastolysis, as mentioned above for pancreatic elastase, hold true for this enzyme.

A serine protease-type elastase has also been isolated from human platelets and is present as a precursor proenzyme.[73,74] Although platelet preparations obtained from platelet-rich plasma are often contaminated by leukocytes, it has been shown that the two enzymes, the platelet-derived elastase-type protease and the leukocyte-derived elastase-type protease, are not identical on the basis of immunological and enzymatic data.[75] Also, platelet preparations devoid of leukocytes exhibit a measurable elastase activity (Figure 11).

The platelet enzyme is liberated from platelets during the aggregation and extrusion reaction and may be involved in the lytic process observed after platelet aggregation on the arterial wall during thrombosis or embolism.[76]

A metallo-protease type enzyme has been isolated from human alveolar macrophages and shown to be active on insoluble elastin, as well as on elastin peptides and synthetic substrates.[77,78] As macrophages have receptors for leukocyte-derived elastase, the results obtained with macrophage extracts may be questionable. The strong increase of the elastase-type protease activity of human alveolar macrophages cultured in vitro, when latex beads are added for phagocytosis, also points to an active biosynthetic increase of this enzyme during the phagocytotic process.[78]

More recently, elastase-type protease(s) were isolated from rat arterial SMC in culture.[79,80] This enzyme was partially purified by affinity chromatography on trialanyl

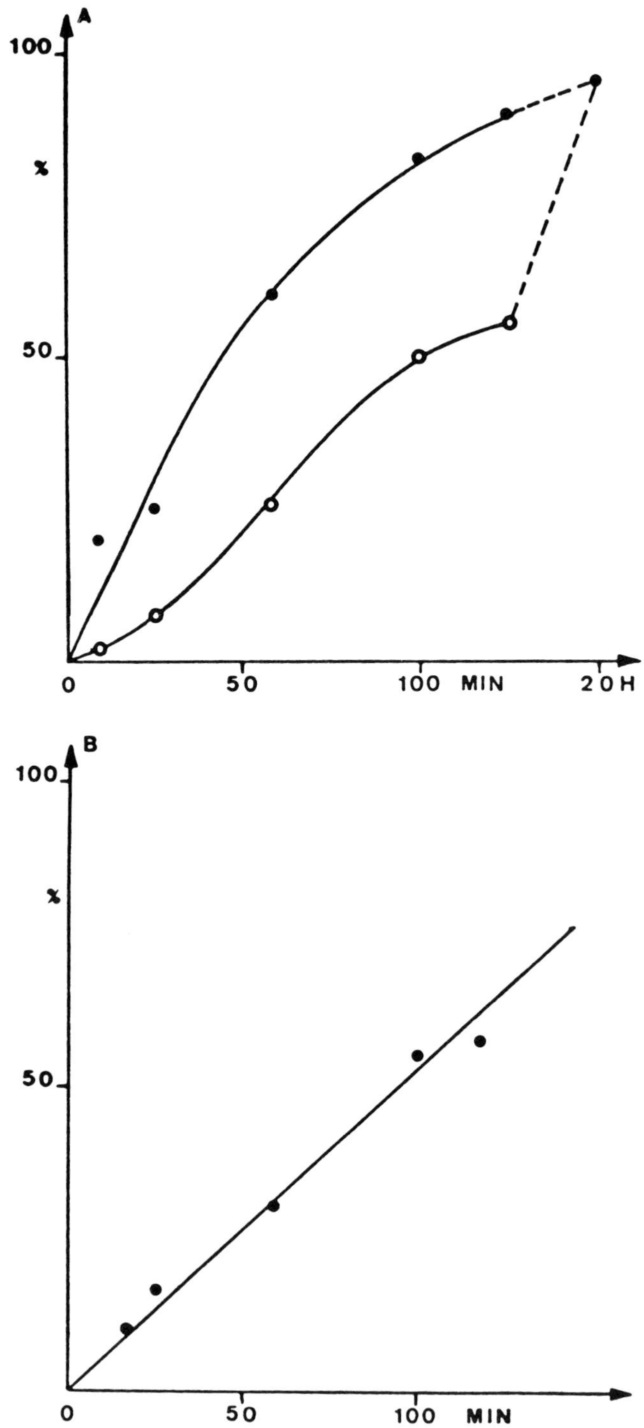

FIGURE 10. Inhibition of human leukocyte elastase (7.5 μg) by α_1-proteinase inhibitor. Enzyme and inhibitor are incubated before adding the substrate, The enzyme is first preadsorbed onto elastic fibers before adding the inhibitor. Abcissa: concentrations of α_2Pi. Ordinates: Percent of residual activity. (From Hornebeck, W. and Schnebli, H. P., *Hoppe Seyler's Z. Physiol. Chem.*, 363, 455, 1982. With permission.)

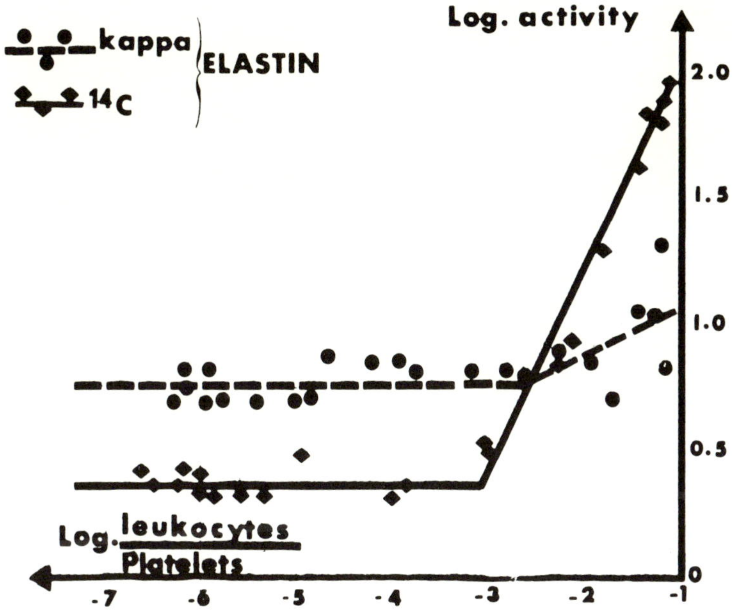

FIGURE 11. Elastase-like activities of platelet suspensions containing different amounts of leukocytes measured on ^{14}C elastin (—) and on κ-elastin (--). (From Hornebeck, W., Pignaud, G., Legrand, Y., and Robert, L., *Clin. Physiol. Biochem.*, 2, 166, 1984. With permission.)

CNBr-Sepharose columns. It possesses a molecular weight estimated by SDS-PAGE and gel permeation of 30 kdaltons and is active on synthetic elastase substrates, as well as on elastins. Its inhibitory profile is consistent with its classification as a serine protease (Table 3).

When the enzyme is studied in SMC cultures, no activity can be detected in an active form in the culture medium. All the activity can be recovered from the cell layer in Triton X-100 extracts. The intracellular enzyme activity increases as a function of the time spent in culture by confluent SMC; this increase can be suppressed by inhibitors of protein synthesis such as cycloheximide added to the culture medium. When the cells are serially subcultured and the enzyme activity determined as a function of passage number, a significant increase can be demonstrated (Figure 12).

Similar experiments have been carried out by adding lipoproteins to the culture medium. When HDL is added in increasing amounts, no increase (on the contrary, some decrease) of the enzyme activity is observed after 12-hr incubation in serum-free medium with the lipoproteins.

When LDL is added in increasing amounts, a strong and significant increase in the biosynthesis of the enzyme occurs.[81] This finding may be significant in respect to the increasing elastase-type activity demonstrated in extracts obtained from post-mortem human aortas as a function of age and also of the degree of atherosclerosis[82] (Figure 13). Although the possibility of LDL penetrating deeply in the intima is now in doubt,[83] it is quite conceivable that LDL-derived lipids do penetrate (perhaps also HDL molecules) all through the medial layers of the aorta. Immunofluorescent demonstration of LDL and of Apo-B in the media of human and experimental animal aortas speaks in favor of this contention.[84]

The age-dependent increase in the biosynthesis of this elastase-type protease bound to the membrane of arterial SMC may be related to its role in atherogenesis.[85] It can be assumed that one of the crucial factors of atherogenesis is a phenotypic modulation

Table 3
INHIBITORY PROFILE OF THE ELASTASE(Suc(Ala)$_3$NA) AND ELASTINOLYTIC (^{3}H INSOLUBLE ELASTIN) ACTIVITIES OF ISOLATED RAT AORTA ELASTASE-TYPE PROTEASE

Enzyme and Inhibitors at the Concentrations Indicated Were Incubated for 2 Hr at Room Temperature Before Determining the Residual Activity on Both Substrates

	Inhibition spectrum (residual activity)		
		Activity	
Inhibition	Concentration	Suc(Ala)$_3$NA	Insoluble elastin
None	—	100	100
DipF	1 m*M*	2.0	0.6
PmsF	1 m*M*	3.5	2.0
EDTA	1 m*M*	47	100
1—10 phenanthroline	1 m*M*	51	100
EDTA + dithiothreitol	2 m*M* (each)	51	22.5
Leupeptin	0.07 m*M*	100	100
Pepstatin A	0.07 m*M*	100	100
Ac(Ala)$_2$ Pro Ala CH$_2$ Cl	0.5 m*M*	00	00
α_2-Antitrypsin	100 m*M*	00	ND

Note: ND, not determined. For other details, see Reference 80.

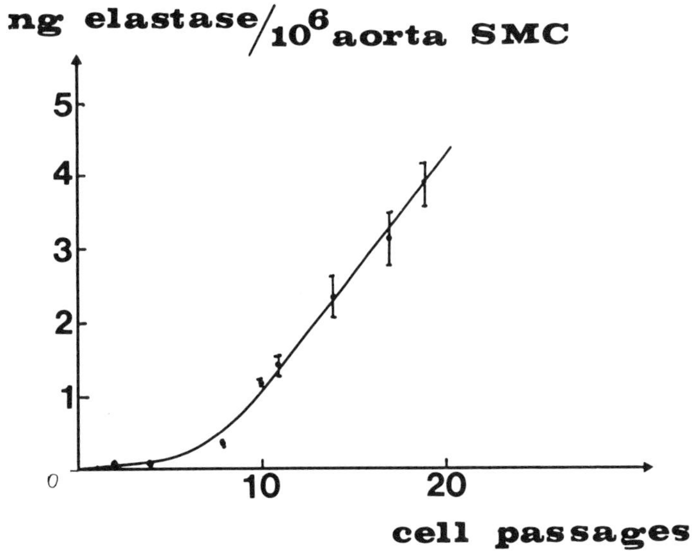

FIGURE 12. Variation of elastase activity as determined on Suc(Ala)$_3$NA of rat aorta SMC as a function of the number of cell passages. Ordinates: elastase activity is expressed as microgram porcine pancreatic elastase equivalents (average value ± s.e.m. as indicated by the bars) per 10^6 viable cells. Abscissas: number of cell passages. (From Hornebeck, W., Bourdillon, M. C., Soleilhac, J. M., and Robert, L., *J. Cell Biol.*, 1985).

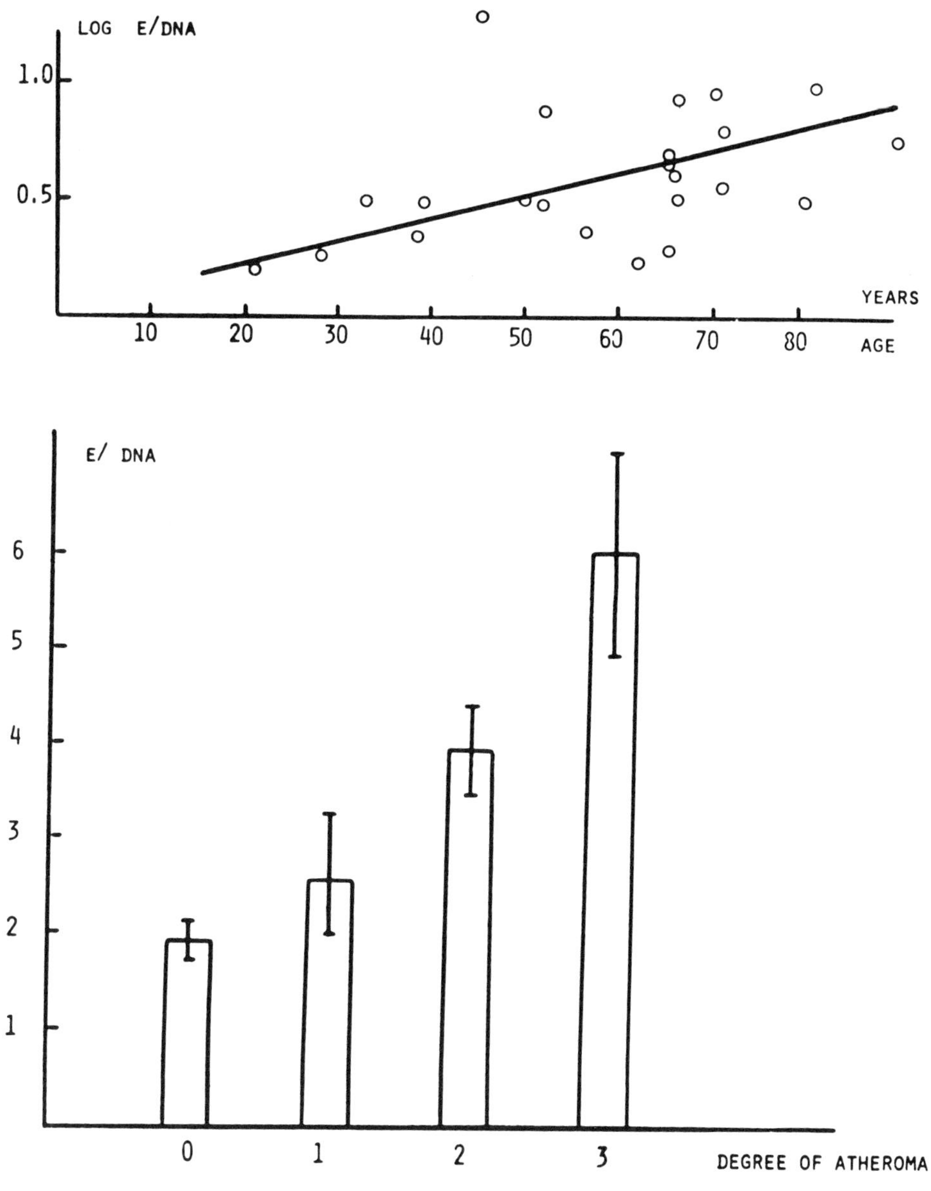

FIGURE 13. Increase of the elastase content of human aorta with age (upper part of graph) and with the degree of atheroma (lower part of graph). The elastase activity of rat extracts is expressed on a DNA basis. (From Hornebeck, W., Derouette, J. C., Roland, J., Chatelet, F., Bouissou, H., and Robert, L., *C.R. Acad. Sci. (Paris)*, 282, 2003, 1976. With permission.)

of SMC, which normally are sessile and contractile, and anchored into neighboring elastic lamellae and thus play an important role in the regulation of blood pressure.[86] As a result of atherogenic stimuli, such as LDL, growth factors (PDGF), or other as yet incompletely understood factors, SMC appear to undergo a "phenotypic change": from sessile and contractile, they become mobile, divide and increase their matrix biosynthetic activity. They migrate towards the intima and secrete extracellular matrix macromolecules, collagen, elastin, and proteoglycans. This is the basic mechanism which seems to be involved in the fibrous cap formation during the atherosclerotic process.[87] This hypothetical mechanism is depicted in Figure 14. The principle of "phenotypic modulation" is described in detail in Volume I, Chapter 4. Therefore, it

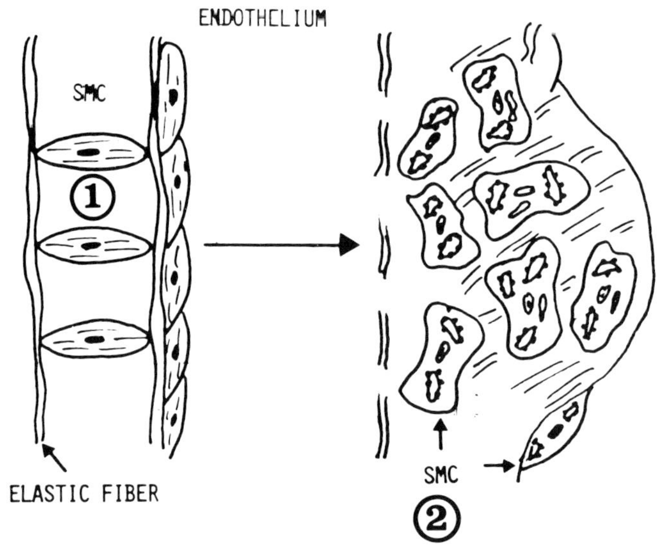

FIGURE 14. Schematic representations of the phenotypic modulation of aortic SMC. (From Robert, L., Chaudiere, J., and Jacotot, B., *Regression of Atherosclerotic Lesions. Experimental Studies and Observations in Humans,* Vol. 79, Manilow, M. R. and Blaton, V. H., Eds., NATO ASI series, 1984, 145. With permission.)

appears probable that this elastase-type protease anchored in the membrane of SMC plays a role in this modified behavior by facilitating the migration of SMC from their original site in the media towards the intima by detaching them from their original site of anchorage and facilitating their passage through the elastic lamellae.

This process may well explain the fragmentation of the elastic lamellae of human aortas as observed with age and during atherosclerosis (see Figure 15). It is, as a matter of fact, a long-standing observation that the subintimal layer, which is hardly detectable in the young lesion-free aortas, increases in thickness progressively by a ''homogenization'' process, including fragmentation of the elastic lamellae, starting from the intima and progressing towards the media, accompanied by the migration of SMC and the formation of fibrous plaques.[8]

Even at sites where no atherosclerotic lesion is observed, this phenomenon is conspicuous and will result in the deposition of a relatively large quantity of type I collagen and the progressive lysis of elastic lamellae (Figure 15).

This lysis of elastic lamellae of the major elastic arteries such as the aorta was shown to be accompanied by a progressive lysis of the elastic fibrils of the papillary dermis, as demonstrated by histochemical procedures in human skin biopsies.[88] Recent studies in our laboratory demonstrate that human skin fibroblasts, as well as fibroblasts of other origin (chick embryo, porcine aortic adventitia), synthesize a metallo-protease which can degrade the elastic fiber system.[89,90] This enzyme is partially secreted in the culture medium and is involved in the lysis of skin elastic fibers in such conditions as *lichen sclerosus et atrophicus.*[61] It is very different in nature both from the pancreatic enzyme and from the SMC enzyme (both being serine proteases) and appears to be involved in the lysis of papillary dermal elastic fibers. A mechanism has to be sought which would coordinate in time these two processes: fragmentation of elastic fibers in the aorta and in the skin. Lipoproteins and mainly LDL are deposited in the dermal connective tissue with age and atherosclerosis both by the determination of Apo-B and of cholesterol.[91] This factor may be the common denominator of this local increase of elastolysis in the atherosclerotic aorta and in the superficial dermis.

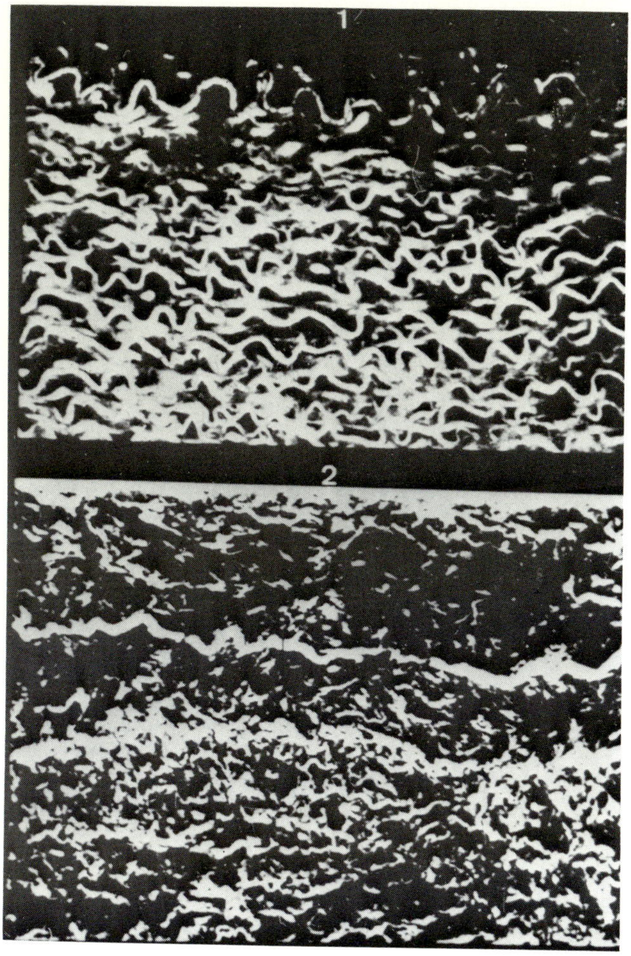

FIGURE 15. On top: Elastic lamellae of a human aorta from a 20-year-old individual. Bottom: Fragmentation of the elastic lamellae in the aorta of a 60-year-old individual. Orcein staining and overexposition to show only the elastic fibers. (Courtesy of Professor H. Bouissou, Toulouse.) (From Robert, L. and Robert, A. M., *Frontiers of Matrix Biology: Biology and Pathology of Elastic Tissues*, Vol. 8, Robert, A. M. and Robert, L., Eds., S. Karger, Basel, 1980, 130. With permission.)

IV. BIOLOGICAL PROPERTIES OF ELASTIN DEGRADATION PRODUCTS

Peptides derived from elastin, either by acid, alkaline, or enzymatic hydrolysis, possess interesting biological properties. One of these properties is a chemotactic action exerted on blood-derived monocyte-macrophages.[92] These experiments were performed using peptides obtained by partial hydrolysis of elastin with pancreatic or leukocyte elastase and also with α-elastin. At 100 $\mu g/m\ell$ elastin digests were generally as active for monocytes as saturating amounts of complement-derived chemotactic activity. These experiments were performed using the Boyden chamber and conclusively demonstrated that elastin-derived peptides may not only attract leukocytes (mainly monocytes) to the site of elastolysis,[93] but also fibroblasts. This process may be important both in the atherosclerotic process and in the development of emphysema as monocytes contain an elastase-type activity.[94] The early contention of Aschoff that blood-derived monocytes enter the arterial wall has recently been confirmed.[45] At least part of the foam cells in the atherosclerotic lesions are derived from blood-derived monocyte-macrophages. This may be due to the attractive action exerted by peptides released during the elastolytic process. Alternatively, and in keeping with the chemotaxis of fibroblasts to elastin peptides, the release of soluble elastin peptides at sites of inflammation may serve as specific signals to attract extracellular matrix-producing cells to assist in remodeling damaged connective tissue. The same may be true in lung alveoli during the degradation of elastin lamellae during the development of emphysema. The liberated elastin peptides may attract more monocyte-macrophage-type cells which themselves can excrete an elastase-type protease which will further degrade elastin and liberate more elastin peptides.

Another important property of elastin-derived peptides is their low but easily demonstrable immunogenicity.[97] When rabbits are immunized with kappa-elastin in complete Freund's adjuvant, a strong sclerotic process develops in the arteries accompanied by massive deposition of calcium salts both intra- and extracellularly.[98] This model of arteriosclerosis is used in our laboratory to study its mechanisms and also as a model for pharmacological studies. It has recently been shown that the development of this arteriosclerotic process can be inhibited by the simultaneous administration of calcitonin.[99] Antielastin peptide antibodies and immune complexes, which are also present in the blood of immunized rabbits, damage the cell membrane of SMC; increasing the outflux of potassium and the influx of calcium and sodium. This strong influx of calcium is inhibited by the administration of calcitonin.[100]

V. REGULATION OF ELASTIN SYNTHESIS AND DEGRADATION

A. In Physiological Conditions

The biosynthesis of elastin starts during the embryonal life and progresses through the early phases of development. Detailed studies carried out on the ontogenesis of rat aorta elastin by Berry et al.[101] showed that the concentric elastic lamellae are deposited quite early during the embryonic life and early phases of postembryonic development, reaching a plateau phase. If destroyed, they are not replaced again. In contrast, the thin elastic fibrils which bridge this concentric elastic pipe system are synthesized continuously during the whole life cycle of the rat. It appears, therefore, that a distinction should be made between the deposition of the concentric lamellae system of the aorta, which would be limited to the embryonic and early postembryonic developmental phases, and the synthesis of elastic fibrils, which would be continuously accomplished by SMC, at least in the rat and probably also in higher vertebrates such as humans, as demonstrated by the presence of elastic fibrils in the atherosclerotic plaque developed even late in life. This could also explain the negative results obtained by earlier investigators, who tried to study the turnover of elastin by in vivo labeling and could not show any significant turnover.[102] If the major portion of aorta elastin is not renewed, with the exception of the fine fibrillar structures, then only turnover studies selectively concerning these different types of elastic structures are meaningful.

Similar considerations concern the elastin network of the papillary dermis, which seems to be progressively destroyed during aging, as well as in an accelerated fashion during the development of arteriosclerosis or diseases such as diabetes.[8] No apparent replacement of this superficial papillary dermal elastic network occurs. However, since the deeper dermal elastic fibers seem to increase with age, this observation has been designated as "senile elastosis".[46]

Ultraviolet light or factors depending on ultraviolet light may also play a role, as shown by the interesting investigations of O'Brien in Sydney, Australia.[103] This inves-

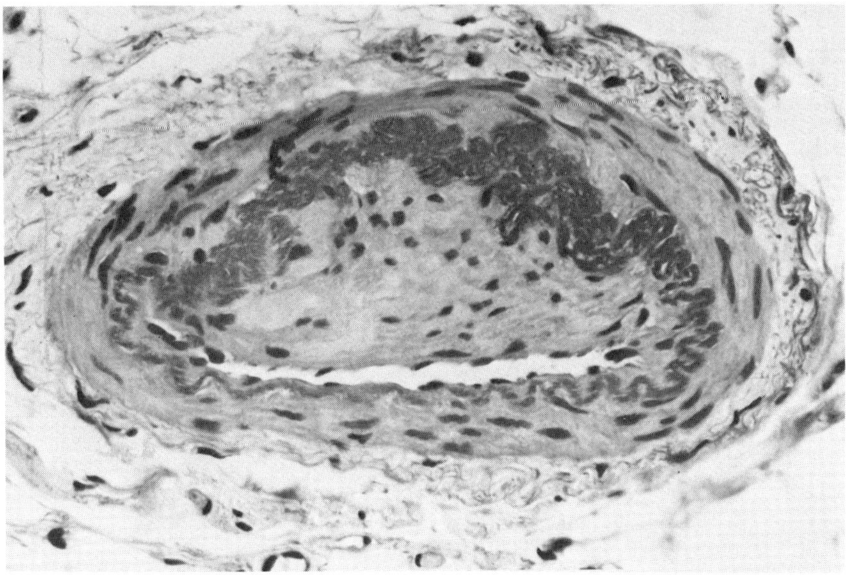

FIGURE 16. A superficial temporal artery showing marked actinic elastotic damage and a more mature, fibrous, atherosclerosis-like plaque. The "weather" lamina is grossly hyperplastic, convoluted, and fibrillary, with typical intense "blue" degeneration (actinic elastotic degeneration) in the original slide. Note continuity of damaged with normal lamina at each lateral edge. The deep wall of vessel appears normal and has a thin, wavy, red-staining lamina in the original. The adventitia also displays actinic elastosis as fine, twisted, bluish fibers. Biopsy specimen aged 80. (Special haematoxylin-buffered eosin; magnification × 465.) (Figure reproduced with permission of the editors of *Clinical Dermatology.)*

tigator showed that biopsies of the temporal artery, obtained in the temporal arteritis myalgia rheumatica syndrome, show a progressive and intensive lysis of the elastic lamina of the external portion while the internal portion, apparently protected by the bloodstream, remains normal (Figure 16). This finding may be related to the demonstration that ultraviolet light can cleave desmosine rings.[104]

Relatively little is known of the factors which regulate the chronology of elastin biosynthesis. Much more is known about factors influencing its degradation (see above). Among the regulating factors, we mentioned already the recent experiments of Mecham et al.,[57,58,60] showing that an elastin-containing matrix can induce elastin biosynthesis in uncommitted fibroblasts derived from ligamentum nuchae.

Another factor incriminated is the pulsatile tension exerted on SMC. Glagov et al. (see Reference 105) cultured aortic SMC on elastin sheets and submitted them to rhythmic pulsations, demonstrating an increase in elastin biosynthesis.

Similar results were reported from our laboratory on SMC of the saphenous vein of dogs after transplantation to an arterial position (in the femoral artery) for several months.[106] After the excision of these veins and incubation in organ culture conditions in the presence of ^{14}C lysine, a strong increase in incorporation into polymeric elastin could be demonstrated.

In contrast to this finding, we point out that although the rhythmic pulsation prevails in the human aorta throughout life, the biosynthesis of elastin does not seem to be activated and the degraded elastic lamellae of the media are not replaced. The oversynthesis of elastic fibers in atherosclerotic plaques does not seem to depend on these rhythmic pulsations, although hemodynamic factors play a role, as demonstrated by the prevalence of atherosclerotic processes at the ostia of vessels leaving the aorta (intercostal arteries) and at other bifurcations.

Table 4
VARIATION OF ELASTASE-TYPE ACTIVITY AND ELASTIN BIOSYNTHESIS IN THE AORTA OF RABBITS FOLLOWING INDUCTION OF ATHEROSCLEROSIS

	Elastase-type activity (Suc-(Ala$_3$)-pNA) ng. panc. el. equivalents per mg DNA	Elastin biosynthesis cpm incorporated in the elastase extract of aorta per mg DNA × 10^{-3}
High cholesterol diet		
Control(7)	60.4[a] ± 9.8	17.3 ± 4.6
Cholesterol(6)	130[a] ± 18.3	20.6 ± 2.6
Ratio cholesterol/control	2.2(S)[b]	1.2
Immunization with κ-elastin peptides		
Control(7)	130[c] ± 23.4	17.1 ± 0.70
κ-Elastin immunized rabbits(7)	434[c] ± 111.2	6.0 ± 2.0
Ratio κ-elastin/control	3.3(S)[b]	0.35(S)[b]

Note: The statistical variations between control and treated animals were evaluated by the Mann-Whitney distribution free test. Average values for the number of animals indicated in parenthesis ± SEM. For other details, see Reference 11.

[a] Determined on $MgCl_2$-extract.
[b] S, significant difference ($p > 0.01$).
[c] Determined on guanidinium-chloride extract.

B. Pharmacological Regulation

Very few drugs are able to influence elastin biosynthesis or degradation. Although elastase inhibitors are widely studied in several laboratories,[107] the biosynthesis of elastase-type enzymes has not been extensively investigated.

We have already mentioned the possibility of decreasing the biosynthesis of SMC elastase-type protease by protein synthesis inhibiting drugs such as cycloheximide. We also mentioned the increased rate of biosynthesis of this enzyme in the presence of LDL-type lipoproteins. More recently, it has been demonstrated that per os administration of colchicine to arteriosclerotic patients over 4 to 6 months results in a significant (about 30%) increase of the density of the elastic fiber network in the skin of these patients.[108] As colchicine is considered to be a microtubule disaggregating agent, activation of biosynthetic processes by colchicine did not appear to be a probable explanation of this in vivo finding. Although colchicine in aortic SMC culture inhibits the synthesis of tropoelastin,[36] the in vivo experiments suggest that its action on elastase synthesis and excretion may predominate. It therefore appears possible that elastin is continuously synthesized by human skin fibroblasts, but its degradation by the fibroblast metallo-protease is much faster than fibrillogenesis.

Recent experiments in our laboratory showed that small amounts of elastin-derived peptides (kappa-elastin) added to rabbit aorta explants maintained in organ culture conditions increase the rate of biosynthesis of extracellular matrix macromolecules. When larger amounts are added, about 10 mg/mℓ, a strong inhibition of this incorporation is observed (unpublished experiments). It appears, therefore, that a feedback type of regulation of elastin biosynthesis by peptides derived from the degradation of elastic fibers is also a conceivable mechanism. It has also been shown[98] that if the aorta of rabbits immunized with kappa-elastin in complete Freund's adjuvant is maintained in explant culture, there is a strong decrease of incorporation of ^{14}C lysine in polymeric elastin as compared to control aorta cultures (Table 4). This is in contrast to the increased incorporation of radioactive precursors in aorta explants obtained from rabbits fed a high cholesterol diet (Table 4).

These findings may be related to the observation that intraperitoneal injection of elastin-derived peptides (kappa-elastin) may protect rabbits against cholesterol-induced atherosclerosis.[109]

VI. PATHOLOGICAL ROLE OF ELASTIN DEGRADATION

The fragmentation and progressive lysis of elastic fibers and laminae can be observed with aging and in an accelerated fashion in the atherosclerotic process in arteries and in emphysema in lung alveoli, as well as in the papillary dermis. It is too early to state if this fragmentation and lysis of elastic fibers is a causative process in the development of these pathological processes or if it can be considered as a side effect. However, the fact that elastin-derived peptides possess important biological properties favors their possible role in the development of the pathologies. The progressive saturation with lipids and calcium salts and fragmentation of elastic laminae in major blood vessels and in skin — and probably in the lung — certainly play an important role in the progressive loss of the functional value of these organs. If one considers the age-dependent decrement of physiological functions as described by Shock,[110] one is struck by the observation that the strongest decrease of these functions with age is in those organs that are relatively rich in elastin. The strongest decrease of these functions is found for the vital capacity of the lungs, where progressive loss of elastin occurs in the aged, when emphysema develops in a relatively large fraction of the population. The next rapid losses are observed in the circulatory system and again point to the possible role of the physicochemical modification and lysis of elastic laminae as possible causative agents in these processes.

It appears therefore legitimate to search for pharmacological agents that could inhibit or slow down these processes and which might be used in the therapy of these age-dependent diseases as atherosclerosis, emphysema, and skin diseases.

VII. CONCLUDING REMARKS

The preceding description of the biosynthesis and degradation of elastic fibers and laminae by SMC and also by fibroblasts can be considered an example of the study at the molecular and cellular level of processes of differentiation, aging, and pathology. The increasing intensity with which these studies are carried out in an increasing number of laboratories can also be considered as a consequence of the manifold important results derived from these studies.

The recent experiments carried out on the characterization of the structural gene(s) of elastin will considerably facilitate studies aimed at understanding the regulation of biosynthesis of these interesting extracellular matrix macromolecules. The recent isolation of several proteases capable of attacking elastin (elastase-type protease) and the study of their mechanisms of activation and inhibition are important assets for the study of mechanisms of pathogenetic processes involved in the development of arterial, skin, and lung diseases and will undoubtedly help in the development of new drugs capable of controlling these diseases.

REFERENCES

1. Garrone, R., Phylogenesis of connective tissue, in *Frontiers of Matrix Biology,* Vol. 5, Robert, L., Ed., S. Karger, Basel, 1978.
2. Labat-Robert, J., Structural glycoproteins of connective tissue, in *Connective Tissue Research: Chemistry, Biology and Physiology,* Deyl, Z. and Adam, M., Eds., Alan R. Liss, New York, 1981, 233.
3. Varma, R. S. and Varma, R., Eds., *Glycosaminoglycans and Proteoglycans in Physiological and Pathological Processes,* S. Karger, Basel, 1982.
4. Sage, E. H. and Gray, W. R., Evolution of elastin structure, in *Elastin and Elastic Tissues. Advances in Experimental Medicine and Biology,* Vol. 79, Sandberg, L., Gray, W. R., and Franzblau, C., Eds., Plenum Press, New York, 1976, 291.
5. Mukherjee, D. P., Hoffman, A. S., and Franzblau, C., The physical properties and molecular structure of ligamentum nuchae elastin, *Biopolymers,* 13, 2447, 1974.
6. Hornebeck, W., Brechemier, D., Bourdillon, M. C., and Robert, L., Isolation and partial characterization of an elastase-like protease from rat aorta smooth muscle cells. Possible role in the regulation of elastin biosynthesis, *Connect. Tissue Res.,* 8, 245, 1981.
7. Robert, L., Bellon, G., and Hornebeck, W., Characterization of different elastases. Their possible role in the genesis of emphysema, *Bull. Eur. Physiopath. Resp.,* 16(Suppl.), 99, 1980.
8. Robert, L. and Robert, A. M., Elastin, elastase and arteriosclerosis, in *Frontiers of Matrix Biology: Biology and Pathology of Elastic Tissues,* Vol. 8, Robert, A. M. and Robert, L., Eds., S. Karger, Basel, 1980, 130.
9. Hornebeck, W. and Legrand, Y., Possible implication of two elastinolyic proteases isolated from tissue aorta and blood platelets in atherosclerosis, in *Frontiers of Matrix Biology: Biology and Pathology of Elastic Tissues,* Vol. 8, Robert, A. M. and Robert, L., Eds., S. Karger, Basel, 1980, 199.
10. Robert, L. and Hornebeck, W., Preparation of insoluble and soluble elastins, in *The Methodology of Connective Tissue Research,* Hall, A., Ed., Joynson-Bruvvers, Oxford, 1976, 81.
11. Jacob, M. P. and Hornebeck, W., Isolation and characterization of insoluble and kappa-elastins, in *Frontiers of Matrix Biology,* Vol. 10, S. Karger, Basel, 1985, 92.
12. Robert, B., Szigeti, M., Derouette, J. C., Robert, L., Bouissou, H., and Fabre, M. T., Studies on the nature of the "microfibrillar" component of elastic fibers, *Eur. J. Biochem.,* 21, 507, 1971.
13. Kadar, A., Robert, B., and Robert, L., Etude biochimique et électromicroscopique de microfibrilles du tissu conjonctif, *Pathol. Biol.,* 21, 97, 1973.
14. Kagan, H. M. and Lerch, R. M., Amidated carboxyl groups in elastin, *Biochim. Biphys. Acta,* 434, 223, 1976.
15. Franzblau, C., Sinex, F. M., Farris, B., and Lampidis, R., Identification of a new cross-linking amino-acid in elastin, *Biochem. Biophys. Res. Commun.,* 21, 575, 1965.
16. Thomas, J., Elsden, D. F., and Partridge, S. M., Degradation products from elastin: partial structure of two major degradation products from the crosslinkages of elastin, *Nature (London),* 200, 651, 1963.
17. Robert, L. and Poullain, N., Etudes sur la structure de l'élastine et le mode d'action de l'élastase. I. Nouvelle méthode de préparation de dérivés solubles de l'élastine, *Bull. Soc. Chim. Biol.,* 45, 1317, 1963.
18. Kornfeld-Poullain, N. and Robert, L., Effects de différents solvants organiques sur la dégradation alcaline de l'élastine, *Bull. Soc. Chim. Biol.,* 50, 759, 1968.
19. Moczar, M., Moczar, E., and Robert, L., Peptides on partial hydrolysis of elastin with aqueous ethanolic potassium hydroxide, in *Frontiers of Matrix Biology: Biology and Pathology of Elastic Tissues,* Vol. 8, Robert, A. M. and Robert, L., Eds., S. Karger, Basel, 1980, 130.
20. Partridge, S. M., Davies, H. F., and Adair, G. S., The chemistry of connective tissues: two soluble proteins derived from partial hydrolysis of elastin, *Biochem. J.,* 61, 11, 1955.
21. Smith, D. W., Weissman, N., and Carnes, W. H., Cardiovascular studies on copper deficient swine. Partial purification of a soluble protein resembling elastin, *Biochem. Biophys. Res. Commun.,* 31, 309, 1968.
22. Sandberg, L. B., Soskel, N. T., and Wolt, T. B., Structure of the elastic fiber: an overview, *J. Invest. Dermatol.,* 79, 128, 1982.
23. Yoon, K., May, M., Goldstein, N., Indik, Z. K., Oliver, L., Boyd, C., and Rosenbloom, J., Characterization of a sheep elastin cDNA clone containing translated sequences, *Biochem. Biophys. Res. Commun.,* 118(1), 261, 1984.
24. Burnett, W., Yoon, K., and Rosenbloom, J., Construction, identification of a chick elastin cDNA clone, *Biochem. Biophys. Res. Commun.,* 99(2), 364, 1981.
25. Saunders, N. A. and Grant, M. E., Elastin biosynthesis in chick embryo arteries, *Biochem. J.,* 221, 393, 1984.

26. Damiano, Y., Tsang, A.-L., Weinbaum, G., Christner, P., and Rosenbloom, J., Secretion of elastin in the embryonic chick aorta as visualized by immunoelectron microscopy, *Collagen Rel. Res.*, 4, 153, 1984.
27. Karr, S. R. and Foster, J. A., Monoclonal antibodies as probes for differentiating tropoelastin a and b, *Collagen Rel. Res.*, 3, 459, 1983.
28. Barrineau, L. L., Rich, C. B., and Foster, J. A., The biosynthesis of tropoelastin in chick and pig tissues, *Connect. Tissue Res.*, 8, 189, 1981.
29. Cheah, K. S. E., Grant, M. E., and Jackson, D. S., Identification of the primary translation product of elastin mRNA, *Connect. Tissue Res.*, 8, 205, 1981.
30. Schwartzbaum, J. E., Tankun, J. W., Lemischka, I. R., and Hynes, R. O., Three different fibronectin mRNAs arise by alternative splicing within the coding region, *Cell*, 35, 421, 1983.
31. Moschetto, Y., De Backer, M., Pizieux, O., Bouissou, H., Pierraggi, M. T., and Julian, M., Evolution de l'elastine d'aortes humaines au cours du vieillissement, *Arterial Wall*, 2, 161, 1974.
32. Tuderman, L., Myllyla, R., and Kivirikko, K. I., Mechanism of the prolyl hydroxylase reaction. I. Role of cosubstrates, *Eur. J. Biochem.*, 80, 341, 1977.
33. Borel, J. P., Macquart, F. X., and Randoux, A., Contrôle hormonal du métabolisme du collagène, *Pathol. Biol.*, 32(7), 795, 1984.
34. Kagan, H. M., Simpson, D. E., and Tseng, L., Substrate-directed modulation of elastin oxidation by lysyl oxidase, *Connect. Tissue Res.*, 8, 213, 1981.
35. Harris, E. D., Rayton, J. K., and De Groot, J. E., A critical role for copper in aortic elastin structure and synthesis, in *Advances in Experimental Medicine*, Sandberg, L. B., Gray, W. R., and Franzblau, C., Eds., Plenum Press, New York, 1977, 543.
36. Uitto, J., Hoffman, H. P., and Prockop, D. J., Synthesis of elastin and procollagen by cells from embryonic aorta. Differences in the role of hydroxyproline and the effects of proline analogues on the secretion of two proteins, *Arch. Biochem. Biophys.*, 173, 187, 1976.
37. Urry, D. W., Molecular perspectives of vascular wall structure and disease: the elastic component, *Perspect. Biol. Med.*, 21, 265, 1978.
38. Derouette, S., Hornebeck, W., Loisance, D., Godeau, G., Cachera, J. P., and Robert, L., Studies on elastic tissue of aorta in aortic dissections and Marfan Syndrome, *Pathol. Biol.*, 29, 539, 1981.
39. Cleary, E. G. and Cliff, W. J., The substructure of elastin, *Exp. Mol. Pathol.*, 28, 227, 1978.
40. Haust, M. D., Fine fibrils of extracellular space (microfibrils). Their structure and role in connective tissue organization, *Am. J. Pathol.*, 1113, 1965.
41. Ross, R. and Bornstein, P., The elastic fiber. The separation and partial characterization of its macromolecular components, *J. Cell Biol.*, 40, 366, 1969.
42. Kadar, A., Bihari-Varga, M., and Csonka, E., The synthesis, transport and excretion of connective tissue macromolecules by smooth muscle cells, *Connect. Tissue Res.*, 8, 175, 1981.
43. Sims, M. R., Ultrastructural analysis of the microfibrillar component of mouse and peridontal oxytalan fibers, *Connect. Tissue Res.*, 13, 59, 1984.
44. Fulmer, H. M. and Lillie, R. D., The oxytalan fiber: a previously undescribed connective tissue fiber, *J. Histochem. Cytochem.*, 6, 425, 1958.
45. Robert, L. and Labat-Robert, J., Le Tissu Conjonctif: les Glycoprotéines de structure, in *Précis de Physiologie Cutanee, J. Meynadier Edit.*, Editions de la Porte Verte, 1980, 175.
46. Frances, C. and Robert, L., Elastin and elastic fibers in normal and pathologic skin, *Int. J. Dermatol.*, 23(3), 166, 1984.
47. Gotte, L., Giro, M. G., Volpin, D., and Horne, R. W., The ultrastructural organization of elastin, *J. Ultrastruct. Res.*, 46, 23, 1974.
48. Urry, D. W., Studies on the conformation and interaction of elastin, in *Arterial Mesenchyme and Arteriosclerosis. Advances in Experimental Medicine and Biology*, Vol. 43, Wagner, W. D. and Clarkson, T. B., Eds., Plenum Press, New York, 1974, 211.
49. Sandberg, L. B., Gray, W. R., Foster, J. A., Torres, A. R., and Alvarez, V. L., Primary structure of porcine tropoelastin, in *Elastin and Elastic Tissues. Advances in Experimental Medicine and Biology*, Vol. 79, Sandberg, L. B., Gray, W. R., and Franzblau, C., Eds., Plenum Press, New York, 1977, 277.
50. Cox, B., Starcher, B., and Urry, D., Coacervation of alpha-elastin results in fibre formation, *Biochim. Biophys. Acta*, 317, 207, 1973.
51. Urry, D. W., What is elastin, what is not, *Ultrastruct. Pathol.*, 4, 227, 1983.
52. Moczar, M., Ouzilou, J., Courtois, Y., and Robert, L., Age-dependence of the biosynthesis of intercellular matrix macromolecules of rabbit aorta in organ culture and cell culture, *Gerontology*, 22, 461, 1976.
53. Franzblau, C. and Faris, B., Synthesis of insoluble elastin in cell and organ culture, *Methods Enzymol.*, 82, 615, 1982.

54. Shibahara, S., Davidson, J. M., Smith, K., and Crystal, R. G., Modulation of tropoelastin production and elastin messenger ribonucleic acid activity in developing sheep lung, *Biochemistry*, 20, 6577, 1981.
55. Mecham, R. P., Lange, G., Madaras, J., and Starcher, B., The elastin synthesis by ligamentum nuchae fibroblasts. Effect of culture conditions and extracellular matrix on elastin production, *J. Cell Biol.*, 90, 332, 1981.
56. Gardner, R., Heng, H., Penner, M., Sedywick, C., and Rucker, R., Elastin accumulation in the chick aorta: effect of 6-hydroxydopamine and deoxycortisone acetate, *Res. Commun. Chem. Pathol. Pharmacol.*, 43(2), 251, 1984.
57. Mecham, R. P., Madaras, J. G., and Senior, R. M., Extracellular matrix specific induction of elastogenic differentiation and maintenance of phenotypic stability in bovine ligament fibroblasts, *J. Cell Biol.*, 98, 1804, 1984.
58. Mecham, R. P., Griffins, G. L., Madaras, J. G., and Senior, R. M., Appearance of chemotactic responsiveness to elastin peptides by developing fetal bovine ligament fibroblasts parallels the onset of elastin production, *J. Cell Biol.*, 98, 1813, 1984.
59. Frisch, S. M. and Werb, Z., Evidence for autoregulation of tropoelastin gene expression in rat aortic smooth muscle cells, *Fed. Proc.*, 42, 1892, 1983.
60. Mecham, R. P., Madaras, J. G., McDonald, J. A., and Ryan, U., Elastin production of cultured calf pulmonary artery endothelial cells, *J. Cell. Physiol.*, 116, 282, 1983.
61. Godeau, G., Frances, C., Hornebeck, W., Brechemier, D., and Robert, L., Isolation and partial characterization of an elastase type protease in human vulva fibroblast: its possible involvement in vulvar elastic tissue destruction of patients with Lichen Sclerosus et Atrophicus, *J. Invest. Dermatol.*, 9, 270, 1982.
62. Claire, M., Jacotot, B., and Robert, L., Characterization of lipids associated with macromolecules of the intercellular matrix of human aorta, *Connect. Tissue Res.*, 4, 61, 1976.
63. Hornebeck, W. and Partridge, S. M., Conformation changes in fibrous elastin due to calcium ions, *Eur. J. Biochem.*, 51, 73, 1975.
64. Jacob, M. P., Hornebeck, W., and Robert, L., Studies on the interaction of cholesterol with soluble and insoluble elastins, *Int. J. Biol. Macromol.*, 5, 275, 1983.
65. Jordan, R. E., Hewitt, N., Lewis, W., Kagan, H., and Franzblau, C., Regulation of elastase catalyzed hydrolysis of insoluble elastin by synthetic and naturally occurring hydrophobic ligands, *Biochemistry*, 13, 3497, 1974.
66. Banga, I. and Balo, J., Elastin and elastase, *Nature (London)*, 171, 44, 1953.
67. Bieth, J., Elastases: structure, function and pathological role, in *Frontiers of Matrix Biology*, Vol. 6, S. Karger, Basel, 1978, 1.
68. Robert, B., Hornebeck, W., and Robert, L., Cinètique hétérogène de l'interation élastine-elastase, *Biochimie*, 56, 239, 1974.
69. Hornebeck, W. and Schnebli, H. P., Effect of different elastase inhibitors on leukocyte elastase preadsorbed to elastin, *Hoppe Seyler's Z. Physiol. Chem.*, 363, 455, 1982.
70. Turino, G. M., Hornebeck, W., and Robert, B., In vivo effects of pancreatic elastase. I. Studies on the serum inhibitors, *Proc. Soc. Exp. Biol. Med.*, 146, 712, 1974.
71. Janoff, A., Purification of human granulocyte elastase by affinity chromatography, *Lab. Invest.*, 29, 458, 1973.
72. Starkey, P. M., Elastase and Cathepsin G. The serine proteases of human neutrophil leukocytes and spleen, in *Proteinases in Mammalian Cells and Tissues*, Barrett, A. J., Ed., North-Holland, Amsterdam, 1977, 57.
73. Robert, B., Legrand, Y., Soria, C., Caen, J., and Robert, L., Etude sur les protéases de plaquettes sanguines humaines: purification d'une elastase, *C.R. Acad. Sci. (Paris)*, 274, 1749, 1972.
74. Legrand, Y., Pignaud, G., Caen, J., Robert, B., and Robert, L., Separation of human blood platelet elastase and pro-elastase by affinity chromatography, *Biochem. Biophys. Res. Commun.*, 63, 224, 1975.
75. Hornebeck, W., Pignaud, G., Legrand, Y., and Robert, L., Differentiation of the elastase-type protease of platelets from other elastases, *Clin. Physiol. Biochem.*, 2, 166, 1984.
76. Legrand, Y., Caen, J., Booyse, F. M., Rafelson, M. E., Robert, B., and Robert, L., Studies on a human blood platelet protease with élastolytic activity, *Biochem. Biophys. Acta*, 309, 406, 1973.
77. Banda, M. J. and Werb, Z., Mouse macrophage elastase. Purification and characterization as a metallo-proteinase, *Biochem. J.*, 193, 589, 1981.
78. De Cremoux, H., Hornebeck, W., Jaurand, M. C., Bignon, J., and Robert, L., Partial characterization of an elastase-like enzyme secreted by human and monkey alveolar macrophages, *J. Pathol.*, 125, 172, 1978.
79. Brechemier, D., Hornebeck, W., Bourdillon, M. C., Blaes, N., Crouzet, B., and Robert, L., Elastase-like proteases in rat aorta smooth muscle cells and fibroblasts, *Artery*, 8(4), 253, 1980.

80. Hornebeck, W., Bourdillon, M. C., Soleilhac, J. M., and Robert, L., Further studies on rat aorta smooth muscle cells elastase activity, in *Extracellular Matrix and Function,* Reddi, A. H., Ed., Alan R. Liss, New York, 1985, 269.
81. Bourdillon, M. C., Soleilhac, J. M., Crouzet, B., Robert, L., and Hornebeck, W., Influcnce of lipoproteins on elastase-type activity of arterial smooth muscle cells in culture, *Cell Biol. Int. Rep.,* 8(5), 415, 1984.
82. Hornebeck, W., Derouette, J. C., Roland, J., Chatelet, F., Bouissou, H., and Robert, L., Corrélation entre l'âge, l'artériosclérose et l'activité élastinolytique de la paroi aortique humaine, *C.R. Acad. Sci. (Paris),* 282, 2003, 1976.
83. Smith, E. B. and Staples, E. M., Distribution of plasma proteins across the human aortic wall. Barrier functions of endothelium and internal elastic lamina, *Atherosclerosis,* 37, 579, 1980.
84. Walton, K. W. and Wiliamson, N., Histological and immunofluorescent studies on the evolution of the human atheromatous plaque, *J. Atheroscler. Res.,* 8, 599, 1968.
85. Leake, D., Hornebeck, W., Brechemier, D., Robert, L., and Peters, T. J., Properties and subcellular localization of elastase-like activities of arterial smooth muscle cells in culture, *Biochem. Biophys. Acta,* 761, 41, 1983.
86. Bader, H., Importance of the gerontology of elastic arteries in the development of essential hypertension, *Clin. Physiol. Biochem.,* 1, 36, 1983.
87. Robert, L., Hornebeck, W., and Robert, A. M., Role of the connective tissue in the arterio-atherosclerotic process. Interest of a cell-matrix directed pharmacology, in *Proc. 6th Int. Symp. on Atherosclerosis,* Vol. 6, Schettler, F. G., Gotto, A. M., Middelhoff, G., Habenicht, A. J. R., and Jurukta, K. R., Eds., Springer-Verlag, Berlin, 1983, 370.
88. Maurel, E., Bouissou, H., Pieraggi, M. T., Julian, M., Moczar, M., and Robert, L., Age-dependent biochemical changes in dermal connective tissue. Relationship to histological and ultrastructural observations, *Connect. Tissue Res.,* 8, 33, 1980.
89. Codogno, P., Hornebeck, W., Goussault, Y., Robert, L., and Aubery, M., Elastase activity in chick embryo fibroblasts. Quantitative changes induced by agents which affect cell functions and variations during embryogenesis, *Cell Biol. Int. Rep.,* 7(6), 433, 1983.
90. Velebny, V., Nogueira, L., Robert, L., and Hornebeck, W., Differentiation between elastase-type activities in medial smooth muscle cells and adventitia fibroblasts of porcine aorta, in preparation, 1985.
91. Bouissou, H., Skin cholesterol and skin apoprotein B in atherosclerosis, *Biomed. Pharmacother.,* 36, 159, 1982.
92. Senior, R. M., Griffins, G. L., and Mecham, R. P., Chemotactic activity of elastin derived peptides, *J. Clin. Invest.,* 66, 859, 1980.
93. Senior, R. M., Griffins, G. L., and Mecham, R. P., Chemotactic responses of fibroblasts to tropoelastin and elastin derived peptides, *J. Clin. Invest.,* 70, 614, 1982.
94. Fine, R., Campbell, M. E., and Collins, J. F., Elastolytic activity of peripheral blood monocytes, *Connect. Tissue Res.,* 13, 27, 1984.
95. Balo, J., Connective tissue changes in atherosclerosis, in *International Review of Connective Tissue Research,* Vol. 1, Hall, D. A., Ed., Academic Press, London, 1963, 241.
96. Gerrity, R. G., The role of the monocyte in atherogenesis. I. Transition of blood borne monocytes into foam cells in fatty lesions, *Am. J. Pathol.,* 103, 181, 1981.
97. Robert, L., Robert, A. M., Moczar, M., and Moczar, E., Constituants macromoléculaires de la paroi artérielle: antigénicité et rôle dans l'athérosclérose, in *Role de la Paroi Artérielle dans l'Athérogénèses,* Colloque CNRS, Paris, 1968, 395.
98. Jacob, M. P., Hornebeck, W., Lafuma, C., Bernaudin, J. F., Robert, L., and Godeau, G., Ultrastructural and biochemical modifications of rabbit arteries induced by immunization with soluble elastin peptides, *Exp. Mol. Pathol.,* 41(2), 171, 1984.
99. Robert, L., Brechemier, D., Godeau, G., Labat, M. L., and Milhaud, G., Prevention of experimental immunoarteriosclerosis by calcitonin, *Biochem. Pharmacol.,* 26, 2129, 1977.
100. Jacob, M. P., Moura, A. M., Tixier, J. M., Lafuma, C., Robert, A. M., Robert, L., and Worcel, M., Prevention by calcitonin of the pathological modifications of the rabbit arterial wall induced by immunization with elastin peptides. Effect on vascular smooth muscle permeability to ions, *Exp. Mol. Pathol.,* 1987, in press.
101. Berry, C. L., Looker, T., and Germain, J., The growth and development of the rat aorta, *J. Anat.,* 113, 1, 1972.
102. Rucker, R. B. and Tinker, D., Structure and metabolism of arterial elastin, in *International Review of Experimental Pathology,* Vol. 17, Richter, G. W. and Epstein, M. A., Eds., Academic Press, New York, 1977, 1.
103. O'Brien, J. P., Destruction of the elastic tissue (elastolysis) as a link between atherosclerosis and the temporal arteritis/polymyalgia rheumatica syndrome, *Pathol. Biol.,* 32(2) 123, 1984.

104. Lamy, F., Baurain, R., Gray, M., and Larochelle, J. F., Photolysis of desmosine and isodesmosine by ultraviolet light, in *Elastin and Elastic Tissues, Advances in Experimental Medicine and Biology,* Vol. 79, Sandberg, L., Gray, W. R., and Franzblau, C., Eds., Plenum Press, New York, 1977, 177.
105. Robert, L. and Moczar, M., Molecular biology of intercellular matrix macromolecules in relation to the cardiovascular system, in *Heart Perfusion, Energetics and Ischemia,* Vol. 62, Dintenfass, L., Julian, D. G., and Seaman, G. V. F., Eds., Pergamon Press, Elmsford, N.Y., 1983, 483.
106. Moczar, M., Bessou, J. P., and Loisance, D., Healing of biodegradable vascular prosthesis. Incorporation ^{3}H-Valine into proteins in the subendothelial scar and host intima-media of rat aorta, *Connect. Tissue Res.,* 12, 33, 1983.
107. Hornebeck, W. and Robert, L., Les inhibiteurs des élastases: utilisation pharmacologique au cours de processus pathologiques du tissu conjontif, in *Pharmacologie Cellulaire et Moléculaire du Tissu Conjonctif, Journées Franco-allamandes de Rhumatologie,* Robert, L. and Grieling, H., Eds., 1984, 327.
108. Godeau, G., Gonnord, G., Wegrowski, J., Pompidou, A., Schoevaert, D., Robert, L., Lagrue, G., and Robert, A. M., Effect of colchicine on atherosclerosis. III. Study of dermal elastic fibers by quantitative histochemistry using automated image analysis, *Clin. Physiol. Biochem.,* 3, 234, 1985.
109. Robert, L., Jacob, M. P., Szemenyei, K., and Robert, A. M., Pharmacological properties of elastin peptides, their action on serum and aorta lipids and on the atherosclerotic process, in *Treatment of Hyperlipoproteinemia,* Carlson, L. A. and Olsson, A. G., Eds., Raven Press, New York, 1984, 185.
110. Shock, N. W., System integration, in *Handbook of the Biology of Aging,* Vol. 1, Finch, C. E. and Hayflick, L., Eds., Van Nostrand Reinhold, New York, 1977, 639.
111. Kadar, A., New concepts of elastic tissue disorders, in *Frontiers of Matrix Biology: Biology and Pathology of Elastic Tissues,* Vol. 8, Robert, A. M. and Robert, L., Eds., S. Karger, Basel, 1980, 54.
112. Robert, L., Chaudiere, J., and Jacotot, B., Interaction between lipids and the intercellular matrix of the arterial wall: its role in the evolution of atherosclerotic lesions, in *Regression of Atherosclerotic Lesions. Experimental Studies and Observations in Humans,* Vol. 79, Manilow, M. R. and Blaton, V. H., Eds., NATO ASI series, 1984, 145.

Chapter 12

EICOSANOID PRODUCTION BY VASCULAR SMOOTH MUSCLE CELLS IN CULTURE

J. Larrue, B. Dorian, J. Bonnet, and H. Bricaud

TABLE OF CONTENTS

I. INTRODUCTION: OXIDATIVE PATHWAYS OF ARACHIDONIC ACID METABOLITES

Eicosanoids constitute a general biological control system including C20 fatty acids as the precursors. Arachidonic acid (AA), the most common of these fatty acids, is normally stored in biological membrane structures and can be released through activation of a hydrolytic system in response to various stimuli. In blood vessels, the metabolism of AA appears to be a key process in the response of vasculature to a number of pathological and pharmacological stimuli, the autacoids formed serving as an important mediator of essential functions, such as platelet aggregation, vascular tone, and cell secretion.

The sequence of events leading to the release of eicosanoids is thought to be initiated by the activation of phospholipases which liberate AA (Figure 1). Then, depending on the availability of active enzymes in the stimulated cells and the nature of the stimulus, AA is converted into different physiologically active compounds (Figure 2), including primary prostaglandins, prostacyclin, and thromboxane A_2. They are formed via a common pathway involving the cyclooxygenase enzyme which converts AA to PGG_2. The endoperoxide is enzymatically converted to PGH_2 which then isomerizes to the primary prostaglandins or is transformed to unstable products, prostacyclin, and TxA_2 by specific enzymes.

AA could also be converted to other compounds of physiological importance: non-cyclized hydroxy acids. The 12-lipoxygenase pathway, which is particularly active in platelets, produces 12-HETE as the major product. A 15-lipoxygenase synthesizes primarily 15-HETE, and a 5-lipoxygenase, found initially in polymorphonuclear cells and macrophages, converts AA to 5-HETE. The formation of these monohydroxy acids occurs via unstable hydroperoxy intermediates. Among them, the 5-HPETE gives rise to a family of compounds, the leukotrienes, through a 5—6 epoxide intermediate, leukotriene A_4. This is converted via a specific hydrolase to leukotriene B_4, or, by a glutation-S-transferase to the sulfido-peptide derivatives, LTC_4 and others.

Since the first reports indicating that blood vessels can synthesize prostaglandins,[1,2] it has been established that prostacyclin (PGI_2) is the major product of arachidonate metabolism by vascular tissue.[3] PGI_2 is more potent than the primary prostaglandins in regulating blood vessel tone and blood platelet aggregation.[45] It is able to modulate cholesterol-ester metabolism in arteries[6,7] and, together with other prostanoids, control cell proliferation.[8]

Prostanoids are not the only arachidonic acid metabolites produced by arteries, and compounds derived from lipoxygenase activities may also be produced.[9,10] The role of these later compounds in regulating vascular functions needs to be clearly elucidated; however, several lines of evidence appear concerning their effects on vascular tone.[10] prostacyclin production,[11,12] blood cell recruitment,[13] smooth muscle cell (SMC) migration,[14] and proliferation.[15] This indicates that, together with prostanoids, they may represent an important factor in the local cell interactions inside the vessels under both physiological and pathological conditions.

Of the various tissues of the vascular wall, the intima has the highest capacity to generate PGI_2,[16] stimulating debate about the relative contributions of endothelial and SMC for PGI_2 production, although its synthesis has been demonstrated in both cell types in culture.[17] Additionally, there have been conflicting reports as to whether vascular cells are able to produce a range of metabolites. Further, the profile of AA metabolism can be substantially altered by changes in the cell environment, particularly those related to pathological processes such as thrombosis or atherosclerosis and, on an experimental point of view, those related to culture conditions. Thus, despite the fact that, in most instances, these mediators are not required to produce a response but

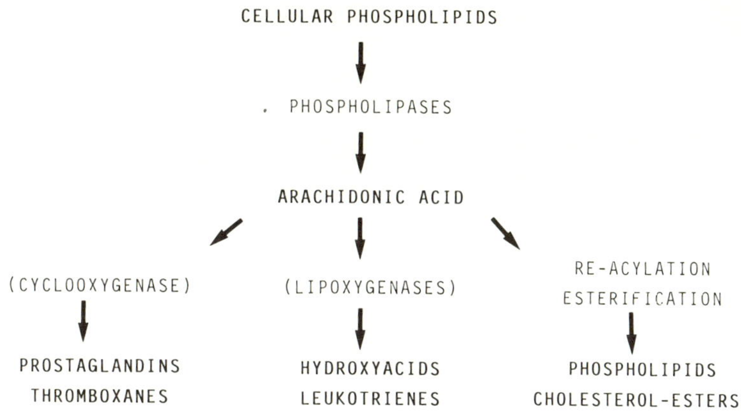

FIGURE 1. General pathways of arachidonic acid metabolism in tissues.

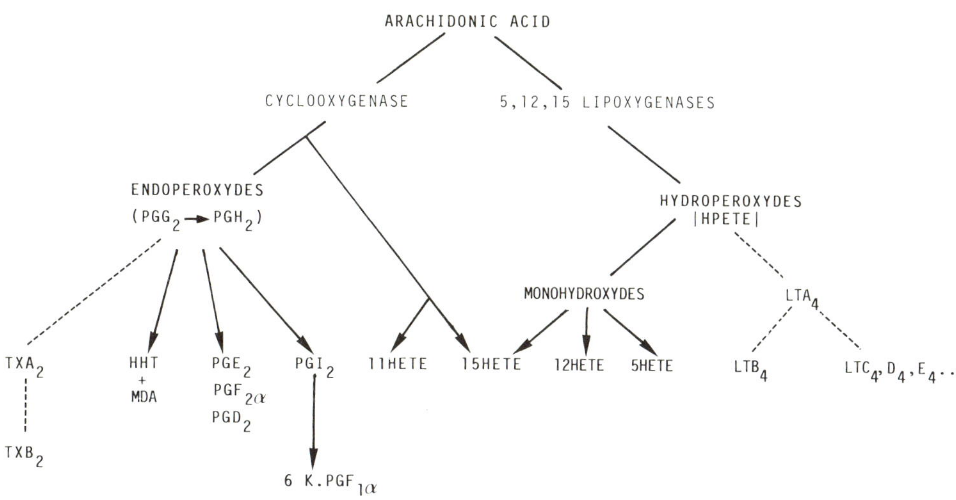

FIGURE 2. Eicosanoid synthesis in vascular SMC. The major product is PGI_2. Full lines refer to recognized pathways under culture conditions. Dotted lines refer to putative pathways.

rather modulate its intensity by amplifying or acting synergistically with other cells and tissue modulators, there is a substantial interest in the knowledge of SMC-eicosanoid production.

In this review, we discuss AA metabolism in cultured vascular SMC, the induction and regulation of eicosanoid synthesis by naturally occurring substances and drugs, and their changes under pathological events related to the atherosclerotic process.

II. ARACHIDONIC ACID METABOLISM IN CULTURED SMOOTH MUSCLE CELLS

A. Influence of Isolation and Culture Conditions

Prostacyclin is the major product of arachidonate metabolism formed by freshly isolated vascular tissues in all mammalian species so far tested.[18] Arteries have been shown to produce more PGI_2 than veins in rabbits,[19] rats,[20] dogs,[21] but such differences were not found in humans.[22] Because prostanoids production also varies along the arterial tree,[23] it is generally difficult to compare the results obtained by different in-

Table 1
CULTURED VASCULAR SMC AND PROSTANOID SYNTHESIS

Species and tissular origin	Ref.
Bovine	
Aorta	28, 48, 50, 53, 55, 57
Guinea pig	
Aorta	15, 36-37, 39
Human	
Umbilical vein	17, 47
Renal artery	17
Abdominal aorta	17
Aorta: thoracic ascending	71
Porcine	
Aorta	24-26, 54, 58
Rabbit	
Aorta	6-8, 70, 88, 90-91
Rat	
Aorta	14, 27, 32, 42, 59-60, 62-63, 69, 89
Mesenteric artery	52

vestigators, and rather large discrepancies appear in the literature concerning both the level and the pattern of prostanoids formed.

Some of the discrepancies undoubtedly arise because investigators have used different vascular segments or different types of cultured cells originating from several anatomical sites and animal species, as summarized in Table 1. Since the amount and the ratio of prostanoids produced by vascular SMC are greatly affected by the conditions used to isolate and culture the cells, it seems that the "history" of cultured cells is of importance. Another reason for discrepancies is that arachidonic acid metabolism has been measured variously by bioassay, radioimmunoassay, or by different chromatographic techniques, including thin-layer chromatography (TLC), high-performance liquid chromatography (HPLC), or gas chromatography-mass spectrometry (GC-MS). Experimental conditions also vary greatly; the most popularly used is the addition of exogenous substrate on either intact cells or cell suspensions. In other cases, cells are treated by different stimulating or inhibiting agents (Table 2) after previous labeling with $[^3H]$ or $[^{14}C]$ AA.

Most of the comparative works on the relative capacity of vascular cells to produce prostaglandins have been done with cells originating from porcine aorta.[24-26] In this species, freshly isolated aortic tissue with or without endothelium present, produce twice as much PGI_2 than PGE_2 during 24 hr of incubation when measured by radioimmunoassay or when incubated with $[^{14}C]$ prostaglandin H_2 or $[^{14}C]$ arachidonate.[24] Isolated endothelial cells synthesize the higher rate of PGI_2 as compared to SMC or fibroblasts from the same artery.[24,25] Since cyclooxygenase activity is known to be a limiting factor in SMC as compared to endothelial cells,[27,28] a lack of cyclooxygenase activity might be considered responsible for the observed differences.

In porcine SMC isolated either by enzymatic digestion or from explant outgrowth, PGE_2 is the predominant prostanoid formed, which suggests that the latter explanation is highly improbable.[24-26] It is possible that some species specificity occurs since SMC obtained from aortic sources of all the other mammalian species studied so far produce essentially PGI_2, at least in primary culture and during the first passages in subcultures.

Indeed, prostanoid formation changes rapidly after isolation and culture mainly because of a decline in prostacyclin synthesis.[24,29] Decreasing PGI_2 production has also

Table 2
REGULATION OF PGI_2 PRODUCTION IN CULTURED VASCULAR SMC

Activators	Ref.
Angiotensin II	47, 53
Bradykinin	47, 53
Fibrinogen degradation products	58
Lipoproteins (HDL, LDL)[a]	83-89
Oestradiol	59
Platelet-derived growth factor (PDGF)	48, 50, 53
Serotonin	48, 53, 55
Thrombin*	61, 63
Inhibitors	
Antiplatelet drugs	18, 94-95
cAMP[a]	43
PGI_2[a]	43
Lipid peroxydes	18, 31, 45, 64, 73, 78
Testosterone	60

[a] See text for discussion.

been reported in fibroblasts and macrophages. The responsible mechanisms are not known but might involve synthesis of hydroperoxy fatty acids, which selectively inhibit PGI_2 synthesis[11] or changes in the cellular oxidant-antioxidant balance.[30,31]

Nevertheless, these hypotheses do not really explain the increase of PGE_2 production observed as a function of cell aging.[32] It is also important to note that rather large variations in PGI_2 production occur between different cell strains from the same vascular origin.[17,24] Finally, eicosanoid production largely depends on the state of the culture (proliferation vs. confluent).

B. Arachidonic Acid Metabolism and Smooth Muscle Cell Proliferation

Vascular SMC in culture, as well as a variety of other cells types, exhibit an activation of prostaglandin production during the exponential phase of growth.[29,33-35] In turn, several exogenously added polyunsaturated fatty acids inhibit the proliferation of cells in culture.[36-38] It has been suggested that this antiproliferative effect is due not only to the conversion of these fatty acids to prostaglandin, but also to their lipoxygenase metabolites.

Whether endogenous eicosanoids are involved in the regulation of cellular proliferation remains to be clearly established since recent results support the hypothesis that cell proliferation may be controlled in part by general peroxidation reactions (see Reference 39 for a review).

When studied in vitro, the PGI_2 synthetic capacity of rabbit artery SMC is higher in the experimental growth phase than at confluency.[34-35] As reported in endothelial and fibroblast-like cells,[33] it seems that this increased PGI_2 production in growing SMC essentially results from an activation of cyclooxygenase rather than PGI_2-synthetase activities. It may be of importance that enhanced PGI_2 formation may occur in vivo in modulated SMC growing in the intima after mechanical injury.[35,40] The fact that nonsteroidal anti-inflammatory drugs that inhibit cyclooxygenase have been found to be potent inhibitors of cell growth by arresting cell cycle in the G_1 phase[41] supports the idea that enhanced prostaglandin production in a given cell type may participate in the induction of growth. In this respect, the effect of exogenously added prostaglandins appears rather contradictory even if concentrations used are generally two to three times the order of magnitude of physiological levels.[15,42] The possibility that exogenous prostaglandin may control its own production from endogenous sources[43] may tentatively explain the apparent discrepancies observed.

In this respect, an interesting approach has been to study the effects of PGE_1 on vascular SMC within 2 days of primary culture.[42] Under these conditions, the cells are known to be in a contractile phenotype. Results indicate that PGE_1 is able to stimulate the modulation of cells from a contractile to synthetic state and to initiate mitosis. By contrast, when added to cells in a modulated state (synthetic phenotype), PGE_1 might control DNA synthesis and inhibit cell proliferation, suggesting a potential dual effect of prostaglandins on vascular SMC that may be relevant in atherosclerosis.

In addition to these variations linked to the biological behavior of vascular SMC, it is necessary to differentiate between the capacity of cells to generate eicosanoids from free arachidonate and from receptor-mediated eicosanoid synthesis.

C. Variables That Affect Arachidonic Acid Metabolism in Vascular Smooth Muscle Cells

The regulation of eicosanoid synthesis by cells in culture has been extensively studied. For details and comprehensive information, the reader is referred to several recent reviews (see Table 2). Here we will first tentatively define the metabolic capacities of vascular SMC, then we will discuss only the variables of physiological importance that may affect eicosanoid synthesis in vascular SMC.

1. Metabolic Capacities of Vascular Smooth Muscle Cells

a. Exogenous Arachidonic Acid Transformation

AA metabolism varies widely in cell culture. The addition of exogenous AA leads to a rapid accumulation of triglycerides or neutral lipids in lipid droplets. Additionally, exogenous AA rapidly incorporates into phospholipids with a relatively selective acylation of phosphorylcholine. Since the fatty acid group in the phospholipids is labile, it is possible to change significantly the phospholipid composition, and the rate of incorporation might constitute a rate limiting factor in the AA transformation by the oxidative cascade.[44]

On the other hand, the concentration of free AA in the incubation medium may lead to the formation of peroxy fatty groups which are inhibitors or destroyers of enzymes in the cascade.[45,46] AA metabolism therefore depends both on the concentration of exogenous fatty acids and its administration as a single dose or long-term infusion.

Most of the initial work has been conducted by incubating vascular SMC with exogenous AA in the micromolar concentration range. Under these conditions, lysed rat aortic SMC synthesize a unique radioactive product identified as 6 Keto PGF_1 alpha.[27] The synthesis appears linear with protein concentration up to 1 mg/mℓ, with an activity of 22 pMol/min/10^6 cells. Later it appears that, as in other species, a range of products may be produced under these experimental conditions, the stable end product 6 Keto PGF_1alpha remaining the major one. For example, human SMC incubated with 5 μM[^{14}C] AA produce several metabolites comigrating with 6 Keto PGF_1 alpha, PGF_2 alpha, PGE_2, and PGD_2, respectively, in several TLC systems.[17] PGI_2 synthetic activity is highly variable and represents values from 1.5 to 30 pM/min/10^6 cells in different cell strains from the same origin. The level of PGI_2 synthesis may approach or sometimes overlap those of endothelial cells from human umbilical vein.[17]

In addition to prostanoids, vascular SMC in culture transform exogenous AA to hydroxylated products, the nature of which is discussed later.

b. Metabolism of Arachidonate from Endogenous Sources

The enzyme-regulated steps in cellular eicosanoid synthesis involve the availability of fatty substrate either released from the cellular lipid stored or originating from extracellular sources of precursors. This is subsequently converted to the endoperoxides or hydroperoxides and, finally, the peroxides are converted to the individual compounds.

The activation of the AA release has been attributed to a number of effectors which appear to potentiate the synthesis of eicosanoids. Among them, it seems that Ca^{2+} may play a central role. The activity of most purified acyl-hydrolases is stimulated by Ca^{2+}. It has therefore been expected that Ca^{2+} has a stimulatory effect on eicosanoid synthesis in cultured cells by increasing the availability of the arachidonate precursor. Indeed, the divalent cation ionophore A_{23187} stimulates eicosanoid synthesis in a number of cultured cells through an activation of Ca^{2+}-dependent phospholipases when exogenous Ca^{2+} is present in the incubation medium. However, the effects of A_{23187} on vascular SMC is somewhat puzzling. A lack of effect has been reported in some vascular SMC strains such as bovine vascular cells, and in vascular SMC the time course of eicosanoid formation following A_{23187} treatment is rather slow compared to endothelial cells.

2. Receptor-Mediated Regulation of PGI_2 Synthesis

Receptors for bradykinin, angiotensin II,[47] serotonin,[48] platelet-derived growth factor (PDGF),[49-50] and others[51-52] have been reported in vascular SMC, and the existence of several cyclooxygenase-sensitive pools of AA that may be differentially sensitive to regulation has been suggested.[52-53] Table 2 summarizes the results, showing a relative specificity of vascular SMC in comparison with endothelial cells.

Prostaglandin production is stimulated by angiotensin II and bradykinin in human umbilical vein SMC. The nanomolar range of minimal bradykinin and angiotensin concentrations that stimulates prostaglandin biosynthesis suggests physiological relevance of this type of response.[47] Later, this effect was confirmed in cells originating from rat mesenteric artery.[52] In this cell type, angiotensin II and vasopressin dose-dependently increase prostaglandin synthesis with a half maximal concentration in the order of 10^{-8} *M*, considerably higher than the concentration of circulating products.

Vasopressin appears to be two to three times as efficient as angiotensin II at maximal effective concentrations. Unlike these vasoconstrictor peptides, norepinephrine has no ability to stimulate prostaglandins. By contrast, both bradykinin and angiotensin II are unable to stimulate prostaglandin synthesis in vascular SMC derived from porcine aorta.[54]

Serotonin, 0.5 μM and above, selectively stimulates the biosynthesis of prostacyclin by bovine aortic SMC in culture. Serotonin stimulates SMC-PGI_2 synthesis through a specific receptor-mediated mechanism involving $5HT_2$ receptors, and the response is calcium-dependent.[55]

Histamine remains ineffective on vascular SMC.[56] The nature of the histamine receptor (H_2 type) may explain the lack of response in these cells, in contrast to the situation occurring in endothelial cells.

The capacity of serum to stimulate PGI_2 synthesis has been reported by several investigators.[50-54] Whether or not this capacity is linked to a phospholipase A_2 stimulating activity or to a greater ability of cells to convert AA to prostanoids remains unknown.[57] Since PDGF has been recognized as a potent activator of PGI_2 production,[50] it appears very likely to be one of the factors involved in the stimulating activity of serum (Figure 3). In addition, several other circulating factors have been recognized as potential stimulators of PGI_2 synthesis,[51,58] among them a heat-labile, nondialyzable factor present in cell-free plasma.[54]

Sex hormones are able to modulate prostaglandin synthesis in vascular SMC. A

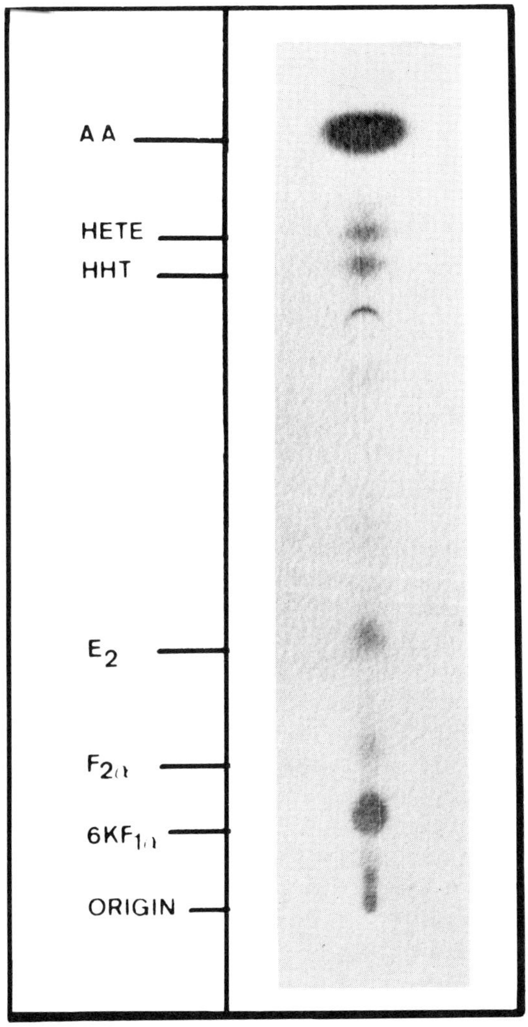

FIGURE 3. Eicosanoid synthesis by vascular SMC. Thin layer chromatographic analysis of the incubation medium of [^{14}C]AA prelabeled rat aortic SMC incubated 3 hr with 5% fetal calf serum. Autoradiography after 3 days of exposition. 6 K F_1 alpha, F_2 alpha, E_2 refer to 6 keto prostaglandin F_1 alpha, prostaglandin F_2 alpha, prostaglandin E_2, respectively. HHT, hydroxy heptadecatrienoic acid; HETE, hydroxy eicosatetraenoic acids; AA, arachidonic acid.

stimulating activity of estradiol has been reported.[59] By contrast, testosterone inhibits PGI_2 formation in rat aortic SMC.[60]

Among the physiological factors potentially involved in the regulation of eicosanoid synthesis in vascular cells, thrombin has been extensively studied. Since the first report of a stimulating effect of thrombin on PGI_2 synthesis by endothelial cells,[61] the effect of this compound on vascular SMC has been debated. To our knowledge, the only vascular SMC responding to thrombin under culture conditions are rat aortic SMC, which under 0.5-IU treatment exhibit an enhanced formation of both prostaglandins and monohydroxy derivatives.[62-63]

In a comparative work conducted on bovine aortic SMC, several agonists were used to stimulate PGI_2 secretion.[53] The level of PGI_2 formed (as measured as 6 Keto PGF_1 alpha in the incubation medium) was raised the same level of magnitude by serotonin, PDGF, fetal-calf serum, the tumor-promoting phorbol-ester - TPA, and the Ca^{2+} ionophore A23187, suggesting that some self-regulation of prostaglandin production may occur, as recently observed in perfused rabbit aorta.[46] In this respect, the interactions between the different eicosanoids may be particularly relevant.[12,64]

3. Lipoxygenase Activities in Vascular Smooth Muscle Cells

The presence of hydroxy fatty acids in arterial tissues has been recognized by several authors.[9,10,65-68] The lipid peroxides are formed in cells and tissues by a number of different mechanisms involving either lipoxygenase, cyclooxygenase-linked cooxidation, or microsomal cytochrome P450 pathways.[39] In contrast, the situation that occurs in cultured vascular SMC remains quite obscure. Early studies report the absence of HETE formation in this particular cell type,[27] but recently several reports demonstrated the formation of monohydroxy fatty acids in cultured cells from arteries of different species. In bovine aortic SMC, hydroxy fatty acid formation occurred from 17% of the total exogenously added [^{14}C] AA. The nature of these compounds is not fully understood.[53]

In rat aorta SMC, the formation of substantial amounts of 15-HETE and 11-HETE has been reported, together with HHT after thrombin treatment of [^{14}C] AA prelabeled cells.[63] These compounds were characterized by GC-MS and appeared to be formed by cyclooxygenase cooxidation mechanisms since their synthesis, together with that of prostacyclin, was inhibited by aspirin and indomethacin. A similar mechanism is suggested for the formation of 15-HPETE, characterized by HPLC, as reported in subcultures of muscle cells from the medial layer of guinea pig aorta incubated 24 hr with labeled [^{14}C] AA.[39] The metabolites that characterize the 12- and 15-lipoxygenase were not identified, and these cells were unable to convert 15-HPETE to corresponding HETE. Additionally, the formation of the malondialdehyde (MDA) was recognized as probably dependent on an increased peroxisomal activity and not linked to the formation of the hydroperoxide.

In contrast to these reports, indirect evidence is given for the formation of the lipoxygenase product 12-HETE in cultured rat aortic SMC treated by partially purified PDGF.[69] In rabbit aortic SMC, the formation of several monohydroxylated derivatives characterized by HPLC and GC-MS has been noted when cell homogenates were challenged by [^{14}C] AA or when prelabeled cells were activated by scraping.[70] Moreover, when homogenates of human aortic SMC were incubated with 10 μM [^{14}C] AA, in addition to the predominant cyclooxygenase derivative, 6 Keto PGF_1 alpha, monohydroxylated derivatives corresponding to 15-HETE, 12-HETE, and 5-HETE, respectively, were characterized.[71] Since, by contrast to 12-HETE and 5-HETE, 15-HETE formation was partially (by 38%) inhibited by indomethacin (30 μM) treatment, its cyclooxygenase origin is, at least in part, likely. The synthesis and the release of these products were confirmed by analyzing the incubation medium of [^{14}C] AA prelabeled SMC treated by the Ca^{2+} ionophore A23187.[71]

Some considerations should be given in interpreting the generation and release of hydroxy fatty acids in cells by adding exogenous AA or after ionophore activation. It is of particular interest that the formation of hydroxylated fatty acids has been recognized from endogenous sources in response to transmembrane physiologic stimuli.[39,63,67] Inhibition experiments remain largely inconclusive, and the metabolic origin of the HETE is sometimes unclear. Despite this, it seems established that appreciable amounts of these compounds originating from several metabolic pathways are synthesized and released by vascular SMC.

Since it must be considered that several inhibitory or activatory interactions between these hydroxy acids and their peroxy precursors and the lipoxygenase pathways occur in several cell types,[12] the relative quantities may be influenced by the modulation of the respective specific lipoxygenases. Moreover, several reports show that incorporation of monohydroxy fatty acids into cellular lipids may depend on the cell type.[72] Whether or not incorporation occurs in SMC remains to be established clearly. Finally, the importance of the role of monohydroxy fatty acids in regulating vascular functions under normal and pathological conditions needs to be clearly elucidated.[39,69-71,73]

In addition to monohydroxy fatty acids, the formation of dihydroxy and peptide-substituted leukotrienes in arteries has been reported.[10,67,68] Whether these leukotrienes originate from vascular cells or from blood cells which are invading the vessel wall remains questionable. Preliminary observations from several laboratories suggest that there may be leukotriene-forming capacities in vascular SMC. The recent evidence showing the formation of 8—15 diHETE in human umbilical vein-endothelial cells in culture strongly supports this possibility.[74]

III. VASCULAR SMOOTH MUSCLE CELL — EICOSANOID PRODUCTION AND THE ATHEROSCLEROTIC PROCESS

One of the most popular models for atherosclerosis suggests that the process is initiated by injury of the endothelium. In response to this injury, platelet activation may occur leading to SMC proliferation, cholesterol influx, and deposition.[75] Under certain circumstances, endoperoxides released from platelets in proximity to vascular cells may be converted to PGI_2 within the vascular wall. In this way, activated platelets may augment vascular PGI_2 formation. It has been suggested that this accounts for the enhancement of the urinary metabolite of PGI_2, the 2—3 dinor 6 Keto PGF_1 alpha, recently observed in human atherosclerosis.[77] Nevertheless, an essential feature of an atherosclerotic vessel is a reduced capacity for PGI_2 synthesis,[78-82] the mechanism of which is essentially unknown.

Experimental, epidemiological, and clinical studies have identified hypercholesterolemia or low-density lipoprotein (LDL) elevation as a major risk factor for atherosclerosis. By contrast, high-density lipoproteins (HDL) exhibit apparent beneficial antiatherogenic effects.

Several mechanisms may be invoked in relating plasma lipoproteins to different aspects of atherosclerosis. Among them, depressed HDL or elevated LDL may cause disturbance in the physiologic balance of prostaglandin production through a variety of pathophysiologic mechanisms.

In this regard, the role of lipoproteins on PGI_2 production has been debated. The direct inhibitory effect of LDL on the endothelium's ability to inhibit platelet aggregation through the synthesis of prostacyclin has been reported as partially counteracted by HDL.[83] When investigated in vitro on the microsomal fraction of pig aorta, a linear negative correlation between the amount of LDL and the PGI_2 synthetase activity was found.[84,85] It has been suggested that the observed inactivation of PGI_2 synthetase is closely associated with lipid peroxides. Nevertheless, the fact that serum lipoproteins were susceptible to peroxidation during the preparation procedure leads to a quite obscure situation.[86] Recently, in contrast to previous results (when lipoproteins were prepared carefully in order to prevent artifactual generation of lipid peroxides), both HDL and LDL were able to stimulate prostaglandin synthesis in several vascular cell types, including SMC.[87-89]

The mechanism of this stimulation may be complex, involving both the lipid and apolipoprotein moieties of the lipoproteins. Lipoproteins (HDL and LDL) may provide arachidonate to cellular phospholipase-sensitive pools accessible to cyclooxygenase,[87-88] and lipoproteins may stimulate the liberation of arachidonate from endogenous cellular stores for prostaglandin synthesis.[89]

The physiological significance of the stimulation of PGI_2 and PGE_2 synthesis in vascular SMC by HDL and LDL remains to be determined. However, it may be of importance to note that PGI_2 activates acid-cholesteryl hydrolases, and PGE_2 inhibits cholesterol ester synthetic activity in cultured SMC.[6-7]

In addition, we have observed that under culture conditions, vascular SMC from atherosclerotic vessels have a reduced capacity to produce PGI_2, and primary prostaglandins from both exogenously added [^{14}C] AA and endogenous sources.[90-91] This defect persists in secondary culture with serial passaging. Taken together, these results make questionable the initial proposal that lipid peroxides in arterial lesions inhibit prostacyclin synthetase. Alternatively, the observation that vascular SMC may produce lipoxygenase-derived hydroperoxides greatly reinforces the hypothesis that eicosanoid synthesis by vascular SMC may induce production of compounds that inhibit cyclooxygenase. This is currently under investigation in several laboratories. In a preliminary experiment, we have observed an enhanced formation of the lipoxygenase-derived product 12-HETE in atherosclerotic cells as compared to control cells, suggesting a balance between cyclooxygenase and lipoxygenase activities in vascular SMC. Another possibility involves the participation of eicosanoids synthesized by circulating cells, or cells which are entering the vascular wall such as macrophages, which produce a wide variety of cyclooxygenase and lipoxygenase-derived compounds.[92-93] The role of these cells and of their eicosanoids in the pathophysiologic events related to atherosclerotic process required further study.

IV. SUMMARY AND CONCLUSIONS

Vascular SMC not only synthesize and release a variety of eicosanoids that exhibit a wide range of biological activities, but are target cells for the same substances. These compounds are extremely potent modulators of physiologic responses in the immediate cell microenvironment by initiating and modulating biochemical reactions. As knowledge of the participation of these products increases in several physiologic and pathologic events, such as (1) regulation of cell interactions at the interface between vascular wall and blood cells and within the vascular wall itself, (2) endothelial-dependent SMC relaxation, (3) SMC migration and proliferation, and (4) cholesterol ester metabolism, the importance of eicosanoids in the pathogenesis of atherosclerosis will become more apparent. As our understanding of the relevant biochemical mechanisms progress, multiple and more specific pharmacological interventions are being developed. While actual results suggest that modulation of eicosanoid production may be beneficial in controlling or preventing vascular SMC disorders, it is not clear, at the moment, which strategy will be most suitable for this pathological situation.[94] As far as atherosclerosis is concerned, much remains to be learned about the physiological actions of eicosanoids and the mechanisms controlling their production in vascular SMC.[95]

Further studies are required, particularly to establish the biological importance of the inhibitory and stimulatory effects of hydroxy- and hydroperoxy fatty acids on eicosanoids synthesis. In this respect, the development of antagonists of the lipoxygenase products could be of considerable value. The potential for altering vascular disorder by manipulating eicosanoid production is particularly exciting and undoubtedly constitutes one of the main interesting areas of biological research.

REFERENCES

1. Tuvemo, T. and Wide, L., Prostaglandin release from the human umbilical artery in vitro, *Prostaglandins,* 4, 689, 1973.
2. Terragano, D. A., Crowshaw, K., Terragano, N. A., and McGiff, J. C., Prostaglandin synthesis by bovine mesenteric arteries and veins, *Circ. Res.,* 36, 76, 1975.
3. Moncada, S., Gryglewski, R., Bunting, S., and Vane, J. R., An enzyme isolated from arteries transforms endoperoxides to an unstable substance that inhibits platelet aggregation, *Nature (London),* 263, 663, 1976.
4. Bunting, S., Gryglewski, R., Moncada, S., and Vane, J. R., Arterial walls generate from prostaglandin endoperoxides a substance (prostaglandin X) which relaxes strips of mesenteric and coeliac arteries and inhibits platelet aggregation, *Prostaglandins,* 12, 897, 1976.
5. Gryglewski, R. J., Bunting, S., Moncada, S., Flower, R. J., and Vane, J. R., Arterial walls are protected against deposition of platelet thrombi by a substance (prostaglandin X) which they make from prostaglandin endoperoxides, *Prostaglandins,* 12, 685, 1976.
6. Hajjar, D. P., Weksler, B. B., Falcone, D. J., Hefton, J. M., Tack-Goldman, K., and Minick, C. R., Prostacyclin modulates cholesteryl ester hydrolytic activity by its effects on cyclic adenosine monophosphate in rabbit aortic smooth muscle cells, *J. Clin. Invest.,* 70, 479, 1982.
7. Hajjar, D. P. and Weksler, B. B., Metabolic activity of cholesteryl esters in aortic smooth muscle cells is altered by prostaglandins I_2 and E_2, *J. Lipid Res.,* 24, 1176, 1983.
8. Smith, D. L., Willis, A. L., and Mahmud, I., Eicosanoid effects on cell proliferation in vitro: relevance to atherosclerosis, *Prost. Leuk. Med.,* 16, 1, 1984.
9. Greenwald, J. E., Bianchine, J. R., and Wong, L. K., The production of the arachidonate metabolite HETE in vascular tissue, *Nature (London),* 281, 588, 1979.
10. Piper, P. J., Letts, L. G., and Galton, S. A., Generation of leukotriene-like substance from porcine vascular and other tissue, *Prostaglandins,* 25, 291, 1983.
11. Salmon, J. A., Smith, D. R., Flower, R. J., Moncada, S., and Vane, J. R., Further studies on the enzymatic conversion of prostaglandin endoperoxides into prostacyclin by porcine aorta microsomes, *Biochim. Biophys. Acta,* 523, 250, 1978.
12. Kuehl, F. A., Dougherty, H. W., and Ham, E. A., Interactions between prostaglandins and leukotrienes, *Biochem. Pharm.,* 23, 1, 1984.
13. Samuelsson, B., Leukotrienes, mediators of immediate hypersensitivity reactions and inflammation, *Science,* 220, 568, 1983.
14. Nakao, J., Ooyama, T., Ito, M., Chang, W. C., and Murota, S., Comparative effect of lipoxygenases products of arachidonic acid on rat aortic smooth muscle cells migration, *Atherosclerosis,* 44, 339, 1982.
15. Huttner, J. J., Gwebu, E. T., Panganamala, R. V., Milo, G. E., Cornwell, D. G., Sharmar, H. M., and Geer, J. C., Fatty acids and their prostaglandin derivatives: inhibitors of proliferation in aortic smooth muscle cells, *Science,* 197, 289, 1977.
16. Moncada, S., Herman, A. G., Higgs, E. A., and Vane, R. J., Differential formation of prostacyclin by layers of the arterial wall. An explanation for the anti-thrombic properties of vascular endothelium, *Thromb. Res.,* 11, 323, 1977.
17. Baenziger, N. L., Becherer, P. R., and Majerus, P. W., Characterization of prostacyclin synthesis in cultured human arterial smooth muscle cells, venous endothelial cells and skin fibroblasts, *Cell,* 16, 967, 1979.
18. Moncada, S., Prostacyclin and arterial wall biology, *Arteriosclerosis,* 2, 193, 1982.
19. Buchanan, M. R., Dejana, E., Cazenave, J. P., Mustard, J. F., and Hirsch, J., Uncontrolled PGI_2, production by whole vessel wall segments due to thrombin generation in vivo and its prevention by heparin, *Thromb. Res.,* 16, 551, 1979.
20. Skidgel, R. A. and Printz, M. P., PGI_2 production by rat blood vessels diminished prostacyclin formation in veins compared to arteries, *Prostaglandins,* 16, 1, 1978.
21. Eldor, A., Hoover, E. L., Pett, S. B., Jr., Gay, W. A., Jr., Alonso, D. R., and Weksler, B. B., Prostaglandin production by arterialized autogenous venous grafts in dogs, *Prostaglandins,* 22, 485, 1981.
22. Moncada, S., Higgs, E. A., and Vane, J. R., Human arterial and venous tissues generate prostacyclin (prostaglandin X) a potent inhibitor of platelet aggregation, *Lancet,* 1, 18, 1977.
23. Hagen, A. A., White, R. P., and Robertson, J. T., Synthesis of prostaglandin and thromboxane B_2 by cerebral arteries, *Stroke,* 10, 306, 1979.
24. Ager, A., Gordon, J. L., Moncada, A. S., Pearson, J. D., Salmon, J. A., and Trevethick, M. A., Effects of isolation and culture on prostaglandins synthesis by porcine aortic endothelial and smooth muscle cells, *J. Cell. Physiol.,* 110, 9, 1982.

25. Ody, C., Seillan, C., and Russo-Marie, F., 6 Keto-PGF_1 alpha, PGE_2, PGF_2 alpha and thromboxane B_2 production by endothelial cells, smooth muscle cells and fibroblasts cultured from piglet aorta, *Biochim. Biophys. Acta,* 712, 103, 1982.
26. Siess, W., Dray, F., Seillan, C., Ody, C., and Russo-Marie, F., Prostanoid synthesis by vascular slices and cultured vascular cells of piglet aorta, *Biochem. Biophys. Res. Commun.,* 99, 608, 1981.
27. Tansik, R. L., Namm, D. H., and White, H. L., Synthesis of prostaglandin 6-Keto PGF_1 alpha by cultured aortic smooth muscle cells and stimulation of its formation in a coupled system with platelet lysates, *Prostaglandins,* 15, 399, 1978.
28. Dewitt, D. L., Day, J. S., Sonnenburg, W. K., and Smith, W. L., Concentration of prostaglandin endoperoxide synthase and prostaglandin I_2 synthase in the endothelium and smooth muscle cell of bovine aorta, *J. Clin. Invest.,* 72, 1882, 1983.
29. Larrue, J., Rigaud, M., Leroux, C., Crockett, R., and Bricaud, H., Prostacyclin synthesis by cultured vascular smooth muscle cells: influence of growth and ageing, *Thromb. Haemost.,* 46(Suppl. I), 38, 1981.
30. Gavino, V. C., Miller, J. S., Ikharebha, S. O., Milo, G. E., and Cornwell, D. G., Effect of polyunsaturated fatty acids and antioxidants on lipids peroxidation in tissue cultures, *J. Lipid Res.,* 22, 763, 1981.
31. Taylor, L., Menconi, M. J., and Polgar, P., The participation of hydroperoxides and oxygen radicals in the control of prostaglandin synthesis, *J. Biol. Chem.,* 258, 6855, 1983.
32. Chang, W. C., Murota, S. I., Nakao, J., and Orimo, H., Age-related decrease in prostacyclin biosynthetic activity in rat aortic smooth muscle cells, *Biochim. Biophys. Acta,* 620, 159, 1980.
33. Ali, A. E., Barrett, J. C., and Eling, T. E., Prostaglandin and thromboxane production by fibroblasts and vascular endothelial cells, *Prostaglandins,* 20, 667, 1980.
34. Larrue, J., Bricaud, H., and Sinzinger, H., Prostacyclin synthesis by proliferative aortic smooth muscle cells, *Vasa,* 13, 311, 1984.
35. Larrue, J., Daret, D., Demond-Henri, J., Allières, C., and Bricaud, H., Prostacyclin synthesis by proliferative aortic smooth muscle cells. A kinetic in vivo and in vitro study, *Atherosclerosis,* 50, 63, 1984.
36. Cornwell, D. G., Huttner, J. J., Milo, G. E., Panganamala, R. V., Sharma, H. M., and Geer, J. C., Polyunsaturated fatty acids, vitamin E, and proliferation of aortic smooth muscle cells, *Lipids,* 14, 194, 1979.
37. Morisaki, N., Sprecher, H., Milo, G. E., and Cornwell, D. G., Fatty acid specificity in the inhibition of cell proliferation and its relationship to lipid peroxidation and prostaglandin biosynthesis, *Lipids,* 17, 893, 1982.
38. Smith, D. L., Willis, A. L., and Mahmud, I., Eicosanoid effects on cell proliferation in vitro: relevance to atherosclerosis, *Prost. Leuk. Med.,* 16, 1, 1984.
39. Morisaki, N., Lindsey, J. A., Stitts, J. M., Zhang, H., and Cornwell, D. G., Fatty acid metabolism and cell proliferation. V. Evaluation of pathways for the generation of lipid peroxides, *Lipids,* 19, 381, 1984.
40. Eldor, A., Falcone, D. J., Hajjar, D. M., Minick, C. R., and Weksler, B. B., Recovery of prostacyclin production by deendothelialized rabbit aorta. Critical role of neointimal smooth muscle cells, *J. Clin. Invest.,* 67, 735, 1981.
41. Bayer, B. M., Kruth, H. S., Vaughan, M., and Beaven, M. A., Arrest of cultured cells in the GI phase of cell cycle by indomethacin, *J. Pharmacol. Exp. Ther.,* 210, 106, 1979.
42. Sjölund, M., Nilsson, J., Palmberg, L., and Thyberg, J., Phenotype modulation in primary cultures of arterial smooth muscle cells. Dual effect of PGE_1, *Differentiation,* 27, 158, 1984.
43. Larrue, J., Dorian, B., Daret, D., Demond-Henri, J., and Bricaud, H., Role of cyclic-AMP in the regulation of prostacyclin synthesis by cultured vascular smooth muscle cells, *Adv. Cyclic Nucleotide Protein Phosphorylation Res.,* 17, 585, 1984.
44. Denning, G. M., Figard, P. H., and Spector, A. A., Effect of fatty acid modification of prostaglandin production by cultured 3T3 cells, *J. Lipid Res.,* 23, 584, 1982.
45. Ham, E. A., Egan, R. W., Soderman, D. D., Gale, P. M., and Kuehl, F. A., Jr., Peroxydase-dependent deactivation of prostacyclin-synthetase, *J. Biol. Chem.,* 254, 2191, 1979.
46. Kent, R. S., Diedrich, S. L., and Whorton, R. A., Regulation of vascular prostaglandin synthesis by metabolites of arachidonic acid in perfused rabbit aorta, *J. Clin. Invest.,* 72, 455, 1983.
47. Alexander, R. W. and Gimbrone, M. A., Jr., Stimulation of prostaglandin E synthesis in cultured human umbilical vein smooth muscle cells, *Proc. Natl. Acad. Sci. U.S.A.,* 73, 1617, 1976.
48. Coughlin, S. R., Moskowitz, M. A., Antoniades, H. N., and Levine, L., Serotonin receptor mediated stimulation of bovine smooth muscle cells prostacyclin synthesis and its modulation by platelet derived growth factor, *Proc. Natl. Acad. Sci. U.S.A.,* 78, 7134, 1981.
49. Heldin, C. H., Westermark, B., and Wasteson, A., Specific receptors for PDGF on cell derived from connective tissue and glia, *Proc. Natl. Acad. Sci. U.S.A.,* 78, 3664, 1981.

50. Coughlin, S. R., Moskowitz, M. A., Zetter, B. R., Antoniades, H. N., and Levine, L., Platelet dependent stimulation of prostacyclin synthesis by platelet derived growth factor, *Nature (London)*, 288, 600, 1980.
51. Hassid, A., Regulation of prostaglandin biosynthesis in cultured cells, *Am. J. Physiol.*, 243, 205, 1982.
52. Hassid, A. and Williams, C., Vasoconstrictor-evoked prostaglandin synthesis in cultured vascular smooth muscle cells, *Am. J. Physiol.*, 245, 278, 1983.
53. Goldstein, S. M., Moskowitz, M. A., and Levine, L., Inhibition of stimulated prostaglandin biosynthesis by retinoic acid in smooth muscle cells, *Cancer Res.*, 44, 120, 1984.
54. MacIntyre, D. E., Pearson, J. D., and Gordon, J. L., Localisation and stimulation of prostacyclin-production in vascular cells, *Nature (London)*, 271, 549, 1978.
55. Coughlin, S. R., Moskowitz, M. A., and Levine, L., Identification of a serotonin type 2 receptor linked to prostacyclin synthesis in vascular smooth muscle cells, *Biochem. Pharmacol.*, 33, 692, 1984.
56. Baenziger, N. L., Fogerty, F. J., Mertz, L. F., and Chernuta, L. F., Regulation of histamine-mediated prostacyclin synthesis in cultured human vascular endothelial cells, *Cell*, 24, 915, 1981.
57. Dejanna, E., de Castellarnau, C., Balconi, G., Olivieri, S., Pietra, A., Barbieri, B., and de Gaetano, G., Recovery of prostacyclin production by cultured bovine smooth muscle cells after aspirin inhibition: effect of serum replacement and concentration in culture medium, *Biochem. Pharmacol.*, 32, 710, 1983.
58. Watanabe, K., Ishida, T., Yoshitomi, F., and Tanaka, K., Fibrinogen degradation products influence PGI_2 synthesis by cultured porcine aortic endothelial and smooth muscle cells, *Atherosclerosis*, 51, 151, 1984.
59. Chang, W. C., Nakao, J., Orimo, H., and Murota, S. I., Stimulation of prostaglandin cyclooxygenase and prostacyclin synthetase activities by oestradiol in rat aortic smooth muscle cells, *Biochim. Biophys. Acta*, 620, 472, 1980.
60. Nakao, J., Chang, W. C., Murota, S. I., and Orimo, H., Testosterone inhibits prostacyclin production by rat aortic smooth muscle cells in culture, *Atherosclerosis*, 39, 203, 1981.
61. Weksler, B. B., Ley, C. W., and Jaffe, E. A., Stimulation of endothelial cell prostacyclin production by thrombin, trypsin and the ionophore A23187, *J. Clin. Invest.*, 62, 923, 1978.
62. Whiting, J., Salata, K., and Bailey, J. M., Aspirin: an unexpected side effect on prostacyclin synthesis in cultured vascular smooth muscle cells, *Science*, 210, 663, 1980.
63. Bailey, J. M., Bryant, R. W., Whiting, J., and Salata, K., Characterization of 11-HETE and 15-HETE, together with prostacyclin as major products of the cyclooxygenase pathway in cultured rat aorta smooth muscle cells, *J. Lipid Res.*, 24, 1419, 1983.
64. Setty, B. N. Y., Jurek, E., Ganley, C., and Stuart, M. J., Effects of hydrogen peroxide on vascular arachidonic acid metabolism, *Prost. Leuk. Med.*, 14, 205, 1984.
65. Powell, W. S., Formation of 6-oxoprostaglandin F_1 alpha, 6,16-dioxoprostaglandin F_1 alpha, and monohydroxyicosatetraenoic acids from arachidonic acid by fetal calf aorta and ductus arteriosus, *J. Biol. Chem.*, 257, 9457, 1982.
66. Powell, W. S., Formation of trihydroxyheptadecenoic acids, monohydroxyicosatetraenoic acids, and prostaglandins from 8, 11, 14-icosatrienoic acid by adult and fetal aorta, *J. Biol. Chem.*, 257, 9465, 1982.
67. Piper, P. J. and Galton, S. A., Generation of LTB_4 and LTE_4 from porcine pulmonary artery, *Prostaglandins*, 28, 905, 1984.
68. Dembinska-Kiec, A., Simmet, T., and Peskar, B. A., Release and vasoconstriction effect of leukotriene C_4-like immunoreactive material in the anaphylactic guinea pig mesenteric vascular bed, *Eur. J. Pharmacol.*, 101, 259, 1984.
69. Nakao, J., Ito, H., Chang, W. C., Koshihara, Y., and Murota, S. I., Aortic smooth muscle cell migration caused by platelet derived growth factor is mediated by lipoxygenase products of arachidonic acid, *Biochem. Biophys. Res. Commun.*, 112, 866, 1983.
70. Larrue, J., Rigaud, M., Razaka, G., Daret, D., Demond-Henri, J., and Bricaud, H., Formation of monohydroxyeicosatetraenoic acids from arachidonic acid by cultured rabbit aortic smooth muscle cells, *Biochem. Biophys. Res. Commun.*, 112, 242, 1983.
71. Larrue, J., Razaka, G., Daret, D., Henri, J., Rigaud, M., and Bricaud, H., Lipoxygenase derived products in cultured human aortic smooth muscle cells, *Adv. Prostaglandin Thromboxane Leukotriene Res.*, 13, 55, 1985.
72. Mayer, B., Rauter, L., Zenzmaier, E., Gleispach, H., and Esterbauer, H., Characterization of lipoxygenase metabolites of arachidonic acid in cultured human skin fibroblasts, *Biochim. Biophys. Acta*, 795, 151, 1984.
73. Turk, J., Wyche, A., and Needleman, Ph., Inactivation of vascular prostacyclin synthetase by platelet lipoxygenase products, *Biochem. Biophys. Res. Commun.*, 95, 1628, 1980.
74. Hopkins, N. K., Oglesby, T. D., Bundy, G. L., and Gorman, R. R., Biosynthesis and metabolism of 15-HPETE by human umbilical vein endothelial cells, *J. Biol. Chem.*, 259, 14048, 1984.

75. Ross, R. and Glomset, J. A., The pathogenesis of atherosclerosis, *N. Engl. J. Med.*, 295, 369, 1976.
76. Marcus, A. J., Weksler, B. B., Jaffe, E. A., and Broekman, M. J., Synthesis of prostacyclin from platelet derived endoperoxides by cultured human endothelial cells, *J. Clin. Invest.*, 66, 979, 1980.
77. Fitzgerald, G. A., Smith, B., Pedersen, A. K., and Brash, A. R., Increased PGI_2 biosynthesis in patients with severe atherosclerosis and platelet activation, *N. Engl. J. Med.*, 310, 1065, 1984.
78. Gryglewski, R. J., Prostacyclin and atherosclerosis, *Trends Pharmac. Sci.*, 1, 164, 1980.
79. D'Angelo, V., Villa, S., Mysliwiec, M., Donati, M. B., and de Gaetano, Z., Defective fibrinolytic and prostacyclin-like activity in human atheromatous plaques [letter], *Thromb. Haemostas.*, 39, 535, 1978.
80. Dembinska-Kiec, A., Gryglewska, T., Zmuda, A., and Gryglewski, R. J., The generation of prostacyclin by arteries and by the coronary vascular bed is reduced in experimental atherosclerosis in rabbits, *Prostaglandins*, 14, 1025, 1977.
81. Sinzinger, H., Silberbauer, K., Feigl, W., Wagner, O., Winter, M., and Auerswald, W., Prostacyclin activity is diminished in different types of morphologically controlled human atherosclerotic lesions, *Thromb. Haemost.*, 42, 803, 1979.
82. Eldor, A., Falcone, D. J., Hajjar, D. P., Minick, C. R., and Weksler, B. B., Diet induced hypercholesterolemia inhibits the recovery of prostacyclin production by injured rabbit aorta, *Am. J. Pathol.*, 107, 186, 1982.
83. Nordoy, A., Svensson, B., Wiebe, D., and Hoak, J. C., Lipoproteins and the inhibitory effect of human endothelial cells on platelet function, *Circ. Res.*, 434, 527, 1978.
84. Beitz, J. and Forster, W., Influence of human low density and high density lipoprotein cholesterol on the in vitro prostaglandin I_2 synthetase activity, *Biochim. Biophys. Acta*, 620, 325, 1980.
85. Beitz, J., Panse, M., Fischer, S., Hora, C., and Forster, W., Inhibition of prostaglandin I_2 (PGI_2) formation by LDL-cholesterol or LDL-peroxides ?, *Prostaglandins*, 26, 885, 1983.
86. Szczeklik, A., Gryglewski, R. J., Domagala, B., Zmuda, A., Martwich, J., Wozny, E., Grywacz, M., Madej, J., and Gryglewska, T., Serum lipoproteins, lipid peroxides and prostacyclin biosynthesis in patients with coronary heart disease, *Prostaglandins*, 22, 795, 1981.
87. Fleisher, L. N., Tall, A. R., Witte, L. D., Miller, R. W., and Cannon, P. J., Stimulation of arterial endothelial cell prostacyclin synthesis by high density lipoproteins, *J. Biol. Chem.*, 257, 6653, 1982.
88. Pomerantz, K. B., Tall, A. R., Feinmark, S. J., and Cannon, P. J., Stimulation of vascular smooth muscle cell prostacyclin and prostaglandin E_2 synthesis by plasma high and low density lipoproteins, *Circ. Res.*, 54, 554, 1984.
89. Larrue, J., Crockett, J., Daret, D., Demond-Henri, J., and Bricaud, H., Modulation of vascular smooth muscle cell prostacyclin synthesis by plasma lipoproteins, *Eur. Heart J.*, 5(Suppl. 1), 159, 1984.
90. Larrue, J., Rigaud, M., Daret, D., Demond, J., Durand, J., and Bricaud, H., Prostacyclin production by cultured smooth muscle cells from atherosclerotic rabbit aorta, *Nature (London)*, 285, 480, 1980.
91. Larrue, J., Leroux, C., Daret, D., and Bricaud, H., Decreased prostaglandin production in cultured smooth muscle cells from atherosclerotic rabbit aorta, *Biochim. Biophys. Acta*, 710, 257, 1982.
92. Moldow, C. F., Neutrophil endothelial interaction, in *Biology of Endothelial Cells*, Jaffe, E. A., Ed., Kluwer Academic, Hingham, Mass., 1984, 286.
93. Goldyne, M. E., Heterogeneity in leucocyte preparations: effects on defining eicosanoid metabolism by human lymphocytes and monocytes, *J. Allergy Clin. Immunol.*, 74, 331, 1984.
94. Weksler, B. B., Prostaglandins and vascular function, *Circulation*, 70(Suppl. 3), 63, 1984.
95. Cannon, P. J., Eicosanoids and the blood vessel wall, *Circulation*, 70, 523, 1984.

Chapter 13

GROWTH AND BIOCHEMICAL PROPERTIES OF AORTIC SMOOTH MUSCLE CELLS FROM CHOLESTEROL-FED RABBITS

Tapio Nikkari, Olli Jaakkola, Olli-Pekka Kallioniemi, Seppo Nikkari, and Kari Pietilä

TABLE OF CONTENTS

I. INTRODUCTION

The development of atherosclerotic lesions involves three processes taking place in the arterial intima: (1) an enhanced proliferation of arterial smooth muscle cells (SMC), (2) an increased rate of synthesis of connective tissue components by the SMC, and (3) an accumulation of lipids in the intima.[1] According to the response-to-injury theory,[1] the enhanced growth of intimal SMC is caused by plasma- or platelet-derived factors gaining entry into the intima as a consequence of endothelial damage and the adherence of platelets to the subendothelium. The monoclonal hypothesis,[2] on the other hand, assumes that atherosclerotic lesions are benign neoplasms originating from single cells that have been transformed by various agents. The observed monotypism in atherosclerotic lesions[1] has also been explained by a selective advantage of growth among a progeny of normal, nontransformed SMC.[3,4]

The response-to-injury theory is supported by data indicating that subcultured vascular SMC can be stimulated to proliferate by the addition of platelet-derived growth factor (PDGF),[5] low-density lipoproteins (LDL),[6] and other serum components. On the other hand, Campbell, Chamley-Campbell, and Ross[3,7] have shown that differentiated, contractile SMC in primary culture do not respond to serum mitogens until after dedifferentiation into a myofilament-poor synthetic phenotype. No factors or mechanisms have so far been identified that could be held responsible for the modulation of contractile medial SMC into synthetic cells capable of migration into the intima and proliferation there. That such a change in phenotype takes place in vivo is suggested by several ultrastructural studies demonstrating the presence in thickened[8-10] and atherosclerotic[3,11-16] intimas of morphologically modified SMC with reduced numbers of myofilaments and increased contents of rough endoplasmic reticulum and mitochondria.

If only the poorly differentiated SMC are capable of proliferation, cells isolated from atherosclerotic vessels should respond more readily to mitogens than those from normal intima-medias. The atherosclerotic cells should also differ biochemically from normal SMC with respect to the composition of cytocontractile proteins, and changes in the contents of these proteins would be likely to occur when normal contractile SMC are allowed to dedifferentiate in culture. Our studies were designed to test these ideas using enzymatically isolated normal and atherosclerotic SMC in primary cultures, in which conditions the cells supposedly still have the same phenotype as in vivo. Another part of the work employed SMC from later passages to examine whether the growth and metabolic properties of completely dedifferentiated atherosclerotic SMC differ from those of corresponding normal cells, as could be expected if the cells represent a transformed or a selected population.

II. INDUCTION OF ATHEROSCLEROSIS

Rabbit aortic atherosclerosis has been used as the model throughout our experiments: young rabbits were fed either a normal rabbit chow (control rabbits) or a chow to which cholesterol had been added as an etheral solution. The cholesterol content of the chow was adjusted to maintain the serum cholesterol level at approximately 40 mmol/ℓ.[17]

In electron microscopy, the alterations in the aortas of rabbits fed cholesterol for 4 months[18] were similar to those described by other authors in the same species.[11,12,14] The thickened intimas contained numerous vacuolated cells, although SMC without lipid inclusions were also present. A large part of the vacuolated cells were SMC because they had basement membranes and numerous plasmalemmal vesicles, but many of them were obviously monocyte-derived, lipid-filled macrophages. Most of the SMC in atherosclerotic intimas differed from the myofilament-filled medial SMC by displaying features of dedifferentiation: a reduced content of myofilaments, located in the periphery of the cell, and a substantial increase in dilated rough endoplasmic reticulum, vesicles, and mitochondria.

After cholesterol feeding for 6 months followed by normal chow for another 6 months, the aortas were covered throughout with lesions that were thicker and more fibrous than those produced by 6 months of cholesterol feeding alone.[19] This is in keeping with previous findings on cholesterol-induced atherosclerosis in the rabbit.[20-22]

III. MORPHOLOGY OF ENZYMATICALLY ISOLATED AORTIC CELLS

Ultrastructurally, the enzyme-dispersed cells from the aortas of the control rabbits were typical differentiated SMC with a high content of myofilaments (Figure 1A). Identification of the cells isolated from the atherosclerotic intima-medias was difficult because basement membranes were removed by the enzyme treatments. A large proportion of the cells were SMC as judged by the presence of myofilaments (Figure 1B), although most of them differed from normal medial SMC by showing signs of dedifferentiation.[18]

Many of the vacuolated cells in the enzyme digests of atherosclerotic aortas lacked all features of SMC, but had Fc-receptors and showed an avid uptake of fluorescent acetyl-LDL (Figure 2), both of which are characteristics of monocyte-macrophages.[25] On the other hand, a sizable portion of the foamy cells had myofilaments and lacked Fc-receptors. Several of these lipid-containing SMC were capable of internalizing acetyl-LDL, which normal SMC are unable to do.[25] This finding accords with previous reports suggesting that "mixed" cells, possessing ultrastructural properties of both SMC and macrophages, are present in atherosclerotic lesions[26,27] and that SMC may acquire some characteristics of macrophages when they become overloaded with lipid.[28]

IV. PRIMARY GROWTH RATES OF THE SMOOTH MUSCLE CELLS

Primary cultures were started either from cells isolated enzymatically[18] or from explants[17] of normal intima-medias or atherosclerotic lesions. When equal numbers of freshly isolated intima-medial cells were seeded into tissue culture flasks, cells from control aortas attached slowly on the culture surface and remained quiescent for 5 to 6 days (Figure 3), which corresponds to the time taken for modulation of contractile SMC into the synthetic phenotype[3,7] (see Volume I, Chapter 4). In contrast, SMC from atherosclerotic aortas spread rapidly on the culture dish and started to divide within 2 days. The macrophage foam cells did not spread on the surface and showed no signs of proliferation.

The almost immediate response of atherosclerotic SMC to serum mitogens was also evident from a rapid uptake of radioactive thymidine and an increase in cell number from the second day onwards (Figure 4), while control cells had a lag period of 5 to 6 days before starting to grow. These results are in good agreement with phase-contrast microscopic observations (Figure 3). Similar differences were noted in explant-derived primary cultures:[17] explants from atherosclerotic intima-medias gave rise to outgrowths sooner and formed larger colonies than those from normal vessels. Grunwald and Haudenschild[29] have reported corresponding findings with explant-derived primary cultures from balloon-injured aortas of rats.

Our results are in accordance with the concept that most SMC in a healthy arterial wall have a differentiated phenotype and are therefore incapable of mitosis, whereas a

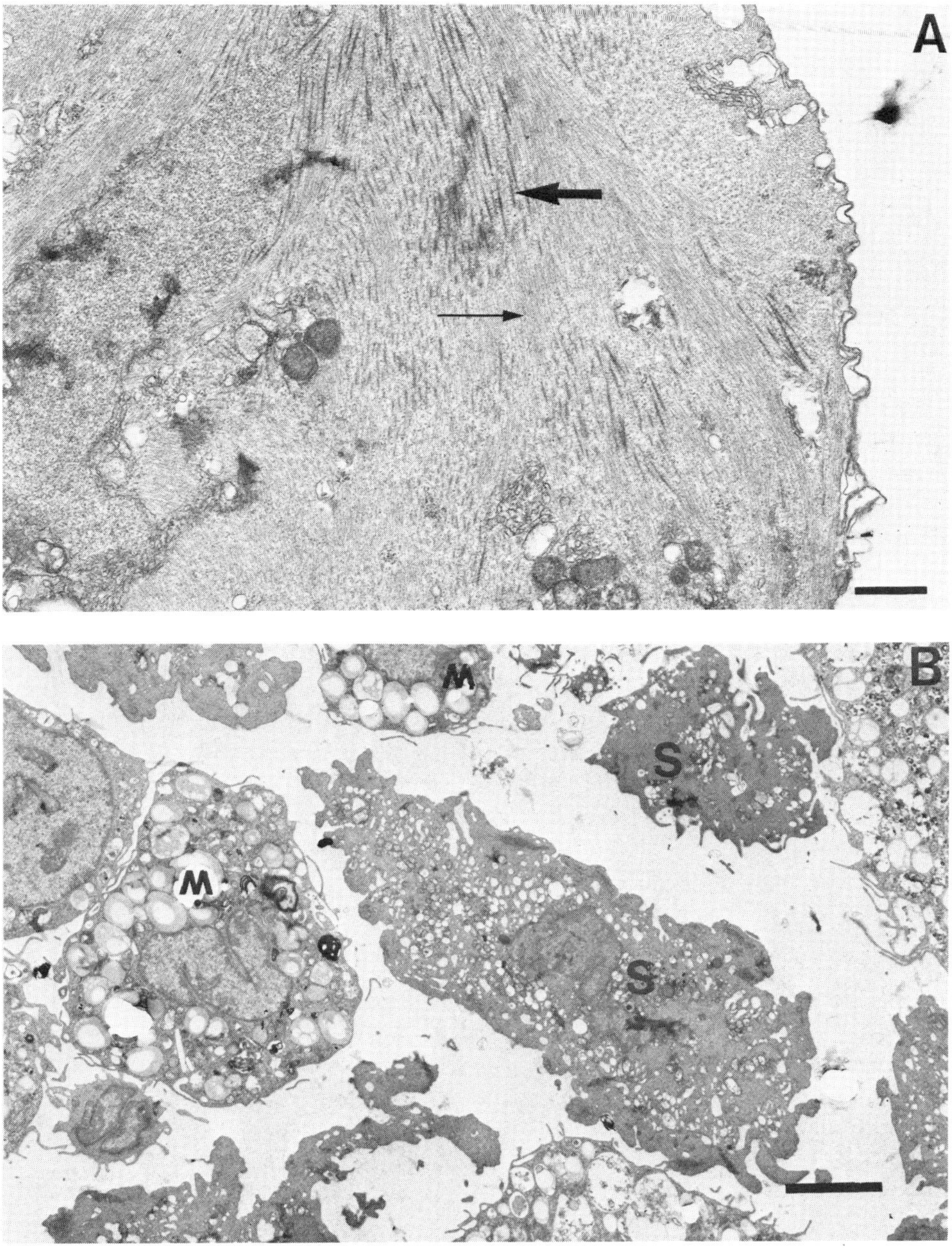

FIGURE 1. (A) Transmission electron micrographs (TEM) of an aortic SMC from a control rabbit immediately after enzyme isolation. Thick arrow, thick filaments; thin arrow, thin filaments. Length of bar, 1 μm. (Magnification × 12,240.) (B) TEM of freshly enzyme-isolated cells from atherosclerotic intima-media of a rabbit fed cholesterol for 4 months. S, cells identified as SMC mainly because they contained myofilaments; M, cells identified as macrophage-foam cells because they had no features of SMC. Length of bar, 5 μm. (Magnification × 2924.) The cells were isolated by collagenase and elastase from small pieces of intima-medias[18] using a modification of the method of Ives.[23]

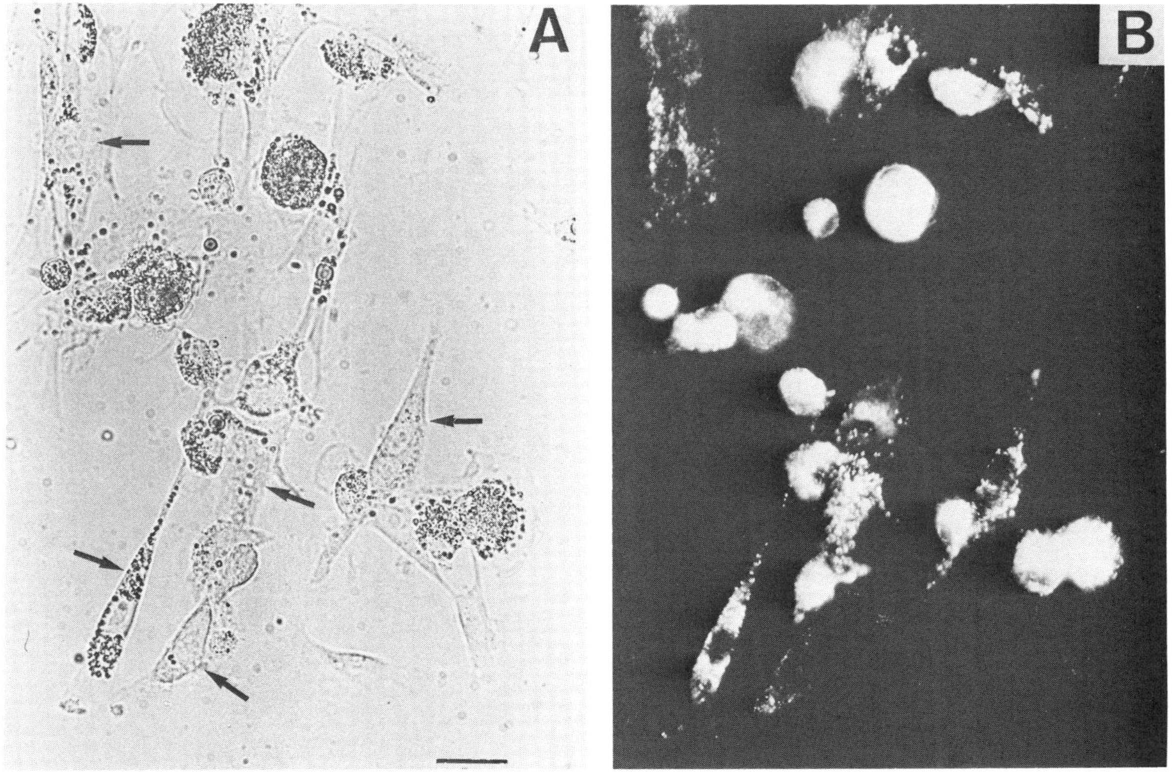

FIGURE 2. Aortic intima-medial cells from a cholesterol-fed rabbit in primary culture in Dulbecco's modification of Eagle's medium (DMEM) containing 10% normal rabbit serum 2 days after enzyme isolation. The cells were incubated with acetyl-LDL, which had been fluorescence-labeled with DiI (3,3′-dioctadecylindocarbocyanine).[24] Phase contrast (A) and fluorescence (B) micrographs of the same field are shown. The foam cells that are morphologically SMC and lack Fc-receptors are marked with arrows. The rest of the cells showing acetyl-LDL uptake were identified as macrophage foam cells on the basis of Fc-receptors, as indicated by their ability to form rosettes with IgG-coated erythrocytes. Bar, 50 μm. (Jaakkola, O., et al., unpublished.)

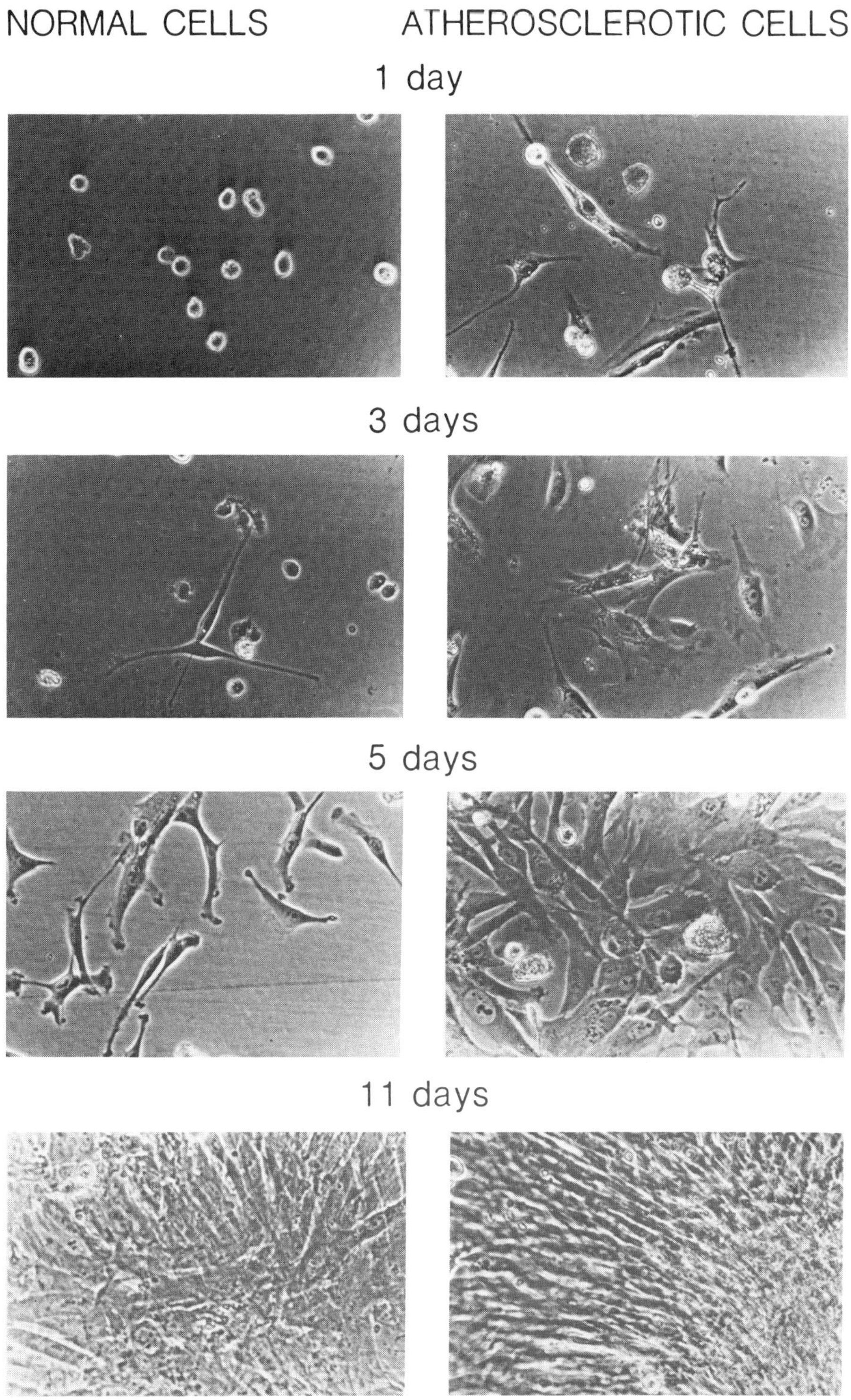

FIGURE 3. A representative series of phase-contrast microscopic pictures of enzyme-isolated cells from control (left) and atherosclerotic (right) rabbits after the indicated times in primary culture in 10% normal rabbit serum. (From Kallioniemi, O.-P., Jaakkola, O., Nikkari, S. T., and Nikkari, T., *Atherosclerosis*, 52, 13, 1984. With permission.)

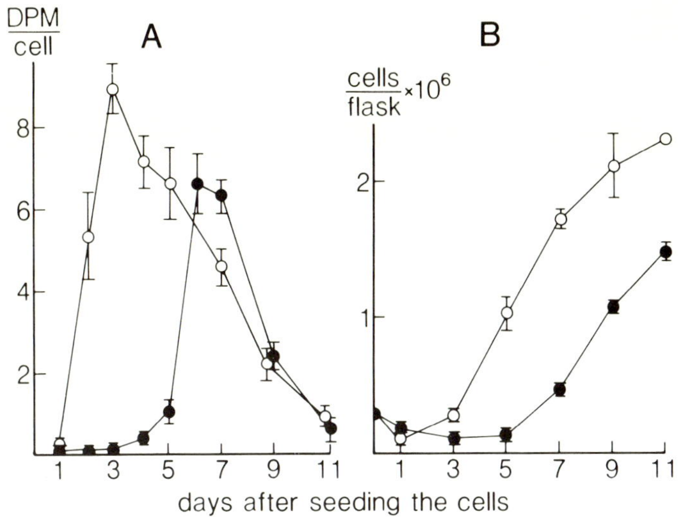

FIGURE 4. (A) Uptake of [3H] thymidine by enzyme-isolated normal (•) and atherosclerotic (O) SMC in primary culture in 10% normal rabbit serum. 1×10^5 cells were seeded into 35-mm dishes. Each point represents the mean (±S.E.M.) of four to six determinations from different animals. (B) Representative growth curves of enzyme-isolated SMC in 10% serum. 3×10^5 cells were seeded into 25-cm^2 tissue culture flasks. Each point is the mean (± range) of duplicate determinations. (From Kallioniemi, O.-P., Jaakkola, O., Nikkari, S. T., and Nikkari, T., *Atherosclerosis,* 52, 13, 1984. With permission.)

substantial portion of SMC in the atherosclerotic aortic wall are in a synthetic state and thus ready to respond to serum mitogens. The factor(s) or mechanism(s) causing the change in the phenotype of the SMC remain unknown. Spontaneous modulation of SMC takes place in culture,[3,7,30,31] and it does not require the presence of serum mitogens.[3,7,32] Dedifferentiation of cultured SMC can be inhibited by a feeder layer of fibroblasts or endothelial cells,[30] an aortic extract,[31] heparin,[31] or cAMP,[30] and its onset is speeded by the addition of purified PDGF[32] and prostaglandin E1.[33] The role of these agents in vivo remains open. Dedifferentiation does not occur in vitro if the cells are seeded in sufficiently dense cultures,[3,31] and a similar mechanism might be operative in the arterial wall after the migration of SMC from the media to the less cellular intima.[3,31] However, it is unclear whether differentiated medial SMC are capable of migration.[34] On the other hand, it is also possible that SMC in atherosclerotic lesions are derived from preexisting foci of intimal SMC.[4]

V. COMPOSITION OF CYTOSKELETAL AND CYTOCONTRACTILE PROTEINS

The altered phenotype of SMC isolated from atherosclerotic intima-medias was also reflected in SDS gel electrophoretic patterns of the cytoskeletal and cytocontractile proteins (Table 1). In comparison with control SMC the atherosclerotic cells had decreased relative contents of myosin, actin, and tropomyosin and increased proportions of the components of the intermediate-sized filaments vimentin and desmin (Table 1). Analogous findings have been obtained by Kocher et al.[35] from rat aortic intimal thickenings: 15 days after a balloon injury the aortic cells contained more vimentin and less actin than normal SMC. The results indicate that dedifferentiation of vascular SMC during atherogenesis leads to an increase in the protein components of the intermediate filaments at the expense of those of the thin and thick filaments. It is interesting that hypertrophy of venous[36] or intestinal[37] smooth muscle has also been reported to be

Table 1
COMPOSITIONS OF CYTOSKELETAL AND CYTOCONTRACTILE PROTEINS IN FRESHLY ISOLATED AORTIC INTIMA-MEDIAL CELLS AND CELLS CULTURED FOR A WEEK

	Freshly isolated cells		Cultured cells	
	Normal n = 4	Atherosclerotic n = 4	Normal n = 4	Atherosclerotic n = 3
Myosin	18.4 ± 4.8	5.0 ± 4.0[a]	2.4 ± 1.5	1.3 ± 0.7[b]
Actin	38.8 ± 3.7	22.4 ± 6.3[c]	27.3 ± 5.8	30.4 ± 5.5[b]
Tropomyosin	9.1 ± 0.7	5.8 ± 0.9[c]	5.2 ± 2.0	5.5 ± 0.4[b]
Vimentin	3.9 ± 0.7	12.9 ± 3.3[c]	12.6 ± 2.3	12.3 ± 0.6[b]
Desmin	0.5 ± 0.2	2.4 ± 0.8[c]	1.4 ± 0.6	1.5 ± 0.3[b]

Note: The results are mean (±S.D.) percents of total Coomassie blue-stained fractions from 20 to 220 kdaltons obtained by densitometry of SDS-polyacrylamide gels. The cells were dissolved directly in an SDS buffer at 100°C for 2 min. N indicates the number of pools, each from two to four rabbits.

[a] $p < 0.05$.
[b] Not significant.
[c] $p < 0.01$.

From Kallioniemi, O.-P., Jaakkola, O., Nikkari, S. T., and Nikkari, T., *Atherosclerosis,* 52, 13, 1984. With permission.

associated with an increase in the number of intermediate filaments quantified morphologically.

The spontaneous dedifferentiation of SMC in vitro has been found to lead to a decrease in the number of thin filaments and in a complete loss of thick filaments and immunologically stainable myosin.[3,30] We confirmed this chemically by following the composition of cytoskeletal and cytocontractile proteins during primary culture of normal SMC. After a week's culture, the contents of myosin, tropomyosin, and actin were significantly lower and those of vimentin and desmin higher than in freshly isolated normal SMC (Table 1). No significant changes took place in the atherosclerotic cells in similar conditions, although there was an insignificant drop of myosin. After a week or longer in culture, the composition of these proteins in normal and atherosclerotic SMC were indistinguishable from each other, which further supports the notion that the compositional differences between freshly isolated normal and atherosclerotic SMC are caused by their different degrees of differentiation in vivo.

VI. GROWTH AND METABOLISM OF SUBCULTURED SMOOTH MUSCLE CELLS

A. Smooth Muscle Cells from Proliferative Lesions

In addition to their earlier start of growth, the enzyme-isolated atherosclerotic SMC grew to higher densities than the cells from normal aortas (Figure 3). Also, explants from atherosclerotic aortas formed larger colonies than those from normal tissue. These observations imply that SMC in atherosclerotic lesions, in addition to being in a modified state and hence rapidly responsive to serum mitogens, also have a higher growth potential than normal SMC. This was clearly proven by our experiments with third-passage, explant-derived SMC.[17] When equal numbers of subcultured atherosclerotic and normal SMC were seeded into tissue culture tubes, the uptake of radioac-

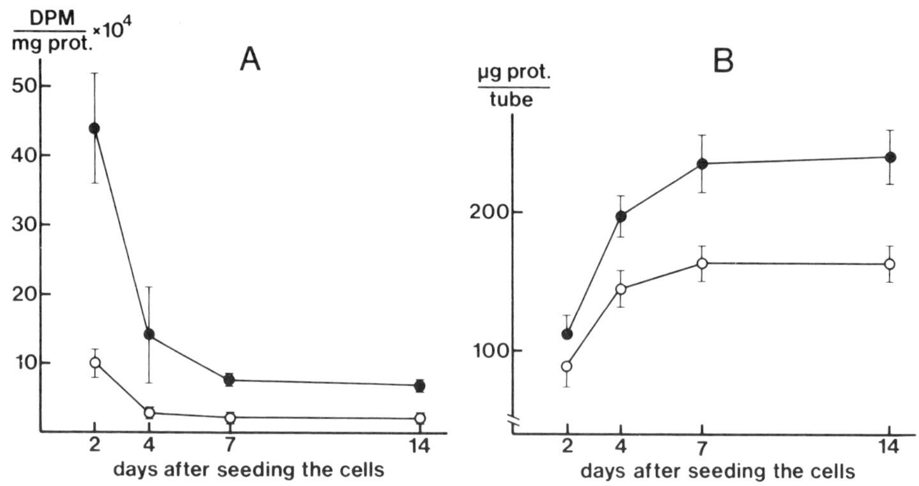

FIGURE 5. The uptake of [3H] thymidine (A) and cell protein (B) in explant-derived, third-passage SMC from normal aortas (○) and from proliferative atherosclerotic lesions (•), produced by feeding rabbits cholesterol chow for 6 months. 3.5×10^4 cells were seeded into 5.5-cm^2 tissue culture tubes and cultured in DMEM containing 10% fetal calf serum. The mean uptake of [3H] thymidine on day 0 was 2.0×10^4 dpm/mg in normal and 1.7×10^4 dpm/mg in atherosclerotic cells. Each point is the mean (±S.D.) of five determinations. (From Pietilä, K. and Nikkari, T., *Atherosclerosis*, 36, 241, 1980. With permission.)

tive thymidine by the atherosclerotic SMC was more than double the uptake by the control SMC, both in the exponential and stationary phases of growth (Figure 5A). Also, the cell protein content of the tubes containing atherosclerotic SMC increased more rapidly and reached higher values than the control tubes, indicating a more rapid growth rate and higher cell density in the cultures of atherosclerotic SMC (Figure 5B). These findings have been substantiated by Hauss et al.,[38,39] who demonstrated that progenies of SMC from rat atheroclerotic aortas proliferate more rapidly in culture than those from healthy aortas and also by Orekhov et al.,[40] who reported that the thymidine indices of intimal cultures from fatty infiltrations and fatty streaks in human aortas are appreciably higher than those of normal tissue.

The third-passage atherosclerotic cells also had an enhanced rate of synthesis of glycosaminoglycans (GAG), particularly sulfated GAG,[41] and total protein and collagen[42] than SMC from healthy aortas (Table 2). These results indicate that after a cholesterol diet of 4 to 6 months, the aortic SMC are in a proliferative and metabolically active state. The high rates of growth and synthesis of GAG and collagen might explain the increase in cellularity and connective tissue taking place during atherogenesis. The sulfated GAG appear to play a role in the accumulation of lipid in the arterial intima by binding LDL.[43] Some reports suggest that the synthesis of either type I or type III collagen is preferentially increased in atherosclerotic SMC.[44,45] In our studies, however, the rates of synthesis of both types were equally enhanced (Figure 6), which agrees with the results of AuMalley and Bricaud.[46]

There was no growth of the atherosclerotic SMC in the absence of serum, and the proliferation rate was proportional to serum concentration;[17] nor were there any differences between the subcultured control and atherosclerotic SMC in ultrastructure, the content of total protein, the amino acid composition of total protein, and some other chemical parameters. A transformation leading to uncontrolled growth or morphologic or gross compositional differences is thus excluded in our work. On the other hand, the faster growth and metabolism of the atherosclerotic SMC that was still pres-

Table 2
SYNTHESIS OF GLYCOSAMINOGLYCANS, TOTAL PROTEIN, AND COLLAGEN BY SUBCULTURED SMC FROM CONTROL AND ATHEROSCLEROTIC AORTAS

	Incorporation of radioactivity into			
	Sulfated GAG[a]	Hyaluronic acid[a]	Collagen[b]	Total protein[b]
Early atherosclerosis[c]				
Lesion cells (n = 6)	198 ± 45	126 ± 27	150 ± 25	139 ± 25
Control cells (n = 6)	100 ± 30	100 ± 19	100 ± 15	100 ± 17
p	<0.001	<0.05	<0.01	<0.01
Late atherosclerosis[d]				
Lesion cells (n = 13)	78 ± 17	138 ± 29	95 ± 17[e]	93 ± 26[e]
Control cells (n = 13)	100 ± 20	100 ± 20	100 ± 19[e]	100 ± 21[e]
p	<0.01	<0.01	ns	ns

Note: The results are expressed as percents of values obtained from simultaneous incubations with control cells.

[a] The cells were incubated with [^{14}C] glucosamine for 24 hr, and the radioactivity was counted in hyaluronic acid and sulfated GAG after their separation with cetyl pyridinium chloride precipitation from the combined medium and trypsin digest of the cell layer.[41]

[b] The cells were incubated with tritiated proline for 6 hr, and the protein-bound hydroxyproline and proline radioactivities were taken to represent collagen and total protein synthesis, respectively.[42]

[c] Cholesterol feeding for 6 months.[17]

[d] Cholesterol feeding for 6 months followed by normal chow for another 6 months.[19]

[e] n = 7.

ent in the third passage can hardly be explained by the action of growth factors carried over by the cells from their original environment. Our results are thus compatible with the concept that a subpopulation of SMC with inherently more active growth potential and metabolism becomes selected during early atherogenesis by some mechanism.[4]

B. Smooth Muscle Cells from Late Lesions

Because mammalian nontransformed cells can undergo only a limited number of divisions,[47] there should be an accelerated senescence of a rapidly proliferating cell population. This idea is in keeping with the findings of our experiments with more advanced atherosclerotic lesions:[19] third-passage SMC from aortic lesions of rabbits fed cholesterol for 6 months and a normal rabbit chow for another 6 months no longer had a higher growth rate as compared to controls (Figure 7), nor were there differences in the synthesis rates of total protein and collagen (Table 2). The synthesis of sulfated GAG was actually lower in the atherosclerotic SMC. These observations might explain why no increases have been found in the growth rates of SMC cultured from advanced human atherosclerotic lesions in comparison to normal tissue.[40,48-50] In fact, in the studies of Ross et al.,[51] SMC from advanced human lesions responded less well to serum than the sublesion cells. The replicative potential of human[52] and murine[53] arterial SMC decreases with the age of the donor. Our data implies that the senescence of SMC from atherosclerotic lesions is also related to the age of the lesions.

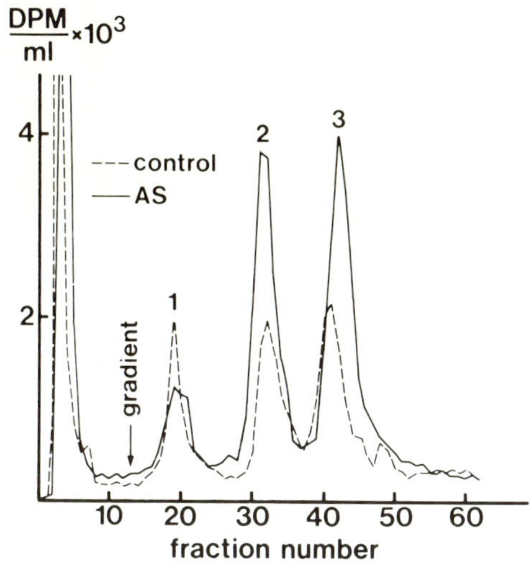

FIGURE 6. DEAE-cellulose chromatograms of radioactive proteins secreted into the incubation medium by atherosclerotic (AS) and control SMC during incubation of the cells with [^{3}H] proline. Peaks (2) and (3) represent procollagens I and III, respectively. The ratios of I to III were 1.33 ± 0.48 in control cells (n = 4) and 1.29 ± 0.40 (n = 4) in atherosclerotic cells. Similar cell densities were used for both incubations. (From Pietilä, K. and Nikkari, T., *Atherosclerosis*, 37, 11, 1980. With permission.)

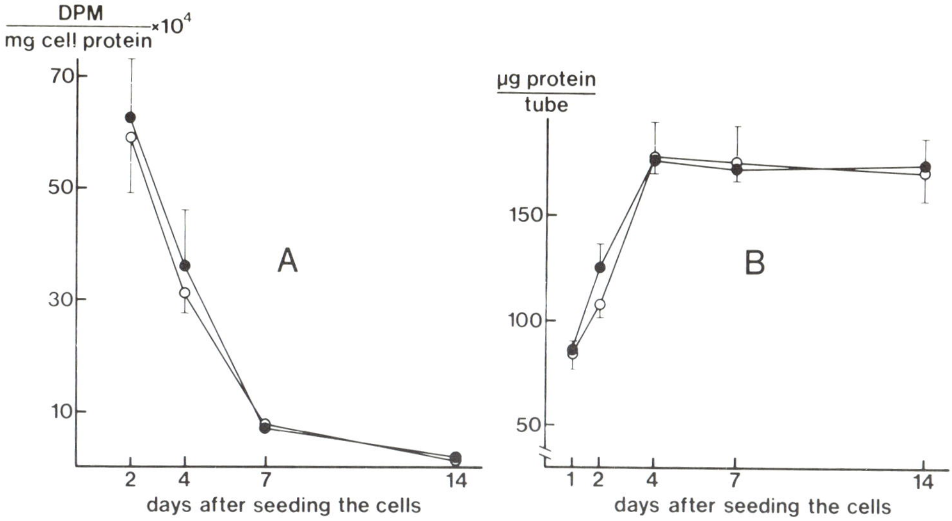

FIGURE 7. The uptake of [3H] thymidine (A) and cell protein (B) in explant-derived, third-passage SMC from normal aortas (O) and from fibrous atherosclerotic lesions (•), produced by feeding rabbits cholesterol chow for 6 months followed by a normal rabbit chow for another 6 months. Conditions were the same as in Figure 5. (From Pietilä, K., Ylä-Herttuala, S., Rantala, I., and Nikkari, T., *Med. Biol.*, 60, 221, 1982. With permission.)

VII. CONCLUSIONS

Our studies show that enzyme-dispersed SMC from the aortas of rabbits fed a cholesterol diet for 4 months proliferate in primary culture without the lag period that normal SMC apparently require for dedifferentiation from a contractile to synthetic phenotype. A sizable portion of SMC isolated from the atherosclerotic intima-medias of cholesterol-fed rabbits were in a dedifferentiated state as judged by their ultrastructure and the composition of cytoskeletal and contractile proteins, indicating a decreased content of thin and thick myofilaments and an increased proportion of intermediate filaments in comparison to myofilament-filled SMC isolated from healthy intima-medias. Corresponding changes in the composition of the cytoskeletal and cytocontractile proteins took place during the spontaneous phenotypic modulation of normal SMC in primary culture. The factor(s) or mechanism(s) causing dedifferentiation during cholesterol feeding in vivo remain speculative.

Our experiments also demonstrate that, in addition to the earlier start of primary growth, the SMC from atherosclerotic lesions have an enhanced subsequent growth rate, which is preserved at least to the third passage and is accompanied by accelerated synthesis rates of GAG, collagen, and other proteins. These properties are no longer related to the phenotypic modulation because the third-passage atherosclerotic SMC did not differ from normal SMC with regard to ultrastructure, contents of the cytoskeletal and cytocontractile proteins, total protein, collagen, and some other constituents. Nor was the enhanced proliferation caused by a transformation since it was serum-dependent and disappeared when the lesion became older. The findings are in agreement with the concept that during cholesterol-induced atherogenesis there is a selection of a cell population with a metabolic advantage either from SMC migrating from the media or from preexisting intimal SMC. It remains to be elucidated to what extent the processes of dedifferentiation and selection depend on each other in vivo.

Subcultured SMC derived from advanced atherosclerotic lesions no longer had the enhanced growth and metabolism typical of cells from earlier lesions. In fact, some synthetic activities of these cells were slower than those of the control SMC. This might be an indication of senescence among the rapidly proliferating atherosclerotic intimal SMC.

ACKNOWLEDGMENTS

The study was supported by a grant from the Research Council for Medicine (Academy of Finland).

REFERENCES

1. Ross, R. and Glomset, J. A., The pathogenesis of atherosclerosis, *N. Engl. J. Med.*, 295, 369 and 420, 1976.
2. Benditt, E. P. and Benditt, J. M., Evidence for a monoclonal origin of human atherosclerotic plaques, *Proc. Natl. Acad. Sci. U.S.A.*, 70, 1753, 1973.
3. Campbell, G. R. and Chamley-Campbell, J. H., Invited review: the cellular pathobiology of atherosclerosis, *Pathology*, 13, 423, 1981.
4. Thomas, W. A. and Kim, D. N., Biology of disease. Atherosclerosis as a hyperplastic and/or neoplastic process, *Lab. Invest.*, 48, 245, 1983.
5. Ross, R., Glomset, J. A., Kariya, B., and Harker, L., A platelet-dependent serum factor that stimulates the proliferation of arterial smooth muscle cells in vitro, *Proc. Natl. Acad. Sci. U.S.A.*, 71, 1207, 1974.

6. Fischer-Dzoga, K., Frazer, R., and Wissler, R. W., Stimulation of proliferation in stationary primary cultures of monkey and rabbit smooth muscle cells. I. Effects of lipoprotein fractions of hyperlipemic serum and lymph, *Exp. Mol. Pathol.*, 24, 346, 1976.
7. Chamley-Campbell, J. H., Campbell, G. R., and Ross, R., Phenotype-dependent response of cultured aortic smooth muscle to serum mitogens, *J. Cell Biol.*, 89, 379, 1981.
8. Buck, R. C., Intimal thickening after ligature of arteries. An electron microscopic study, *Circ. Res.*, 9, 418, 1961.
9. Geer, J. C., Fine structure of human aortic intimal thickening and fatty streaks, *Lab. Invest.*, 14, 1764, 1965.
10. Veress, B., Kadar, A., and Jellinek, H., Ultrastructural elements in experimental intimal thickening. I. Electron microscopic study of the development and cellular elements of intimal proliferation, *Exp. Mol. Pathol.*, 11, 200, 1969.
11. Parker, F., An electron microscopic study of experimental atherosclerosis, *Am. J. Pathol.*, 36, 19, 1960.
12. Buck, R. C., Lesions in the rabbit aorta produced by feeding a high cholesterol diet followed by a normal diet. An electron microscopic study, *Br. J. Exp. Pathol.*, 43, 236, 1962.
13. Thomas, W. A., Jones, R., Scott, R. F., Morrison, E., Goodale, F., and Imai, H., Production of early atherosclerotic lesions in rats characterized by proliferation of "modified smooth muscle cells", *Exp. Mol. Pathol.*, Suppl. 1, 40, 1963.
14. Parker, F. and Odland, G. F., A correlative histochemical, biochemical and electron microscopic study of experimental atherosclerosis in the rabbit aorta with special reference to the myo-intimal cell, *Am. J. Pathol.*, 48, 197, 1966.
15. Scott, R. F., Jones, R., Daoud, A. S., Zumbo, O., Coulston, F., and Thomas, W. A., Experimental atherosclerosis in rhesus monkeys. II. Cellular elements of proliferative lesions and possible role of cytoplasmic degeneration in pathogenesis as studied by electron microscopy, *Exp. Mol. Pathol.*, 7, 34, 1967.
16. Lee, K. T., Lee, K. J., Lee, S. K., Imai, H., and O'Neal, R. M., Poorly differentiated subendothelial cells in swine aortas, *Exp. Mol. Pathol.*, 13, 118, 1970.
17. Pietilä, K. and Nikkari, T., Enhanced growth of smooth muscle cells from atherosclerotic rabbit aortas in culture, *Atherosclerosis*, 36, 241, 1980.
18. Kallioniemi, O.-P., Jaakkola, O., Nikkari, S. T., and Nikkari, T., Growth properties and composition of cytoskeletal and cytocontractile proteins in aortic cells isolated and cultured from normal and atherosclerotic rabbits, *Atherosclerosis*, 52, 13, 1984.
19. Pietilä, K., Ylä-Herttuala, S., Rantala, I., and Nikkari, T., Characterisation of cells cultured from advanced atherosclerotic lesions of the rabbit, *Med. Biol.*, 60, 221, 1982.
20. Constantinides, P., Booth, I., and Carlson, G., Production of advanced cholesterol atherosclerosis in the rabbit, *Arch. Pathol.*, 70, 712, 1960.
21. Frazer, R., Vesselinovitch, D., and Wissler, R. W., New interpretations of lipoproteins and arterial lesions of cholesterol-fed rabbits, *Pathology*, 8, 57, 1976.
22. Vesselinovitch, D., Animal models of atherosclerosis. Their contributions and pitfalls, *Artery*, 5, 193, 1979.
23. Ives, H. E., Schultz, G. S., Galardy, R. E., and Jamieson, J. D., Preparation of functional smooth muscle cells from the rabbit aorta, *J. Exp. Med.*, 148, 1400, 1978.
24. Pitas, R. E., Innerarity, T. L., Weinstein, J. N., and Mahley, R. W., Acetoacetylated lipoproteins used to distinguish fibroblasts from macrophages in vitro by fluorescence microscopy, *Arteriosclerosis*, 1, 177, 1981.
25. Pitas, R. E., Innerarity, T. L., and Mahley, R. W., Foam cells in explants of atherosclerotic rabbit aortas have receptors for β-very low density lipoproteins and modified low density lipoproteins, *Arteriosclerosis*, 3, 2, 1983.
26. Geer, J. C., McGill, H. C., and Strong, J. P., The fine structure of human atherosclerotic lesions, *Am. J. Pathol.*, 38, 263, 1961.
27. Haust, M. D., The nature of bi- and trinuclear cells in atherosclerotic lesions in man. Ultrastructural studies of aortic fatty dots and streaks, *Atherosclerosis*, 36, 365, 1980.
28. Fowler, S., Shio, H., and Haley, N. J., Characterization of lipid-laden aortic cells from cholesterol-fed rabbits. IV. Investigation of macrophage-like properties of aortic cell populations, *Lab. Invest.*, 41, 372, 1979.
29. Grünwald, J. and Haudenschild, C., Intimal injury in vivo activates vascular smooth muscle cell migration and explant outgrowth in vitro, *Arteriosclerosis*, 4, 183, 1984.
30. Chamley, J. H., Campbell, G. R., McConnel, J. D., and Gröschel-Stewart, U., Comparison of vascular smooth muscle cells from adult human, monkey and rabbit in primary culture and in subculture, *Cell Tissue Res.*, 177, 503, 1977.
31. Chamley-Campbell, J. H. and Campbell, G. R., What controls smooth muscle phenotype? *Atherosclerosis*, 40, 347, 1981.

32. Thyberg, J., Palmberg, L., Nilsson, J., Ksiazek, T., and Sjolund, M., Phenotype modulation in primary cultures of arterial smooth muscle cells: on the role of arterial platelet-derived growth factor, *Differentiation,* 25, 156, 1983.
33. Sjölund, M., Nilsson, J., Palmberg, L., and Thyberg, J., Phenotype modulation in primary cultures of arterial smooth-muscle cells. Dual effect of prostaglandin E1, *Differentiation,* 27, 158, 1984.
34. Webster, W. S., Bishop, S. P., and Geer, J. C., Experimental aortic intimal thickening. I. Morphology and source of intimal cells, *Am. J. Pathol.,* 76, 245, 1974.
35. Kocher, O., Skalli, O., Bloom, W. S., and Gabbiani, G., Cytoskeleton of rat aortic smooth muscle cells. Normal conditions and experimental intimal thickening, *Lab. Invest.,* 50, 645, 1984.
36. Berner, P. F., Somlyo, A. V., and Somlyo, A. P., Hypertrophy-induced increase of intermediate filaments in vascular smooth muscle, *J. Cell Biol.,* 88, 96, 1981.
37. Gabella, G., Hypertrophic smooth muscle. IV. Myofilaments, intermediate filaments and some mechanical properties, *Cell Tissue Res.,* 201, 277, 1979.
38. Hauss, W. H., Mey, J., and Schulte, H., Effect of risk factors and antirheumatic drugs on the proliferation of aortic wall cells, *Atherosclerosis,* 34, 119, 1979.
39. Hauss, W. H., The role of arterial wall cells in atherogenesis, *Cardiovasc. Res. Cent. Bull. (Houston),* 17, 75, 1980.
40. Orekhov, A. N., Kosykh, V. A., Repin, V. S., and Smirnov, V. N., Cell proliferation in normal and atherosclerotic human aorta. II. Autoradiographic observation on deoxyribonucleic acid synthesis in primary cell culture, *Lab. Invest.,* 48, 749, 1983.
41. Pietilä, K., Ylä-Herttuala, S., Jaakkola, O., and Nikkari, T., Metabolism of glycosaminogycans and lipids in smooth muscle cells from atherosclerotic rabbit aortas in culture, *Atherosclerosis,* 37, 449, 1980.
42. Pietilä, K. and Nikkari, T., Enhanced synthesis of collagen and total protein by smooth muscle cells from atherosclerotic rabbit aortas in culture, *Atherosclerosis,* 37, 11, 1980.
43. Vijayagopla, P., Srinivasan, S. R., Radhakrishnamurthy, B., and Berenson, S., Interaction of serum lipoproteins and a proteoglycan from bovine aorta, *J. Biol. Chem.,* 256, 8234, 1981.
44. McCullach, K. G., Pattrick, M., and Harvey, G., Hypercholesterolemia induced changes in collagen and elastin synthesis in experimental atherosclerosis, in *Abstracts of the 6th Colloquium of the Federation of European Connective Tissue Clubs,* Paris, 1978, 251.
45. Larrue, J., Daret, D., Demond, J., and Bricaud, H., Normal and pathological rabbit aortic cells in culture: determination of growth and collagen polymorphism, in *Abstracts of the 6th Colloquium of the Federation of European Connective Tissue Clubs,* Paris, 1978, 249.
46. AuMalley, M. and Bricaud, H., Collagen synthesis in organ culture of normal and atherosclerotic aortas, *Atherosclerosis,* 39, 1, 1981.
47. Hayflick, L., The limited in vitro lifetime of human diploid cells strains, *Exp. Cell Res.,* 37, 614, 1965.
48. Moss, N. S. and Benditt, E. P., Human atherosclerotic plaque cells and leiomyoma cells. Comparison of in vitro growth characteristics, *Am. J. Pathol.,* 78, 175, 1975.
49. Björkerud, S. and Ekroth, R., The growth of human atherosclerotic and non-atherosclerotic aortic intima and media in vitro, *Artery,* 8, 329, 1980.
50. Eskin, S. G., Sybers, H. D., Lester, J. W., Navarro, L. T., Gotto, Jr., A. M., and DeBakey, M. E., Human smooth muscle cells cultured from atherosclerotic plaques and uninvolved vessel wall, *In Vitro,* 17, 713, 1981.
51. Ross, R., Wight, T. N., Strandness, E., and Thiele, B., Human atherosclerosis. I. Cell constitution and characteristics of advanced lesions of the superficial femoral artery, *Am. J. Pathol.,* 114, 79, 1984.
52. Bierman, E. L., The effect of donor age on the in vitro life span of cultured human arterial smooth-muscle cells, *In Vitro,* 14, 951, 1978.
53. Martin, G. M., Ogburn, C. E., and Wight, T. N., Comparative rates of decline in the primary cloning efficiencies of smooth muscle cells from the aging thoracic aorta of two murine species of contrasting maximum life span potentials, *Am. J. Pathol.,* 110, 236, 1983.

Chapter 14

LIPOPROTEIN AND CHOLESTEROL METABOLISM IN CULTURED ARTERIAL SMOOTH MUSCLE CELLS

John F. Oram, Alan Chait, and Edwin L. Bierman

TABLE OF CONTENTS

I. INTRODUCTION

Interest in cholesterol metabolism of arterial smooth muscle cells (SMC) evolved out of studies indicating that this cell type is one of the major precursors of the arterial "foam" cell believed to accumulate in the early stages of the developing atherosclerotic lesion. Analysis of the lipid composition of these cells revealed that their foamy appearance is due to massive intracellular accumulation of lipid droplets that contain mostly cholesteryl ester. It became apparent that insight into the cellular mechanisms underlying atherosclerosis would require a thorough understanding of the biochemical processes involved in regulation of cholesterol homeostasis in arterial SMC.

II. CELLULAR PATHWAYS OF CHOLESTEROL METABOLISM

Cholesterol is used by arterial SMC as a structural component of membranes. It cannot be utilized as an energy source, nor can it be degraded by cells. Modest fluctuations in membrane free cholesterol content alters membrane fluidity and affects membrane function, including the activities of membrane-bound enzymes and transport systems. Since cholesterol is poorly soluble in water, microcrystals of cholesterol can form within cells when the free cholesterol concentration exceeds the absorptive capacity of membranes. At very low cholesterol concentrations, the ability of cells to form membranes becomes limited, and cell growth is disturbed. Therefore, for normal cell function, the level of cellular free cholesterol must be maintained within narrow limits.

Studies with many different types of cultured cells, including arterial SMC demonstrated that cells possess at least four distinct pathways that operate to maintain cell cholesterol homeostasis. Two of these pathways function to deliver free cholesterol to cells, and two function to remove excess free cholesterol from cellular compartments (Figure 1). One of the delivery and one of the removal pathways involve the interaction of plasma lipoproteins with specific receptors on the cell surface. The receptor responsible for delivery of cholesterol to cells binds the major cholesterol-carrying lipoprotein in the plasma, low-density lipoprotein (LDL), and regulates the rate at which lipoprotein cholesterol is transported into cells. The receptor responsible for removal of cholesterol from cells reversibly binds another class of lipoprotein, high-density lipoprotein (HDL), and regulates the rate at which cellular cholesterol is transported out of cells to lipoproteins. Since both of these receptor pathways utilize lipoproteins as either a source or an acceptor of cellular cholesterol, they represent "exogenous" delivery and removal pathways. The "endogenous" pathways contain microsomal enzymes that either provide cholesterol by synthesizing it from acetyl units (delivery) or convert excess free cholesterol to its esterified form for storage as lipid droplets (removal).

A. Exogenous Delivery Pathway

The exogenous pathway for delivery of cholesterol to cells is a series of steps involving binding of LDL to cell-surface receptors, the internalization of LDL-receptor complexes, and the eventual degradation of most of the LDL particles by cellular lysosomes (Figure 2). The amount of LDL cholesterol delivered to cells is modulated by the number of receptors on the cell surface.

The cellular mechanisms involved in the biosynthesis and processing of LDL receptors have been characterized extensively by Brown, Goldstein, and colleagues (see References 1 and 2 for reviews). The LDL receptor is synthesized in the rough endoplasmic reticulum as a precursor glycoprotein that has an apparent molecular weight of 120,000. Shortly after synthesis, the N- and O-linked carbohydrates undergo modification and lengthening, respectively, so that the mature receptor exhibits an apparent molecular weight of 160,000. The mature receptor is transported to the cell surface and

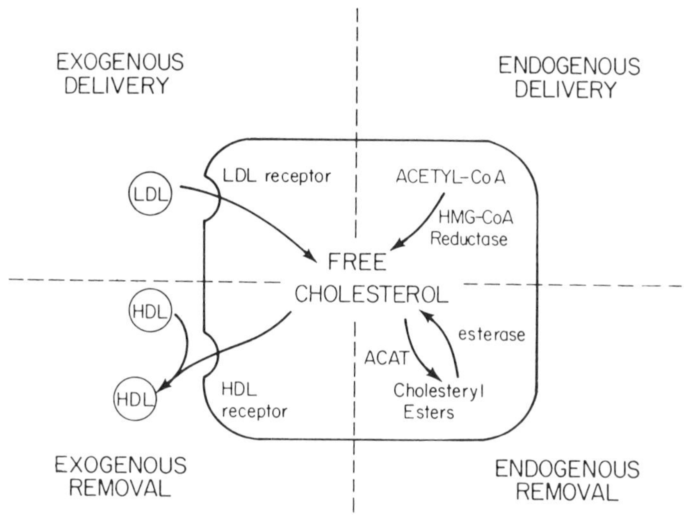

FIGURE 1. Schematic representation of the four major pathways of cholesterol metabolism in arterial SMC.

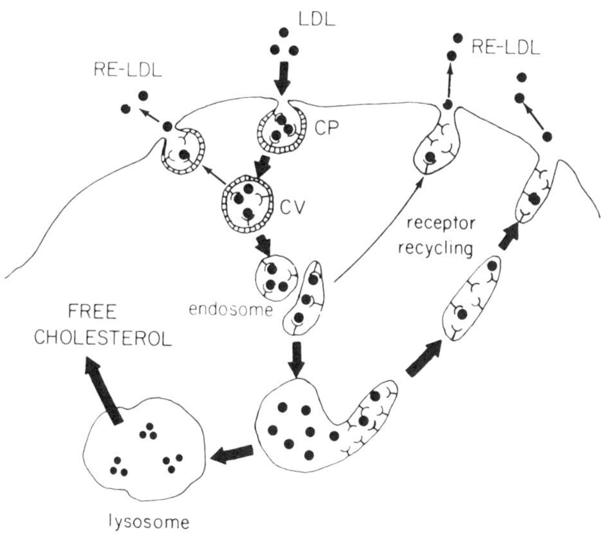

FIGURE 2. The LDL-receptor pathway. RE-LDL, retroendocytosis of LDL; CP, coated pits; CV, coated vesicles.

inserted in the plasma membrane so that all but 72 of its 839 amino acids extend into the extracellular space. The binding sites that recognize the two ligands for the receptor, apoproteins B and E, are located within the NH_2-terminal 322 amino acids. The 50 amino acids at the COOH-terminal end project into the cytoplasm of the cell, and the adjacent 22 amino acids span the plasma membrane. A unique feature of the LDL receptor is that it contains an ~350-amino-acid domain located between the membrane-spanning and the ligand-binding segments that bear a strong homology to the precursor for the epidermal growth factor (EGF), a peptide that stimulates the growth of epidermal cells. This homology implies that the LDL receptor and EGF evolved from the same ancestral gene, underscoring the functional coupling of stimulation of cell growth with the supply of exogenous cholesterol for cell membrane synthesis.

In the presence of LDL in the extracellular fluid, the receptors in the plasma membrane rapidly become occupied with LDL particles, and the receptor-LDL complexes migrate to specialized invaginations of the plasma membrane called "coated pits" that contain an abundance of the protein clathrin (Figure 2). Within minutes, the receptor-LDL complexes are internalized, and the coated pits become coated vesicles. The vesicles then lose their clathrin coat and fuse together to form endosomes. The internal microenvironment of endosomes then becomes acidic due to the action of membrane-associated proton pumps. When the intravesicular pH drops below pH 6.0, LDL dissociates from its receptor. At this stage, LDL particles and receptors part company, with the bulk of the LDL being directed towards lysosomes for complete degradation, and most of the receptors return to the cell surface for reutilization. One LDL receptor can be reutilized 150 times during its life span of 30 hr, making one round trip from the cell surface to inside the cell and back to the cell surface every 12 min.

Although most of the LDL particles internalized by the receptor pathway eventually reaches lysosomes where they are degraded, a portion of the internalized LDL returns to the surface and is released from the cell by a process termed "retroendocytosis".[3-5] This process (Figure 2) appears to represent the resurfacing of endocytotic vesicles that contain LDL either free in solution or still bound to its receptor. Upon fusion of the vesicular membrane with the plasma membrane, the LDL is released intact back into the extracellular fluid. Although the LDL released from cells by retroendocytosis does not undergo degradation, modest changes in the physical properties of the particles may occur during their transit through the cell. As discussed later, these changes may have important implications in atherogenesis.

B. Endogenous Delivery Pathway

Cultured arterial SMC possess a multienzyme pathway that catalyzes the synthesis of cholesterol from acetyl CoA. The rate-controlling step in this pathway is the enzyme 3-hydroxy-3-methylglutaryl coenzyme A reductase (HMG-CoA reductase), which converts HMG-CoA to mevalonic acid. Studies with cultured Chinese hamster ovary cells have indicated that HMG-CoA reductase is a 97,000 molecular-weight protein, containing 887 amino acid residues, that is embedded in the endoplasmic reticulum of the cell (reviewed in Reference 1). The enzyme is divided into two domains. The first domain contains the NH_2-terminal 339 amino acids and the membrane binding segment of the enzyme. The interaction of cholesterol with this domain modulates the rate of degradation of the enzyme and plays an important role in the feedback regulation of cholesterol biosynthesis.[6] The second domain, the COOH-terminal 548 amino acid, projects into the cytoplasm and contains the catalytic site of the enzyme. Most of the cholesterol synthesized by the HMG-CoA reductase pathway is transported vectorally to the plasma membrane, possibly within vesicular membranes formed from the endoplasmic reticulum.[7,8]

C. Exogenous Removal Pathway

In addition to receptors for LDL, it appears that cultured arterial SMC also contain receptors for HDL.[9,10] In contrast to the function of the LDL receptor, the HDL receptor acts to facilitate removal of cholesterol from cells. The molecular structure of the HDL receptor is currently unknown; however, it has unique properties that enable it to specifically interact with the major apoproteins in HDL, apo A-I and apo A-II, with very high affinity (K_d for HDL particles of $\sim 10^{-8}$ *M*).[10-12]

Although some of the receptor-bound HDL protein appears to become internalized by cultured cells, most of the HDL is released back into the extracellular fluid intact rather than directed towards lysosomes for complete degradation.[9,10] This reversible association allows for HDL to sequester cholesterol and remove it from the cell. It is

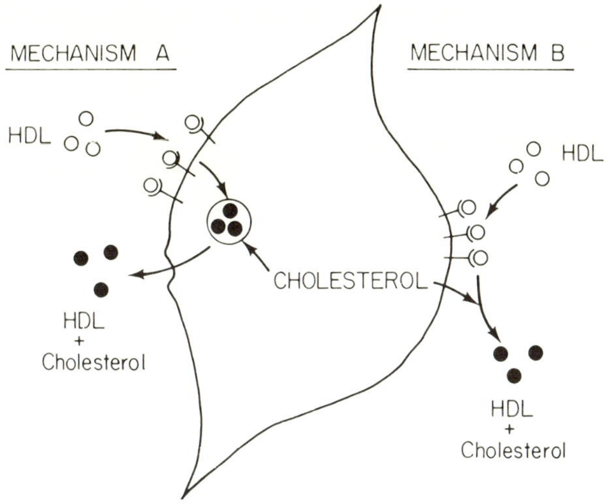

FIGURE 3. Possible mechanism for receptor-mediated transport of cholesterol from SMC to HDL.

not yet known how the interaction of HDL with its receptor promotes removal of cholesterol from cells. One hypothesis is that receptor binding of HDL leads to internalization and resurfacing of receptor-HDL complexes in a manner similar to the retroendocytosis process described earlier for the LDL receptor pathway[13] (mechanism A, Figure 3). Retroendocytosis of HDL could target HDL to specific intracellular pools of excess cholesterol. Alternatively, rather than promoting internalization of HDL, receptor binding may act to concentrate HDL particles at the cell surface where it can sequester cholesterol that diffuses from the plasma membrane into the aqueous layer[14] (mechanism B, Figure 3).

D. Endogenous Removal Pathway

Cultured SMC have the ability to store excess cholesterol in the form of cholesteryl esters. The size of this ester pool is modulated by the activities of two enzymes: acyl coenzyme A: cholesterol acyltransferase (ACAT) and neutral cholesteryl esterase. The ACAT enzyme catalyzes the esterification of cholesterol with long-chain fatty acyl CoA, predominantly oleolyl CoA. Hydrolysis of the cholesteryl esters is catalyzed by a microsomal esterase. This dual enzyme system appears to serve two functions in the cell. One is to provide a storage reservoir of cholesterol that can be remobilized when the cells need free cholesterol for membrane synthesis. The second function is to protect cells from overaccumulation of potentially harmful free cholesterol by converting it to its esterified form.

III. REGULATION OF CELL CHOLESTEROL HOMEOSTASIS

The four major cellular pathways of cholesterol metabolism work together to keep the free cholesterol content within a narrow range, providing enough cholesterol for membrane synthesis but not in amounts large enough to endanger the cell. Thus, under culture conditions where cells are quiescent and the medium concentration of sterol is low, the cholesterol delivery and removal pathways are relatively inactive. However, culture conditions can be established to at least transiently perturb the cell cholesterol content of cells, invoking marked changes in the activities of the different regulatory pathways. These conditions involve varying the nutritional and hormonal composition of the tissue culture medium in order to alter both the availability of exogenous sterol and the cellular requirements for cholesterol.

A. Cholesterol Depletion

When cultured cells are stimulated to grow in the absence of an exogenous source of sterol, the activity of both the endogenous and exogenous delivery pathways are increased.[1,15-18] Similar effects occur when quiescent cells are incubated with medium containing particles such as HDL_3 that remove cholesterol from cells.[19,20] Conversely, the activities of these two pathways are suppressed when sterols, either in the form of LDL or cholesterol dissolved in ethanol, are added to cholesterol-deficient medium.[1]

Regulation of the exogenous delivery pathway occurs at the level of transcription of the LDL receptor gene.[1] When cells are deprived of cholesterol, there is a marked increase in the cellular content of the species of mRNA that encodes the LDL receptor protein. As a result, cholesterol depletion leads to synthesis of new LDL receptors and an increase in the concentration of receptors on the cell surface, causing increased binding and internalization of LDL particles. Once enough LDL cholesterol is delivered to cells to satisfy cellular needs, synthesis of new LDL receptors is suppressed, and existing receptors are degraded by the cell.

The relative activity of the endogenous delivery pathway is modulated by both the amount and activity of HMG-CoA reductase. The amount of enzyme is induced in response to cholesterol depletion by at least two mechanisms.[1] First, transcription of the reductase gene is stimulated, leading to increased biosynthesis of enzyme. Second, the rate of degradation of preexisting reductase is inhibited. Since binding of cholesterol to reductase accelerates its rate of degradation,[6] the removal of cholesterol from cells leads to a suppressed degradation rate and an increase in the amount of enzyme. In addition to long-term modulation of the amount of reductase enzyme, enzyme activity is acutely regulated by a phosphorylation/dephosphorylation mechanism.[21-23] Cholesterol depletion of cells converts the inactive phosphorylated form of the reductase to the active dephosphorylated form, increasing the rate of cholesterol synthesis within the cell.[24]

B. Cholesterol Excess

Since the cholesterol delivery pathways of cultured arterial SMC undergo feedback regulation, delivery of cholesterol through these pathways does not lead to accumulation of excessive amounts of cholesterol in cells. However, when cells are exposed to medium containing nonlipoprotein cholesterol in ethanol[10] or high concentrations of LDL,[25] cholesterol is delivered to cells by processes that do not involve receptors and therefore are not down-regulated when the cell cholesterol content increases. The excess cellular cholesterol that accumulates under these conditions leads to up-regulation of both the endogenous and exogenous removal pathways.

When cultured arterial SMC accumulate excess cholesterol, the concentration of HDL receptors on the cell surface increases.[10] By increasing the reversible binding of HDL to the cell surface, this regulatory process facilitates the removal of cholesterol from cells. The mechanism by which excess cellular cholesterol increases the number of cell-surface HDL receptors is not yet known; however, it appears to be due to increased transcription of a gene that codes for either the HDL receptor itself or some other protein that is involved in receptor function. This conclusion is based on studies demonstrating that treatment of cells with inhibitors of both RNA[26] and protein[10,27,28] synthesis can block the increased receptor binding of HDL that occurs when cells are loaded with cholesterol.

The activity of the endogenous removal pathway is enhanced in response to overaccumulation of cellular free cholesterol by several mechanisms that activate ACAT, the enzyme that catalyzes esterification of free cholesterol (reviewed in Reference 29). These regulatory mechanisms are still poorly understood, but they may involve modulation of enzyme activity in response to alterations in the cholesterol and phospholipid composition of microsomal membranes.[30-32] In addition, the enzyme appears to be regulated by a phosphorylation/dephosphorylation mechanism.[33] In direct opposition to regulation of HMG-CoA reductase, cholesterol loading of cells leads to conversion of the inactive dephosphorylated form of the enzyme to the active phosphorylated form. The enhanced ACAT activity that accompanies accumulation of free cholesterol in cells may also be due to increased synthesis of enzyme.[30]

In contrast to ACAT, the neutral cholesterol esterase activity is not regulated by the cholesterol content of the cell. Therefore, it is unlikely that the esterase functions as a regulatory enzyme in the endogenous removal of cellular free cholesterol. However, regulation of this enzyme may play an important role in the mobilization of stored pools of cholesteryl esters when the cellular demand for free cholesterol is increased. There is evidence that the neutral cholesteryl esterase of arterial cells has properties similar to the hormone-sensitive triglyceride lipase of adipose tissue, in that it is activated by a cAMP-dependent protein kinase and is under hormonal control.[34] Whether hormonal regulation of the esterase influences cell cholesterol homeostasis in arterial SMC remains to be established.

C. Effect of Growth Factors

The stimulation of cell growth triggers a need for increased supply of cholesterol for membrane synthesis. Both exogenous and endogenous pathways of cell cholesteryl metabolism are affected by mitogenesis. Thus, an increase in the delivery pathways and an inhibition of removal pathways would be predicted to result from stimulation by mitogens. Many of these events have indeed been demonstrated in vitro using a variety of mitogens.

1. Platelet-Derived Growth Factor

The platelet-derived growth factor (PDGF) has been most extensively used to perturb cell cholesterol homeostasis. The earliest events following exposure to PDGF are stimulation of protein kinase activities and the phosphatidyl inositol cycle, which occur within minutes of exposure to the mitogen. Within 4 hr of PDGF exposure, cholesterol synthesis is increased.[15,17] This is followed shortly by stimulation of LDL receptor activity[15,18] due largely to an increase in the number of receptors on the surface of the arterial SMC.[15] Thus, within 6 hr of stimulation by PDGF, both endogenous and exogenous delivery pathways of cholesterol are stimulated. These events precede the onset of DNA synthesis by several hours and occur many hours before actual cell division.

Delivery of cholesterol to the cell via LDL receptor-independent mechanisms also is increased. Uptake of LDL that has been reductively methylated, to the extent that its binding to the LDL receptor is inhibited, is increased by PDGF,[35] presumably in part by stimulation of fluid pinocytosis[36] or possibly by stimulation of low-affinity binding sites for this lipoprotein.[37] Further evidence that LDL receptor-independent pathways are enhanced by PDGF comes from studies using mutant fibroblasts that lack LDL receptors. The small rate of nonreceptor-mediated uptake and degradation of LDL by these cells was enhanced by PDGF exposure, although to a much lesser extent than that seen in cells that contained LDL receptors.[35]

Recent studies also have demonstrated that the pathways for cholesterol removal may be influenced by PDGF. Exposure of cells to PDGF is associated with a reduction in the number of HDL receptors, accompanied by a decrease in HDL-mediated efflux of cholesterol from cells.[38] These events also occur before the onset of cell division.

Thus, preparation for cell division is accompanied by a series of events that are aimed at maximizing cholesterol availability to the cell. Loss of cholesterol is minimized by down-regulation of HDL receptor activity, and uptake is facilitated by stimulation of both LDL receptor-dependent and receptor-independent uptake of exogenous cholesterol, while endogenous cholesterol synthesis is stimulated simultaneously.

2. Other Growth Factors

These effects of growth factors on cell cholesterol homeostasis are likely to be universal since other mitogens that have been tested exert similar effects. Other mitogens such as EGF and fibroblast growth factor (FGF) appear to stimulate LDL receptor activity in skin fibroblasts in proportion to their mitogenic strength for these cells.[35,39] Similarly, EGF, FGF, insulin-like growth factor (IGF), and insulin all have been shown to inhibit HDL receptor activity.[38,40] It therefore appears that a general effect of mitogens is stimulation of cholesterol delivery pathways and inhibition of cholesterol removal pathways, thereby maximizing the availability of cholesterol required for synthesis of new membranes during cell division.

D. Effect of Hormones

Several hormones also affect cell cholesterol homeostasis in cultured cells. Most of these studies have been performed using cultured skin fibroblasts, but where studies also have been carried out using arterial SMC, similar results have been found.

Insulin, in doses that span the physiological range, stimulates both the exogenous and endogenous pathways of cholesterol delivery. The binding, uptake, and degradation of LDL are increased after as little as 4-hr exposure to insulin in vitro, due to an increase in the number of LDL receptors on the surface of these cells.[41] Cell cholesterol synthesis also is stimulated by insulin.[41,42] While studies of the effect of insulin on ACAT activity have not been reported, recent findings in our laboratory suggest that insulin leads to a reduction in HDL receptor activity.[40] Thus, the effects of insulin on cell cholesterol homeostasis resemble those of PDGF, although the degree of stimulation of cholesterol delivery is far greater with PDGF.

The physiological significance of these effects of insulin on cell cholesterol homeostasis is unknown. However, it is conceivable that the effect of insulin on cell cholesterol homeostasis relates to its weak mitogenic effect on cells which may be exerted through its interaction with the IGF receptor. Nonetheless, these in vitro observations have been shown to occur in vivo. LDL catabolism in vivo is stimulated by both endogenous and exogenous insulin. Endogenous hyperinsulinemia that results from the administration of total parenteral nutrition leads to an increase in the fractional catabolic rate of LDL.[43] Further, the infusion of exogenous insulin with sufficient glucose to maintain euglycemia, results in an acceleration of LDL fractional catabolic rate and also leads to increased LDL degradation by freshly isolated circulating mononuclear cells,[44] indicative of elevated LDL receptor activity in cells in vivo.

Thyroid hormones appear to exert similar effects. Triidothyronine, at physiological concentrations, stimulates receptor-mediated LDL uptake and degradation in cultured skin fibroblasts.[45] No effects of the hormone were observed in cells derived from subjects with the syndrome of resistance to thyroid hormones.[46] Once again, an in vivo counterpart of these in vitro observations has been demonstrated. LDL catabolism is delayed in subjects with hypothyroidism.[47] This catabolic defect was shown to revert towards normal upon replacement with thyroid hormones,[48] an improvement due to enhanced catabolism by both LDL-receptor-mediated and non-LDL-receptor-mediated pathways.

Glucocorticoids, which in general are catabolic to cells, have opposite effects to insulin and thyroid hormones on cell cholesterol homeostasis. Hydrocortisone, at physiological concentrations, does not affect LDL binding but reduces the internalization of this lipoprotein, such that its degradation and delivery of cholesterol to cells is inhibited.[49] Hydrocortisone also leads to inhibition of cholesterol synthesis,[50] indicating that the activities of both the endogenous and exogenous delivery pathways are suppressed by this hormonc.

E. Effect of Hypoxia

Considerable confusion exists concerning the effect of oxygen tension on cell cholesterol homeostasis and content. Some of this confusion may emanate from the O_2 tension routinely used in most tissue culture laboratories; arterial SMC are usually grown in a mixture of 5% CO_2 and 95% air (i.e., approximately 20% O_2). However, cells of the intima and media of the artery wall appear to be exposed to much lower oxygen tension in vivo.[51,52] An oxygen tension equivalent to 5% O_2 would more closely simulate in vivo conditions, yet use of 5% O_2 usually is referred to as "hypoxia." It is likely, therefore, that in experiments in which cells are exposed to 20% oxygen, the cells are actually hyperoxic relative to their natural state.

While some studies have failed to show differences in LDL and lipid metabolism by cells grown in either low (4 to 5%) or high (usually 20%) O_2, others have shown marked differences.[53,54] LDL uptake was originally shown to be increased in cells grown for several weeks in 5% O_2 relative to that in cells grown in 20% O_2. Conversely, LDL degradation was lower in the cells grown in the lower O_2 concentration,[53] suggesting that impaired LDL catabolism resulted in intracellular accumulation of this lipoprotein. These studies have subsequently been confirmed and extended to show that the increased cell-associated LDL that was seen under the lower O_2 conditions could also in part be attributed to reduced retroendocytosis of LDL.[54]

Cholesterol synthesis may also be affected by the oxygen tension of the tissues. Cholesterol synthesis is increased in rat arterial SMC grown in 20% relative to 5% O_2 despite an absence of effect on LDL uptake in the same study.[55] A small increase in unesterified cholesterol, accompanied by a large increase in cholesterol ester content (i.e., with lipid composition similar to that of foam cells), has been demonstrated in rabbit arterial SMC that had been cultured at low oxygen tension in serum from hyperlipidemic cholesterol and fat-fed rabbits, but not in normolipidemic rabbit serum.[56] These findings imply that large amounts of exogenous cholesterol must be present for cholesterol to accumulate intracellularly at low O_2 tensions, consistent with in vivo studies that demonstrate accelerated atherosclerosis in hyperlipidemic animals maintained under hypoxic conditions.[57] To date, no studies have been reported on the effects of O_2 concentrations on the pathways of removal of cholesterol from cells.

Thus, "hypoxia" appears to influence cell cholesterol homeostasis so as to favor cholesterol accumulation and foam cell formation, possibly by a reduction in catabolic pathways and retroendocytosis. "Hypoxia" also has been shown to be associated with enhanced proliferation of diploid cells,[58] including arterial SMC,[59] which may result in stimulation of both exogenous and endogenous pathways of cholesterol delivery and inhibition of cholesterol removal from cells. However, as pointed out earlier, the use of the term "hypoxia" may be inappropriate for arterial SMC, which normally are exposed to much lower O_2 concentrations in vivo. Thus, the normoxic condition might actually favor cholesterol accumulation by these cells.

IV. ABNORMALITIES OF CELL CHOLESTEROL HOMEOSTASIS

A. Genetic

1. LDL Receptor Abnormalities

The availability of genetic mutant strains of skin fibroblasts in which the LDL receptor is absent or functionally impaired has allowed for extensive characterization of the role of the LDL receptor in cell cholesterol homeostasis. Although the lack of arterial specimens from patients with homozygous familial hypercholesterolemia has precluded detailed study of cultured arterial SMC devoid of LDL receptors, it is likely that they would share similar characteristics with receptor-negative fibroblasts.

Multiple mutations of the LDL receptor locus in familial hypercholesterolemia disrupts the transport and processing of the receptor protein.[60] To date, seven such mutations have been described, all of which are associated with the clinical manifestations of familial hypercholesterolemia and with absent or defective LDL receptor activity demonstrable in vitro. In the absence of functional LDL receptors, exogenous cholesterol transported in LDL fails to be taken up by absorptive endocytosis. Thus, LDL in the incubation medium is not taken up and degraded intralysosomally with subsequent liberation of the exogenous cholesterol for use by the cell. Exposure of such cells to LDL fails to lead to inhibition of cholesterol synthesis or stimulation of ACAT-mediated cholesterol esterification such as occurs with cells that contain LDL receptors. Under these circumstances, cholesterol used by receptor-negative fibroblasts for growth and cell division is derived primarily from endogenous synthesis. Thus, when cholesterol synthesis is inhibited by the use of inhibitors of HMG CoA reductase, the loss of both exogenous and endogenous sources of cholesterol result in rapid cell death.[61]

2. Cholesterol-Ester Storage Diseases

The LDL pathway also can be affected by genetic defects of the lysosomal cholesterol ester hydrolase that results in lysosomal degradation of LDL cholesterol esters. In Wolman's disease and cholesterol ester storage disease, there is total absence or 95 to 99% reduction in the activity of this lysosomal enzyme, respectively. Binding and uptake of LDL by cells derived from patients with these genetic disorders is normal. Lysosomal degradation of LDL apoprotein occurs, but the cholesteryl esters are not hydrolyzed.[62] Thus, they accumulate intralysosomally and have the fatty acid pattern of LDL cholesteryl esters rather than cholesteryl oleate that results from postlysosomal reesterification of cholesterol.

B. Induced Abnormalities of Cell Cholesterol Homeostasis

1. Enzyme Inhibitors

Inhibitors of three enzymes crucial to the maintenance of cell cholesterol homeostasis (i.e., HMG-Co A reductase, ACAT, and lysosomal cholesterol esterase) have been studied. Since the discovery that compactin[63] and, more recently, mevinolin[64] can specifically inhibit sterol synthesis by direct inhibition of HMG-Co A reductase, these agents have been widely used to perturb cell cholesterol homeostasis. Compactin is an extremely potent competitive inhibitor of this enzyme, which is the rate-limiting enzyme in cholesterol synthesis, and when given to arterial SMC in culture, compactin inhibits cholesterol biosynthesis in a highly specific fashion. This leads to up-regulation of LDL receptors to ensure an adequate supply of cholesterol to the cell. Inhibition of HMG-CoA reductase will lead to cell death in the absence of an exogenous supply of cholesterol.[61,65]

Weak bases such as chloroquine and methylamine inhibit lysosomal acid hydrolase activities, including acid cholesterol esterase, presumably by elevating the pH of lysosomes beyond the optimum for enzyme activity.[2,66] This inhibition, in association with an apparent blockage of fusion of endosomes with lysosomes, leads to a build-up of undegraded LDL cholesterol ester in the cells. Similar to the genetic disorders of cholesterol-ester storage described earlier, the fatty acid composition of the accumulated cholesterol ester reflects that in the original LDL particle, which is largely cholesterol linoleate. In contrast, cholesterol oleate is usually deposited when cholesterol ester delivered to the cell via LDL is normally degraded in lysosomes and the cholesterol is subsequently reesterified with oleic acid by action of the ACAT enzyme. Thus the cholesterol ester fatty acid composition of the accumulated lipid in SMC-derived foam cells serves to distinguish prelysosomal from postlysosomal mechanisms.

A variety of inhibitors of the cholesterol esterifying enzyme (ACAT) have been studied. Progesterone[67] and other sterol derivatives, such as analogues of 7-ketocholesterol[67] and 22-hydroxycholesterol,[68] can inhibit ACAT activity in cultured cells. New synthetic agents (e.g., Sandoz compound 58-035),[69] as well as the drug chlorpromazine,[70] are potent inhibitors of the ACAT enzyme in arterial SMC and can completely suppress the incorporation of oleic acid into cholesterol esters. These inhibitors will block the stimulation of ACAT activity in response to LDL cholesterol delivery. By promoting an increase in the intracellular free cholesterol pool, use of these inhibitors can lead to up-regulation of HDL receptors and down-regulation of LDL receptors.[28]

2. Alteration of Endocytosis

Receptor-mediated endocytosis of LDL can be inhibited by agents that affect the transport and fusion of vesicles and the targeting of LDL to lysosomes. These agents include weak bases (such as chloroquine and methylamine), as well as ionophores (such as monensin) that block acidification of endosomes.[2] This blockage leads to impaired delivery of LDL to lysosomes by two mechanisms. First, the elevated pH of the intravesicular fluid prevents the dissociation of LDL from its receptor that appears to be necessary for targeting of LDL to lysosomes. Second, the fusion of vesicles with each other and with lysosomes also appears to be inhibited. Thus, in the presence of weak bases and ionophores, intracellular transport of LDL to lysosomes is inhibited, and the regurgitation of LDL from cells via retroendocytosis is enhanced several-fold[2,4] (see Figure 2).

Although weak bases and ionophores appear to have similar effects on endosome function, their overall effects on receptor-mediated uptake of LDL by cells are markedly different. Within minutes after exposure of cells to an ionophore such as monensin, recycling of LDL receptors from within the cell to the cell surface is inhibited.[2] Therefore, receptor-mediated uptake of LDL by cells is quickly arrested when monensin is added to the culture medium, and cells accumulate very little LDL. However, at concentrations that inhibit lysosomal function, weak bases such as chloroquine have little effect on recycling of LDL receptors.[4,66] Thus, when cultured cells that have high levels of LDL receptors are exposed to medium containing LDL plus chloroquine, LDL enters cells by receptor-mediated endocytosis but is not degraded in lysosomes. Since the lysosomal hydrolysis of LDL sterols is inhibited by the presence of chloroquine, internalization of LDL does not lead to rapid suppression of receptor synthesis, and the rate of uptake of LDL is sustained over long periods of time. Consequently, massive amounts of LDL sterol accumulate in lysosomal and prelysosomal compartments. Under these conditions, retroendocytosis of intact LDL particles represents the major pathway by which cells rid themselves of excess LDL.[4,5] The possibility that alteration of endosomal and lysosomal function could produce changes in the LDL particle prior to regurgitation from the cell remains to be tested.

Receptor-mediated endocytosis can also be inhibited at the level of internalization of receptor-LDL complexes. Agents that interrupt the cytoskeleton of cells, such as colchicine[71] and cytochalasin B,[72] inhibit endocytosis of LDL. Internalization of receptor-bound LDL can be inhibited by short-term treatment of cells with sulfhydryl blocking agents, such as *N*-ethylmaleimide.[73]

3. Inhibition of Receptor Binding of Lipoproteins

The interaction of lipoproteins with their cell-surface receptors can be altered using methods designed to modify the activity of either the cell-surface receptor or the lipoprotein components that interact with the receptor. The binding activity of the LDL receptor is abolished by treatment of intact cells with low concentrations of pronase.[74] Since LDL binding is calcium-dependent, addition of calcium chelators such as EDTA to the culture medium leads to reduced receptor binding of LDL.[74] In contrast to the LDL receptor, the HDL receptor is not calcium-dependent and is insensitive to mild pronase treatment; methods to directly alter the binding activity of the HDL receptor have not as yet been reported.

Receptor binding activity of lipoproteins can be altered by selective chemical modification of their apoproteins. Covalent attachment of N,N-dimethyl-1,3-propanediamine to LDL produces a polycationic lipoprotein that binds extensively to nonspecific, negatively charged sites on the cell surface, from which it is internalized by cells via a receptor-independent process.[75] In the presence of cationized LDL, SMC amass large quantities of LDL-derived sterols, since the rate of uptake of lipoprotein is not modulated by feedback mechanisms. Studies using chemical modification of specific amino acids of LDL apoprotein demonstrated that receptor binding of LDL is mediated by arginine and lysine residues.[76] Therefore, binding of LDL is inhibited when lysine residues are acetylated, acetoacetylated, or reductively methylated, and arginine residues are modified by cyclohexanedione treatment.[74,76] Modification of lysine and arginine residues of the apoproteins in HDL have little effect on the interaction of HDL with its receptor.[77] However, treatment of HDL with tetranitromethane, an agent that nitrates tyrosine residues but also promotes cross-linking of apoproteins, abolishes the receptor binding activity of HDL and inhibits its ability to facilitate transport of cholesterol from cells.[77]

V. RELATION OF LDL AND HDL PATHWAYS IN ARTERIAL SMOOTH MUSCLE CELLS TO ATHEROSCLEROSIS

Since atherosclerosis is associated with the development of foam cells derived from both SMC and macrophages in the arterial wall,[78] the conversion of normal cells to cholesterol ester-rich foam cells must involve a perturbation of cell cholesterol homeostasis. This could involve alterations of (1) delivery of cholesterol to cells via both LDL receptor-mediated pathways and nonreceptor-mediated cholesterol delivery, (2) abnormalities of cholesterol synthesis and cell cholesterol processing, and (3) impairment of cell cholesterol removal.

A. Receptor-Mediated Cholesterol Delivery

LDL receptor-mediated cholesterol delivery to arterial SMC can play a role in atherogenesis, but since atherogenesis is accelerated in vivo under conditions associated with an absence of LDL receptor function (homozygous familial hypercholesterolemia and the Watanabe rabbit), LDL receptors are not obligatory for its development. In fact, the LDL receptors on hepatic cells appear to be antiatherogenic since they function to promote removal of LDL from plasma and are involved in the maintenance of normal levels of plasma LDL.[74] However, in the presence of normally functioning LDL receptors on arterial SMC, increases in plasma LDL cholesterol levels should result in increased flux of LDL into cells via the receptor-mediated pathway. If it exceeds the rate of egress of cholesterol from cells, this increased flux could promote atherogenesis. Growth factors potentially involved in atherogenesis (e.g., PDGF and insulin) could enhance this process by stimulating LDL receptor activity.

Alterations in the composition of LDL can also influence the way LDL is processed by arterial SMC. All forms of hypertriglyceridemia are associated with altered LDL composition, i.e., an increase in LDL core triglyceride with a reciprocal reduction in cholesteryl ester. These LDL deliver less cholesterol per particle to cells and therefore are unable to down-regulate cell cholesterol synthesis effectively.[79,80] Such altered LDL are common in uncontrolled diabetes.[80] Other forms of altered LDL, such as the glycosylated LDL found in increased concentrations in diabetes mellitus, bind poorly to the LDL receptor and presumably deliver cholesterol via other pathways and to other cells.[81]

B. LDL Receptor-Independent Cholesterol Delivery

As discussed earlier, the exogenous and endogenous pathways in delivery of cholesterol to cells undergo feedback regulation. Thus, in the presence of abundant LDL in the incubation medium, the activities of the LDL receptor and cholesterol biosynthesis pathways are suppressed. As a result, the exogenous and endogenous pathways have limited capacities to deliver cholesterol to cells. However, arterial SMC appear to accumulate cholesteryl esters in vivo and are one of the precursor cells of the arterial wall foam cell.[78] Furthermore, they are capable of accumulating cholesteryl esters in vitro, particularly after exposure to high concentrations of LDL derived from animals fed diets rich in saturated fat and cholesterol.[82-84] These findings raise the possibility that uptake and accumulation of cholesteryl esters by arterial SMC may be via LDL receptor-independent mechanisms or possibly via low-affinity binding sites that recognize LDL.

Further evidence that LDL uptake and cell cholesteryl ester accumulation can occur other than via the LDL receptor pathway is obtained from studies using LDL that had been reductively methylated to prevent its recognition by the LDL receptor. Under these circumstances, cholesteryl ester accumulation by arterial SMC equaled that seen after exposure to native LDL.[25] Both normal and LDL receptor-negative strains of fibroblasts accumulated cholesteryl esters to similar extents after exposure to high levels of LDL.[25] Thus, interaction of LDL with its receptor does not appear to be a requirement for cellular accumulation of cholesteryl esters.

The extent to which the LDL-receptor-independent pathways of cholesterol uptake contribute to LDL degradation in vivo can be derived from studies in which LDL that has been treated to minimize receptor-dependent uptake is injected into man or experimental animals and from comparison of LDL fractional catabolic rates in patients with heterozygous and homozygous familial hypercholesterolemia with normal controls. From such studies, it appears that a considerable fraction (20 to 50%) of LDL may be catabolized via LDL receptor-independent pathways. However, since the pool size of LDL is markedly increased in familial hypercholesterolemia and in the WHHL rabbit, an animal model of human familial hypercholesterolemia, it is likely that the absolute rates of catabolism via these LDL receptor-independent pathways are actually increased substantially when circulating LDL levels are elevated (Table 1).

It is in these circumstances of reduced LDL receptor activity, elevated plasma LDL levels, and increased absolute catabolic rates via LDL receptor-independent mechanism that atherosclerosis is most pronounced. Thus, these LDL receptor-independent pathways may play important roles in the pathogenesis of atherosclerosis and accumulation of cholesterol within cells.

C. Modification of LDL by Arterial Smooth Muscle Cells

There has been a recent interest in modifications of LDL that inhibit the uptake of the lipoprotein by the LDL receptor pathway on fibroblasts and arterial SMC, but which facilitate their uptake by the scavenger receptor on macrophages, the other pre-

Table 1
LDL RECEPTOR-DEPENDENT AND RECEPTOR-INDEPENDENT CATABOLISM OF LDL

	Percent of FCR		Relative	Percent of ACR	
	RD	RI	pool size	RD	RI
Normal (man and rabbit)	67	33	×	0.67×	0.33×
FH heterozygote	50	50	2×	×	×
FH homogygote			4×	0	4×
or WHHL rabbit	0	100	20×	0	20×

Note: FH, familial hypercholesterolemia; FCR, fractional catabolic rate; ACR, absolute catabolic rate = FCR × pool size; RD, LDL receptor-dependent; RI, LDL receptor-independent.

cursor of the arterial wall foam cell. The earliest modifications of LDL that facilitated their uptake by macrophages included acetylation and acetoacetylation.[74,76] Malondialdehyde-modified LDL was the first form of modified LDL described that had potential biological significance[85] since it could potentially occur in vivo as a result of platelet aggregation. Subsequently, both endothelial cells[86,87] and arterial SMC[86-88] in culture have been shown to modify LDL. These biological modifications appear to result from a free radical-mediated process that leads to lipid peroxidation.[87] This process is dependent on the presence of the transition metals Cu[88,89] or Fe[88] and can be inhibited by several chelators of these metal ions. The reactive oxygen species that initiates these reactions may differ from one cell type to another. However, unstimulated human and monkey arterial SMC appear to generate substantial amounts of the superoxide anion,[90] a reactive oxygen species that hitherto has been shown to be present in the extracellular environment only of phagocytic cells such as neutrophils and monocytes.

Superoxide derived from arterial SMC initiates a free radical chain reaction that results in lipid peroxidation and, by mechanisms as yet undetermined, also leads to proteolysis of the LDL apoprotein and to enhanced electrophoretic mobility. Such cell-modified LDL are then taken up at enhanced rates by cultured macrophages[86,88-89] and could thereby facilitate lipid accumulation and foam cell formation in macrophages (steps 1 and 3, Figure 4). Phospholipase A_2 activity, which may be an intrinsic part of the LDL particle, appears to be a necessary component of a similar LDL modification that occurs after exposure to endothelial cells, since inhibitors of phospholipase A_2 prevent lipid peroxidation, apoprotein B degradation, and increased uptake by macrophages.[91]

Since cell-modified LDL is taken up by LDL receptors to a reduced extent, it is conceivable that its uptake by LDL receptor-independent pathways could be facilitated in SMC of the artery wall (step 4, Figure 4). Thus, LDL that has been modified by oxidation by arterial SMC could potentially result in lipid accumulation in these cells as well.

It is not known if arterial cells in vivo can modify LDL in a manner similar to that which has been demonstrated in serum-free conditions in vitro, particularly since antioxidants and free radical scavengers are likely to be present in interstitial fluids. However, the abundance of SMC relative to the small volume of interstitial fluid in the artery wall suggests that sufficient superoxide could be generated to initiate LDL modification. In fact, the appearance of LDL with enhanced electrophoretic mobility in interstitial fluid derived from subcutaneous sponge implants of rabbits,[92] the presence of lipid peroxides in circulating lipoproteins of animals and human subjects with dia-

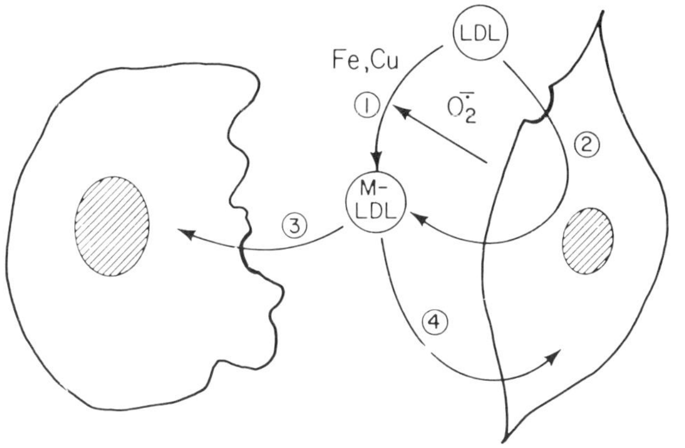

FIGURE 4. Production and metabolism of arterial SMC-modified LDL (M-LDL). (1) Modification of LDL by superoxide generated from SMC; (2) modification of LDL during its transit through the retroendocytosis branch of the LDL-receptor pathway; (3) uptake of modified LDL by scavenger receptors on macrophages; (4) uptake of modified LDL by LDL-receptor-independent mechanisms in SMC.

betes mellitus,[93,94] and the finding of lipid peroxides in atherosclerotic plaques support the contention that such changes do occur in vivo and may be involved in atherogenesis. Although high levels of unbound metal ions are not thought to occur in vivo, a recent report shows that superoxide generated by a xanthine oxidase model system can liberate free iron from ferritin.[95] This raises the intriguing possibility that the sequence of events that has been demonstrated to occur in vitro could indeed occur in the microenvironment of the artery wall and play a role in foam cell formation and atherogenesis.

In addition to being modified by factors released from cells, it is likely that LDL undergoes modification during its transit through the retroendocytosis pathway of arterial smooth muscle (step 2, Figure 4). Studies have demonstrated that a portion of the LDL released from cultured cells by retroendocytosis has altered size and density.[4,5] Although not tested as yet, it is possible that these altered particles bind to scavenger receptors and promote lipid accumulation in macrophages.

In addition to producing altered LDL particles that directly bind to scavenger receptors on macrophages, arterial SMC may also produce LDL particles that have an enhanced ability to form complexes with other extracellular macromolecules. These complexes may contribute to atherogenesis by accumulating in the extracellular environment of the artery wall, where they are scavenged by macrophages. An example of possible complex formation is the interaction of LDL with proteoglycans, major components of the arterial wall extracellular matrix that are synthesized and secreted by artery wall cells, including SMC. It has been postulated that complex formation between LDL and proteoglycans is a major factor contributing to the lipid accumulation in the artery wall that occurs during atherogenesis.[96,97] It remains to be established whether alteration of LDL by SMC enhances this process.

D. HDL-Mediated Cholesterol Removal

Population studies have consistently demonstrated a strong inverse correlation between plasma levels of HDL cholesterol and risk for coronary heart disease. Since low levels of HDL cholesterol in the plasma and increased deposition of cholesteryl esters in cells of the artery wall are two hallmarks of atherosclerosis, it has been postulated that at least some forms of this disease may represent defective removal of cholesterol from arterial cells by HDL. A defect in this process could reflect either a deficiency in the quantity or receptor binding activity of HDL or an abnormality in some step in the HDL receptor pathway of cells.

Several familial disorders of HDL have been identified where apoprotein AI, the major protein component of HDL, is either absent in the plasma or exists in very low concentrations (see Reference 98 for review). Subjects with these disorders develop premature atherosclerosis, possibly due to diminished capacity of cells to secrete excess cellular cholesterol via the HDL receptor pathway. It is also possible that alteration in the apoprotein and lipid composition of the HDL particle may affect receptor-HDL interactions and HDL-mediated cholesterol transport from cells. Studies comparing HDL_3 particles isolated from the plasma of normal and diabetic subjects, with or without hypertriglyceridemia, demonstrated that the ability of HDL to interact with the HDL receptor on cultured fibroblasts varies significantly between individuals and is affected by factors that appear to be independent of either the lipid or total protein composition of the HDL particles.[99] It is not yet known how important these factors are in determining relative risk for development of premature atherosclerosis.

The HDL receptor pathway has only recently gained attention as a major process involved in modification of cell cholesterol homeostasis, and data concerning possible genetic defects in this pathway is not yet available. Based on studies with other receptor systems, including that for LDL, it can be predicted that mutations in the genes for protein involved in the HDL receptor pathway will eventually be identified. These mutations may interrupt the normal cell cholesterol transport process, leading to retention of cholesterol by cells and to enhanced atherogenesis.

ACKNOWLEDGMENTS

The authors' research has been supported by NIH grants AM 02456, HL 18645, HL 31194. Alan Chait is an Established Investigator of the American Heart Association.

REFERENCES

1. Goldstein, J. L. and Brown, M. S., Progress in understanding the LDL receptor and HMG-CoA reductase, two membrane proteins that regulate plasma cholesterol, *J. Lipid Res.*, 25, 1450, 1984.
2. Brown, M. S., Anderson, R. G. W., and Goldstein, J. L., Recycling receptors: the roundtrip itinerary of migrant membrane proteins, *Cell*, 32, 663, 1983.
3. Aulinskas, T. H., van der Westhuyzen, D. R., Bierman, E. L., Gevers, W., and Coetzee, G. A., Retro-endocytosis of low density lipoproteins by cultured bovine aortic smooth muscle cells, *Biochim. Biophys. Acta*, 664, 225, 1981.
4. Aulinskas, T. H., Oram, J. F., Bierman, E. L., Coetzee, G. A., Gevers, W., and van der Westhuyzen, D. R., Retro-endocytosis of low density lipoprotein by cultured human skin fibroblasts, *Arteriosclerosis*, 5, 45, 1985.
5. Greenspan, P. and St. Clair, R. W., Retroendocytosis of low density lipoprotein. Effect of lysosomal inhibition on the release of undegraded ^{125}I-low density lipoprotein of altered composition from skin fibroblasts in culture, *J. Biol. Chem.*, 259, 1703, 1984.
6. Gil, G., Faust, J. R., Chin, D. J., Goldstein, J. L., and Brown, M. S., Membrane-bound domain of HMG-CoA reductase is required for sterol-enhanced degradation of the enzyme, *Cell*, 41, 249, 1985.
7. Lange, Y. and Matthies, H. J. G., Transfer of cholesterol from its site of synthesis to the plasma membrane, *J. Biol. Chem.*, 254, 14624, 1985.

8. Kaplan, M. R. and Simoni, R. D., Transport of cholesterol from the endoplasmic reticulum to the plasma membrane, *J. Cell Biol.*, 101, 446, 1985.
9. Biesbroeck, R., Oram, J. F., Albers, J. J., and Bierman, E. L., Specific high-affinity binding of high density lipoprotein to cultured human skin fibroblasts and arterial smooth muscle cells, *J. Clin. Invest.*, 71, 525, 1983.
10. Oram, J. F., Brinton, E. A., and Bierman, E. L., Regulation of high density lipoprotein receptor activity in cultured human skin fibroblasts and human arterial smooth muscle cells, *J. Clin. Invest.*, 72, 1611, 1983.
11. Brinton, E. A., Oram, J. F., Chen, C.-H., Albers, J. J., and Bierman, E. L., Apoprotein specificity of the HDL receptor on cultured human fibroblasts, *Arteriosclerosis*, 5, 536a, 1984.
12. Fidge, N. H. and Nestel, P. J., Identification of apolipoproteins involved in the interaction of human high density lipoprotein$_3$ with receptors on cultured cells, *J. Biol. Chem.*, 260, 3570, 1985.
13. Schmitz, G., Robenek, H., Lohmann, V., and Assmann, G., Interaction of high density lipoproteins with cholesteryl ester-laden macrophages: biochemical and morphological characteristics of cell surface receptor binding, endocytosis, and resecretion of high density lipoproteins by macrophages, *EMBO J.*, 4, 613, 1985.
14. Rothblat, G. M. and Phillips, M. C., Mechanism of cholesterol efflux from cells. Effects of acceptor structure and concentration, *J. Biol. Chem.*, 257, 4775, 1982.
15. Chait, A., Ross, R., Albers, J. J., and Bierman, E. L., Platelet-derived growth factor stimulates low density lipoprotein receptor activity, *Proc. Natl. Acad. Sci. U.S.A.*, 77, 4084, 1980.
16. Witte, L. D. and Cornicelli, J. A., Platelet-derived growth factor stimulates low density lipoprotein receptor activity in cultured human fibroblasts, *Proc. Natl. Acad. Sci. U.S.A.*, 77, 5962, 1980.
17. Habenicht, A. J., Glomset, J. A., and Ross, R., Relation of cholesterol and mevalonic acid to the cell cycle in smooth muscle and Swiss 3T3 cells stimulated by platelet-derived growth factor, *J. Biol. Chem.*, 255, 5134, 1980.
18. Witte, L. D., Cornicelli, J. A., Miller, R. W., and Goodman, D. S., Effect of platelet-derived growth and endothelial cell-derived growth factors on the low density lipoprotein receptor pathway in cultured human fibroblasts, *J. Biol. Chem.*, 257, 5392, 1982.
19. Oram, J. F., Albers, J. J., Cheung, M. C., and Bierman, E. L., The effects of subfractions of high density lipoprotein on cholesterol efflux from cultured fibroblasts. Regulation of low density lipoprotein receptor activity, *J. Biol. Chem.*, 256, 8358, 1981.
20. Oram, J. F., Effects of high density lipoprotein subfractions on cholesterol homeostasis in human fibroblasts and arterial smooth muscle cells, *Arteriosclerosis*, 3, 420, 1983.
21. Brown, M. S., Brunschede, G. Y., and Goldstein, J. L., Inactivation of 3-hydroxy-3-methylglutaryl coenzyme A reductase *in vitro*. An adenine nucleotide-dependent reaction catalyzed by a factor in human fibroblasts, *J. Biol. Chem.*, 250, 2502, 1975.
22. Goodwin, C. D. and Margolis, S., Cyclic AMP-sensitive activation of hepatic sterol synthesis and 3-hydroxy-3-methylglutaryl coenzyme A reductase, *J. Lipid Res.*, 6, 747, 1978.
23. Beg, Z. H., Stonik, J. A., and Brewer, H. B., Characterization and regulation of reductase kinase, a protein kinase that modulates the enzymic activity of 3-hydroxy-3-methylglutaryl coenzyme A reductase, *Proc. Natl. Acad. Sci. U.S.A.*, 76, 4375, 1979.
24. Scallen, T. J. and Sanghvi, A., Regulation of three key enzymes in cholesterol metabolism by phosphorylation/dephosphorylation, *Proc. Natl. Acad. Sci. U.S.A.*, 50, 2477, 1983.
25. Chait, A., Bierman, E. L., and Ross, R., Non-LDL receptor mediated uptake and accumulation of cholesteryl esters by arterial smooth muscle cells, *Arteriosclerosis*, 4, 536A, 1984.
26. Oram, J. F., Chait, A., and Bierman, E. L., Upregulation of HDL binding to fibroblasts by cholesterol treatment is inhibited by actinomycin D, unpublished results.
27. Brinton, E. A., Kenagy, R. D., Oram, J. F., and Bierman, E. L., Regulation of high density lipoprotein binding activity of aortic endothelial cells by treatment with acetylated low density lipoprotein, *Arteriosclerosis*, 5, 324, 1985.
28. Aulinskas, T. H. and Oram, J. F., Regulation of high density lipoprotein receptor activity in cultured fibroblasts. Effects of inhibition of acyl coenzyme A: cholesterol acyltransferase, *Arteriosclerosis*, 5, 535a, 1984.
29. Suckling, K. E. and Stang, E. F., Role of acyl-CoA: cholesterol acyltransferase in cellular cholesterol metabolism, *J. Lipid Res.*, 26, 647, 1985.
30. Brecher, P. and Chan, C. T., Properties of acyl-CoA-Cholesterol O-acyltransferase in aortic microsomes from atherosclerotic rabbits, *Biochim. Biophys. Acta*, 617, 458, 1980.
31. Mathur, S. N. and Spector, A. A., Effect of liposome composition on the activity of detergent-solubilized acylcoenzyme A: cholesterol acyltransferase, *J. Lipid Res.*, 23, 692, 1983.
32. Synouri-Vrettakou, S. and Mitropoulos, K. A., Acyl-coenzyme A:cholesterol acyltransferase. Transfer of cholesterol to its substrate pool and modulation of activity, *Eur. J. Biochem.*, 133, 299, 1983.
33. Gavey, K. L., Trujillo, D. L., and Scallen, T. N., Evidence for phosphorylation/dephosphorylation of rat liver acyl-CoA:cholesterol acyltransferase, *Proc. Natl. Acad. Sci. U.S.A.*, 80, 2171, 1983.

34. Hajjar, D. P., Minick, C. R., and Fowler, S., Arterial neutral cholesteryl esterase. A hormone-sensitive enzyme distinct from lysosomal cholesteryl esterase, *J. Biol. Chem.*, 258, 192, 1983.
35. Chait, A., Ross, R., Albers, J. J., and Bierman, E. L., Stimulation of low density lipoprotein receptor activity by platelet derived growth factor, *Clin. Res.*, 28, 517A, 1980.
36. Davies, P. F. and Ross, R., Mediation of pinocytosis in cultured arterial smooth muscle and endothelial cells by platelet-derived growth factor, *J. Cell. Biol.*, 79, 663, 1978.
37. Brown, M. S. and Goldstein, J. D., Lipoprotein metabolism in the macrophage: implications for cholesterol deposition in atherosclerosis, *Annu. Rev. Biochem.*, 52, 223, 1983.
38. Oppenheimer, M. J., Oram, J. F., and Bierman, E. L., Down-regulation of high density lipoprotein receptor activity in cultured fibroblasts by platelet-derived growth factor, *Clin. Res.*, 33, 14a, 1985.
39. Davies, P. F. and Kerr, C., Modification of low density lipoprotein metabolism by growth factors in cultured vascular cells and human skin fibroblasts, *Biochim. Biophys. Acta*, 712, 26, 1982.
40. Oppenheimer, M. J., Oram, J. F., and Bierman, E. L., Insulin-induced down-regulation of high density lipoprotein receptor activity in cultured fibroblasts, *Diabetes*, 34, 64a, 1985.
41. Chait, A., Bierman, E. L., and Albers, J. J., Low density lipoprotein receptor activity in cultured human skin fibroblasts: mechanism of insulin-induced stimulation, *J. Clin. Invest.*, 64, 1309, 1979.
42. Bathena, S. J., Avigan, J., and Schreiner, M. E., Effect of insulin on sterol and fatty acid synthesis and hydroxymethylglutaryl CoA reductase activity in mammalian cells grown in culture, *Proc. Natl. Acad. Sci. U.S.A.*, 71, 2174, 1974.
43. Chait, A., Foster, D., Miller, D. G., and Bierman, E. L., Acceleration of low density lipoprotein turnover in man by total parenteral nutrition, *Proc. Soc. Exp. Biol. Med.*, 168, 97, 1981.
44. Mazzone, T., Foster, D., and Chait, A., *In vivo* stimulation of low density lipoprotein degradation by insulin, *Diabetes*, 33, 333, 1984.
45. Chait, A., Bierman, E. L., and Albers, J. J., Regulatory role of triiodothyronine in the degradation of low density lipoprotein by cultured human skin fibroblasts, *J. Clin. Endocrinol. Metab.*, 48, 887, 1979.
46. Chait, A., Kanter, R., Kenny, M., and Green, W., Defective thyroid hormone action in fibroblasts cultured from subjects with the syndrome of resistance to thyroid hormone, *J. Clin. Endocrinol. Metab.*, 54, 767, 1982.
47. Walton, K. W., Scott, P. J., Dykes, P. W., and Davies, J. S., The significance of alterations in serum lipids in thyroid dysfunction. II. Alterations of the metabolism and turnover of ^{131}I low density lipoproteins in hypothyroidism and thyrotoxicosis, *Clin. Sci.*, 29, 217, 1965.
48. Thompson, G. R., Soutar, A. K., Spengel, E. A., Jadhav, A., Gavigan, S. J., and Myant, N. B., Defects of receptor-mediated low density lipoprotein catabolism in homozygous familial hypercholesterolemia, *Proc. Natl. Acad. Sci. U.S.A.*, 78, 2591, 1981.
49. Henze, K., Chait, A., Albers, J. J., and Bierman, E. L., Hydrocortisone decreases the internalization of low density lipoprotein in cultured human fibroblasts and arterial smooth muscle cells, *Eur. J. Clin. Invest.*, 13, 177, 1983.
50. Henze, K., Kuchodkar, B. J., Chait, A., Albers, J. J., and Bierman, E. L., The effect of hydrocortisone on cholesterol metabolism of cultured human skin fibroblasts, *Biochim. Biophys. Acta*, 666, 199, 1981.
51. Niinikoski, J., Heughan, C., and Hunt, T. K., Oxygen tension in the aortic wall of normal rabbits, *Atherosclerosis*, 17, 353, 1973.
52. Heughan, C., Niinikowski, J., and Hunt, T. K., Oxygen tension in lesions of experimental atherosclerosis of rabbits, *Atherosclerosis*, 7, 361, 1973.
53. Albers, J. J. and Bierman, E. L., The effect of hypoxia on uptake and degradation of low density lipoproteins by cultured human arterial smooth muscle cells, *Biochim. Biophys. Acta*, 424, 422, 1976.
54. Filipovic, I. and Buddecke, E., Metabolism of homologous lipoproteins in cultured bovine aortic smooth muscle cells as influenced by hypoxia, *Artery*, 4, 243, 1978.
55. Kuehl, K. S. and Holloway, P. W., Lipoprotein uptake by vascular smooth muscle cells of the rat cultured in 5% or 20% oxygen, *Cell Tissue Res.*, 233, 453, 1983.
56. Tsukitani, M., Okamoto, R., and Fukuzaki, H., Effect of hypoxia on cholesterol accumulation in cultured rabbit aortic smooth muscle cells, *Atherosclerosis*, 52, 167, 1984.
57. Okamata, R., Hatani, M., Tsukitani, M., Suehiro, A., Fujuo, M., Imai, N., Takano, S., Watanabe, Y., and Fukuzaki, H., The effect of oxygen on the development of atherosclerosis in WHHL rabbits, *Atherosclerosis*, 47, 47, 1983.
58. Packer, L. and Fuehr, K., Low oxygen concentration extends the lifespan of cultured human diploid cells, *Nature (London)*, 267, 423, 1977.
59. Bierman, E. L. and Albers, J. J., Lipoprotein uptake and degradation by human arterial smooth muscle cells in tissue culture, *Ann. N. Y. Acad. Sci.*, 275, 199, 1976.
60. Tolleshaug, H., Hobgood, K. K., Brown, M. S., and Goldstein, J. L., The LDL receptor locus in familial hypercholesterolemia multiple mutations disrupt transport and processing of a membrane receptor, *Cell*, 32, 941, 1983.

61. Goldstein, J. L., Helgeson, J. A., and Brown, M. S.,Inhibition of cholesterol synthesis with compactin renders growth of cultured cells dependent on the low density lipoprotein receptor, *J. Biol. Chem.*, 254, 5403, 1979.
62. Brown, M. S., Sobhani, M. K., Brunschede, G. Y., and Goldstein, J. L., Restoration of a regulatory response to low density lipoprotein in acid lipase deficient human fibroblasts, *J. Biol. Chem.*, 251, 3277, 1976.
63. Brown, M. S., Faust, J. R., Goldstein, J. L., Kaneko, L., and Endo, A., Induction of 3-hydroxy-3-methylglutaryl coenzyme A reductase activity in human fibroblasts incubated with compactin (ML-236B), a competitive inhibitor of the reductase, *J. Biol. Chem.*, 253, 1121, 1978.
64. Alberts, A. W., Chen, J., Kuron, G., Hunt, V., Huff, J., Hoffman, C., Rothrock, J., Lopez, M., Joshua, H., Harris, E., Patchett, A., Monaghan, R., Currie, S., Stapley, E., Alberts-Schonberg, G., Hensen, O., Hirshfield, J., Hoogsteen, K., Liesch, J., and Springer, J., Mevinolin: a highly potent competitive inhibitor of hydrocymethylglutaryl-coenzyme A reductase and a cholesterol-lowering agent, *Proc. Natl. Acad. Sci. U.S.A.*, 77, 3957, 1980.
65. Brown, M. S. and Goldstein, J. L., Suppression of 3-hydroxy-3-methylglutaryl coenzyme A reductase activity and inhibition of growth of human fibroblasts by 7-ketocholesterol, *J. Biol. Chem.*, 249, 7306, 1974.
66. Goldstein, J. L., Brunschede, G. Y., and Brown, M. S., Inhibition of the proteolytic degradation of low density lipoprotein in human fibroblasts by chloroquine, concanavalin A, and Triton WR 1339, *J. Biol. Chem.*, 250, 7854, 1975.
67. Goldstein, J. L., Faust, J. R., Dygos, J. H., Chorvat, R. J., and Brown, M. S., Inhibition of cholesterol ester formation in human fibroblasts by an analogue of 7-ketocholesterol and by progesterone, *Proc. Natl. Acad. Sci. U.S.A.*, 75, 1877, 1981.
68. Bates, S. R., Jett, C., and Miller, J. E., Prevention of the hyperlipidemic serum or LDL-induced cellular cholesterol ester accumulation by 22-hydroxycholesterol and its analogue, *Biochim. Biophys. Acta*, 753, 281, 1983.
69. Ross, A. C., Go, K. J., Heider, J. G., and Rothblat, G. H., Selective inhibition of acyl coenzyme A:cholesterol acyltransferase by compound 58-035, *J. Biol. Chem.*, 259, 815, 1984.
70. Bell, E. P., Effect of chlorpromazine on lipid metabolism in aortas from cholesterol fed rabbits and normal rats in vitro: inhibition of sterol esterification and modification of phospholipid synthesis, *Exp. Mol. Pathol.*, 38, 336, 1983.
71. Ostlund, R. E., Jr., Pfleger, B., and Schonfeld, G., Role of microtubules in low density lipoprotein processing by cultured cells, *J. Clin. Invest.*, 63, 75, 1979.
72. Miller, N. E. and Yin, J. A., Effects of cytochalasin B on low-density lipoprotein metabolism by cultured human fibroblasts, *Biochim. Biophys. Acta*, 530, 145, 1978.
73. Brown, M. S. and Goldstein, J. L., Analysis of a mutant strain of human fibroblasts with a defect in the internalization of receptor-bound low density lipoprotein, *Cell*, 9, 663, 1976.
74. Brown, M. S., Kovanen, P. T., and Goldstein, J. L., Regulation of plasma cholesterol by lipoprotein receptors, *Science*, 212, 628, 1981.
75. Basu, K. S., Anderson, R. G. W., Goldstein, J. L., and Brown, M. S., Metabolism of cationized lipoproteins by human fibroblasts, *J. Cell Biol.*, 74, 119, 1977.
76. Mahley, R. W., Innerarity, J. L., Rall, S. C., Jr., and Weisgraber, K. H., Plasma lipoproteins: apolipoprotein structure and function, *J. Lipid Res.*, 25, 1277, 1984.
77. Brinton, E. A., Oram, J. F., Chen, C. H., Albers, J. J., and Bierman, E. L., Ligand characterization of the HDL receptor in cultured fibroblasts, *Arteriosclerosis*, 3, 491a, 1983.
78. Ross, R., Atherosclerosis: a problem of the biology of the arterial wall cells and their interaction with blood components, *Arteriosclerosis*, 1, 293, 1981.
79. Chait, A., Eisenberg, S., Steinmetz, A., Albers, J. J., and Bierman, E. J., Low density lipoproteins modified by lipid transfer protein have altered biological activity, *Biochim. Biophys. Acta*, 795, 314, 1984.
80. Hiramatsu, K., Bierman, E. L., and Chait, A., Metabolism of low density lipoprotein from patients with diabetic hypertriglyceridemia by cultured human skin fibroblasts, *Diabetes*, 34, 8, 1985.
81. Steinbrecher, U. P. and Witztum, J. L., Glycosylation of low density lipoprotein to an extent comparable to that seen in diabetes slows their catabolism, *Diabetes*, 33, 130, 1983.
82. Chen, R. M. and Fischer-Dzoga, K., Effect of hyperlipemic serum lipoproteins on the lipid accumulation and cholesterol flux of rabbit aortic medial cells, *Atherosclerosis*, 28, 339, 1979.
83. Bates, S. R., Accumulation and loss of cholesterol esters in monkey arterial smooth muscle cells exposed to normal and hyperlipemic serum lipoproteins, *Atherosclerosis*, 32, 165, 1979.
84. St. Clair, R. W. and Leigh, M. A., Differential effects of isolated lipoproteins from normal and hypercholesterolemic rhesus monkeys on cholesterol esterification and accumulation in arterial smooth muscle cells in culture, *Biochim. Biophys. Acta*, 530, 279, 1978.

85. Fogelman, A. M., Shechter, I., Seager, J., Hokum, M., Child, J. S., and Edwards, P. A., Malondialdehyde alteration of low density lipoproteins leads to cholesterol ester accumulation in human monocyte-macrophages, *Proc. Soc. Natl. Acad. Sci. U.S.A.,* 77, 2214, 1980.
86. Henriksen, T., Mahoney, F. M., and Steinberg, D., Enhanced macrophage degradation of biologically modified low density lipoproteins, *Arteriosclerosis,* 3, 149, 1983.
87. Morel, D. W., Di Corletto, P., and Chisolm, G. M., Endothelial and smooth muscle cells alter low density lipoproteins in vitro by free radical oxidation, *Arteriosclerosis,* 4, 357, 1984.
88. Heinecke, J. W., Rosen, H., and Chait, A., Iron and copper promote modification of low density lipoprotein by human arterial smooth muscle cells, *J. Clin. Invest.,* 74, 1890, 1984.
89. Steinbrecher, U. P., Parthasarathy, S., Leake, D. S., Witztum, J. L., and Steinberg, D., Modification of low density lipoproteins by endothelial cells involves lipid peroxidation and degradation of low density lipoprotein phospholipids, *Proc. Natl. Acad. Sci. U.S.A.,* 81, 3883, 1984.
90. Heinecke, J. W., Baker, L., Rosen, H., and Chait, A., Mechanism of free radical modification of low density lipoprotein by arterial smooth muscle cells, *Clin. Res.,* 33, 570A, 1985.
91. Parthasarathy, S., Steinbrecher, U. P., Batnell, J., Witztum, J. L., and Steinberg, D., Essential role of phospholipase A_2 activity in endothelial cell-induced modification of low density lipoprotein, *Proc. Natl. Acad. Sci. U.S.A.,* 82, 3000, 1985.
92. Raymond, T. L. and Reynolds, S. A., Lipoproteins of the extravascular space: alterations in low density lipoproteins of interstitial inflammatory fluid, *J. Lipid Res.,* 24, 113, 1983.
93. Higuchi, Y., Lipid peroxides and L-tocopherol in rat streptozotocin-induced diabetes mellitus, *Acta Med. Okayama,* 36, 165, 1982.
94. Nishigaki, I., Hagihara, M., Tsunekawa, H., Maseki, M., and Yagi, K., Lipid peroxide levels in serum lipoprotein fractions of diabetic patients, *Biochem. Med.,* 25, 373, 1981.
95. Thomas, C. E., Morehouse, L. A., and Aust, S. D., Ferritin and superoxide-dependent lipid peroxidation, *J. Biol. Chem.,* 260, 3275, 1985.
96. Hollander, W., Unified concept on the role of acid mucopolysaccharides and connective tissue proteins in the accumulation of lipids, lipoproteins, and calcium in the atherosclerotic plaque, *Exp. Mol. Pathol.,* 25, 106, 1976.
97. Vijayagopal, P., Srinivasan, S. R., Radhakrishnamurthy, B., and Berenson, G. S., Interaction of serum lipoproteins and a proteoglycan from bovine aorta, *J. Biol. Chem.,* 256, 8234, 1981.
98. Schaefer, E. J., Clinical, biochemical, and genetic features in familial disorders of high density lipoprotein deficiency, *Arteriosclerosis,* 4, 303, 1984.
99. Brinton, E. A., Oram, J. F., and Bierman, E. L., The effect of hypertriglyceridemia and diabetes on high density lipoprotein interaction with cultured human fibroblasts, submitted for publication.

Chapter 15

VASCULAR CELL INTERACTIONS IN VITRO: ALTERED SMOOTH MUSCLE LDL METABOLISM INDUCED BY CO-CULTURE WITH ENDOTHELIAL CELLS

Peter F. Davies and George A. Truskey

TABLE OF CONTENTS

I. INTRODUCTION

The individual cells within all differentiated mammalian tissues, including blood vessels, are in communication with each other via either humoral interactions or contact-mediated mechanisms. Such arrangements presumably exist to maintain homeostasis during normal physiological conditions and to allow for the coordination of tissue responsiveness to external, nonpathological stimuli. In tissue culture, and to a limited extent in situ, interactions between the normal resident cells of blood vessels — endothelium and smooth muscle cells (SMC) — and transient residents derived from the blood (monocyte-derived macrophages, polymorphonuclear leukocytes, and lymphocytes) have been recently documented.[1-10] The close apposition of endothelial cells and SMC in vivo suggested to us that both normal vascular homeostasis and pathophysiological developments may involve communication between these cell populations. We, therefore, began in 1980 a study of endothelial cell-SMC interactions with respect to two characteristics of SMC behavior which are relevant to early atherogenesis: cell proliferation (growth control) and lipoprotein metabolism. In order to maintain a high degree of manipulative control of cell interactions, tissue culture systems were devised to allow humoral[3,4] — and more recently, contact-mediated[8,11] — interactions to occur. In this chapter, we review the effects of endothelial-SMC co-culture upon low-density lipoprotein (LDL) metabolism in vascular SMC, present a kinetic analysis of LDL metabolism under such conditions, and discuss the mechanisms which may be responsible.

II. CO-CULTURE OF SMOOTH MUSCLE AND ENDOTHELIAL CELLS

A. Co-Culture System

A co-culture system has been devised which utilizes microcarrier culture techniques and offers significant advantages over coplating of mixed cultures,[12] Rose chamber systems,[13] or slide preparations sharing the same medium.[14] Relatively large numbers of microcarrier-borne cells can be introduced into co-culture because of the increased surface area available for anchorage-dependent cells, and cell numbers can readily be increased or decreased. As shown in Figure 1, a shallow plastic cylinder was reversibly attached to the underside of a petri dish lid. The lower end was closed by a silicone-treated nylon net (1 μm pore size), and microcarrier-cells were loaded into the cylindrical chamber. When the lid was placed on a culture dish, the lower part of the chamber was submerged in culture medium. An SMC population was grown conventionally on the culture dish surface. Thus, the culture medium was shared by both cell populations, thereby allowing humoral interchange between them without direct cell contact. (Further information about microcarrier culture and co-culture is in Chapter 3 of this volume and in References 15 and 16). Bovine aortic endothelial cells were isolated and propagated using conventional techniques[17,18] and grown to confluence on microcarriers, as previously described.[15] Bovine aortic SMC were obtained from explants by the methods of Ross[19] and were in subcultures 1, 2, or 3 at the time of these experiments. Cells were plated at 5×10^4 cells per 35-mm dish in 10% Dulbecco's Modified Eagle's Medium containing 10% calf serum (DME). After 48 hr, the cells were washed with Hank's Balanced Salt Solution (HBSS) and the medium replaced with 5% (v/v) plasma-derived serum (PDS) in DME to arrest cell growth. PDS was prepared according to the methods of Vogel et al.[20] For studies involving lipoprotein metabolism, SMC were deprived of LDL by preincubation in a medium deficient in both lipoproteins and growth factors — designated lipoprotein-deficient, growth factor-depleted medium (LPDM).

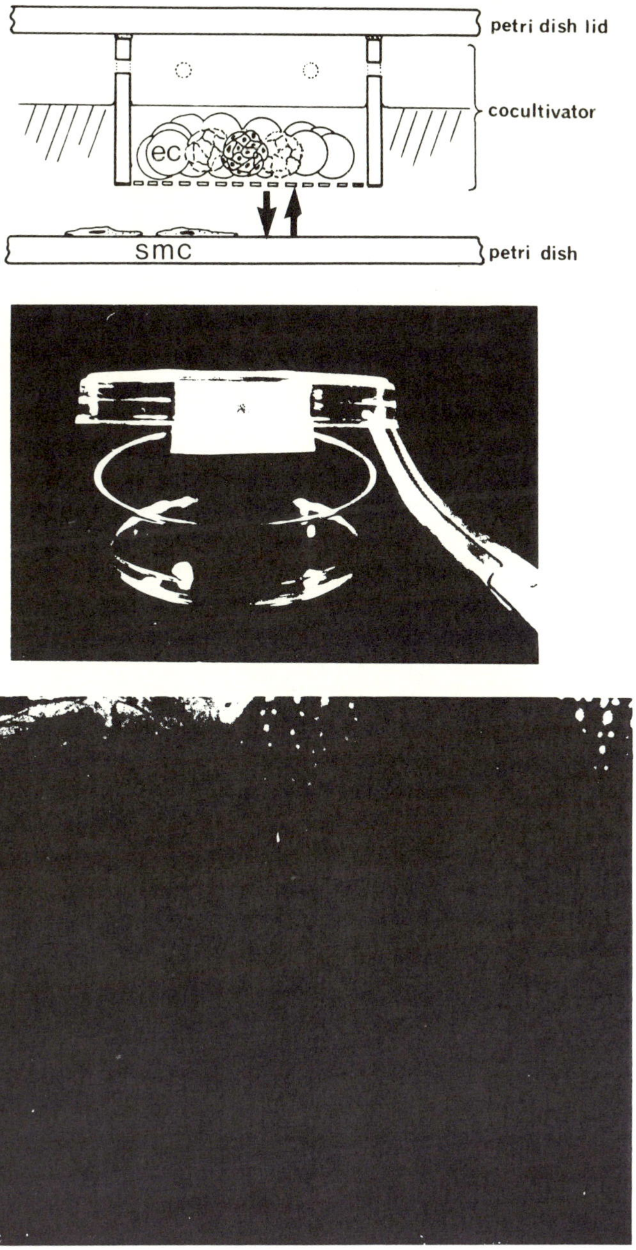

FIGURE 1. Diagram and photograph of a co-culture attachment for 35 mm diameter petri dishes. Microcarrier cultures of endothelial cells are retained in the attachment, while SMC are grown on the dish surface. The lower photograph shows a reconstruction from three photographs taken through the system vertically. (Hematoxylin.) (From Davies, P. F. and Kerr, C., *Exp. Cell Res.*, 141, 455, 1982. With permission.)

B. Co-Culture Protocol for LDL Metabolism

Binding, internalization, and degradation of ^{125}I-LDL were determined using standard procedures.[21] Single cultures of quiescent SMC or co-cultures of SMC and endothelial cells were separately preincubated with 5% LPDM for 48 hr. A schematic of this protocol is shown in Figure 2. The two cell populations were then brought together

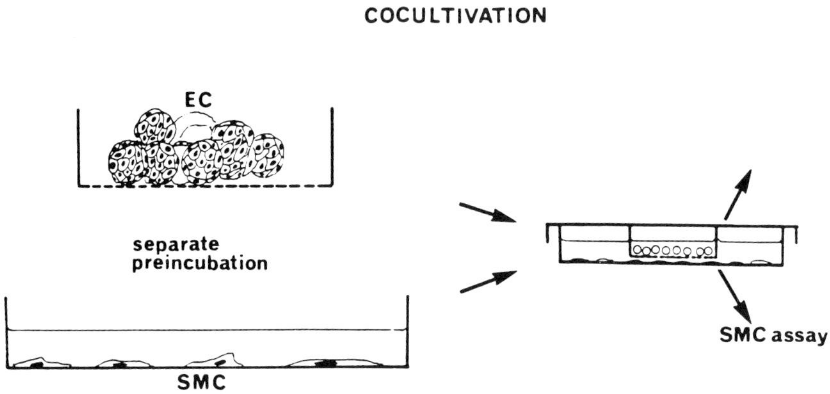

FIGURE 2. Protocol for receptor studies using co-culture. Endothelial cells and SMC were preincubated separately in LPDM. The two-cell populations were then brought together in co-culture, after which ^{125}I-LDL was added. The SMC population was assayed separately from the endothelial cells for LDL metabolism.

for varying lengths of time depending on the experiment, after which the co-culture baskets were removed along with the endothelial cells. The SMC were then incubated with ^{125}I-LDL at 37°C for periods appropriate to each experiment. At the end of the experiment, the dishes were rapidly chilled to 4°C and the medium removed for determination of LDL degradation, while the cells were processed for LDL binding and internalization. In all experiments, receptor-independent LDL binding, internalization, and degradation were determined by incubation with excess (500 μg/mℓ unlabeled LDL). Receptor-mediated metabolism was determined by subtracting receptor-independent metabolism from total LDL metabolism. Cell-free dishes were incubated with ^{125}I-LDL in parallel to the above, and the amount degraded was subtracted from the specific and nonspecific contributions.

C. Microcarrier-Bound Endothelial Cells

Bovine aortic endothelial cells readily grow to confluence on solid plastic microcarriers. We have extensively characterized these cells and found that they are identical to cells grown on plastic dishes in terms of cell growth, morphological appearance, ultrastructural characteristics, and prostaglandin I_2 production.[15] At confluence there are between 150 and 200 cells per bead.

D. Growth Stimulation of SMC by Endothelial Cells

Following exposure to purified mitogens, SMC and fibroblasts metabolize an increased mass of LDL by the receptor-mediated pathway.[22-24] These changes in LDL metabolism coincide with stimulation of cells into the growth cycle. Endothelial cell-conditioned medium contains at least two endothelial-derived mitogens which stimulate SMC and fibroblast proliferation.[25] Warren of our laboratory has studied the growth of bovine SMC co-cultured with bovine aortic endothelial cells. In these experiments, incubation in 2% PDS for 72 hr arrested cell growth. Thereafter, dishes receiving fresh PDS plus co-culture with either endothelial cells or with more SMC expressed different responses in terms of growth. As shown in Figure 3, co-culture of SMC with microcarrier-bound SMC or with empty beads did not stimulate SMC growth. Co-culture of SMC with microcarrier-bound endothelial cells, however, resulted in a significant stimulation of SMC growth. By varying the number of microcarriers, the effects of endothelial cell mass on the growth of SMC was studied. There were significant

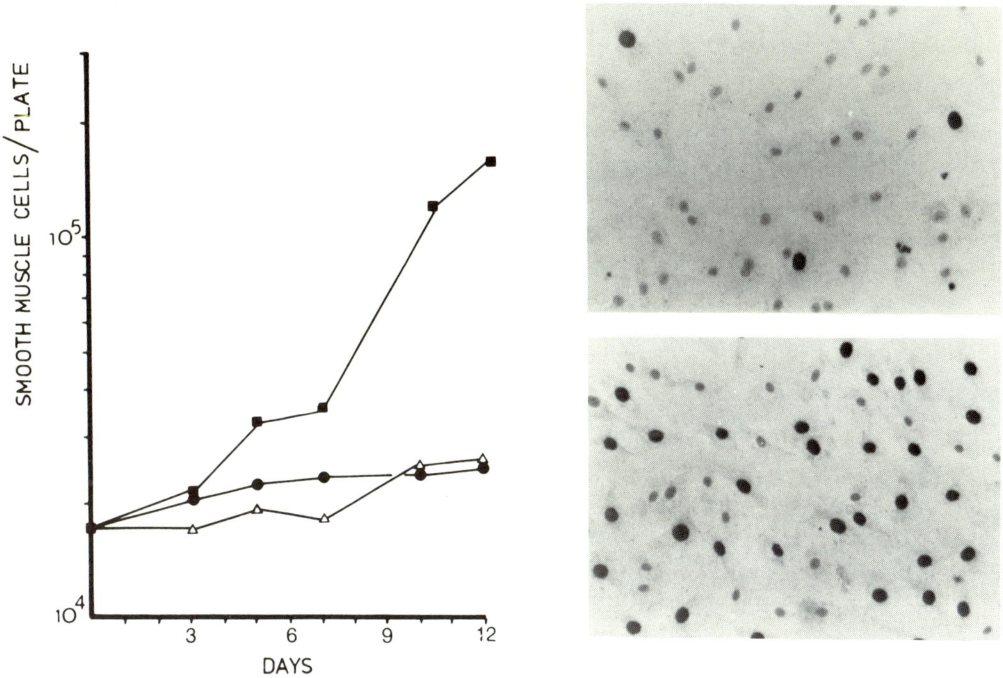

FIGURE 3. Mitogenic effects upon SMC by co-culture with endothelial cells. At day 0, all dishes received fresh 2% PDS, after which SMC were co-cultured with equal numbers of microcarrier-bound confluent endothelial cells (■) or SMC (●)or empty microcarriers (△). SMC numbers were determined by a Coulter Counter on the days indicated. ^{3}H-thymidine autoradiographs of SMC co-cultured with microcarrier-bound SMC (upper panel) or endothelial cells (lower panel) for 48 hr in 2% PDS. Endothelial: SMC ratio = 1.0. (Reproduced from *The Journal of Cell Biology,* 1985, Vol. 101, pp. 871-879, by copyright permission of The Rockefeller University Press.)

increases in SMC number with increasing endothelial cell mass, whereas growth increased only slightly as the mass of SMC on microcarriers increased (Figure 4). Note that 0.1 mg cell protein is equal to approximately 2.3×10^5 endothelial cells and 3.0×10^5 SMC.

By least squares linear regression, the data were fit to the following lines:

$$\text{Endothelial cell co-culture} \qquad y = 23.6 \times 10^4\, x + 6.4 \times 10^4 \qquad (1)$$

$$\text{Smooth muscle cell co-culture} \qquad y = 4.5 \times 10^4\, x + 6.2 \times 10^4 \qquad (2)$$

where x is the mass (mg) of endothelial cells or SMC on microcarriers and y is the number of SMC. The correlation coefficients are 0.89 and 0.66, respectively, for endothelial cell and SMC co-culture with monolayers of target SMC. The slope in Equation 1 is statistically significant ($p < 0.025$) whereas the slope in Equation 2 is not ($p >$ 0.20).

In the above studies, SMC co-cultured with endothelial cells were stimulated to proliferate, resulting in an increase of cell numbers. Similar experiments in the presence of lipoprotein-deficient medium, however, stimulated DNA synthesis in SMC, but the cells were unable to complete the cell cycle probably because of a limited supply of exogenous sterols which prevented completion of mitosis.[27] DNA synthesis was measured using ^{3}H-thymidine autoradiography.[28] As shown in Table 1, SMC incubated

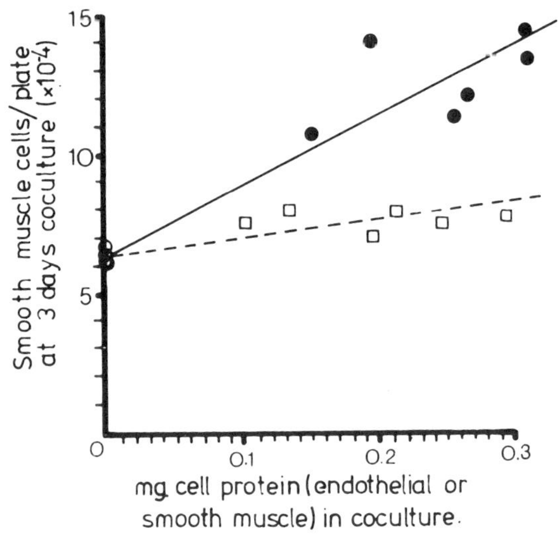

FIGURE 4. Effects of increasing numbers of endothelial cells upon SMC growth. Increasing numbers of confluent microcarrier-bound endothelial cells (•) or microcarrier-bound SMC (□) were co-cultured with 5 × 10⁴ SMC for 3 days in 2% PDS at which time SMC numbers were counted. (Reproduced from *The Journal of Cell Biology*, 1985, Vol. 101, pp. 871-879, by copyright permission of The Rockefeller University Press.)

Table 1
^{3}H-THYMIDINE LABELING[a] OF SMC IN CO-CULTURE WITH ENDOTHELIAL CELLS OR IN ENDOTHELIAL CELL-CONDITIONED MEDIUM

Culture conditions	Percent labeled nuclei (±SD)[b] 20 hr	45 hr
Endothelial cell co-culture	—	63.4 ± 4.4
SMC co-culture	—	4.6 ± 3.2
Endothelial cell-conditioned media	62.3 ± 5.4	39.5 ± 3.5
SMC-conditioned media	2.1 ± 0.1	0.9 ± 0.1
SMC alone	2.3 ± 0.4	2.3 ± 0.1

[a] Continuous exposure to ^{3}H-thymidine.
[b] Determined by autoradiography.

alone, co-cultured with other SMC, or incubated with SMC-conditioned medium exhibited a low level of ^{3}H-thymidine labeling, indicating that the cells were quiescent. In contrast, co-culture with endothelial cells or incubation with endothelial cell-conditioned medium stimulated a significant percentage of the cells to synthesis DNA. These results are consistent with the growth studies performed by Warren.

E. Endothelial Cell-Specific Stimulation of SMC LDL Metabolism

Endothelial cell-SMC co-culture stimulated receptor-mediated metabolism of LDL by bovine SMC, as shown in Table 2. This table also demonstrates that endothelial

Table 2
EFFECT OF CO-CULTURE AND CELL-CONDITIONED MEDIA ON LDL METABOLISM BY SMC[a]

Culture conditions	ng ^{125}I-LDL protein/mg cell protein/4 hr (± SD)		
	Bound	Internalized	Degraded
Endothelial cell co-culture	37.3 ± 0.5	489 ± 34	285 ± 19
Endothelial cell-conditioned media	31.4 ± 6.8	592 ± 89	521 ± 64
SMC-conditioned media	5.0 ± 2.2	84.5 ± 1.1	49.6 ± 20.1
LPDM control	6.7 ± 5.6	93.0 ± 8.8	28.7 ± 8.6
Summary of Three Experiments			
SMC in LPDM (control)	19.9 ± 6.6	127 ± 22	58.8 ± 28.9
Endothelial cell co-culture	48.0 ± 16.5	481 ± 66	396 ± 43

[a] SMC were cultured under the conditions indicated for 41 hr after which ^{125}I-LDL was added for the final 4 hr.

cell-conditioned medium stimulated smooth muscle LDL metabolism, whereas SMC-conditioned medium had no effect. The average stimulation for three experiments is also summarized in Table 2. It should be noted that in co-culture, LDL binding and degradation are stimulated to a greater extent than internalization, suggesting that an increase in the number of cell surface receptors is not the only metabolic response. This observation will be considered later in the section on kinetic analysis.

The data presented thus far are consistent with endothelial-derived growth factor stimulation of LDL metabolism in SMC where passage through the cell cycle modulates the expression of LDL receptors on SMC and fibroblasts.

F. Co-Culture vs. Conditioned Medium

LDL metabolism by SMC incubated with microcarrier-bound endothelial cells or endothelial cell-conditioned medium has been investigated (Figure 5). In order to maintain cell-to-volume ratios similar to those in co-culture, conditioned medium was obtained by incubating 5×10^5 microcarrier-endothelial cells with 2.5-mℓ, 5% LPDM per 35 mm petri dish for 48 hr. The conditioned medium was then diluted 1:1 with 5% LPDM. After the indicated time of incubation, the SMC were incubated with 10 μg/mℓ ^{125}I-LDL for 2 hr ± an excess of unlabeled LDL for determination of nonspecific metabolism. LDL binding, internalization, and degradation were stimulated by 16-hr co-culture or by conditioned medium. As time of exposure increased, the difference between LDL metabolism in SMC control experiments vs. that in co-culture and conditioned medium experiments became greater. For SMC treated with endothelial cell-conditioned medium, stimulation of LDL metabolism began to level off by 46 hr, suggesting depletion of growth factors. Co-culture of SMC and endothelial cells, however, resulted in a continued increase of LDL metabolism throughout the duration of the experiment, perhaps because of continuous production of endothelial cell-derived growth factors. Although the results suggest that co-culture is at least as potent as conditioned medium in stimulating LDL metabolism, direct comparison of co-culture and conditioned medium is difficult. Conditioned medium represents an end point in growth factor production by the endothelial cells, whereas, in co-culture, growth factor production is initially zero and increases linearly with time.[29] At the beginning of the experiment presented in Figure 5, those SMC which received endothelial cell-conditioned medium were, in effect, exposed to the cumulative amount of growth factor

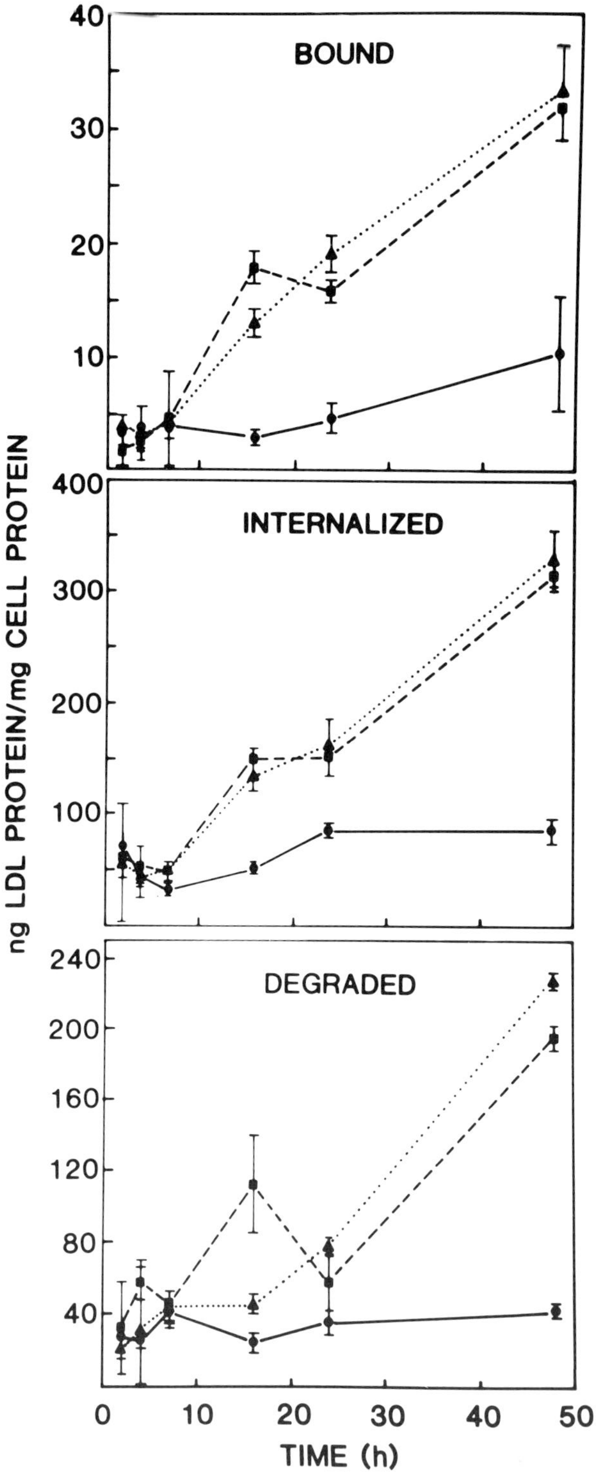

FIGURE 5. Time-course of the effects of endothelial cell-conditioned medium (■---■) or endothelial cell-SMC co-culture (▲.....▲) upon LDL metabolism in SMC. SMC alone (•——•). (See text for details of experiment.)

produced after 48 hr. This is in contrast to SMC co-cultured with endothelial cells that were initially exposed to low concentrations of growth factor. Yet the changes in LDL metabolism by SMC exposed to co-culture or conditioned medium were very similar. This suggests that either very low concentrations of endothelial cell-derived growth factors are required to stimulate LDL metabolism, or additional cell-cell interactions occur.

To account for differences in production of growth factor, conditioned medium has also been obtained by coincubating SMC and microcarrier-endothelial cells in 5% LPDM for 48 hr. After the incubation, this "co-culture conditioned medium" was diluted 50% with 5% LPDM before SMC were incubated with it for periods ranging from 8 to 72 hr. At the end of the incubations, the medium was removed and replaced with the same medium containing ^{125}I-LDL. The cells were then incubated for 4 hr at 37°C, after which receptor-mediated LDL metabolism was determined. The results of a representative experiment are presented in Figure 6. Conditioned medium derived from endothelial cell-SMC co-culture gave results which were identical to those for endothelial cell-conditioned medium alone.

G. Effect of Endothelial Cell Number on SMC LDL Metabolism

The stimulation of smooth muscle LDL metabolism following co-culture with endothelial cells was analyzed with respect to the ratio of cells in co-culture. Bovine aortic SMC were incubated with varying amounts of endothelial cells for 48 hr. At the end of incubation, SMC were washed and incubated with ^{125}I-LDL for 4 hr, after which receptor-mediated binding, internalization, and degradation were measured. As shown in Figure 7, as the number of endothelial cells increased, LDL metabolism by SMC also increased. A plateau was reached at approximately 0.15 mg endothelial cell protein (corresponding to 3×10^5 endothelial cells). Data were fit to the following empirical function:

$$y = y_o + \frac{a_1 x}{x + a_2} \tag{3}$$

where y is the amount of LDL bound, internalized, or degraded per milligram SMC; x is the mass of endothelial cells; y_o is the amount of LDL bound, internalized, or degraded per milligram SMC in the absence of endothelial cells; and a_1 and a_2 are empirical constants. For internalized and degraded LDL, the half-saturation value, a_2, is between 0.08 and 0.09 mg endothelial cell protein, corresponding to 1.9 to 2.1×10^5 endothelial cells in co-culture.

III. KINETIC ANALYSIS OF LDL METABOLISM

The stimulation of LDL metabolism in SMC co-cultured with endothelial cells is attributable in part to an increase in the number of receptors. This is consistent with changes of LDL metabolism in SMC and fibroblasts following exposure to PDGF. If this were the only effect, it would be expected that internalization and degradation would increase proportionately. In order to examine these changes in more detail, kinetic models were developed[30] that were used to determine rate constants.

Figure 8 shows LDL metabolism in SMC in co-culture with endothelial cells at increasing concentrations of LDL. Binding and degradation appear to increase to a greater extent than internalization.

Schematically, the interaction of LDL with its receptor on SMC and subsequent metabolic fate in the cell can be described as

$$\text{LDL} + \text{Rec} \underset{k_{-1}}{\overset{k_1}{\rightleftarrows}} \text{LDL}-\text{Rec} \xrightarrow{k_2} \text{LDL}_{int} \xrightarrow{k_3} \text{LDL}_d \tag{4}$$

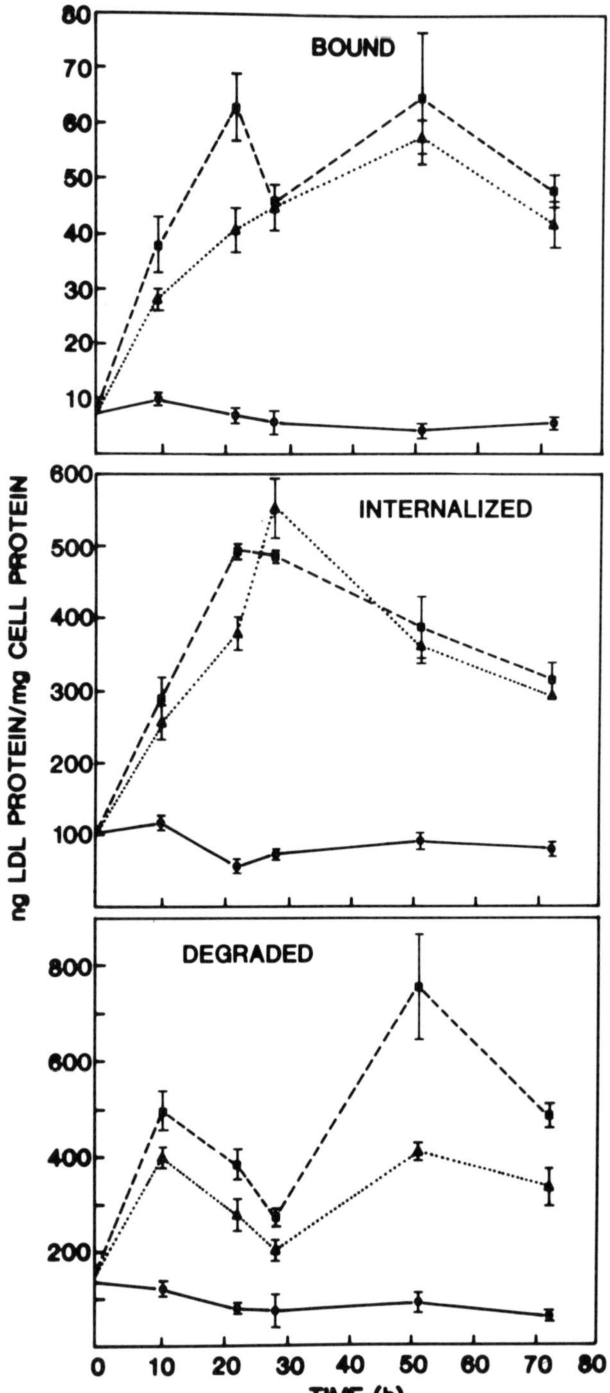

FIGURE 6. A comparison of LDL metabolism by SMC incubated with either endothelial cell-conditioned medium (■---■) or co-culture-conditioned medium derived from endothelial cells-SMC (▲.....▲). SMC alone (•——•).

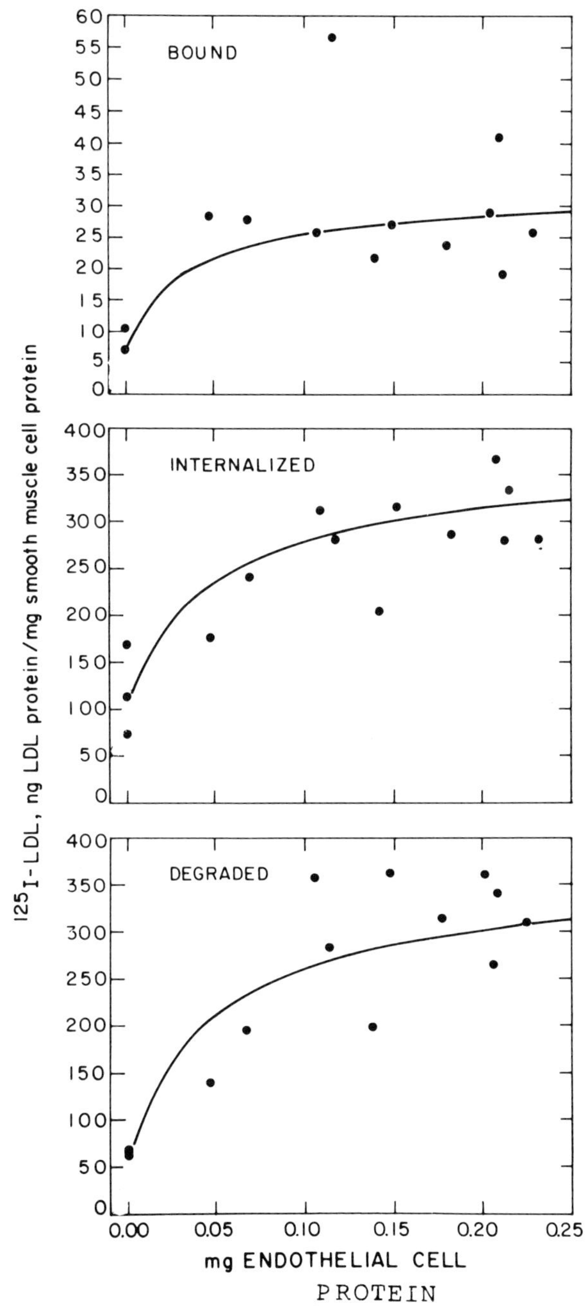

FIGURE 7. Influence of increasing numbers of co-cultured endothelial cells upon SMC high-affinity binding, internalization, and degradation of ^{125}I-LDL. 2 × 10^5 SMC were incubated in co-culture with increasing numbers of confluent microcarrier-bound endothelial cells. After 48 hr, 10 μg ^{125}I-LDL were added for 4 hr, after which LDL metabolism was determined in the SMC. Note that 0.1 mg endothelial cell protein is equivalent to approximately 2 × 10^5 cells. (Reproduced from *The Journal of Cell Biology*, 1985, Vol. 101, pp. 871-879, by copyright permission of The Rockefeller University Press.)

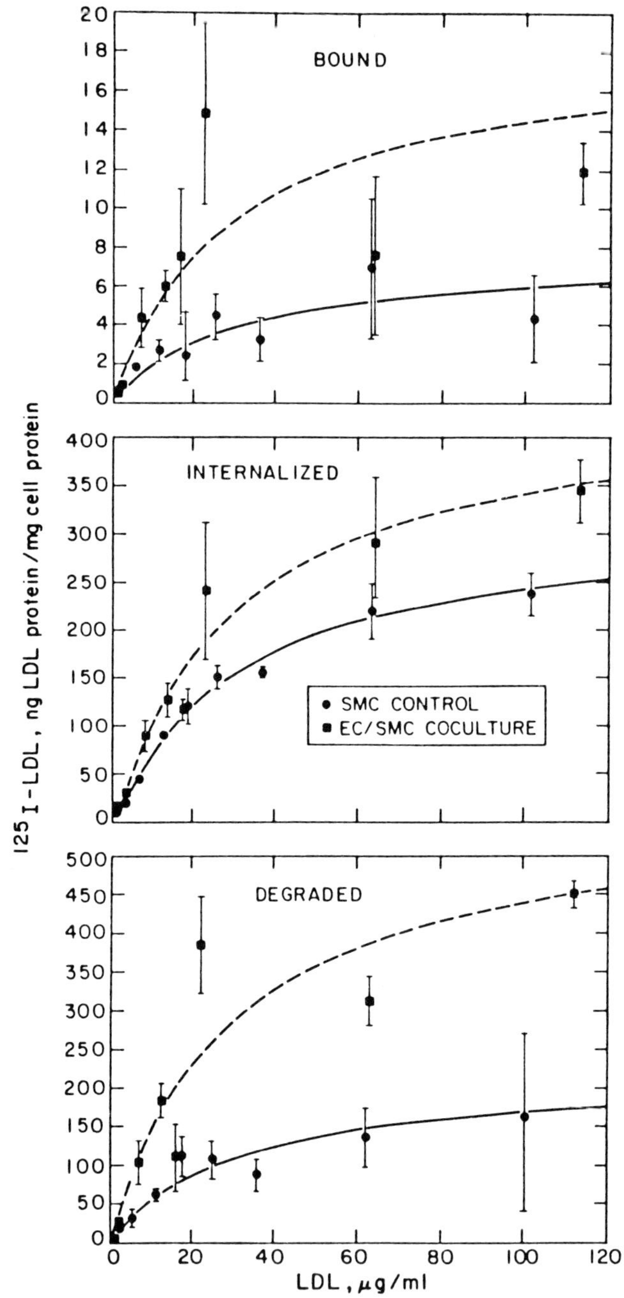

FIGURE 8. Relation of high-affinity binding, internalization, and degradation of ^{125}I-LDL in SMC to the concentration of LDL in single cultures of SMC (•——•) and co-cultures of endothelial cells with SMC (■---■).

where LDL is the free concentration of LDL (μg/mℓ) and Rec, LDL-Rec, LDL_{int}, and LDL_d represent the free receptor, LDL-receptor complex, internalized LDL, and degraded LDL, respectively (ng/mg). Ligand binding is a reversible, bimolecular reaction with association constant K_1 (mℓ μg^{-1} min^{-1}) and dissociation constant k_{-1} (min^{-1}). The rate of internalization is first order in cell surface-bound LDL with rate constant k_2 (min^{-1}), and the rate of degradation is first order for intracellular LDL with rate constant k_3 (min^{-1}).

Material balances on bound, internalized, and degraded LDL yield

$$\frac{d[LDL\text{–}Rec]}{dt} = k_1[LDL_o]\,[Rec] - (k_{-1} + k_2)\,[LDL\text{–}Rec] \tag{5}$$

$$\frac{d[LDL_{int}]}{d+} = k_2[LDL\text{–}Rec] - k_3[LDL_{int}] \tag{6}$$

$$\frac{d[LDL_d]}{d+} = k_3[LDL_{int}] \tag{7}$$

$[LDL_0]$ represents the concentration of labeled LDL added at the beginning of the experiment and is essentially constant throughout. The total number of receptors is constant and is equal to the sum of free and ligand-bound receptors:

$$[R_T] = [LDL\text{–}Rec] + [Rec] \tag{8}$$

A constant of interest is K_{int}:

$$K_{int} = \frac{k_{-1} + k_2}{k_1} \tag{9}$$

K_{int} is the ratio of the rate constants for LDL − Rec dissociation and internalization to the rate constant for binding. It is analogous to the half-saturation constant defined in Michaelis-Menten kinetics;[28] k_{-1} is negligible relative to k_2.[31]

Equations 5 to 8 are a set of linear first-order ordinary differential equations and were solved by standard methods. The rate constants k_1, k_2, and k_3, plus R_T and K_{int} were determined by simultaneous, nonlinear regression of data for bound, internalized, and degraded LDL using a Bayesian parameter estimation of multiresponse data.[32]

Table 3 shows the rate constants for SMC LDL metabolism following co-culture. The major effect of co-culture was to more than double the total number of LDL receptors expressed by SMC (average threefold increase; range two- to sevenfold). In addition, there were changes in the major rate constants for LDL metabolism. The association rate constant, k_1, for LDL receptor binding decreased in co-culture, indicating that binding occurred 33% more slowly than in single culture (range 15 to 38%). The rate constant for receptor-mediated endocytosis of LDL, k_2, decreased 42% in co-culture (range 21 to 49%). The overall affinity of LDL for its receptor K_{int}, however, was unchanged because K_{int} is derived from a ratio of k_2/k_1. In contrast, the rate of degradation of LDL, k_3, was increased 51% in co-culture (range 33 to 74%). In co-culture, therefore, LDL was internalized less efficiently but was degraded more efficiently. The value of such a kinetic approach to these studies is primarily twofold: (1) assessment of the effects of endothelial cells upon SMC LDL metabolism at 37°C instead of 4°C, where measurements are restricted to determination of binding alone and (2) the identification of a rate-limiting step of LDL metabolism in SMC, i.e., the

Table 3
KINETIC ANALYSIS[a] OF LDL METABOLISM IN CULTURED ARTERIAL SMC AT 37°C

Kinetic parameter	SMC, single culture	Endothelial cells-SMC, co-culture[b]	Change (%) Mean	Change (%) Range
Total numbers of LDL receptors per cell, R_T	8,323 (± 5,066)	27,234 (±8424)	+220[c]	112—457
Binding association constant, k_1 (mℓ μg^{-1} min^{-1})	1.79×10^{-2}	1.20×10^{-2}	−33[d]	15—38
Internalization rate constant, k_2 (min^{-1})	0.506	0.294	−42[d]	21—49
Degradation rate constant, k_3 (min^{-1})	5.1×10^{-3}	7.7×10^{-3}	+51[d]	33—74
Affinity constant for LDL receptor, K_{int} (μg mℓ$^{-1}$)	27.1	28.5	Unchanged	

[a] Calculated at 37°C using a Bayesian parameter estimation with simultaneous regression of bound, internalized, and degraded LDL.
[b] Endothelial cell-to-SMC ratio, 1:0.
[c] Significantly different from single culture, $p < 0.001$.
[d] Significantly different from single culture, $p < 0.01$.

internalization process. The latter indicates that an investigation of the cell biology of coated vesicle formation using a variety of cell biological probes during receptor-mediated endocytosis of LDL in this system might be fruitful.

IV. GROWTH FACTOR-INDEPENDENT STIMULATION OF LDL METABOLISM

As discussed above, growth factors secreted by endothelial cells are responsible, in part, for the stimulation of LDL metabolism. Endothelial cell-derived growth factors are believed to have molecular weights in the range 25,000 to 40,000.[29] In order to separate growth factor-dependent stimulation of LDL metabolism from the effect of lower-molecular-weight, nonmitogenic agents, the co-culture system was modified (Figure 9). The mesh was replaced with a dialysis membrane of low-molecular-weight cutoff (3500 daltons). Tests using a variety of ^{125}I-labeled proteins ranging in molecular weight from 6000 (insulin) to 66,200 (albumin) indicated that >95% of the trichloroacetic acid precipitable radioactivity was retained in the upper chamber of the co-culture apparatus. Interposition of the dialysis membrane between microcarrier-endothelial cells and target SMC successfully blocked DNA synthesis, as measured by ^{3}H-thymidine autoradiography (Figure 10). Table 4 presents data on LDL metabolism in the same apparatus. Although replacement of the mesh by a dialysis membrane prevented growth factors from reaching SMC, their LDL metabolism was still significantly stimulated. The increase averaged approximately 50% of the stimulation observed if dialysis membrane were absent (i.e., regular co-culture conditions).

In order to determine whether conditioned medium from endothelial cells also contained factors which stimulate LDL metabolism in SMC in the absence of cell growth, the following experiments were performed. Endothelial cell-conditioned medium (ECCM) was prepared by incubating LPDM with confluent endothelial cells for 72 hr. Part of the ECCM was concentrated fivefold while the remainder was diluted 1:1 with

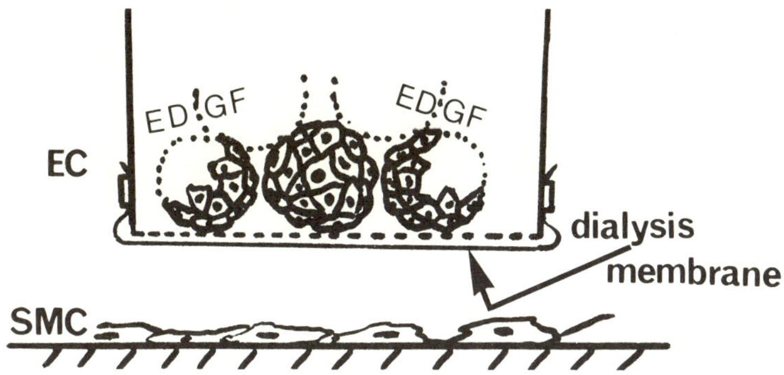

FIGURE 9. Modification of the co-culture apparatus to contain endothelial-derived mitogens (EDGF) in the cylindrical chamber. A dialysis membrane (molecular weight cutoff = 3500 daltons) was placed between the two cell populations.

unconditioned medium. One milliliter of either concentrated or diluted ECCM was placed in the co-culture cylinder separated from SMC by dialysis membrane. As shown in Figure 11, there was no significant stimulation of SMC LDL metabolism. In the same experiment, unconcentrated ECCM added directly to SMC stimulated LDL binding, internalization, and degradation by 238, 360, and 560%, respectively (mitogenic response; 65% labeled cells). Thus, the ability of co-culture to stimulate LDL metabolism in SMC in the absence of a mitogenic response contrasted sharply with the failure of endothelial-conditioned medium to do so even when concentrated fivefold. These results suggest that the sharing of culture medium by both cell types is necessary for enhanced LDL metabolism by SMC in the absence of cell proliferation and imply that either an unstable product of endothelial cells may influence LDL metabolism or that reciprocal communication between endothelial cells and SMC is required to activate the mechanism.

V. DOES CELL-DERIVED NH_4^+ INFLUENCE LDL METABOLISM?

Witte et al.[9] have shown that the mass of LDL bound and internalized in fibroblasts increases, together with the number of high-affinity surface receptors for LDL, following exposure to porcine ECCM. Surprisingly, however, degradation of LDL in the lysosomal system of the fibroblast was significantly inhibited, a response opposite to that observed when fibroblasts were exposed to purified mitogen.[23] Cornicelli et al.[33] subsequently showed that NH_4^+ produced by porcine endothelium was responsible for the lysosomotropic effects. In co-culture of bovine endothelial cells with bovine SMC, we observed no inhibition of lysosomal degradation of LDL, and the rate constant for degradation was significantly increased, as shown above. In order to reconcile our results with the reports concerning the porcine system, we have examined LDL metabolism in relation to NH_4^+ levels in the bovine system using endothelial cell-conditioned and SMC-conditioned media.[34]

NH_4^+ concentrations in conditioned media were determined by reductive amination of α-ketoglutaric acid catalyzed by L-glutamate dehydrogenase. Decrease in absorbance at 340 nm due to oxidation of NADH was proportional to NH_4^+ concentration.[35] Media conditioned by endothelial cells, SMC or endothelial cell-SMC co-culture were collected after 48 hr incubation. The number of cells used to condition the media were similar to those reported by Cornicelli et al.[33] The initial concentration of glutamine in the medium was 2 m*M*, the same concentration used by Cornicelli et al. Total NH_4^+

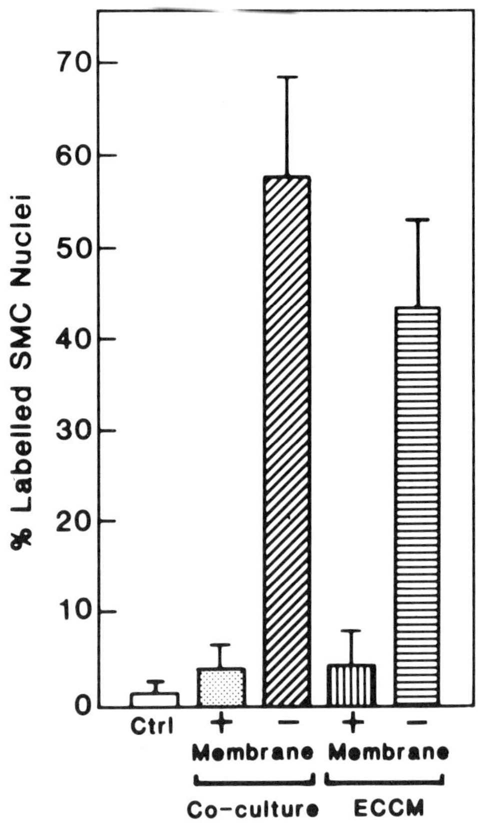

FIGURE 10. Effectiveness of dialysis membrane interposed between endothelial cells and SMC in preventing endothelial-derived growth factors from reaching the SMC. Single culture of SMC □; co-culture with confluent endothelial cells with dialysis membrane between the cell populations ▩; co-culture with endothelial cells, membrane absent ▨; sevenfold concentrated endothelial cell-conditioned medium, membrane present ▥; unconcentrated endothelial cell-conditioned medium, membrane absent ▤. ^{3}H-thymidine incubation for 24 hr. (Reproduced from *The Journal of Cell Biology,* 1985, Vol. 101, pp. 871-879, by copyright permission of The Rockefeller University Press.)

concentration and that due to cell-specific production of ammonia are shown in Table 5. Bovine endothelial cells produced very little NH_4^+, whereas bovine SMC produced significantly more. Nevertheless, NH_4^+ concentrations were much less than those obtained by Cornicelli et al. following 48-hr incubation with porcine endothelial cells. The low levels of NH_4^+ are consistent with the absence of any inhibition of LDL degradation.

NH_4^+ is a potent lysosomotropic agent which appears to inhibit the activity of proteolytic enzymes by raising the lysosomal pH.[36] If significant quantities were produced by endothelial cells in vitro or in vivo, inhibition of lysosomal degradation of macromolecules internalized by receptor-mediated endocytosis might result. This could influence transendothelial transport of blood proteins, as well as their subsequent uptake by vascular SMC. We found no evidence that bovine endothelial cells produced more

Table 4
GROWTH FACTOR-INDEPENDENT STIMULATION OF LDL METABOLISM BY ENDOTHELIAL CELLS IN CO-CULTURE

Culture conditions	ng ^{125}I-LDL protein/mg cell protein/4 hr[a]		
	Bound	Internalized	Degraded
Endothelial cell/SMC co-culture	10.4	142.3	180.7
Endothelial cell/SMC co-culture (+ dialysis membrane)	7.4	135.2	117.0
LPDM control	3.5	81.5	73.7

[a] ^{125}I-LDL metabolism was determined during the final 4 hr of 48-hr exposure to the various culture conditions. Data compiled from three experiments (n = 15).

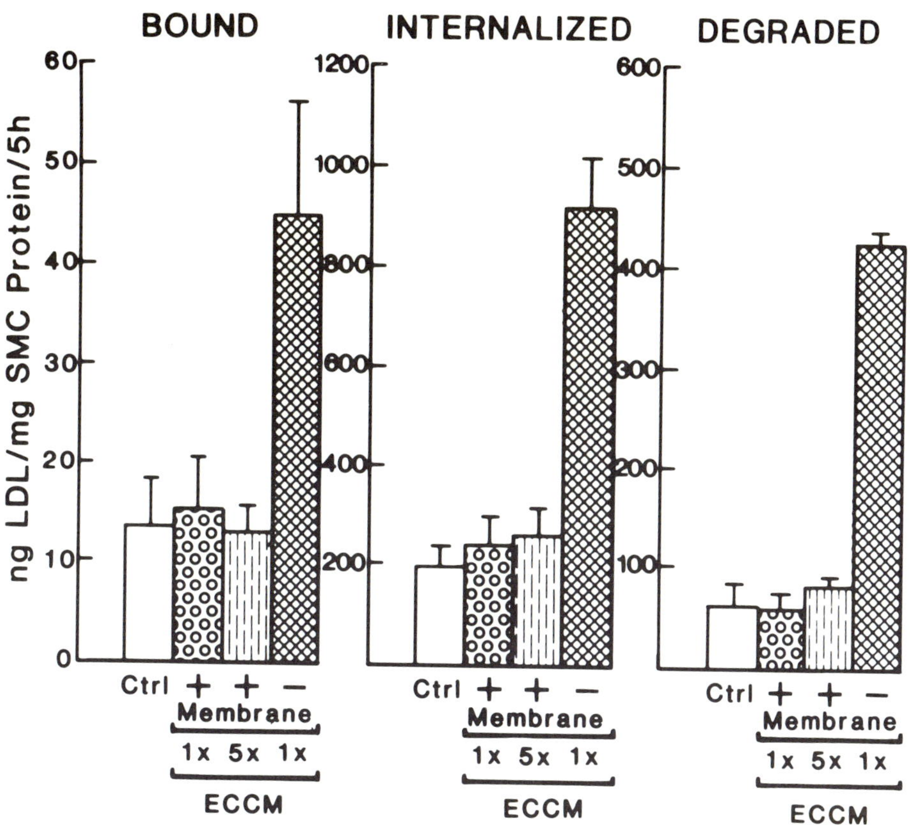

FIGURE 11. Absence of mitogen-independent stimulation of LDL metabolism in SMC incubated with endothelial cell-conditioned medium. SMC cultured alone □; SMC cultured with unconcentrated endothelial cell-conditioned medium ░ or fivefold concentrated endothelial cell-conditioned medium ▥ placed in the upper chamber of the co-culture apparatus and separated by a dialysis membrane. A fourth group of SMC was directly exposed to unconcentrated endothelial cell-conditioned medium ▨ 24 hr later ^{125}I-LDL was added for 5 hr, after which specific LDL metabolism in the SMC was determined. (From Davies, P. F., Truskey, G. A., Warren, H. B., O'Connor, S. E., and Eisenhaure, B. E., *J. Cell Biol.*, 101, in press. With permission.)

Table 5
NH_4^+ PRODUCTION BY ENDOTHELIAL CELLS AND SMC

	mM NH_4^+ after in medium 48 hr	
	Spontaneous	Cell-generated
Endothelial/SMC co-culture	0.41	0.10
Endothelial-conditioned medium	0.40	0.22
SMC-conditioned medium	0.41	1.25
5% LPDM at 4°C	0.20	—

NH_4^+ into conditioned medium than did SMC. Furthermore, medium incubated alone also produced a measurable quantity of NH_4^+ (0.45 m*M* after 72 hr). It seems likely that the origins of the low NH_4^+ concentrations noted in this study were a combination of spontaneous breakdown of glutamine in the medium, as well as cell-mediated glutamine breakdown. In the culture medium, glutamine spontaneously decomposes to pyrrolidine-carboxylic acid and NH_4^+ at pH 7.4. The decomposition reaction is first order in glutamine concentration, and at 37°C the rate constant is 0.0048 hr^{-1}. In the cell, ammonia is derived from the metabolism of glutamine to glutamic acid in the presence of glutaminase. At physiological pH, ammonia is present, largely as NH_4^+. Although renal epithelial cells and porcine endothelial cells appear to produce significant amounts of ammonia,[37,38] bovine endothelial cells do not, and it appears likely that any lysosomotropic influence of NH_4^+ upon LDL degradation in the bovine culture system is negligible. We do not yet know, however, whether human endothelial cells produce significant amounts of NH_4^+ in culture.

VI. EXPERIMENTAL SUMMARY

The experimental results reported in this chapter can be summarized as follows:

1. Bovine aortic endothelial cells co-cultured with bovine SMC stimulated LDL metabolism in the SMC.
2. Kinetic analysis of SMC LDL metabolism revealed that increased LDL receptor number (two- to sevenfold) was a major driving force of enhanced LDL endocytosis and degradation, but that the internalization process was the rate-limiting step.
3. Concomitant stimulation of the SMC cell cycle by endothelial cell-derived growth factors was in part responsible for stimulated LDL metabolism.
4. When co-culture was set up under conditions which prevented endothelial-derived mitogens from reaching the SMC, there was no stimulation of cell growth, but there remained a significant increase in LDL metabolism in SMC. This endothelial cell-dependent, nonmitogenic stimulation of SMC LDL metabolism is currently under investigation.
5. Bovine endothelial cells do not produce significant amounts of lysosomotropically relevant NH_4^+, in contrast to porcine endothelial cells.

VII. DISCUSSION

The complexity of interactions between cells of the vessel wall, as well as interactions between resident cells, the extracellular matrix, and blood-borne cells can conveniently be analyzed in vitro. In the co-culture system described in this chapter, endothelial cells and SMC are bathed in the same solution, allowing bidirectional humoral interactions to occur between the two cell populations. In contrast, transfer of signals via conditioned medium is unidirectional.

Confluent endothelial cells stimulated SMC growth and LDL metabolism. The results were consistent with stimulation of LDL metabolism, in part, by endothelial cell-derived growth factors. DiCorleto and associates[25] have described endothelial-derived mitogens as consisting of at least two distinct proteins that are biochemically separable and immunologically distinct. Using a radioreceptor assay, they have demonstrated that one of these mitogens is a platelet-derived growth factor (PDGF)-like protein constitutively secreted into serum-containing or serum-free medium. Fox and DiCorleto[29] have recently presented evidence that the PDGF-like protein production rate may substantially increase in injured cells. Detection of mRNA for PDGF in endothelial cells was recently made possible through the discovery that there is considerable sequence homology between one of the two chains of PDGF and the simian sarcoma virus transforming protein (p28 sis).[39,40] Thus, endothelial transcription of PDGF can be detected by hybridization of ^{32}P-labeled c-sis DNA probe.[41] This experimental approach can be used to study the expression of the PDGF-encoding gene in endothelial cells. The production rate of endothelial cell-derived growth factors in culture is approximately 0.69 ng/10^6 cells per hour and is constant for up to 3 weeks.[29] At half-maximal stimulation of LDL metabolism, 2.0×10^5 endothelial cells produce about 6.6 ng of growth factor after 48 hr (i.e., at the time of the assay for LDL metabolism) at a concentration of 2.6 ng/mℓ. From the data of Witte et al.[9], half-maximal stimulation of binding occurs with 10% endothelial cell-conditioned medium. The conditioned medium was prepared with about 10^7 endothelial cells incubated in 10 mℓ 5% LPDS for 72 hr. The cumulative amount of growth factor produced was 497 ng, and the concentration initially present in 10% conditioned medium was 5.0 ± 1.4 ng/mℓ. Within the errors inherent in this calculation, these values are quite similar. Nevertheless, this calculation is a rough approximation which ignores substantial degradation of growth factor by SMC.[42] It is interesting to note that these values correspond to the concentration of PDGF required to cause half-maximal binding to the PDGF receptor[43] and half-maximal LDL metabolism.

The primary response of SMC to the presence of endothelial cells was an increase in the number of LDL receptors. Increases in the receptor number ranged from two- to sevenfold, a variability partly due to variations in endothelial cell number, as well as to variations in the expression of receptors. Literature estimates for the number of PDGF receptors per cell ranges from 7200 on bovine SMC[44] to 79,000 on monkey SMC.[45] Furthermore, PDGF receptors increase with subculture.[44]

In addition to mitogen-dependent stimulation of LDL metabolism, up to 70% of total stimulation may be attributable to low-molecular-weight factors which are non-mitogenic. Since growth factor-independent stimulation of LDL metabolism was not observed with endothelial cell-conditioned medium, the agent(s) must either be short-lived or require cell-cell interactions to be produced. Bounds can be placed on the half-life of any biologically active molecule in this system. The absence of a growth factor-independent response in endothelial cell-conditioned medium may be due to a molecule with a short half-life. Processing of conditioned medium for addition to SMC requires about 1 hr. If the low-molecular-weight species is not active in conditioned medium, its half-life must be no more than 30 min. The low-molecular-weight agent is active in co-culture where the endothelial cells are separated from SMC by 1 mm. Typical diffusion coefficients for low-molecular-weight solutes in water range from 5×10^{-6} cm²/sec for sucrose (342 g/mol) to 2×10^{-6} cm²/sec for inulin (4000 g/mol), and the characteristic time required for these solutes to diffuse 1 mm ranges from 30 to 83 min. These diffusion times are greater than the upper limit of the half-life of any active low-molecular-weight solute. It is thus unlikely that a short-lived intermediate is responsible for growth factor-independent stimulation of LDL metabolism. This line of reasoning implies a requirement for cell-cell interactions. A plausible scheme consistent with the data would be that endothelial cells may alter a molecule produced or modified by SMC. The biologically activated molecules may then cause SMC to increase their production of LDL receptors. Based upon diffusion times, at least 1 hr in co-culture is required before activation of SMC. We are currently investigating this hypothesis.

VIII. ENDOTHELIAL CELL-SMC INTERACTIONS IN THE VESSEL WALL

The proximity of endothelial cells to vascular SMC, particularly in smaller vessels,[46] suggests that their interactions are important for maintenance of normal blood vessel physiology and that perturbation of such interactions in large elastic and muscular distributing arteries may play a role in the initiation and development of atherosclerosis. During early atherogenesis, a continuous endothelium remains in place over the developing lesion,[47,48] suggesting that endothelial cell-vessel wall interactions may play some part in the development of the lesion. Early events in atherogenesis include the proliferation of intimal SMC and the intracellular accumulation in intimal SMC and monocyte-derived macrophages of large amounts of esterified cholesterol, the sterol ring of which is derived primarily from plasma LDL.[49] Thus, the SMC growth cycle and cellular LDL metabolism are linked, as has been demonstrated in cells exposed to purified mitogens,[22-24] to mitogen-containing, cell-conditioned media,[1,9,25] and in cocultures.[3,4] The demonstration that endothelial cells synthesize and secrete a PDGF-like mitogen on the one hand, and yet also produce a heparin-like inhibitor of connective tissue cell growth on the other,[2] raises the probability that intercellular communication may be a major mechanism for regulating cell proliferation. Alterations in LDL metabolism, while in part linked to the cell cycle, also appeared to be significantly influenced by nonmitogenic endothelial cell factors. It is conceivable, therefore, that endothelial cells can modify the metabolism of lipoproteins by intimal SMC without influencing SMC proliferation. What these factors are, or how they may be regulated, is not known at the present time. Possible candidates for such effects include prostacyclin, other prostaglandins, and endothelial-derived relaxing factor (EDRF). Prostacyclin has been shown to influence the activities of several intracellular enzymes involved in cholesterol metabolism[50] and is under investigation in this laboratory for any effects upon LDL receptor-mediated endocytic pathways. EDRF, required for certain vasodilator-induced relaxation responses in arterial tissue, has a half-life of seconds.[51] Using elevation of cGMP in cultured SMC as an assay for EDRF activity in a co-culture system,[8] we have demonstrated that the time required for EDRF diffusion from the endothelium to the SMC far exceeds the half-life of the molecule, and thus EDRF (at least in its assayable form) cannot be responsible for stimulated LDL metabolism in cultured SMC.

Recently, Campbell et al.[52] have drawn attention to the question of how cell phenotype may influence SMC interactions with lipoproteins. They showed that contractile SMC typical of those in the arterial media bind much lower amounts of a range of lipoproteins, whereas phenotypically distinct, synthetic-state cells, which are capable of extensive proliferation, bind much more lipoprotein and accumulate cholesteryl esters in their cytoplasm. These findings are consistent with the accumulation of lipid in intimal (synthetic, proliferative) SMC which occurs in vivo. These results are an important consideration in studies of endothelial-SMC interactions because SMC phenotype is subject to modulation by endothelial cells[53] (see Chapter 4).

It is clear from in vitro studies that endothelial cells can produce both mitogens for SMC and inhibitors of SMC proliferation. In a simplistic scenario of the vessel wall, growth inhibitory factors would normally dominate, and few SMC would be found in the cell cycle. Under conditions which favor increased expression of endothelial cell-derived growth factors, however, the balance may be altered towards SMC proliferation and, *inter alia,* altered lipoprotein metabolism. The factors which may regulate such cell interactions are currently the subject of intense investigation.

ACKNOWLEDGMENTS

We are most grateful to our collaborators in these studies, Dr. Henry Warren, Susan O'Connor, and Barbara Eisenhaure. This work is supported by grants HL-24612 and HL-22602 from the National Heart Lung and Blood Institute of the National Institutes of Health.

REFERENCES

1. Gajdusek, C., DiCorleto, P. E., Ross, R., and Schwartz, S. M., An endothelial cell-derived growth factor, *J. Cell Biol.,* 85, 467, 1980.
2. Castellot, J. J., Addonizio, M., Rosenberg, R., and Karnovsky, M. J., Cultured endothelial cells produce a heparin-like inhibitor of smooth muscle cell growth, *J. Cell Biol.,* 90, 372, 1981.
3. Davies, P. F. and Kerr, C., Cocultivation of vascular endothelium and smooth muscle cells using microcarrier techniques, *Exp. Cell Res.,* 141, 455, 1982.
4. Davies, P. F., Truskey, G. A., Warren, H. B., O'Conner, S. E., and Eisenhaure, B. E., Metabolic cooperation between vascular endothelial cells and smooth muscle cells in coculture: changes in low density lipoprotein metabolism, *J. Cell Biol.,* 101, 871, 1985.
5. Furchgott, R. F. and Zawadzki, J. V., The obligatory role of endothelium in the relaxation of arterial smooth muscle by acetylcholine, *Nature (London),* 288, 373, 1980.
6. Stein, O., Halperin, G., and Stein, Y., Interaction between macrophages and aortic smooth muscle cells. Enhancement of cholesterol esterification in smooth muscle cells by media of macrophages incubated with acetylated LDL, *Biochim. Biophys. Acta,* 665, 477, 1981.
7. Henriksen, T., Mahoney, E. M., and Steinberg, D., Enhanced macrophage degradation of biologically modified LDL, *Arteriosclerosis,* 3, 149, 1983.
8. Ganz, P., Davies, P. F., Leopold, J., Gimbrone, M. A., Jr., and Alexander, R. W., Shorthand long term interactions of endothelium and vascular smooth muscle in coculture: effects on cyclic GMP production, *Proc. Natl. Acad. Sci. U.S.A.,* 83, 3552, 1986.
9. Witte, L. D., Cornicelli, J. A., Miller, D., and Goodman, D. S., Effects of platelet-derived and endothelial cell-derived growth factors on the LDL receptor pathway in cultured human fibroblasts, *J. Biol. Chem.,* 257, 5392, 1982.
10. Bevilacqua, M. P., Pober, J. S., Majeau, G. R., Cotran, R. S., and Gimbrone, M. A., Jr., Interleukin 1 induces biosynthesis and cell surface expression of procoagulant activity in human vascular endothelial cells, *J. Exp. Med.,* 160, 618, 1984.
11. Davies, P. F., Ganz, P., and Diehl, J. S., Reversible microcarrier-mediated junctional communication between endothelial and smooth muscle cell monolayer: an in vitro model of vascular cell interactions, *Lab. Invest.,* 85, 710, 1985.
12. Cook, R. D. and Peterson, E. R., The growth of smooth muscle and sympathetic ganglia in organotypic tissue cultures. Light and electron microscopy, *J. Neurol. Sci.,* 22, 25, 1974.
13. Chamley, J. H. and Campbell, G. R., Trophic influences of sympathetic nerves and cyclic AMP on differentiation and proliferation of isolated smooth muscle cells in culture, *Cell Tissue Res.,* 161, 497, 1975.

14. Harel, L., Jullien, M., and DeMonti, M., Diffusible factor(s) controlling density inhibition of 3T3 cell growth: a new approach, *J. Cell. Physiol.*, 96, 327, 1978.
15. Davies, P. F., Microcarrier culture of vascular endothelium, *Exp. Cell Res.*, 134, 365, 1981
16. Davies, P. F., Microcarrier cultures in vascular endothelial research, *Dev. Biol. Stand.*, 50, 125, 1982.
17. Gimbrone, M. A., Jr., Culture of vascular endothelium, in *Progress in Hemostasis and Thrombosis.*, Spaet, T. H., Ed., Grune & Stratton, New York, 1976, 1.
18. Davies, P. F., Rennke, H. G., and Cotran, R. S., Influence of molecular charge upon the endocytosis and intracellular fate of peroxidase activity in cultured arterial endothelium, *J. Cell Sci.*, 49, 69, 1981.
19. Ross, R., The smooth muscle cell. II. Growth of smooth muscle in cultured and formation of elastin fibers, *J. Cell Biol.*, 50, 172, 1971.
20. Vogel, A., Raines, E., Kariya, B., Rivest, M.-J., and Ross, R., Coordinate control of 3T3 cell proliferation by platelet-derived growth factor and plasma components, *Proc. Natl. Acad. Sci. U.S.A.*, 75, 2810, 1978.
21. Goldstein, J. L., Basu, S. K., Brunschede, G. Y., and Brown, M. S., Release of LDL from its cell surface receptor by sulfated glycosaminoglycans, *Cell*, 7, 85, 1976.
22. Chait, A., Ross, R., Albers, J. J., and Bierman, E. L., Platelet-derived growth factor stimulates activity of LDL receptors, *Proc. Natl. Acad. Sci. U.S.A.*, 77, 4084, 1980.
23. Witte, L. D. and Cornicelli, J. A., Platelet-derived growth factor stimulates low density lipoprotein receptor activity in cultured human fibroblasts, *Proc. Natl. Acad. Sci. U.S.A.*, 77, 5962, 1980.
24. Davies, P. F. and Kerr, C., Modification of LDL metabolism by growth factors in cultured vascular cells and human skin fibroblasts. Dependence on duration of exposure, *Biochim. Biophys. Acta*, 712, 26, 1982.
25. DiCorleto, P. E., Cultured endothelial cells produce multiple growth factors for connective tissue cells, *Exp. Cell Res.*, 153, 167, 1984.
26. Warren, H. B., O'Conner, S. E., Eisenhaure, B. E., and Davies, P. F., Coculture of vascular endothelium and smooth muscle cells: effects of heparin on smooth muscle cell proliferation, *J. Cell Biol.*, 97, 87a, 1983.
27. Quesney-Huneens, V., Galick, H. A., Siperstein, M. D., Erickson, E. K., Spencer, T. A., and Nelson, J. A., The dual role of mevalonate in cells, *J. Biol. Chem.*, 258, 378, 1982.
28. Davies, P. F. and Ross, R., Mediation of pinocytosis in cultured arterial smooth muscle and endothelial cells by platelet-derived growth factor, *J. Cell Biol.*, 79, 663, 1978.
29. Fox, P. L. and DiCorleto, P. E., Regulation of production of a platelet-derived growth factor-like protein by cultured bovine aortic endothelial cells, *J. Cell. Physiol.*, 121, 298, 1984.
30. Truskey, G. A., Colton, C. K., and Davies, P. F., Kinetic analysis of receptor-mediated endocytosis and lysosomal degradation in cultured cells, *Ann. N.Y. Acad. Sci.*, 439, 349, 1984.
31. Goldstein, J. L. and Brown, M. S., The low density lipoprotein pathway and its relation to atherosclerosis, *Annu. Rev. Biochem.*, 46, 897, 1977.
32. Box, G. E. and Draper, N. R., The Bayesian estimation of common parameters from several responses, *Biometrika*, 52, 355, 1965.
33. Cornicelli, J. A., Witte, L. D., and Goodman, D. S., Inhibition of LDL degradation in cultured human fibroblasts induced by endothelial cell-conditioned medium, *Arteriosclerosis*, 3, 560, 1983.
34. Truskey, G. A. and Davies, P. F., Effects of ammonium ion from bovine endothelial cells upon low density lipoprotein degradation in cultured vascular smooth muscle cells, *Cell Biol. Int. Rep.*, 9, 323, 1985.
35. Dewan, J. G., The L-glutamic dehydrogenase of animal tissues, *Biochem. J.*, 32, 1378, 1938; Sigma Diagnostic Kit 170-UV, Sigma Chemical Co., St. Louis, Mo.
36. Tycko, B., Keith, C., and Maxfield, F. R., Rapid acidification of endocytic vesicles containing asialoglycoprotein in cells of human hepatoma line, *J. Cell Biol.*, 97, 1762, 1983.
37. Butler, M., Inanura, T., Thomas, J., and Thilly, W. G., High yields from microcarrier cultures by medium perfusion, *J. Cell Sci.*, 61, 351, 1983.
38. Glacken, M. W. and Sinskey, A. J., Ammonia production and glutamine metabolism of cultured mammalian cells, *Biotechnol. Bioeng.*, in press, 1985.
39. Waterfield, M. D., Scrace, G. T., Whittle, N., Stroobant, P., Johnsson, A., Wasteson, A., Westermark, B., Heldin, C. M., Huang, J. S., and Deuel, T. F., Platelet-derived growth factor is structurally related to the putative transforming protein p28 sis of simian sarcoma virus, *Nature (London)*, 304, 35, 1983.
40. Doolittle, R. F., Hunkapiller, M. W., Hood, L. E., Devare, S. G., Robbins, K. C., Aaronson, S. A., and Antoniades, H. N., Simian sarcoma virus onc-gene, v-sis, is derived from the gene(s) encoding a platelet-derived growth factor, *Science*, 221, 275, 1983.
41. Barrett, T. B., Gajdusek, C. M., Schwartz, S. M., McDougall, J. K., and Benditt, E. P., Expression of the sis gene by endothelial cells in culture and in vivo, *Proc. Natl. Acad. Sci. U.S.A.*, 81, 6772, 1984.

42. Heldin, C. H., Wasteson, A., and Westermark, B., Interaction of platelet-derived growth factor with its fibroblast receptor, *J. Biol. Chem.*, 257, 4216, 1982.
43. Stiles, C. D., The molecular biology of platelet-derived growth factor, *Cell*, 33, 653, 1983.
44. DiCorleto, P. E. and Bowen-Pope, D., Cultured endothelial cells produce a platelet-derived growth factor-like protein, *Proc. Natl. Acad. Sci. U.S.A.*, 80, 1919, 1983.
45. Bowen-Pope, D. and Ross, R., Platelet-derived growth factor. II. Specific binding to cultured cells, *J. Biol. Chem.*, 257, 5161, 1982.
46. Rhodin, J. A. G., The ultrastructure of mammalian arterioles and precapillary sphincters, *J. Ultrastruct. Res.*, 18, 181, 1967.
47. Davies, P. F., Reidy, M. A., Goode, T. B., and Bowyer, D. E., Scanning electron microscopy in the evaluation of endothelial integrity of the fatty streak lesion of atherosclerosis, *Atherosclerosis*, 25, 125, 1976.
48. Goode, T. B., Davies, P. F., Reidy, M. A., and Bowyer, D. E., Aortic endothelial cell morphology observed in situ by scanning electron microscopy during atherogenesis in the rabbit, *Atherosclerosis*, 27, 235, 1977.
49. Ross, R., Atherosclerosis: a problem of the biology of vessel wall cells and their interaction with blood components. Duff memorial lecture, *Atherosclerosis*, 1, 293, 1981.
50. Hajjar, D. P. and Weksler, B. B., Metabolic activity of endothelial cells and aortic smooth muscle is altered by prostaglandins I_2 and E_2, *J. Lipid Res.*, 24, 1176, 1983.
51. Griffith, T. M., Edwards, D. H., Lewis, M. J., Newby, A. C., and Henderson, A. H., The nature of endothelium-derived vascular relaxant factor, *Nature (London)*, 308, 645, 1984.
52. Campbell, J. H., Reardon, M. F., Campbell, G. R., and Nestel, P. J., Metabolism of atherogenic lipoproteins by smooth muscle cells of different phenotype in culture, *Arteriosclerosis*, 5, 318, 1985.
53. Chamley-Campbell, J. H. and Campbell, G. R., What controls smooth muscle phenotype? *Atherosclerosis*, 40, 347, 1981.

Chapter 16

BIOCHEMICAL PHARMACOLOGY OF NORADRENERGIC, SEROTONIN, AND HISTAMINE RECEPTOR SYSTEMS IN VASCULAR SMOOTH MUSCLE

A. Bobik

TABLE OF CONTENTS

I. INTRODUCTION

Until relatively recently, receptor responses of vascular smooth muscle could only be investigated by measuring contractile or relaxation responses of intact vessel strips or rings. Although this approach has proved to be extremely useful in characterizing the different types of receptors mediating contracture and relaxation, it has given no insight into how the binding of a drug or hormone to a receptor transmits a signal from the cell surface to the interior of the cell ("transmembrane signaling"), thereby initiating a biochemical or physical response. This approach also gave no insight as to how receptor proteins might differ in their molecular properties. The simple concept originally proposed by Clark[1] that a receptor system consists of at least two components, a recognition site or receptor [R] to which a drug or hormone [H] binds which in some way couples to a biochemical effector system [E] to elicit a response could not be proven[1] (see Equation 1).

$$A + R - E \rightarrow AR - E \rightarrow \text{[Biochemical Response]} \rightarrow \rightarrow \rightarrow \text{Tissue Response} \quad (1)$$

With the advent of new biochemical approaches, developed over the past 10 to 15 years, it has now become possible to gain some insight into how the interaction of drugs or hormones with specific membrane receptors elicit biochemical responses that may ultimately result in contracture and relaxation of blood vessels. Contracture mediated by noradrenaline, serotonin, and histamine is thought to be due to receptor activation of phosphatidylinositol hydrolysis with the formation of *myo*-inositol-1,4,5-triphosphate, which releases calcium from the endoplasmic reticulum. Receptor-mediated relaxation is thought to be due to activation of adenylate cyclase. The aim of this article is to present a brief overview of the methods used and studies carried out which have increased our understanding, at a biochemical level, of how noradrenaline, serotonin, and histamine responses are initiated in vascular smooth muscle and to highlight areas requiring further study.

II. PREPARATION OF SMOOTH MUSCLE CELL CULTURES

The three main methods currently used to obtain cultured vascular smooth muscle to study the properties of noradrenergic, serotonin, and histamine receptors and the mechanism by which they transmit signals from the cell surface to the cell's interior ("transmembrane signaling") are briefly described below. Each has its merits and limitations, and many factors need be considered to ensure that the most appropriate culture system is chosen.

A. Primary Contractile State Smooth Muscle

Morphologically well-differentiated, contractile-state, vascular smooth muscle in primary culture may be obtained from major vessels such as the aorta or mesenteric arteries of young rabbits or rats by stripping the intima and media from longitudinally cut sections of the vessel with forceps. The strips of vascular smooth muscle are incubated with gentle shaking in collagenase, after which the collagenase is removed and tissue rinsed with Medium 199 to remove endothelial cells. The tissue is resuspended in collagenase and reincubated for about 1 hr. The resulting suspension of single cells is centrifuged at low speed and the pelleted cells resuspended in Medium 199 containing 5% fetal calf serum. The cells are normally seeded at a density of 1.5×10^6 cells per 5 mℓ into plastic dishes and grown in culture for 4 to 5 days. The resulting culture consists primarily of contractile state smooth muscle cells (SMC) attached to plastic dishes.

Primary contractile vascular SMC are probably the most appropriate in vitro system currently available to examine the properties of receptors and their transmembrane signaling mechanisms in vessels. However, this type of culture is only infrequently used in biochemical studies since the amount of usable tissue is small. Little et al.[2] have used contractile aortic smooth muscle of rabbits in primary culture to examine the properties of the β-adrenoceptor-adenylate cyclase system. Cyclic AMP determinations using standard radioimmunoassays as well as measurements of adenylate cyclase and phosphodiesterase activities could easily be performed when cultures were prepared from six young (6- to 8-week-old) rabbits. However, receptor binding studies which require far greater amounts of particulate protein are relatively difficult to perform on this quantity of cell protein. To partially overcome this problem, Bobik et al.[3] have reduced the seeding density of rabbit aortic cells to between 0.5 and 1×10^6 and stimulated cell division by adding 2 m*M* glutamine to the culture medium. Under these conditions, the cells rapidly divide to confluency. Providing the number of cell divisions required to reach confluency is five or less, confluent monolayers rapidly revert from a predominately synthetic state smooth muscle to the contractile phenotype. The culture time required to obtain contractile SMC by this method varies from about 7 to 10 days. Using this modified culturing procedure, the tissue obtained from six young rabbits is sufficient to carry out complete receptor-radioligand binding isotherms.[3] Primary cultures of rat aortic smooth muscle have been prepared by similar methods.[4,5]

B. Explant-Derived Smooth Muscle

Aortic smooth muscle derived from explants of dissected inner media of aorta from a number of mammalian species has also been used to examine receptor binding properties and transmembrane signaling mechanisms. Cells obtained by this procedure exist predominantly in the synthetic phenotype and differ not only in their morphological characteristics from smooth muscle *in situ*, but also in many of their biochemical characteristics.[6] Cultures of smooth muscle in the synthetic phenotype have also been obtained from immature guinea pig aorta, rabbit and rat aorta.[7-9] In general, the method used to obtain these cells involves incubating 1 mm^3 sections of dissected inner media of thoracic aorta in smooth plastic petri dishes containing Dulbecco's modified essential medium. The tissue explants are grown in culture for between 1 to 4 weeks, with medium changes every 2 days. Upon reaching confluency, the explant cells are digested with 0.05% trypsin-0.5 m*M* EDTA and reseeded at densities approaching 2.5×10^6 cells per dish. These cells normally reach confluency after about 4 days in culture. These "first-generation" subcultured cells may either be used for experimentation at this stage or subcultured further to increase the yield of cell protein. No formal comparisons have been carried out between these "synthetic" vascular SMC and those in the "contractile" phenotype to determine the extent, if any, to which membrane receptor binding properties might have changed, either in their ability to bind receptor ligands or affect transmembrane signaling mechanisms. However, the overall data suggests that the synthetic phenotype of vascular smooth muscle possesses receptor systems similar to those present in the contractile phenotype and which respond, at least qualitatively, in a manner similar to cultured smooth muscle in the contractile phenotype and smooth muscle in blood vessels. The major reason to use such cultures is when experiments require large amounts of protein material that cannot normally be obtained using primary culture techniques.

C. Clonal Smooth Muscle Cell Lines

Relatively few permanent clonal cell lines are available to study receptors and receptor transmembrane signaling systems. It should be remembered that while continuous SMC lines are convenient to use (because of the relatively large amount of tissue which can be obtained from such cultures), the results of studies with such lines may not be directly applicable to vascular smooth muscle because in most instances their precise origin is not known. The most commonly used cell line has been the BC3H-1 clone derived from an intracranial tumor induced in one offspring of a C3H mouse injected with nitrosoethylurea when 15 days pregnant.[10,11] The cell line has several morphological, electrical, and pharmacological properties in common with vascular smooth muscle. However, it also has some properties characteristic of striated muscle.[11] Despite the close similarity of many of its properties to those of vascular smooth muscle, its tissue of origin is not known. The BC3H-1 clone has been primarily used to study the properties of α_1- and β_2-adrenoceptors in relation to phosphatidylinositol turnover and adenylate cyclase activation.[10,12,13] Several other SMC lines derived from rat aorta have also been described.[14,15] To date they have not been used in studies on membrane receptors and their transduction mechanisms.

III. MEASUREMENT OF SURFACE MEMBRANE RECEPTORS

The many practical aspects of carrying out receptor binding studies have been previously reviewed in detail.[16] In general, most of the receptor-radioligand binding studies performed in cultured smooth muscle have been carried out by binding an iodinated [^{125}I] or tritiated [^{3}H] receptor ligand to homogenates or particulate protein under equilibrium conditions. The unbound receptor radioligand is most frequently separated from membrane bound radioligand by rapid filtration under vacuum. This rapid filtration technique can be used with most of the currently available receptor radioligands used to quantitate noradrenergic, serotonin, and histamine receptors, since their affinity constants for the respective receptors usually exceed 10^8 *M*.

With the increasing availability of receptor radioligands that differ from each other predominantly in their physicochemical characteristics, it is now possible in some instances not only to measure the different receptor subtypes on SMC, but also to gain greater insights as to the proportion of receptors of the same subtype within the different environs of the membrane. Hertel et al.[17] have recently demonstrated that cells desensitized to catecholamines contain two populations of β-adrenoceptors in the light vascular fraction of cell homogenates. [^{3}H] CGP-12177, a polar β-adrenoceptor radioligand, detected approximately one third of the receptors measured by the more lipophilic compound [^{125}I] iodopindolol. Receptor sites not accessible to [^{3}H] CGP-12177 could be unmasked by incubating the vesicular fraction with alamethacin, an antibiotic possessing channel-forming ability and causing free access of polar compounds across membranes. Hydrophilic receptor radioligands can also be used to measure receptors and examine their properties on intact cultured cells. In general, cells grown in culture are loosened from culture plates by a 2-min incubation with 0.02% EDTA in phosphate-buffer saline prior to suspension in physiological buffer saline. Equilibrium binding radioreceptor assays can be carried out using the cell suspensions in an identical manner to those utilizing membrane preparations. Under these conditions, the hydrophilic β-adrenoceptor ligand [^{3}H] CGP-12177 has been shown to be displaced from both cultured intact cells and membranes in an identical stereospecific manner by adrenoceptor agonist and antagonist drugs.[18] Sher and Clementi used [^{3}H] CGP-12177 to determine the rate at which β-adrenoceptors are lost from the surface of BC_3H-1 muscle cells during exposure to isoprenaline.[19] The recent availability of [^{125}I] iodopindolol, a relatively hydrophilic β-adrenoceptor ligand, which appears to bind to all cell membrane β-adrenoceptors, should also be an invaluable tool for examining the properties of these receptors in cultured vascular smooth muscle.[20]

Attempts have also been made to quantitate α_1-adrenoceptors on BC3H-1 SMC with the α_1-selective adrenoceptor ligand [^{3}H] prazosin.[21] Comparisons between the relative potencies of adrenergic agonists and antagonists to displace [^{3}H] prazosin from cells and membrane preparations demonstrated large disparities in the abilities of adrenoceptor agonist drugs to displace [^{3}H] prazosin from the two preparations. It would appear that the hydrophobic properties of [^{3}H] prazosin may limit its ability to quantitatively detect α_1-adrenoceptors on the surface membrane of intact cells.

Photoaffinity labeling of membrane receptors of cultured vascular SMC has only recently been reported.[22] The α_1 selective radioligand, 4-amino-6,7-diemthoxy-2-[4-5-(4-azido-3-[^{125}I] iodophenyl) pentanoyl]-1-piperazinyl] quinazoline (^{125}IAPDQ), was covalently linked to α_1-adrenoceptors present in membrane preparations of vascular smooth muscle originating from rabbit aorta during ultraviolet irradiation of membrane-bound radioligand. In the future, photoaffinity labeling of membrane receptors on cultured smooth muscle will be useful in aiding the isolation of pure receptor proteins.

IV. MEASUREMENT OF CYCLIC AMP AND ADENYLATE CYCLASE ACTIVITY

A. Cyclic AMP

Increases in cyclic AMP content in vascular SMC upon exposure to various receptor agonists, e.g., isoprenaline, serotonin, and histamine have been reported in a number of culture systems.[2,23-25] In order to achieve close to maximal increases in cyclic AMP during activation of adenylate cyclase by β-adrenoceptor or serotonin receptor agonists, the length of exposure to such compounds should be relatively short, between 3 and 5 min. The precise time interval chosen is usually a practical compromise between the ability of the experimenter to rapidly handle the required number of culture plates and minimizing the extent of any receptor desensitization that reduces ensuing cyclic AMP levels.[2,25] The rises in cyclic AMP content following activation of adenylate cyclase by histamine tend to be maximal after about 20 min.[25] In a recent study of the effects of isoprenaline on cyclic AMP content in cultured rabbit aortic smooth muscle, cyclic AMP content in the cells reached peak levels approximately 5 min after adding isoprenaline and thereafter decline.[2] Addition of phosphodiesterase inhibitors to the incubation medium does not appear to affect the rate of this decline.[24] Cyclic AMP accumulation in smooth muscle is normally measured after homogenizing the cells in 10% trichloroacetic or related acid to precipitate cell proteins, followed by ion exchange chromatography of the tissue extract on Dowex AG-50 and barium sulfate precipitation.[26] This procedure removes all interfering nucleotides, enabling cyclic AMP content to be measured by a cyclic AMP protein-binding method or commercial radioimmunoassay kit.[24,27] The recovery of cyclic AMP throughout its isolation and purification is monitored by adding tracer amounts of [^{3}H] cyclic AMP with the homogenizing acid.

B. Adenylate Cyclase Activity

Potential factors which might influence the magnitude of hormone or drug stimulation of adenylate cyclase activity in broken cell preparations of smooth muscle have been recently reviewed.[28] Only limited studies have been reported on the measurement of adenylate cyclase activity in cultured vascular smooth muscle.[2,25,29] Histamine, serotonin, and β-adrenoceptor agonists are all potent activators of adenylate cyclase. Little et al.[2] demonstrated that isoprenaline could elevate basal adenylate cyclase up to fivefold, a level which compared well with peak increases in cyclic AMP concentrations, observed when intact cells were exposed to this drug. This increase in adenylate cyclase activity represented 40% of the activity obtained with 10 mM sodium fluoride. Luchins and Makman reported that histamine and serotonin also had similar effects on adenylate cyclase activity measured in vitro and cyclic AMP content in intact cells.[25]

In all these instances adenylate cyclase stimulation by receptor agonists was obtained in crude cell homogenates prepared by manual homogenization with a glass homogenizer. When membranes were isolated from cell homogenates, the magnitude of β-adrenoceptor stimulation by isoprenaline is reduced from about fivefold to onefold or less.[71] This reduction in the sensitivity of adenylate cyclase to β-adrenoceptor stimulation was not due to the lack of guanyl nucleotides or any apparent reduction in β-adrenoceptor concentration. Sodium fluoride activation of adenylate cyclase through the guanyl nucleotide regulatory proteins was unaffected. This current difficulty in achieving a level of stimulation by β-adrenoceptor agonists in purified membrane preparations similar to that achieved in cell homogenates is probably the major reason why receptor regulated adenylate cyclase in vascular smooth muscle is so poorly characterized.

V. MEASUREMENT OF PHOSPHATIDYLINOSITOL AND ITS METABOLITES

α-Adrenoceptors, histamine H_1, and serotonin receptors appear to exert their effects by altering the rate of metabolism of phosphatidylinositol to yield intermediate metabolites that act as second messengers in much the same way as does cyclic AMP. The two metabolites which appear to be most important as potential second messengers are *myo*-inositol-1,4,5-triphosphate (IP_3) and diacylglycerol (Figure 1). IP_3 and diacylglycerol are formed concomitantly from phosphatidyl-4,5-biphosphate following activation of the phosphodiesterase, phospholipase C.[30] Phosphatidylinositol-4,5-bisphosphate is produced by the sequential actions of the ATP-requiring enzymes, phosphatidylinositol kinase and phosphatidyl-4-phosphate kinase on phosphatidylinositol.[31] The action of phospholipase C on phosphatidylinositol can also contribute to cellular diacylglycerol content.[32]

IP_3 has many of the attributes expected of a calcium mobilizing second messenger.[31,33,34] Diacylglycerol has been shown to enhance the activity of protein kinase C, a calcium and phospholipid-dependent protein kinase, by increasing its affinity for calcium.[35] Diacylglycerol kinase further metabolizes diacylglycerol to phosphatidic acid. It has been suggested that phosphatidic acid might increase calcium flux across cell membranes by acting as a calcium ionophore.[36] Most of this recent knowledge concerning IP_3 and diacylglycerol has been obtained from experiments in hepatocytes, blowfly salivary glands, and rat parotid glands (for reviews, see References 32 and 33).

Information on phosphatidylinositol metabolism in vascular smooth muscle has been limited to measuring either [^{32}P] or [^{3}H] phosphatidylinositol turnover in intact vessel segments and cultured aortic smooth muscle during activation of α_1-adrenoceptors, serotonin, or histamine H_1 receptors.[3,37-40] Bobik et al.[3] demonstrated that α_1-adrenoceptor activation by adrenaline increased [^{32}P] phosphatidylinositol turnover in cultured rabbit aortic SMC; α_1-adrenoceptor activation also increased the turnover of [^{32}P] phosphatidic acid in these cells.[71] Both effects could be antagonized by phentolamine or the selective α_1-adrenoceptor antagonist prazosin. [^{32}P] Orthophosphate added to the culture medium is also converted to a small extent to phospholipids which co-migrate on silica gel thin layer chromatography with phosphatidylcholine and phosphatidylethanolamine. The turnover of these phospholipids, measured as changes in the specific activity of [^{32}P]-labeled phospholipids, was not affected by α_1-adrenoceptor stimulation.

Somewhat more detailed studies on the effects of α_1-adrenoceptor activation on the incorporation of [^{3}H] inositol into phosphatidylinositol have been carried out on BC3H-1 muscle cells.[13] Phenylephrine stimulated the incorporation of [^{3}H] inositol into chloroform-extractable phospholipids in a concentration-dependent manner. The

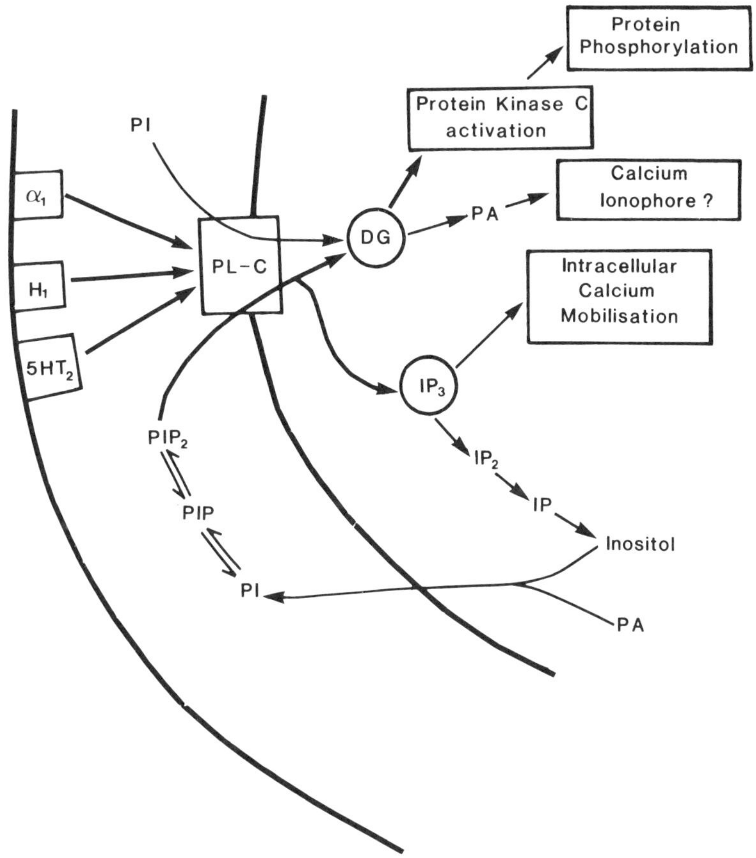

FIGURE 1. Major sequence of events leading to the production of myo-inositol-1,4,5-triphosphate (IP_3) and diacylglycerol (DG) during activation of α_1-adrenoceptors (α_1), histamine receptors (H_1), and serotonin receptors (5-HT_2). Other abbreviations: PL-C, phospholipase C; PI, phosphatidylinositol; PA, phosphatidic acid; IP_2 , myo-inositol-1,4-bisphosphate; IP, myo-inositol-1-phosphate; PIP, phosphatidylinositol-4-phosphate; PIP_2, phosphatidylinositol-4,5-bisphosphate.

rate of [^{3}H]phosphatidylinositol-4,5-bisphosphate hydrolysis by phospholipase C was also determined indirectly by measuring the accumulation of [^{3}H]inositol-1,4,5-triphosphate, following inhibition of its dephosphorylation with lithium chloride. Increases in [^{3}H] inositol-1-phosphate were observed 30 min. after adding phenylephrine to the medium; 5 min after adding phenylephrine there appeared to be no detectable increase in cellular [^{3}H]inositol-1-phosphate or [^{3}H]inositol-1,4-diphosphate. The cellular content of [^{3}H] inositol-1,4,5-triphosphate also appeared unaffected during a 5-min exposure to phenylephrine. The inability to detect significant rises in [^{3}H]inositol-1,4,5-triphosphate at a time when the mobilization of intracellular [^{45}Ca] calcium is close to maximum suggests that local rather than whole cell concentrations of [^{3}H]inositol-1,4,5-triphosphate should be measured. In cultured vascular smooth muscle this could be achieved indirectly by measuring the degradation of [^{32}P]phosphatidylinositol-4,5-bisphosphate in response to receptor activation in the different subcellular fractions rather than in intact cells. Such an approach has recently been used to localize and quantitate vasopressin-stimulated hydrolysis of phosphoinositides in rat hepatocytes.[41]

VI. β ADRENOCEPTORS

β-Adrenoceptors have been identified by direct radioligand binding techniques in several cultured SMC systems.[2,42,43] Although in all instances these receptors are linked to adenylate cyclase, there are differences between tissues in their ability to respond to β-adrenoceptor stimulation. For example, in subcultured calf-aortic smooth muscle, maximal β-adrenoceptor stimulation doubles basal levels of cyclic AMP.[25] Cyclic AMP content of rabbit aortic smooth muscle in primary culture is elevated fourfold upon exposure to high concentrations of isoprenaline.[2] Similar elevations in intracellular cyclic AMP levels have also been reported in cultured cerebrovascular smooth muscle.[29] However, at least 20-fold elevations in cyclic AMP levels occur when cultured smooth muscle derived from explants of rat aorta are exposed to β-adrenoceptor agonists.[24] At present, it is not known whether the above-mentioned differences between the various smooth muscle cultures are due to the different species used to obtain the smooth muscle or whether it is due to differences in smooth muscle phenotype.

β-Adrenoceptors activating adenylate cyclase in vascular smooth muscle are of the β_2-subtype. In cultured cerebrovascular smooth muscle the $\beta_2$selective adrenoceptor antagonist, butoxamine, as well as nonselective β-adrenoceptor antagonists are potent inhibitors of β-adrenoceptor-mediated increases in adenylate cyclase activity.[29] β_1 Selective antagonists are ineffective in inhibiting these increases in enzyme activity. β_2 Adrenoceptors also appear to increase the rate of efflux of ^{86}Rb from BC3H-1 cell cultures previously loaded with ^{86}Rb.[44] Evidence for β_2-adrenoceptor participation in this response was based on catecholamines stimulating this efflux with the following order of potency: isoprenaline > adrenaline ≫ noradrenaline, as opposed to β_1-adrenoceptor responses where adrenaline and noradrenaline are approximately equipotent. Radioligand binding studies have also characterized smooth muscle β-adrenoceptors as being predominantly of the β_2-subtype.[12,42] The rank order of potency of agonists in competing for [^{125}I] iodocyanopindolol binding sites was (−)-isoprenaline > (−)adrenaline ≫ (−)noradrenaline. The concentration dependence of competing ligands in displacing [^{125}I] iodocyanopindolol indicated that agonists were binding to both low- and high-affinity sites and that guanyl triphosphate (GTP) reduces the overall apparent affinity of these agonists. The β_2-adrenoceptor antagonist zinterol bound only to one class of [^{125}I]cyanopindolol binding site in a manner consistent with there being a single population of β_2-adrenoceptor sites on BC3H-1 cells.[12] Binding sites for [^{125}I]-iodocyanopindolol on rabbit aortic SMC cultures have also been shown to possess properties expected of β-adrenoceptors.[2] Thus the evidence to date indicates that vascular smooth muscle β_2-adrenoceptors are linked through guanine nucleotide stimulatory proteins to the catalytic unit of adenylate cyclase. The affinity of the receptor for β-adrenergic agonists can be modulated by GTP through the guanine nucleotide regulatory unit. This modulation of receptor affinity by the guanine nucleotide regulatory unit appears to be an important mechanism by which the responsiveness of the β-adrenoceptor-adenylate cyclase system can be regulated.

Prolonged exposure of vascular SMC to β-adrenoceptor agonists rapidly reduces their ability to subsequently respond to β-adrenoceptor stimulation.[2,24] The magnitude of this loss in the ability to respond to β-adrenoceptor agonists (desensitization) is dependent both on the concentration of agonist to which the cells are exposed and the length of exposure. β-Adrenoceptor-mediated desensitization of vascular smooth muscle has been shown to be associated with a reduction in the concentration of β-adrenoceptor binding sites within the cell membrane.[2] A rapid loss of β-adrenoceptors has also been reported following exposure of the BC3H-1 SMC.[45] Using the radioligand [^{3}H]CGP-12177, which specifically binds to surface membrane receptors of intact cells, it was shown that β-adrenoceptors disappeared from the surface of the membrane at a rate which is dependent upon the concentration of isoprenaline to which the cells were exposed. Reducing the incubation temperature greatly attenuates this loss of receptor numbers. This loss of surface β-adrenoceptors was not accompanied by any loss of α_1-adrenoceptors or cholinergic surface receptors. The actual mechanism by which β-adrenoceptors are lost from the membrane surface of vascular smooth muscle has not been investigated. It is not known whether receptor loss is a direct consequence of receptor occupancy by an agonist or initiated by the rise in cyclic AMP. In frog erythrocytes, where β-adrenoceptors appear to be affected in a similar manner to those in vascular smooth muscle, surface membrane β-adrenoceptors are internalized and appear to be concentrated in lysosomes. Internalization of receptors may be prevented by compounds which inhibit transglutaminase-Ca^{2+}-dependent enzymes which cross-link proteins by forming isopeptide bonds between lysine and glutamine residues of any two proteins.[46,47] Following loss of β-adrenoceptors from the membrane surface of vascular smooth muscle, receptors are replenished at a relatively slow rate suggesting that, rather than receptors simply being recycled, protein synthesis is required.[2]

Relatively few studies have been carried out to examine the effects of circulating hormones, disease and age on β-adrenoceptor sensitivity in cultured vascular smooth muscle. Voliser et al.[23] demonstrated that the reduced β-adrenoceptor responsiveness described in blood vessels of old rats can also be demonstrated in rat aortic smooth muscle grown in culture. Part of the loss in β-adrenoceptor responsiveness could be prevented in these rats by dietary restriction. The effects of hypertension on vascular smooth muscle β-adrenoceptors has also recently been examined in culture.[24] The ability of vascular smooth muscle, derived from spontaneously hypertensive rats and WKY controls, to increase cyclic AMP concentrations during β-adrenoceptors stimulation was similar.

VII. α-ADRENOCEPTORS

Biochemical evidence to date suggests that cultured vascular smooth muscle possess α_1- and α_2-adrenoceptors with properties similar to those found on intact vessels.[3,8,48-51] Both primary and subcultured vascular smooth muscle derived from rabbit thoracic aorta bind the α_1 selective adrenoceptor ligand [^{125}I]HEAT with high affinity. Adrenergic agonists and antagonists compete with [^{125}I]HEAT for binding to cell membranes in the order (−)-epinephrine > (−)-norepinephrine > (+)-epinephrine > isoprenaline and prazosin > phentolamine > yohimbine. Agonist competition curves indicate that binding occurs in a reversible manner to a single site.[3,8,52]

Somewhat more complex competition between α_1-agonists and [^{3}H]prazosin have been reported in studies on intact cells.[21] At 37°C adrenaline, noradrenaline, and phenylephrine exhibited shallow competition curves with Hill coefficients less than one. Furthermore, norepinephrine inhibited only about 70% of [^{3}H]prazosin binding with a potency 4 to 22 times lower than observed in particulate membrane preparations. Although the precise reason for the discrepancy between α_1 selective radioligand binding to membrane preparations and intact cells is not known, it is possible that due to the lipophilicity of [^{3}H]prazosin, it is detecting endocytic vesicles containing α_1-adrenoceptors (endosomes).[53] Hydrophilic α-adrenoceptor agonists such as noradrenaline will only compete with [^{3}H]prazosin for surface membrane receptors. The availability of more hydrophilic α_1-selective adrenoceptor ligands should help to resolve this problem.

Recently the α_1-adrenoceptor of subcultured rabbit aortic smooth muscle has been isotopically labeled with the photoaffinity probe [^{125}I]APDQ (4-amino-6,7-dimethoxy-2-[4-[5-(4-azido-3-[^{125}I]iodophenyl)-pentanoyl]-1-piperazinyl]quinazoline.[22] Photoincorporation of [^{125}I]APDQ could be inhibited by adrenergic agonists and antagonists in a manner which was consistent with the radiolabel covalently attaching to an α_1-adrenoceptor. [^{125}I]APDQ labeled a protein with a molecular weight of approximately 85 kdaltons. Occasionally, two minor proteins with molecular weights of approximately 65 and 42 kdaltons also appeared to be labeled. These lower-molecular-weight proteins appear to be degradation products rather than subunits of the α_1-adrenoceptor since their formation could be inhibited by protease inhibitors. The 85-kdalton, α_1-adrenoceptor protein of vascular SMC appears similar in molecular weight and binding characteristics to α_1-adrenoceptor proteins identified in spleen, lung, and cerebral cortex. Photoaffinity labeling of the α_1-adrenoceptor of vascular smooth muscle will in the future greatly assist the isolation and characterization of this protein.

It is generally believed that in vascular smooth muscle there are many more α_1-adrenoceptors than necessary to provoke maximal contracture. Calculations from studies using rabbit aorta and dibenamine to antagonize responses to noradrenaline and adrenaline suggested that only one third of the adrenoceptor pool appeared to be necessary to initiate maximum contractile effects.[54,55] This concept of "spare" α_1-adrenoceptors has recently been examined, using BC3H-1 cells. Ambler et al.[13] examined the relationship between α_1-adrenoceptor number and the activation by α-adrenoceptor agonists of [$^{45}Ca^{2+}$] calcium efflux from BC3H-1 cells, as well as the enhancement of [^{3}H]inositol incorporation into phosphatidylinositol. Graded reductions in cell receptor numbers were obtained by alkylating receptors with phenoxybenzamine. Residual "active" receptors were quantitated with [^{3}H]prazosin. In this instance, the extent of receptor inactivation by phenoxybenzamine was inversely related to [$^{45}Ca^{2+}$] calcium efflux initiated by α-adrenoceptor agonists, suggesting no receptor reserve for this response. Similar results were obtained for α-adrenoceptor enhancement of [^{3}H]inositol incorporation into phosphatidylinositol.[13,56]

When α_1-adrenoceptors on rabbit aortic smooth muscle are reduced by chronically exposing the cells to high concentrations of noradrenaline, there is also a roughly equivalent reduction in the magnitude of activation of [^{32}P]phosphatidylinositol turnover induced by adrenaline.[3] Taken together, these studies suggest that the α_1-adrenoceptor is a monomeric rather than oligomeric protein and that α_1-adrenergic phosphatidylinositol and calcium responses are proportional to the number of sites occupied by adrenergic agonists. These results suggest that there are no spare α_1-adrenoceptors initiating the immediate biochemical responses, but, rather, that submaximal amounts of α_1-mediated released calcium are probably sufficient to initiate maximum contracture. Fluorimetric techniques utilizing calcium-induced quin 2 fluorescence in cultured vascular smooth muscle will help to increase our understanding of α-mediated calcium release and contracture.[57]

Little is known about physiological and environmental factors which might affect the number or properties of α_1-adrenoceptors on vascular smooth muscle. α_1-Adrenoceptors on cultured rabbit aortic smooth muscle have been shown to slowly "down-regulate" by a reduction in their numbers during prolonged exposure to α_1-adrenoceptor agonists.[3,8] This reduction in receptor number occurs without any apparent alteration in its affinity for adrenergic agonists or antagonists. Simultaneously with this slow-down regulation, there is also a reduction in the ability of the cells to increase [^{32}P]phosphatidylinositol turnover during exposure to adrenaline.[3] Basal levels of [^{32}P]phosphatidylinositol turnover are unaffected. This effect of adrenergic agonists on α_1-adrenoceptors in cultured smooth muscle is somewhat different to what has been observed in vivo. Chronic infusion of adrenaline into rats resulted in a reduction in the apparent affinity of the receptor for α_1-adrenergic agonists rather than any reduction in receptor number.[58]

It is not known whether this difference is due to species difference between the rabbit and rat or whether adrenaline is in some way influencing other metabolic or hormone pathways in vivo which indirectly influence the properties of the α_1-adrenoceptor. Taken together, these experiments suggest that α_1-adrenoceptor properties may be influenced by high circulating concentrations of noradrenaline and adrenaline, which explain why catecholamine-induced vascular reactivity in patients with pheochromocytoma is greatly attenuated. It is not known precisely how α_1-adrenoceptor numbers are reduced in vascular smooth muscle. α_1-Adrenoceptor numbers can also be reduced by cycloheximide.[12,59] The time course of loss of receptors is similar to that observed when cells are exposed to α_1-adrenoceptor agonists.[3,8] This close similarity between the rate of receptor loss induced by high concentrations of α_1-agonists or by inhibiting protein synthesis suggests that regulation of these receptors by α_1-adrenoceptor agonists could be via regulation of their production rather than any recycling or enhanced degradation phenomenon. This hypothesis remains to be tested.

α_2-Adrenoceptor binding sites have also been shown to be present on vascular smooth muscle.[49,51,60] These receptors differ from α_1-adrenoceptors in their ability to bind various adrenergic agonists and antagonists. The actual ratio of the number of α_1- to α_2-adrenoceptor can differ from vessel to vessel.[49] In canine aorta and the femoral artery there appears to be about twice as many α_1- as there are α_2-adrenoceptors, while in the mesenteric and renal arteries their concentration is similar. It is not known whether these differences are due to differences in sympathetic innervation between the vessels or due to the smooth muscle per se. α_2-Adrenoceptors have only recently been identified by [^{3}H]clonidine binding to membranes isolated from cultured vascular smooth muscle.[48] These receptors do not appear to exert any inhibitory affect on either basal- or β-adrenoceptor-stimulated adenylate cyclase activity. The mechanism by which they transmit their signal across the cell membrane remains to be elucidated.

VIII. SEROTONIN AND HISTAMINE RECEPTORS

A. Serotonin Receptors

Serotonin (5-HT) is a potent modulator of vascular muscle tone. In the main, it activates vasoconstrictor mechanisms but can also induce vasodilatation. Its ability to induce vasoconstriction or vasodilatation depends upon the type of vessel being examined, the species from which the vessel was obtained, and the experimental conditions used.[61-64] Generally speaking, serotonin-induced contracture appears to be mediated by its interaction with 5-HT_2 receptors.[66,67] However, in the basilar artery of the dog, contracture appears to be mediated by 5-HT_1 receptors.[68] The interaction of serotonin with 5-HT_2 receptors activates phosphatidylinositol metabolism and calcium gating mechanisms.[65] Intracellular levels of free calcium have been shown to be increased in cultured rat aortic smooth muscle upon exposure to serotonin.[57] Stimulation of 5-HT_2 receptors also increases prostacyclin synthesis, as measured by the accumulation of its stable metabolite 6-Keto PGF_1.[66,67] This response exhibits great specificity for serotonin, since other indole-containing molecules such as melatonin, 5-hydroxytryptophan and *N*-acetyl-serotonin do not stimulate prostacyclin synthesis. The partial serotonin agonists quipazine and *N*-(α, α, α-trifluoro-*n*-tolyl)piperazine induce small elevations in 6-Keto PGF_1 content. Dexamethasone, a drug which inhibits deacylation of phospholipids antagonizes the effects of serotonin on prostacyclin synthesis. This suggests that activation of the 5-HT_2 receptor promotes phospholipid deacylation in vascular smooth muscle. It has been suggested that the increase in prostacyclin synthesis induced by serotonin may represent a "turn off" mechanism that terminates serotonin-induced contracture.[66] Desensitization of 5-HT_2 receptor-mediated contracture has been reported in rat portal vein.[62] In the future it will be of interest to examine the above hypothesis, as well as the potential role of 5-HT_2 receptor numbers in the desensitization phenomenon. The recent availability of the 5-HT_2 selective receptor ligand,

N_1-methyl-2-[^{125}I]-LSD should enable investigators to examine at a receptor level, factors which are known to affect receptor vascular smooth muscle responses and also to investigate the molecular properties of 5-HT_2 receptors.[68]

5-HT receptors on vascular smooth muscle appear to be coupled to adenylate cyclase. Serotonin induces a concentration-dependent rise in cyclic AMP content in cultured calf-aorta smooth muscle.[25] Peak increases in cyclic AMP content occur between three and 5 min after the addition of serotonin and then progressively decline in a manner which suggests that the receptor may desensitize. The effect of serotonin on cyclic AMP content can be mimicked by 5-hydroxy-*N*-methyltryptamine and 5-methoxytryptamine. Other tryptamines such as *N*-methyltryptamine and *N*-acetyl-5-hydroxytryptamine are ineffective. This serotonin response cannot be antagonized by most of the classical 5-HT_2 receptor antagonists. Pizotifen, cyproheptadine, cinanserin, molindone, and lysergic acid diethylamide are ineffective. Methylsergide appears to be an exception, inhibiting the rise in cyclic AMP by 40%. Since increases in cyclic AMP content in vascular smooth muscle are closely associated with vasodilatation, it is tempting to suggest that serotonin receptors coupled to adenylate cyclase may be of the 5-HT_1 subtype. Further studies are required to confirm this suggestion.

B. Histamine Receptors

The circulating effects of histamine are mediated by both histamine H_1 and H_2-receptors. These two receptor systems can act either in concert or opposite one another and their interaction determines whether the local response to histamine results in relaxation or contracture.[69] The H_2-receptor-mediated vasodilator response correlates well with the rise in cyclic AMP content in cultured calf aorta smooth muscle.[25] Histamine initiates a rapid time-dependent increase in cyclic AMP content in these cells which can be antagonized by the H_2-receptor antagonists metiamide and cimetidine, but not by H_1-receptor antagonists. In addition, the H_2-receptor agonists dimaprit and 4-methylhistamine are more potent than the H_1-receptor agonists, 2-methylhistamine in stimulating cyclic AMP accumulation. H_1-receptor activation stimulates phosphatidylinositol metabolism, an effect consistent with it initiating contracture of vascular smooth muscle.[40] This effect of histamine could be mimicked by 2-(2-aminoethyl)thiazole, a H_1-receptor-selective agonist. It is inhibited by H_1-selective antagonists. Histamine has also been reported to stimulate prostaglandin E synthesis in cultured umbilical vein SMC.[70] It will be of interest to determine whether prostaglandin E production contributes to the vasodilator effects of adenylate cyclase or antagonizes the vasoconstrictor effects of H_1-receptor activation. Further studies on the characterization of H_1 and H_2-receptors in cultured vascular smooth muscle by radioligand ligand receptor binding techniques combined with studies on cyclic AMP, phosphatidylinositol metabolism, and prostaglandin synthesis should greatly clarify the mechanisms by which these receptors transmit signals across the cell membrane to induce contracture and relaxation.

IX. CONCLUSIONS

Studies on the mechanisms by which noradrenaline, serotonin, and histamine regulate cyclic AMP and phosphatidylinositol metabolism in cultured vascular smooth muscle are increasing our understanding of how these receptors transmit messages across cell membranes to initiate contracture, relaxation, or alterations in cell metabolism. α_1 Adrenoceptors, histamine H_1-receptors and serotonin 5-HT_2-receptors all stimulate phosphatidylinositol turnover and also induce contraction. β_2 Adrenoceptors, histamine H_2-receptors, and serotonin receptors all increase cyclic AMP levels and initiate relaxation. It will be important in the future to understand how the various classes of receptors, as well as their subtypes, are regulated in intact cells. It will also be important to examine the role of new potential intracellular messengers, particularly the phosphatidylinositol metabolites, thought to be involved in calcium mobilization. The use of cultured vascular smooth muscle, together with the increasing availability of highly selective receptor radioligands, methods for measuring various potential intracellular messengers and calcium mobilization, should help us attain these goals.

REFERENCES

1. Clark, A. J., General pharmacology, in *Heffter's Handbook der Experimentellen Pharmakologie,* Band IV, Erg., Berlin, 1937.
2. Little, P. J., Campbell, J. H., Skews, H., and Bobik, A., Mechanism of isoprenaline induced desensitization of rabbit aortic smooth muscle β-adrenoceptor responses, *Clin. Exp. Pharmacol. Physiol.,* 11, 503, 1984.
3. Bobik, A., Campbell, J. H., and Little, P. J., Desensitization of the $alpha_1$ adrenoceptor system in vascular smooth muscle, *Biochem. Pharmacol.,* 33, 1143, 1984.
4. Harder, D. R. and Sperelakis, N., Action potential generation in reaggregates of rat aortic smooth muscle cells in primary culture, *Blood Vessels,* 16, 186, 1979.
5. Gunther, S., Alexander, R. W., Atkinson, W. J., and Gimbrone, M. A., Functional angiotensin II receptors in cultured vascular smooth muscle cells, *J. Cell Biol.,* 92, 289, 1982.
6. Fowler, S., Shio, H., and Wolinsky, H., Subcellular fractionation and morphology of calf aortic smooth muscle cells, *J. Cell Biol.,* 75, 166, 1977.
7. Ross, R., The smooth muscle cell. II. Growth of smooth muscle in culture and formation of elastic fibers, *J. Cell Biol.,* 50, 172, 1971.
8. Wikberg, J. E. S., Akers, M., Caron, M., and Hagen, P.-D., Norepinephrine-induced down regulation of $alpha_1$ adrenergic receptors in cultured rabbit aortic smooth muscle cells, *Life Sci.,* 33, 1409, 1983.
9. Anand-Srivastava, M. B., Franks, D. J., Cantin, M., and Genest, J., Presence of 'Ra' and 'P'-site receptors for adenosine coupled to adenylate cyclase in cultured vascular smooth muscle cells, *Biochem. Biophys. Res. Commun.,* 108, 213, 1982.
10. Brown, R. D., Berger, K. D., and Taylor, P., α_1-Adrenergic receptor activation mobilises cellular Ca^{2+} in a muscle line, *J. Biol. Chem.,* 259, 7554, 1984.
11. Schubert, D., Harris, A. J., Devine, C. E., and Heinemann, S., Characterisation of a unique smooth muscle line, *J. Cell Biol.,* 61, 398, 1974.
12. Hughes, R. J., Boyle, M. R., Brown, R. D., Taylor, P., and Insel, P. A., Characterisation of coexisting $alpha_1$ and $beta_2$ adrenergic receptors on a cloned muscle cell line, BC3H-1, *Mol. Pharmacol.,* 22, 258, 1982.
13. Ambler, S. K., Brown, R. D., and Taylor, P., The relationship between phosphatidylinositol metabolism and mobilisation of intracellular calcium elicited by $alpha_1$-adrenergic receptor stimulation in BC3H-1 muscle cells, *Mol. Pharmacol.,* 26, 405, 1984.
14. Kimes, B. W. and Brandt, B. L., Characterisation of two putative smooth muscle cell lines from rat thoracic aorta, *Exp. Cell Res.,* 98, 349, 1976.
15. Owen, N. E., Regulation of Na/K/Cl cotransport in vascular smooth muscle cells, *Biochem. Biophys. Res. Commun.,* 125, 500, 1984.
16. Bennett, J. P., in *Methods in Binding Studies in Neurotransmitter Receptor Binding,* Jamamura, H. I., et al., Eds., Raven Press, New York, 1978, 57.
17. Hertel, C., Stachelin, M., and Perkins, J. P., Evidence for intravascular β-adrenergic receptors in membrane fractions from desensitized cells: binding of the hydrophilic ligand CGP-12177, only in the presence of alamethicin, *J. Cycl. Nucleot. Prot. Phosphor. Res.,* 9, 119, k1983.
18. Stachelin, M., Simons, P., Jaeggi, K., and Wigger, N., CGP-12177, a hydrophilic β-adrenergic receptor radioligand reveals high affinity binding of agonists to intact cells, *J. Biol. Chem.,* 258, 3496, 1983.
19. Sher, E. and Clementi, F., Agonist-induced internalisation of the β-adrenergic receptor in a smooth muscle cell line, *Biochem. Biophys. Res. Commun.,* 124, 863, 1984.
20. Linden, J., Patel, A., Spanier, A. M., and Weglecki, W. B., Rapid agonist-induced decrease of ^{125}I-pindolol binding to β-adrenergic receptors, *J. Biol. Chem.,* 259, 15115, 1984.
21. Sladeczek, F., Bockaert, J., and Manger, J.-P., Differences between agonist and antagonist binding to $alpha_1$ adrenergic receptors of intact and broken cell preparations, *Mol. Pharmacol.,* 24, 392, 1983.

22. Leeb-Lundberg, L. M. F., Dickinson, K. E. J., Heald, S. L., Wikberg, J. E. S., Hagen, P.-O., DeBernardis, J. F., Winn, M., Arendsen, D. L., Lefkowitz, R. J., and Caron, M. G., Photoaffinity labeling of mammalian alpha$_1$-adrenergic receptors, *J. Biol. Chem.*, 259, 2579, 1984.
23. Voliser, L., West, C. D., Chase, A. R., and Green, L., Beta adrenergic receptor sensitivity in cultured vascular muscle cells: effect of age and of dietary restriction, *Mech. Ageing Dev.*, 21, 283, 1983.
24. Nabika, T., Velletri, P. A., Igawa, T., Yamori, Y., and Lovenberg, W., Comparison of cyclic AMP accumulation and morphological changes induced by β-adrenergic stimulation of cultured vascular smooth muscle cells and fibroblasts, *Blood Vessels*, 22, 47, 1985.
25. Luchins, A. R. and Makman, M. H., Presence of histamine and serotonin receptors associated with adenylate cyclase in cultured calf-aorta smooth muscle cells, *Biochem. Pharmacol.*, 29, 3155, 1980.
26. Bobik, A., Campbell, J. H., Carson, V., and Campbell, G. R., Mechanism of isoprenaline-induced refractoriness of the β-adrenoceptor-adenylate cyclase system in chick embryo cardiac cells, *J. Cardiovasc. Pharmacol.*, 3, 541, 1981.
27. Tovey, K. C., Oldham, K. G., and Whelan, I. A. M., A simple direct assay of cyclic AMP in plasma and other biological samples using an improved binding technique, *Clin. Chim. Acta*, 56, 221, 1974.
28. Krall, J. F., Fortier, M., and Korenmann, S. G., Smooth muscle cyclic nucleotide biochemistry, in *Biochemistry of Smooth Muscle*, Vol. 3, Stephens, N. L., Ed., CRC Press, Boca Raton, Fla., 1984, 89.
29. Wroblenewska, B., Spatz, M., Merkel, N., and Bembry, J., Cerebrovascular smooth muscle culture. II. Characteristics of adrenergic receptors linked to adenylate cyclase, *Life Sci.*, 34, 783, 1984.
30. Burgess, G. M., Godfrey, P. P., McKinney, T. S., Berridge, M. J., Irvine, R. F., and Putney, J. W., Jr., The second messenger linked receptor activation to internal Ca release in liver, *Nature (London)*, 309, 63, 1984.
31. Joseph, S. K., Thomas, A. P., Williams, R. J., Irvine, R. F., and Williamson, J. R., *Myo*-inositol 1,4,5-triphosphate: a second messenger for the hormonal mobilization of intracellular Ca^{2+} in liver, *J. Biol. Chem.*, 259, 3077, 1984.
32. Majerus, P. W., Wilson, D. B., Connolly, T. M., Bross, T. E., and Neufield, E. J., Phosphoinositide turnover provides a link in stimulus-response coupling, *Trends Biochem. Sci.*, 10, 168, 1985.
33. Williamson, J. R., Cooper, R. H., Joseph, S. K., and Thomas, A. P., Inositol triphosphate and diacylglycerol as intracellular second messengers, *Am. J. Physiol.*, 248, C203, 1985.
34. Leyfred, M. A. and Wells, W. W., Subcellular incorporation of ^{32}P into phosphoinositides and other phospholipids in isolated hepatocytes, *J. Biol. Chem.*, 259, 7659, 1984.
35. Nishizuka, Y., The role of protein kinase C in surface signal transduction and turnover promotion, *Nature (London)*, 308, 693, 1984.
36. Ohsako, S. and Deguchi, T., Stimulation by phosphatidic acid of calcium influx and cyclic GMP synthesis in neuroblastoma cells, *J. Biol. Chem.*, 256, 10945, 1981.
37. Legan, E., Chernow, B., Parrillo, J., and Roth, B. L., Activation of phosphatidylinositol turnover in rat aorta by alpha$_1$-adrenergic receptor stimulation, *Eur. J. Pharmacol.*, 110, 389, 1985.
38. Zeleznikar, R. J., Quist, E. E., and Drewes, L. R., An alpha$_1$-adrenergic receptor-mediated phosphatidylinositol effect on canine cerebral vessels, *Mol. Pharmacol.*, 24, 163, 1983.
39. Villalobos-Molina, R. and Garcia-Sainz, J. A., H_1-Histaminergic activation stimulates phosphatidylinositol labeling in rabbit aorta, *Eur. J. Pharmacol.*, 90, 457, 1983.
40. Roth, B. L., Nakaki, T., Chuang, D. M., and Costa, E., Aortic recognition sites of serotonin (5HT) are coupled to phospholipase C and modulate phosphatidylinositol turnover, *Neuropharmacology*, 23, 1223, 1983.
41. Leyfred, M. A. and Wells, W. W., Subcellular site and mechanism of vasopressin-stimulated hydrolysis of phosphoinositides in rat hepatocytes, *J. Biol. Chem.*, 259, 7666, 1984.
42. Mauger, J.-P. and Worcel, M., Relationship between the (−)-[^{3}H]-dihydroalprenolol binding to β-adrenoceptors and transmembrane ^{86}Rb efflux of the BC3H1 nonfusing muscle cell line, *Br. J. Pharmacol.*, 68, 731, 1980.
43. Norris, J. S., Garnier, D. J., Brown, F., Popovich, K., and Cornett, L. E., Characterization of an adenylate cyclase coupled β_2-adrenergic receptor in a smooth muscle human cell line, *J. Receptor Res.*, 3, 623, 1983.
44. Mauger, J.-P., Moura, A.-M., and Worcel, M., Pharmacology of the adrenoceptors and cholinoceptors of the BC3H1 nonfusing cell line, *Br. J. Pharmacol.*, 64, 29, 1978.
45. Sher, E. and Clementi, F., Agonist-induced internalisation of the β-adrenergic receptor into a smooth muscle cell line, *Biochem. Biophys. Res. Commun.*, 124, 863, 1984.
46. Chaung, D.-M., β-Adrenergic receptor internalisation and processing: role of transglutaminase and lysosomes, *Mol. Cell Biochem.*, 58, 79, 1984.
47. Riggrani, A., Vernalione, F., and Robinson, G. A., Loss and restoration of sensitivity to catecholamines in cultured BHK cells: influence of dansylcadavarine, *Soc. Neurosci. Abstr.*, 6, 534, 1980.
48. Wroblewska, B., Spatz, M., and Bembry, J., Binding studies of alpha$_2$-adrenergic receptors in cultured cerebrovascular smooth muscle cells, *Soc. Neurosci. Abstr.*, 234, 699, 1984.

49. Bobik, A., Identification of alpha adrenoceptor subtypes in dog arteries by [^{3}H]yohimbine and [^{3}H]prazosin, *Life Sci.*, 30, 219, 1982.
50. Bobik, A. and Anderson, W. P., Influence of sympathectomy on alpha$_2$ adrenoceptor binding sites in canine blood vessels, *Life Sci.*, 33, 331, 1983.
51. Drew, G. M. and Whiting, S. B., Evidence for two distinct types of post synaptic alpha-adrenergic receptors in vascular smooth muscle in vivo, *Br. J. Pharmacol.*, 67, 207, 1979.
52. Colucci, W. S., Brock, T. A., Gimbrone, M. A., and Alexander, R. W., Regulation of alpha$_1$ adrenergic receptor coupled calcium flux in cultured vascular smooth muscle cells, *Hypertension*, 6, 1, 1984.
53. Rome, L. H., Curling receptors, *Trends Biochem. Sci.*, 10, 151, 1985.
54. Nickerson, M., Non-equilibrium drug antagonism, *Pharmacol. Rev.*, 9, 246, 1957.
55. Furchgott, R. F., Pharmacology of vascular smooth muscle, *Pharmacol. Rev.*, 7, 183, 1955.
56. Brown, R. D., Berger, K. D., and Taylor, P., Alpha$_1$-adrenergic receptor activation mobilises cellular calcium Ca^{2+} in a muscle cell line, *J. Biol. Chem.*, 259, 7554, 1984.
57. Nabika, T., Velletri, P. A., Lovenberg, W., and Beaven, M. A., Increase in cytosolic calcium and phosphoinositide metabolism induced by angiotensin II and [Arg]vasopressin in vascular smooth muscle cells, *J. Biol. Chem.*, 260, 4661, 1985.
58. Colucci, W. S., Gimbrone, A., and Alexander, R. W., Regulation of the postsynaptic alpha-adrenergic receptor in rat mesenteric artery, *Circ. Res.*, 48, 104, 1981.
59. Manger, J.-P., Sladeczek, F., and Bockaert, J., Characteristics and metabolism of alpha$_1$-adrenergic receptors in a nonfusing muscle cell line, *J. Biol. Chem.*, 287, 875, 1982.
60. Weiss, R. J., Webb, R. C., and Smith, C. B., Alpha-2 adrenoreceptor on arterial smoth muscle: selective labeling by [^{3}H]clonidine, *J. Pharmacol. Exp. Ther.*, 225, 599, 1983.
61. Black, J. L., French, R. J., and Mylecharana, E. J., Receptor mechanisms for 5-hydroxytryptamine in rabbit arteries, *Br. J. Pharmacol.*, 74, 619, 1981.
62. Lemberger, H. F., Mason, N., and Cohen, M. L., 5-HT$_2$ receptors in the rat portal vein: desensitization following cumulative serotonin addition, *Life Sci.*, 35, 71, 1984.
63. Peroutka, S. J., Tolner, M. D. J., and Allen, G., Serotonin-induced contracture of canine basilar artery mediated by 5-HT$_1$ receptors, *Brain Res.*, 259, 327, 1983.
64. Edrinsson, L., Hardeto, J. E., and Owman, C., Pharmacological analysis of 5-hydroxytryptamine receptors in isolated intracranial and extracranial vessels of the cat and man, *Circ. Res.*, 42, 143, 1978.
65. Berridge, M., Phosphatidylinositol metabolism and calcium gating in a 5-HT receptor system, in *Drug Receptors and Their Effectors*, Birdsall, N.-J., Ed., MacMillan, London, 1981, 75.
66. Coughlin, S. R., Moskowitz, M. A., Antoniades, H. N., and Levine, L., Serotonin receptor-mediated stimulation of bovine smooth muscle cell prostacyclin and its modulation by platelet-derived growth factor, *Proc. Natl. Acad. Sci. U.S.A.*, 78, 7134, 1981.
67. Coughlin, S. R., Moskowitz, M. A., and Levine, L., Identification of a serotonin type 2 receptor linked to prostacyclin synthesis in vascular smooth cells, *Biochem. Pharmacol.*, 33, 692, 1984.
68. Hoffman, B. J., Karpa, M. D., Lever, J. R., and Hartig, P. R., N_1-Methyl-2-[^{125}I]LSD ([^{125}I]MIL), a preferred ligand for serotonin 5-HT$_2$ receptors, *Eur. J. Pharmacol.*, 110, 147, 1985.
69. Angus, J., Bobik, A., and Korner, P. I., Effects of histamine bolus injections and continuous infusions on the H_1 and H_2-receptors in the hind limb vessels of the rabbit, *Clin. Exp. Pharmacol. Physiol.*, 4, 303, 1977.
70. Alexander, R. W. and Gimbrone, M. A., Stimulation of prostaglandin E synthesis in cultured human umbilical vein smooth muscle cells, *Proc. Natl. Acad. Sci. U.S.A.*, 73, 1617, 1976.
71. Little, P. J. and Bobik, A., unpublished.

Chapter 17

INNERVATION OF SMOOTH MUSCLE IN CULTURE

Julie H. Campbell and Gordon R. Campbell

TABLE OF CONTENTS

I. SYMPATHETIC NEURONS IN CULTURE

Dissociated sympathetic neurons in culture are normal ultrastructurally and electrophysiologically,[1] possess functional muscarinic cholinergic receptors, and retain the ability to release noradrenaline via a stimulus-secretion coupling mechanism.[2-4] In the presence of nonneuronal cells, dissociated neurons from the newborn rat superior cervical ganglion grown for 3 weeks or longer have resting potentials, passive electrical properties, and action potentials generally reported for principal neurons of the superior cervical ganglion of adult rats.[5] Frequently the action potential is followed by a prolonged after-hyperpolarization, whose properties suggest the presence of potassium channels controlled by calcium ions. When the neurons are grown in the absence of nonneuronal cells, the action potentials are similar, but the prolonged after-hyperpolarization is rarely seen, and the neurons usually discharge repetitively in response to a steady depolarization.

A. Nerve Growth Factor

The hormone nerve growth factor (NGF) has marked effects on the survival, growth, and differentiation of sympathetic neurons in culture[6-7] and like other growth factors and hormones, induces rapid and delayed responses. The rapid responses include the uptake of metabolites such as uridine and glucose,[8-10] while the delayed responses include polymerization of microtubules, stimulation of two enzymes involved in catecholamine biosynthesis,[10] production of neurites, and long-term maintenance of cell viability.[11] Dissociated newborn rat sympathetic neurons, in the absence of NGF or other cell types, do not survive for more than 1 day in culture; however, in the presence of increasing levels of NGF, there is increased survival with saturation at 0.5 μg/mℓ 7S NGF.[12] Low concentrations of NGF (such as occur in plasma) elicit maximum axon formation from these cells, but it is high concentrations (as occur in some effector organs) that induce maximal cell survival and tyrosine hydroxylase activity.[13] Therefore, in vivo, NGF from the two sources may subserve different regulatory functions in the developing neuron; that is, circulating NGF may stimulate neurite elaboration, while target organ NGF may aid survival. However, the increased survival of dissociated sympathetic neurons in the presence of target or accessory (i.e., Schwann) cells is not due solely to production of NGF by these cells, as the cell-derived activity is not blocked by antibodies to NGF.[14]

B. Modulation of Neuronal Transmitters

Each neuron possesses the potential ability to synthesize the complete enzymatic machinery for all transmitter substances. The particular transmitter that appears at the end of differentiation is determined by external trophic factors released from certain cells that trigger the expression of the appropriate genetic program.[15] Thus, it is possible to influence the transmitter produced in populations of developing autonomic neurons in vivo by transplantation of neural crest cells to foreign sites.[16-17]

In cell culture, dissociated sympathetic neurons from newborn rats grown in the absence of nonneuronal cells are predominantly adrenergic and synthesize, store, release, and take up noradrenaline while acetylcholine synthesis is negligible.[18] However, if the same neurons are grown in the presence of nonneuronal cells from ganglia or the heart or in a medium conditioned by them, the cultures synthesize significant amounts of acetylcholine, as well as catecholamines. If sufficiently high concentrations of conditioned medium are used, the cultures become predominantly cholinergic.[19-22] Differential survival and selection of subclasses of the neuronal population have been ruled out, indicating that the conditioned medium acts by altering the differentiated fate of individual neurons. The development of cholinergic characteristics in adrenergic neurons is age-dependent as there is a marked decrease in the ability of sympathetic ganglion explants taken from rats older than 2 to 5 days to develop choline acetyltransferase activity in culture.[23-25] This suggests that most sympathetic neurons may become committed to a certain neurotransmitter at a critical stage and lose their ability to respond to alternative instructions after that time.

A major question is why in culture is it possible through conditioning with nonneuronal cells from ganglia or from target tissues to induce virtually all of the neurons to become cholinergic, whereas in vivo, despite the potential presence of a cholinergic-inducing factor in nonneuronal cells in the ganglia and in tissues to which nerve processes grow, only about 5% are cholinergic? Cholinergic-inducing signals selectively localized in a target which receives sympathetic cholinergic innervation would explain why only some neurons become cholinergic, and indeed it has been found that targets normally receiving cholinergic innervation (skeletal and heart muscle) are far better at "cholinergic-conditioning" the culture medium than a target receiving only adrenergic innervation (liver).[26] However, cell types not known to receive synapses at all (fibroblasts, glia) can also cholinergically condition medium. NGF from either the blood supply to the ganglia or transported retrogradely from the target tissue cannot be involved, as NGF stimulates both adrenergic and cholinergic differentiation.[27] One possibility is that the influence of the preganglionic synapses is to prevent the neurons of the sympathetic ganglia from becoming cholinergic since prolonged depolarization of sympathetic neurons in culture prevents the large increase in the acetylcholine/catecholamine ratio caused by the conditioned medium from nonneuronal cells.[28] However, transection of the preganglionic nerve trunk of the young rat in vivo does not result in an increase in the intrinsic choline acetyltransferase activity of the ganglion.[29] Therefore, the role of preganglionic input remains equivocal.

The synthetic glucocorticoid dexamethasone and corticosterone, the naturally occurring glucocorticoid in rats, prevents the development of cholinergic properties in sympathetic neurons in culture.[30] The influence of the glucocorticoids is apparently on the nonneuronal cells to alter selectively the production or liberation of a factor that induces neuronal cholinergic development, rather than a direct effect on the nerves.[31] However, reduction of circulating glucocorticoids in vivo by adrenalectomy does not lead to an increase in cholinergic properties in the superior cervical ganglion.[32]

II. TROPIC INFLUENCE OF EFFECTOR ORGANS ON NERVE FIBER GROWTH

The term "trophic" as applies to the autonomic system denotes an influence on maintenance or survival, whereas "tropic" implies an influence on directional growth. The tropic influence of effector organs on nerve fiber growth in vivo is not understood. However, in culture the growth and direction of both sympathetic and parasympathetic nerves can be influenced by gradients of diffusable agents.

A. Sympathetic Nerves

The best studied case is the influence of NGF on sympathetic and sensory nerve fiber growth. Regenerating neurities in culture grow preferentially towards a capillary tube filled with NGF,[33-34] and processes from dissociated neurons grow preferentially into adjacent chamber compartments containing NGF.[35] With semisolid matrices of agar and culture medium, orientation of nerve tips from dissociated neurons occurs up a defined gradient of NGF as far as 23 mm from the NGF source.[36]

Using a tissue source of NGF, growth stimulation of sympathetic and sensory nerves occurs on the side of the ganglion explant opposite an explant of NGF-producing mouse sarcoma 1 to 2 mm distant.[37] Sympathetic nerve fiber growth is stimulated towards explants of tissue normally densely innervated by sympathetic nerves (caudal artery, atrium, vas deferens) but not towards explants of tissues normally sparsely innervated (aorta, uterus, distal ureter)[37-41] (see also References 27 and 34). The "attraction" effect is evident as soon as the nerve fibers emerge from the sympathetic ganglion explant and occurs over a distance of 2 mm. NGF is synthesized by smooth muscle tissues in culture,[42] but whether an NGF gradient is responsible for the direct outgrowth is uncertain. The amount of NGF is higher in tissues which become densely innervated by sympathetic nerves,[43-44] but the "attraction" and growth stimulatory effects in culture are sometimes but not always blocked by the presence of antibodies to NGF.[34,40] There is a growth stimulatory effect of heart on ciliary ganglia neurons which are not responsive to NGF,[34,45-46] but heart has no effect on spinal cord neurons which are unresponsive to NGF.[39]

A tropic effect of NGF in vivo is demonstrated by the original experiments of Bueker[47] and of Levi-Montalcini and her colleagues.[48-49] More recently, it has been shown that intracerebral injection of NGF causes a highly abnormal growth of sympathetic axons into the spinal cord of developing mice and rats, with postganglionic axons from thoracic and cervical sympathetic ganglia running cephalad in the spinal cord and brain stem toward the region of NGF injection.[50] This leaves no doubt that NGF can exert a tropic influence on sympathetic nerves.

B. Parasympathetic Nerves

There is some evidence to suggest that parasympathetic nerves are "attracted" by their normal targets in vivo and in vitro.[46,51-55] The survival and development of parasympathetic nerves in culture require co-culture with target tissues[56-58] or growth in target-organ conditioned medium[55,59-60] or with tissue homogenates.[61-65]

It remains to be shown that NGF or other diffusible chemical agents contribute a tropic stimulus in normal development. Other possible mechanisms for eliciting directed growth in vivo can be inferred from the fact that growing axons in vitro are very sensitive to mechanical factors and may be affected by differential adhesiveness of the surfaces over which they grow.[66-68] Finally, there is some evidence for recognition of specific surface molecules by developing neurons.[69]

III. TROPHIC INFLUENCE OF SYMPATHETIC NERVES ON SMOOTH MUSCLE

There are several reports suggesting a trophic influence of sympathetic nerves on smooth muscle in vitro. Thus, in primary cultures of dissociated newborn guinea pig ureter, long processes grow from intrinsic nonadrenergic neurons to form close and long-lasting associations with reformed muscle chains.[70] Where this occurs, the muscle chains commence spontaneous contraction about 13 days in advance of muscle chains without nerve fibers, and their contractions are considerably stronger and more rapid. Nerve fiber growth from extrinsic sympathetic ganglia into clumps of partially dispersed guinea pig vas deferens stimulates the formation of gap junctions between muscle cells and the formation of foci of synchronous contractions;[71] the rate and strength of contraction in explants of mouse intestine in culture are enhanced by the presence of extrinsic sympathetic ganglion neurons;[72] and denervation atrophy of skeletal muscle is prevented by the presence, but not necessarily innervation, of explants of sympathetic ganglia.[73]

A trophic influence of autonomic nerves on smooth muscle in culture is further demonstrated by the delay of 3 to 7 days in spontaneous phenotypic modulation from the contractile to synthetic state and subsequent proliferation of isolated smooth muscle cells from the guinea pig vas deferens and rabbit aorta and ear artery.[71,74] A similar delay in modulation and proliferation occurs when the cells are grown in the presence of a crude extract of homogenized sympathetic ganglia, indicating that the trophic influence of sympathetic neurons on smooth muscle cells (SMC) is chemically mediated.[74-75]

IV. FORMATION OF FUNCTIONAL JUNCTIONS IN CULTURE

A. Interactions Between Sympathetic Nerves and Isolated Smooth Muscle Cells

The initial interactions between sympathetic nerve fibers and isolated SMC have been observed with time-lapse microcinematography.[70,74,76-77] There is no obvious "attraction" from a distance of the nerve fibers to the single cells, with chance contacts occurring through random growth. Once a nerve growth cone encounters a cell, it halts in its growth and palpates the cell for about 50 min. The nerve fiber then appears to be able to distinguish whether or not the cell is a suitable target to innervate. That is, contact with a fibroblast or smooth muscle cell from a normally sparsely innervated organ (ureter, aorta) leads to a transitory relationship lasting no longer than a few hours, whereas contact with mature SMC from a normally densely innervated organ (vas deferens, ear artery) leads to an association that lasts for days or weeks. The association may be complex, with many fine fibers plexusing over the cell, or may consist of a single varicose fiber running along the length of the cell. Receptor sites for noradrenaline or acetylcholine on the muscle cells do not appear to be involved in the process of nerve-muscle recognition since the presence of propranolol or hyoscine does not inhibit the formation of nerve-muscle associations in culture.[78]

B. Ultrastructure of Nerve-Muscle Associations

The associations that form between sympathetic nerve fibers and isolated smooth muscle cells from the guinea pig vas deferens closely resemble the in vivo situation with a separation of 100 Å and no specialization of either nerve or muscle.[77] The separation between sympathetic nerves and isolated SMC from rabbit ear artery is 100 to 500 Å.[74] This is considerably less than the minimum 5000-Å separation that occurs in vivo with this tissue[79] and may be due to the absence of connective tissue elements in the culture situation. The associations that form between sympathetic nerve fibers and SMC in mouse intestinal explants have a separation of 200 to 300 Å,[72] whereas those between nerves and muscle cells of rat iris explants are generally no closer than 3000 Å.[80]

C. Functional Junctions

Nerve fibers from explants of sympathetic and ciliary ganglia form functional junctions in culture with explants and single cells of smooth muscle from the rat iris sphincter pupillae and guinea pig vas deferens and taenia coli.[80-81] Stimulation of the ganglia evoke contractions of the smooth muscle which are potentiated by the cholinesterase inhibitor neostigmine and blocked by the muscarinic antagonist hyoscine, demonstrating that in these cases the transmitter eliciting the effect is acetylcholine.

However, electrophysiological studies performed on microcultures (300 to 500 μm in diameter) of solitary sympathetic neurons plated on cardiac muscle from the newborn rat have shown that some neurons inhibit, some excite, and others first inhibit, then excite, the cardiac muscle.[82] Application of drugs has provided evidence for secretion of acetylcholine by the first group, catecholamines by the second, and both acetylcholine and catecholamines by the third. Ultrastructurally, the cholinergic endings contain small agranular vesicles, the adrenergic endings small granular vesicles, and the dual function endings mainly agranular vesicles, with an occasional granular vesicle[22] (see also References 21 and 83). Excitatory cholinergic synapses form between dissociated sympathetic neurons in culture in a medium permissive for proliferation of nonneuronal cells[84] and between dissociated sympathetic neurons and rat skeletal myotubes.[85]

Ciliary ganglia from newborn rabbits (which normally make exclusively cholinergic muscarinic connections with SMC) form cholinergic nicotinic junctions with chick skeletal muscle in culture, indicating that the character of the muscle and not that of the neuron determines the pharmacological nature of the neuromuscular junctions.[86] However, unlike spinal cord-skeletal muscle junctions in culture, innervation of skeletal muscle by the ciliary ganglia does not provide the support to maintain cross-striations, suggesting that recognition of a cell as an appropriate target and its functional innervation does not automatically lead to adequate neurotrophic support of the cell.

REFERENCES

1. Kim, S. U., Warren, K. G., and Kalia, M., Tissue culture of adult human neurons, *Neurosci. Lett.*, 11, 137, 1979.
2. Greene, L. A., Sytkowski, A. J., Vogel, Z., and Nirenberg, M. W., α-Bungarotoxin used as a probe for acetylcholine receptors of cultured neurones, *Nature (London)*, 243, 163, 1973.
3. Obata, K., Transmitter sensitivities of some nerve and muscle cells in culture, *Brain Res.*, 73, 71, 1974.
4. Greene, L. A. and Rein, G., Release of norepinephrine from neurons in dissociated cell cultures of chick sympathetic ganglia via stimulation of nicotinic and muscarinic acetylcholine receptors, *J. Neurochem.*, 30, 579, 1978.
5. O'Lague, P. H., Potter, D. D., and Furshpan, E. J., Studies on rat sympathetic neurons developing in cell culture. I. Growth characteristics and electrophysiological properties, *Dev. Biol.*, 67, 384, 1978.
6. Levi-Montalcini, R. and Angeletti, P. U., Nerve growth factor, *Physiol. Rev.*, 48, 534, 1968.
7. Varon, S. and Adler, R., Nerve growth factors and control of nerve growth, *Curr. Top. Dev. Biol.*, 16, 207, 1980.
8. Horii, Z. I. and Varon, S., Nerve growth factor action on membrane permeation to exogenous substrates in dorsal root ganglionic dissociates from the chick embryo, *Brain Res.*, 124, 121, 1977.
9. Skaper, S. D., Bottenstein, J. E., and Varon, S., Effects of nerve growth factor on cyclic AMP levels in embryonic chick dorsal root ganglia following factor deprivation, *J. Neurochem.*, 32, 1845, 1979.
10. Thoenen, H., Angeletti, P. U., Levi-Montalcini, R., and Kettler, R., Selective induction by nerve growth factor of tyrosine hydroxylase and dopamine-β-hydroxylase in the rat superior cervical ganglia, *Proc. Natl. Acad. Sci. U.S.A.*, 68, 1598, 1971.
11. Levi-Montalcini, R., The nerve growth factor: its role in growth, differentiation and function of the sympathetic adrenergic neuron, *Prog. Brain Res.*, 45, 235, 1976.
12. Chun, L. L. Y. and Patterson, P. H., Role of nerve growth factor in the development of rat sympathetic neurons *in vitro*. I. Survival, growth and differentiation of catecholamine production, *J. Cell Biol.*, 75, 694, 1977.
13. Hill, C. E. and Hendry, I. A., Differences in sensitivity to nerve growth factor of axon formation and tyrosine hydroxylase induction in cultured sympathetic neurons, *Neurosci.*, 1, 489, 1976.
14. Varon, S., Skaper, S. D., and Manthorpe, M., Trophic activities for dorsal root and sympathetic ganglionic neurons in media conditioned by Schwann and other peripheral cells, *Dev. Brain Res.*, 1, 73, 1981.
15. Burnstock, G., Do some nerve cells release more than one transmitter? *Neurosci.*, 1, 239, 1976.
16. Le Douarin, N. M. and Teillet, M. A., Experimental analysis of the migration and differentiation of neuroblasts of the autonomic nervous system and of neuroectodermal mesenchymal derivatives, using a biological cell marking technique, *Dev. Biol.*, 41, 162, 1974.
17. Le Douarin, N. M., Renaud, D., Teillet, M. A., and Le Douarin, G. H., Cholinergic differentiation of presumptive adrenergic neuroblasts in interspecific chimeras after heterotropic transplantations, *Proc. Natl. Acad. Sci. U.S.A.*, 72, 728, 1975.
18. Mains, R. E. and Patterson, P. H., Primary cultures of dissociated sympathetic neurones. I. Establishment of long term growth in culture and studies of differentiated properties, *J. Cell Biol.*, **59**, 329, 1973.
19. Patterson, P. H. and Chun, L. L. Y., The influence of non-neuronal cells on catecholamine and acetylcholine synthesis and accumulation in cultures of dissociated sympathetic neurons, *Proc. Natl. Acad. Sci. U.S.A.*, 71, 3607, 1974.

20. Patterson, P. H. and Chun, L. L. Y., The induction of acetylcholine synthesis in primary cultures of dissociated rat sympathetic neurons. I. Effects of conditioned medium, *Dev. Biol.*, 56, 263, 1977.
21. Johnson, M., Ross, D., Meyers, M., Rees, R., Bunge, R., Wakshull, E., and Burton, H., Synaptic vesicle cytochemistry changes when cultured sympathetic neurones develop cholinergic interactions, *Nature (London)*, 262, 308, 1976.
22. Landis, S. C., Developmental changes in the neurotransmitter properties of dissociated sympathetic neurons: a cytochemical study of the effects of medium, *Dev. Biol.*, 77, 349, 1980.
23. Hill, C. E. and Hendry, I. A., Development of neurons synthesizing noradrenaline and acetylcholine in the superior cervical ganglion of the rat in vivo and in vitro, *Neurosci.*, 2, 741, 1977.
24. Ross, D., Johnson, M., and Bunge, R., Development of cholinergic characteristics in adrenergic neurones is age dependent, *Nature (London)*, 267, 536, 1977.
25. Johnson, M. I., Ross, C. D., and Bunge, R. P., Morphological and biochemical studies on the development of cholinergic properties in cultured sympathetic neurons. II. Dependence on postnatal age, *J. Cell Biol.*, 84, 692, 1980.
26. Patterson, P. H., Environmental determination of neurotransmitter function, *Trends Neurosci.*, 1, 126, 1978.
27. Coughlin, M. D., Dibner, M. D., Boyer, D. M., and Black, I. B., Factors regulating development of an embryonic mouse sympathetic ganglion, *Dev. Biol.*, 66, 513, 1978.
28. Walicke, P. A., Campenot, R. B., and Patterson, P. H., Determination of transmitter function by neuronal activity, *Proc. Natl. Acad. Sci. U.S.A.*, 74, 5767, 1977.
29. Hill, C. E. and Hendry, I. A., The influence of preganglionic nerves on the superior cervical ganglion of the rat, *Neurosci. Lett.*, 13, 133, 1979.
30. McLennan, I. S., Hill, C. E., and Hendry, I. A., Glucocorticosteroids modulate transmitter choice in developing superior cervical ganglion, *Nature (London)*, 283, 206, 1980.
31. Fukada, K., Hormonal control of neurotransmitter choice in sympathetic neurone cultures, *Nature (London)*, 287, 553, 1980.
32. Hill, C. E., Hendry, I. A., and McLennan, I. S., Factors influencing transmitter type in sympathetic ganglion cells, in *Histochemistry and Cell Biology of Autonomic Neurons, SIF Cells and Paraneurons*, Eränkö, O., Soinila, S., and Päivärinta, H., Eds., Raven Press, New York, 1980, 69.
33. Charlwood, K. A., Lamont, D. M., and Banks, B. E. C., Apparent orienting effects produced by nerve growth factor, in *Nerve Growth Factor and its Antiserum*, Zaimis, E., Ed., Athlone Press, London, 1972, 102.
34. Ebendal, T. and Jacobson, C.-O., Tests of possible role of NGF in neurite outgrowth stimulation exerted by glial cells and heart explants in culture, *Brain Res.*, 131, 373, 1977.
35. Campenot, R. B., Local control of neurite development by nerve growth factor, *Proc. Natl. Acad. Sci. U.S.A.*, 74, 4516, 1977.
36. Letourneau, P. C., Chemotactic response of nerve fiber elongation to nerve growth factor, *Dev. Biol.*, 66, 183, 1978.
37. Levi-Montalcini, R., Meyer, H., and Hamburger, V., *In vitro* experiments on the effects of mouse sarcomas 180 and 37 on the spinal and sympathetic ganglia of the chick embryo, *Cancer Res.*, 14, 49, 1954.
38. Chamley, J. H., Goller, I., and Burnstock, G., Selective growth of sympathetic nerve fibers to explants of normally densely innervated autonomic effector organs in tissue culture, *Dev. Biol.*, 31, 362, 1973.
39. Chamley, J. H. and Dowel, J. J., Specificity of nerve fibre "attraction" to autonomic effector organs in tissue culture, *Exp. Cell Res.*, 90, 1, 1975.
40. Rawdon, B. B. and Dockray, G. J., Directional growth of sympathetic nerve fibres *in vitro* towards enteric smooth muscle and heart from mice with congenital aganglionic colon and their normal littermates, *Dev. Brain Res.*, 7, 53, 1983.
41. Southwell, B. R., Chamley-Campbell, J. H., and Campbell, G. R., Tropic interactions between sympathetic nerves and vascular smooth muscle, *J. Autonom. Nerv. Syst.*, 13, 343, 1985.
42. Barth, E.-M., Korsching, S., and Thoenen, H., Regulation of nerve growth factor synthesis and release in organ cultures of rat iris, *J. Cell Biol.*, 99, 839, 1984.
43. Johnson, D. G., Gorden, P., and Kopin, I. J., A sensitive radioimmunoassay for 7S nerve growth factor antigens in serum and tissues, *J. Neurochem.*, 18, 2355, 1971.
44. Korsching, S. and Thoenen, H., Nerve growth factor in sympathetic ganglia and corresponding target organs of the rat: correlation with density of sympathetic innervation, *Proc. Natl. Acad. Sci. U.S.A.*, 80, 3513, 1983.
45. Ebendal, T. and Jacobson, C.-O., Tissue explants affecting extension and orientation of axons in cultured chick embryo ganglia, *Exp. Cell Res.*, 105, 379, 1977b.
46. Ebendal, T., Stage-dependent stimulation of neurite outgrowth exerted by nerve growth factor and chick heart in cultured embryonic ganglia, *Dev. Biol.*, 72, 276, 1979.

47. Bueker, E. D., Implantation of tumors in the hindlimb field of the embryonic chick and the developmental response of the lumbosacral nervous system, *Anat. Rec.*, 102, 369, 1948.
48. Levi-Montalcini, R., Effects of mouse tumor transplantation on the nervous system, *Ann. N.Y. Acad. Sci.*, 55, 330, 1952.
49. Levi-Montalcini, R. and Hamburger, V., A diffusible agent of mouse sarcoma producing hyperplasia of sympathetic ganglia and hyperneurotization of viscera in the chick embryo, *J. Exp. Zool.*, 123, 223, 1953.
50. Menesini Chen, M. G., Chen, J. S., and Levi-Montalcini, R., Sympathetic nerve fibers ingrowth in the central nervous system of neonatal rodent upon intracerebral NGF injections, *Arch. Ital. Biol.*, 116, 53, 1978.
51. Coughlin, M. D., Early development of parasympathetic nerves in the mouse submandibular gland, *Dev. Biol.*, 43, 123, 1975.
52. Coughlin, M. D., Target organ stimulation of parasympathetic nerve growth in the developing mouse submandibular gland, *Dev. Biol.*, 43, 140, 1975.
53. Coughlin, M. D. and Rathbone, M. P., Factors involved in the stimulation of parasympathetic nerve outgrowth, *Dev. Biol.*, 61, 131, 1977.
54. Coughlin, M. D., Bloom, E. M., and Black, I. B., Characterization of a neuronal growth factor from mouse heart-cell-conditioned medium, *Dev. Biol.*, 82, 56, 1981.
55. Helfand, S. L., Smith, G. A., and Wessells, N. K., Survival and development in culture of dissociated parasympathetic neurons from ciliary ganglia, *Dev. Biol.*, 50, 541, 1976.
56. Hooisma, J., Slaaf, D. W., Meeter, E., and Stevens, W. F., The innervation of chick striated muscle fibers by the chick ciliary ganglion in tissue culture, *Brain Res.*, 85, 79, 1975.
57. Nishi, R. and Berg, D. K., Dissociated ciliary ganglion neurons *in vitro:* survival and synapse formation, *Proc. Natl. Acad. Sci. U.S.A.*, 74, 5171, 1977.
58. White, W. B. and Bennett, M. R., The survival and development of cholinergic neurons in the presence of striated muscle *in vitro*, *Brain Res.*, 159, 379, 1978.
59. Bennett, M. R. and Nurcombe, V., The survival and development of cholinergic neurons in skeletal muscle conditioned media, *Brain Res.*, 173, 543, 1979.
60. Varon, S., Manthorpe, M., and Adler, R., Cholinergic neuronotrophic factors. I. Survival, neurite outgrowth and choline acetyltransferase activity in monolayer cultures from chick embryo ciliary ganglia, *Brain Res.*, 173, 29, 1979.
61. Ebendal, T., Belew, M., Jacobson, C.-O., and Porath, J., Neurite outgrowth elicited by embryonic chick heart: partial purification of the active factor, *Neurosci. Lett.*, 14, 91, 1979.
62. McLennan, I. S. and Hendry, I. A., Parasympathetic neuronal survival induced by factors from muscle, *Neurosci. Lett.*, 10, 269, 1978.
63. McLennan, I. S. and Hendry, I. A., Influence of cardiac extracts on cultured ciliary ganglia, *Dev. Neurosci.*, 3, 1, 1980.
64. Tuttle, J. B., Suszkiw, J. B., and Ard, M., Long-term survival and development of dissociated parasympathetic neurons in culture, *Brain Res.*, 183, 161, 1980.
65. Bonyhady, R. E., Hendry, I. A., Hill, C. E., and McLennan, I. S., Characterization of a cardiac muscle factor required for the survival of cultured parasympathetic neurones, *Neurosci. Lett.*, 18, 197, 1980.
66. Letourneau, P. C., Possible roles for cell-to-substratum adhesion in neuronal morphogenesis, *Dev. Biol.*, 44, 77, 1975.
67. Letourneau, P. C., Cell-to-substratum adhesion and guidance of axonal elongation, *Dev. Biol.*, 44, 92, 1975.
68. Sidman, R. L. and Wessells, N. K., Control of direction of growth during elongation of neurites, *Exp. Neurol.*, 48, 237, 1975.
69. Moscona, A. A., Cell recognition in embryonic morphogenesis and the problem of neuronal specificities, in *Neuronal Recognition*, Barfondes, S. H., Ed., Plenum Press, New York, 1976, 205.
70. Chamley, J. H. and Campbell, G. R., Isolated ureteral smooth muscle cells in culture. Including their interaction with intrinsic and extrinsic nerves, *Cytobiologie Z. Exp. Zellforsch.*, 11, 358, 1975.
71. Chamley, J. H., Campbell, G. R., and Burnstock, G., Dedifferentiation, redifferentiation and bundle formation of smooth muscle cells in tissue culture: the influence of cell number and nerve fibres, *J. Embryol. Exp. Morphol.*, 32, 297, 1974.
72. Cook, R. D. and Peterson, E. R., The growth of smooth muscle and sympathetic ganglia in organotypic tissue cultures (light and electron microscopy), *J. Neurol. Sci.*, 22, 25, 1974.
73. Crain, S. M. and Peterson, E. R., Development of neural connections in culture, *Ann. N.Y. Acad. Sci.*, 228, 6, 1974.
74. Chamley, J. H. and Campbell, G. R., Tissue culture: interaction between sympathetic nerves and vascular smooth muscle, in *Vascular Neuroeffector Mechanisms*, Proc. 2nd Int. Symp., Odense, Bevan, J. A., Burnstock, G., Johansson, B., Maxwell, R. A., and Nedergaard, O. A., Eds., S. Karger, Basel, 1976, 10.

75. Chamley, J. H. and Campbell, G. R., Trophic influence of sympathetic nerves and cyclic AMP on differentiation and proliferation of isolated smooth muscle cells in culture, *Cell Tissue Res.*, 161, 497, 1975.
76. Mark, G. E., Chamley, J. H., and Burnstock, G., Interactions between autonomic nerves and smooth and cardiac muscle cells in tissue culture, *Dev. Biol.*, 32, 194, 1973.
77. Chamley, J. H., Campbell, G. R., and Burnstock, G., An analysis of the interactions between sympathetic nerve fibres and smooth muscle cells in tissue culture, *Dev. Biol.*, 33, 344, 1973.
78. Campbell, G. R., Chamley, J. H., and Burnstock, G., Lack of effect of receptor blockers on the formation of long-lasting associations between sympathetic nerves and cardiac muscle cells *in vitro*, *Cell Tissue Res.*, 187, 551, 1978.
79. Bevan, J. A., Bevan, R. D., Purdy, R. E., Robinson, C. P., Su, C., and Waterson, J. G., Comparison of adrenergic mechanisms in an elastic and a muscular artery of the rabbit, *Circ. Res.*, 30, 541, 1972.
80. Hill, C. E., Purves, R. D., Watanabe, H., and Burnstock, G., Specificity of innervation of iris musculature by sympathetic nerve fibres in tissue culture, *Pfluegers Arch.*, 361, 127, 1976.
81. Purves, R. D., Hill, C. E., Chamley, J. H., Mark, G. E., Fry, D. M., and Burnstock, G., Functional autonomic neuromuscular junctions in tissue culture, *Pfluegers Arch.*, 350, 1, 1974.
82. Furshpan, E. J., MacLeish, P. R., O'Lague, P. H., and Potter, D. D., Chemical transmission between rat sympathetic neurons and cardiac myocytes developing in micro-cultures: evidence for cholinergic, adrenergic, and dual-function neurons, *Proc. Natl. Acad. Sci. U.S.A.*, 73, 4225, 1976.
83. Johnson, M. I., Ross, C. D., Meyers, M., Spitznagel, E. L., and Bunge, R. P., Morphological and biochemical studies on the development of cholinergic properties in cultured sympathetic neurons. I. Correlative changes in choline acetyltransferase and synaptic vesicle cytochemistry, *J. Cell Biol.*, 84, 680, 1980.
84. O'Lague, P. H., Obata, K., Claude, P., Furshpan, E. J., and Potter, D. D., Evidence for cholinergic synapses between dissociated rat sympathetic neurons in cell culture, *Proc. Natl. Acad. Sci. U.S.A.*, 71, 3602, 1974.
85. Nurse, C. A. and O'Lague, P. H., Formation of cholinergic synapses between dissociated sympathetic neurons and skeletal myotubes of the rat in cell culture, *Proc. Natl. Acad. Sci. U.S.A.*, 72, 1955, 1975.
86. Stevens, W. F., Slaaf, D. W., Hooisma, J., Magchielse, T., and Meeter, E., Target recognition and synapse formation by ciliary-ganglion neurons in tissue culture, *Biochem. Soc. Trans.*, 6, 487, 1978.

Chapter 18

VASOACTIVE HORMONE RECEPTOR EXPRESSION IN CULTURED VASCULAR SMOOTH MUSCLE CELLS

Michael A. Gimbrone, Jr. and R. Wayne Alexander

TABLE OF CONTENTS

I. INTRODUCTION

The vascular actions of hormones, such as angiotensin II and norepinephrine, are mediated primarily through interactions with specific receptors in vascular smooth muscle cells (VSMC). Expression of these receptors by VSMC in different vascular beds and their coupling to cellular contractile mechanisms thus potentially have important implications for normal vascular physiology and the pathophysiology of hypertension. Although pharmacological and biochemical studies in whole animals and excised vascular tissues have helped to identify and characterize receptors for a number of vasoactive substances, until recently, the cellular localization of these receptors, biochemical correlates of their activation, and factors regulating their expression in VSMC have not been well defined, in part due to the structural complexity of blood vessels. Selective isolation and in vitro cultivation of the cellular components of blood vessels has provided a useful approach to this problem.[1-10]

In this chapter, we briefly summarize the efforts of our laboratories over the last 5 years to study vasoactive hormone receptors in cultured VSMC. We review the approach we have taken for isolating *functional* VSMC from muscular, resistance-type arteries and other sources and their use for studies of the mechanisms of receptor expression, regulation, and activation-response coupling at the cellular level. The related cell biology issue of *phenotypic modulation* in cultured VSMC and its potential relevance to such studies is also considered.

II. ISOLATION AND CULTURE OF FUNCTIONAL VSMC

Historically, large fibroelastic arteries, such as the aorta and its proximal branches, have been the preferred sources of VSMC for culture.[2,6,7] Primarily this was due to their relative accessibility and the anatomical fact that the inner one third of the medial layer of these vessels normally does not contain other cell types. In addition, VSMC from aortic media explants typically undergo a series of morphological and biochemical changes in culture which mimic certain events observed in the development of atherosclerotic lesions, thus potentially providing a useful in vitro model for this disease process.[11-13] These phenotypic changes, which include increased proliferative and biosynthetic activity, as well as ultrastructural and biochemical alterations in cytoskeletal elements, also are correlated with decreased contractile responsiveness to various vasoactive hormones (reviewed in Chamley-Campbell et al.).[9] In general, the tendency for explant-cultured, large-vessel VSMC to undergo such changes has limited their usefulness for in vitro studies of vasoactive hormone action.

As an approach to this problem, we have applied the technique of enzymatic dissociation[4,6,7] to the rat mesenteric arterial arcade, a highly reactive, smooth-muscle-rich, resistance-type vascular bed, to isolate a population of viable, functionally intact VSMC for culture.[14] By various morphological, immunochemical, and biochemical criteria, these VSMC cultures are essentially free of contamination by other cell types (e.g., endothelial cells and fibroblasts) and exhibit features characteristic of VSMC in situ.[14] In parallel studies with homogenates prepared from the same vascular source,[15,16] we have documented the presence of specific, high-affinity binding sites for certain vasoactive hormones of interest, including angiotensin II (Ang II), thus providing a direct basis for in vivo/in vitro comparisons. In our initial studies,[16-20] as discussed in detail below, we documented the retention of specific high affinity Ang II binding sites in VSMC isolated from rat mesenteric artery which had proliferated in response to serum growth factors and had undergone certain morphologic changes consistent with phenotypic modulation.[9] Furthermore, at least a portion of these cellular Ang II binding sites were functional receptors, as evidenced by the stimulation of

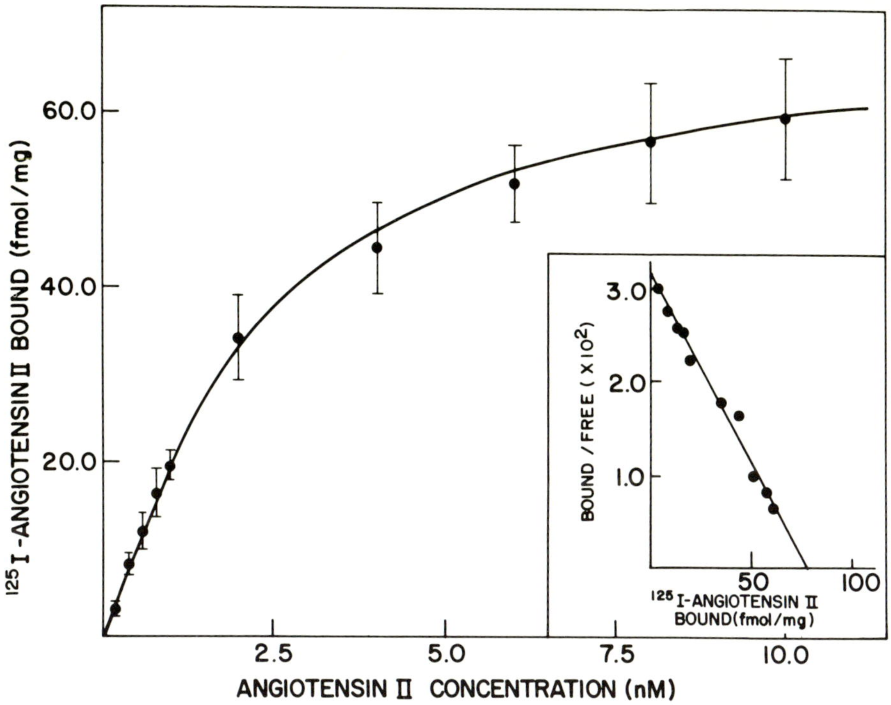

FIGURE 1. Saturation binding curve of ^{125}I-angiotensin II to suspended, intact rat mesenteric arterial SMC after 7 days in culture. Each point represents the mean ±1 SD from five experiments. The inset shows the Scatchard analysis of this data and demonstrates that ^{125}I-angiotensin II binds to a single class ($K_D = 2.8 \pm 0.2$ n*M*) of saturable ($B_{max} = 81.5 \pm 5.0$ fmol/mg) binding sites. (Reproduced from *The Journal of Cell Biology*, 1982, Vol. 92, pp. 289-298, by copyright permission of The Rockefeller University Press.)

myosin light chain phosphorylation and visible cellular contraction at physiological concentrations of Ang II.[17-19] In addition, these cultures produce prostaglandins in response to Ang II[19] and have a catecholamine- and prostaglandin-stimulated adenylate cyclase system.[20] Therefore, despite their altered morphologic appearance (principally their cytoskeletal ultrastructure[14]) important biochemical steps in receptor-activation-contraction coupling appear to be retained in these cultured rat mesenteric artery VSMC, thus making them a potentially useful in vitro model. Although these initial studies focused on the Ang II receptor system in rat mesenteric artery VSMC in primary culture, we have applied a similar enzymatic dissociation method[14,21,22] to obtain VSMC from rat and rabbit aorta. These VSMC from rat and rabbit aorta continue to express biochemically coupled Ang II and α-adrenergic receptors, respectively, even after serial propagation in culture, although they typically do not undergo visible contraction (see later).

III. RECEPTOR EXPRESSION IN CULTURED VSMC

A. Angiotensin II Receptor Expression in Rat VSMC

As mentioned earlier, primary cultures of enzymatically dissociated rat mesenteric arterial VSMC express ^{125}I-Ang II binding sites which have characteristics of saturability and specificity expected of physiologic Ang II receptors[14,15] (Figures 1 and 2). Ang II receptor expression in the mesenteric VSMC is stable for at least 20 days in primary culture.[14] These cells, however, do not lend themselves readily to extensive subcultur-

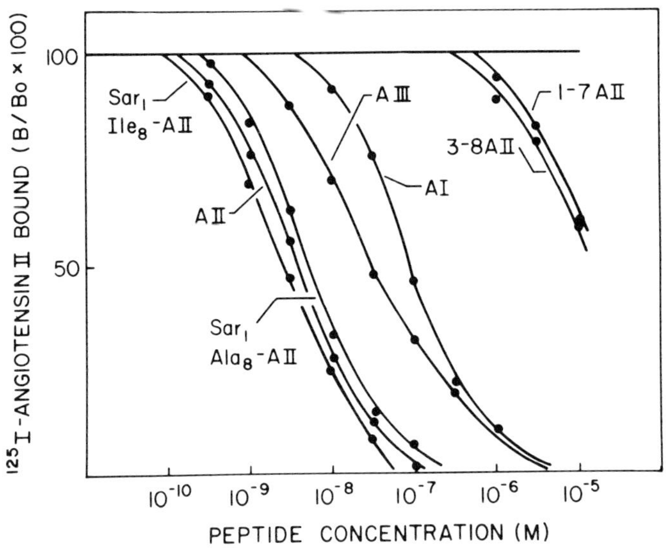

FIGURE 2. Specificity of ^{125}I-angiotensin II binding sites in cultured rat mesenteric arterial SMC. The order of potency of Ang II (A-II), Ang III (AIII), Ang I (AI) and the synthetic analogues sarcosine$_1$, isoleucine$_8$-Ang II (Sar$_1$ Ile$_8$ AII) and sarcosine$_1$, alanine$_8$-Ang II (Sar$_1$ Ala$_8$ AII) is identical with that expected from pharmacologic experiments in intact vessels. The physiologically inactive hexapeptide and heptapeptide interact with the receptors only at very high concentrations. (Reproduced from *The Journal of Cell Biology,* 1982, Vol. 92, pp. 289-298, by copyright permission of The Rockefeller University Press.)

ing. In contrast, the enzymatically dissociated rat aortic VSMC not only can be passaged extensively, but also continue to express Ang II receptors in relatively high density after 20 to 25 subcultures. The density of Ang II receptors in the aortic VSMC (primary and passaged) is generally higher than in the mesenteric arterial VSMC (100 — 150 × 10^3 sites per cell [unpublished observations] vs. 40 — 45 × 10^3 sites per cell,[14] respectively).

B. Biological Correlates of Angiotensin II Binding to VSMC

Ang II receptors in cultured VSMC are functional and are coupled to several intracellular biochemical events likely related to the contractile response in vivo. These events include the breakdown of membrane phospholipids, cation (Ca^{++} and Na^+) translocation, and protein phosphorylation.

C. Angiotensin II-Mediated Phosphoinositide Breakdown in VSMC

It has been known for many years that certain hormones stimulate the turnover of phosphatidylinositol in cell membranes.[23] Michell in 1975 suggested that the breakdown of the phosphorylated derivative of PI, phosphatidylinositol 4,5 bisphosphate (PIP_2) plays a pivotal role in calcium mobilization for a variety of hormones (reviewed in Reference 25). The breakdown of PIP_2 by hormonal activation of phospholipase C results in the generation of both the water-soluble inositol trisphosphate (IP_3), which releases Ca^{++} from intracellular stores[25] and the lipophylic Sn 1,2-diacylglycerol (DAG) which acts as a second messenger to activate the phospholipid, Ca^{++}-dependent enzyme protein kinase C (reviewed in Reference 26). Recent evidence suggests that phosphoinositide breakdown is one of the earliest consequences of Ang II receptor activation in cultured vascular smooth muscle. Thus, Ang II stimulates the rapid (<5 sec) break-

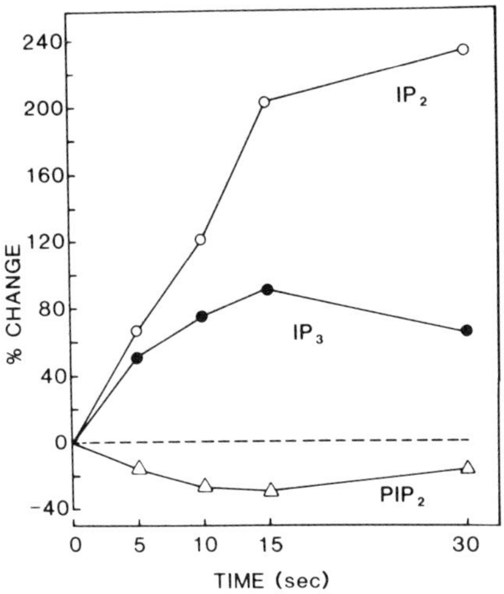

FIGURE 3. Time course of Ang II-mediated changes in phosphoinositide metabolism in subcultured rat aortic SMC. Cells were labeled with $^{32}P_i$ (60 min) for determination of phosphatidylinositol 4,5 bisphosphate (PIP_2) or with [^3H]-myosinositol (48 hr) for determination of inositol trisphosphate (IP_3) or inositol bisphosphate (IP_2). Ang II concentration was 100 n*M*. (From Alexander, R. W., Brock, T. A., Gimbrone, M. A., Jr., and Rittenhouse, S. E., *Hypertension,* 7, 447, 1985. By permission of the American Heart Association.)

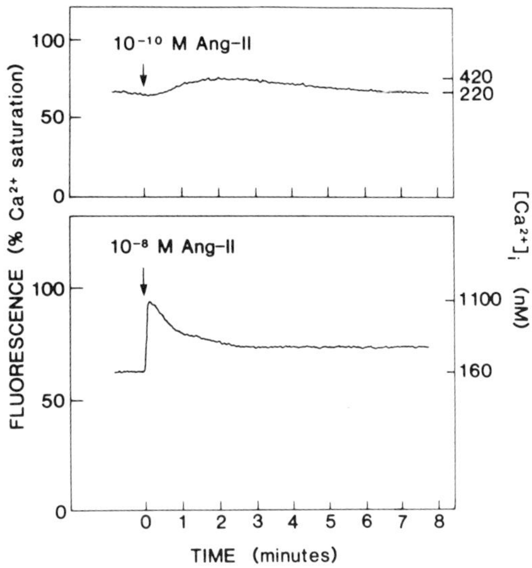

FIGURE 4. Ang II induced changes in cytosolic-free Ca^{++} in cultured rat aortic SMC as measured with quin 2. Upper panel shows the typical fluorescence response to 10^{-10} *M* Ang II, while lower panel shows to response to 10^{-8} *M*. The calculated values for $[Ca^{2+}]_i$ are indicated at the right. (From Brock, T. A., Alexander, R. W., Ekstein, L. S., Atkinson, W. J., and Gimbrone, M. A., Jr., *Hypertension,* 7(3), 105, 1984. By permission of the American Heart Association.)

down of PIP_2 to IP_3 (Figure 3).[27] IP_3 formation is concentration-dependent with detectable increases noted at Ang II concentrations of less than 1 n*M*.[27] Ang II also stimulates the formation of DAG, but, unlike IP_3 which has returned toward basal concentrations after 2 to 5 min,[27] increased DAG levels are sustained for at least 20 min.[28] It is likely that the source of DAG shifts from PIP_2 at early (<2 min) time points to PI at later times.[28] These data raise the possibility that DAG, possibly by stimulating protein kinase C, is involved in the sustained, tonic contractile response in intact blood vessels. Protein kinase C-mediated mechanisms are operative in Ang II-mediated responses in VSMC, as will be discussed later.

D. Angiotensin II-Mediated Cation (Ca^{++} and Na^+) Translocation in VSMC

A major consequence of agonist-induced contraction in blood vessels is the transient elevation of cytosolic-free calcium.[29] We have utilized the Ca^{++} sensitive tetracarboxylate dye, quin 2, to characterize Ang II-induced changes in cytosolic-free Ca in VSMC. Ang II causes a rapid (onset <5 sec), concentration-dependent increase $[Ca^{++}]_i$ in VSMC (Figure 4).[21] The EC_{50} for Ang II for this response is ∼0.5 n*M*.[21] The peak $[Ca^{++}]_i$ is not sustained, but gradually falls back toward, but usually not to, baseline over the next 5 to 10 min. In the absence of extracellular calcium, the peak response is modestly attentuated, but $[Ca^{++}]_i$ rapidly returns to basal values.[21] Studies with VSMC loaded with $^{45}Ca^{++}$ showed that Ang II induces a rapid efflux of calcium from the cell.[30] Taken together, these data are consistent with the formulation that Ang II induces the rapid release, probably via IP_3, of Ca^{++} from intracellular storage sites that most likely are in the endoplasmic reticulum. The resulting increase in $[Ca^{++}]_i$ is likely associated

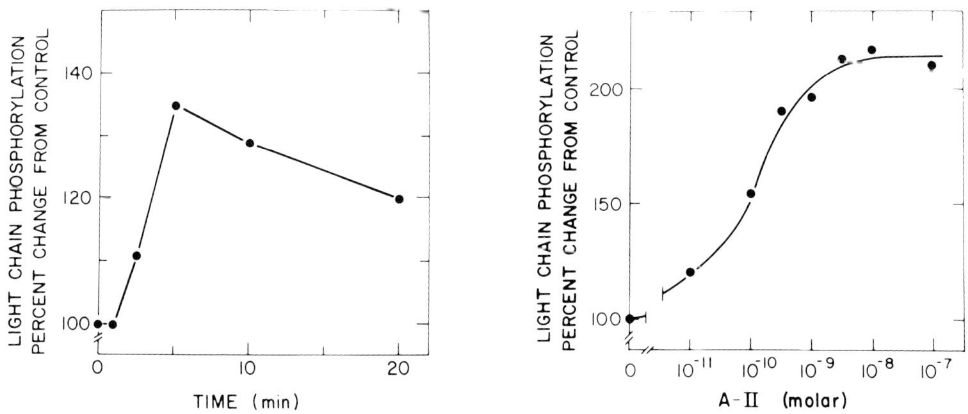

FIGURE 5. Time and concentration dependence of the Ang II-induced phosphorylation of the myosin light chain in cultured rat mesenteric arterial SMC. Left panel demonstrates the rapid phosphorylation and the spontaneous dephosphorylation of the myosin light chain induced by 0.1 n*M* Ang II. Right panel illustrates the concentration-response relationship for Ang II-mediated phosphorylation measured at 4 min. (From Anderson, J. M., Gimbrone, M. A., Jr., and Alexander, R. W., *J. Biol. Chem.*, 256, 4693, 1981. With permission.)

with activation of calcium-calmodulin-dependent mechanisms, including activation of myosin light chain kinase[31] and plasma membrane Ca^{++} pumps.[32] The pumping of Ca^{++} out of the cell is probably an important mechanism accounting for the transient nature of the high $[Ca^{++}]_i$ after initial agonist stimulation since there is evidence that, in the continued presence of agonist, intracellular storage sites do not refill until desensitization or tachyphylaxis has occurred.[43]

Ang II also stimulates Na^+ influx into cultured rat aortic SMC.[33] The mechanisms and implications of this influx have not been delineated. However, since diacylglycerol is produced and protein kinase C is presumably activated by Ang II, the Na^+ influx may represent activation of a protein kinase C activated Na^+/H^+ antiport.[34] The alkalinization of the cytosol which might result from the activity of this putative cation exchanger could be important in controlling the activity of pH-sensitive processes involved in tonic responses of vascular smooth muscle to agonists. In addition, the Na^+ influx could be important in Na^+/Ca^{++} exchange mechanisms.

E. Protein Phosphorylation in Cultured VSMC

Regulation of protein function by phosphorylation is a general mechanism of physiologic control of a wide variety of cellular processes. There are at least three major general classes of protein kinases which are thought to be involved in vascular smooth muscle function, and there is evidence that each is expressed in cultured VSMC. Calcium-calmodulin-dependent protein kinases mediate phosphorylation reactions involved in control of cellular functions by calcium mobilizing hormones, such as Ang II. Myosin light chain kinase, which phosphorylates the myosin light chain of vascular smooth muscle (thus initiating contraction), is a calcium-calmodulin-dependent enzyme. Ang II stimulates phosphorylation of the myosin light chain, which is time- and concentration-dependent (Figure 5).[17] This phosphorylation is inhibited by the calmodulin inhibitor chlorpromazine.[17] The second group of protein kinases is cAMP-dependent and mediates vasodilator function of hormones stimulating adenylate cyclase. The myosin light chain kinase is inhibited by cAMP, and dibutryl cAMP inhibits myosin light chain phosphorylation in VSMC. Protein kinase C is a Ca^{++} and phosphatidyl-serine dependent kinase which is activated by diacylglycerol produced by the phospholipase C-mediated hydrolysis of phosphoinositides.[26] Protein kinase C is acti-

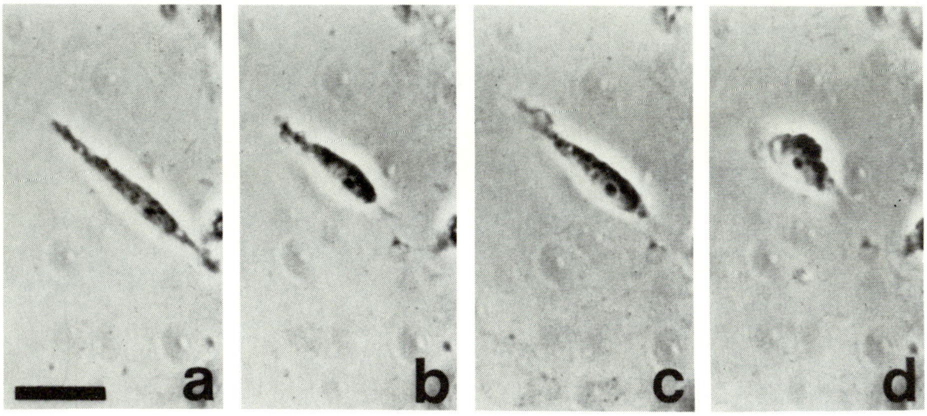

FIGURE 6. Phase contrast photomicrographs of contractile response of isolated rat mesenteric artery VSMC in primary culture (bar = 20 μm). (a) Control medium; (b) 1 min after infusion of 10 n*M* Ang II — cell has shortened to 65% of original length; (c) 10 min washout with control medium — note partial relaxation; (d) 3 min after rechallenge with 10 n*M* Ang II — note further shortening. (Reproduced from *The Journal of Cell Biology,* 1982, Vol. 92, pp. 289-298, by copyright permission of The Rockefeller University Press.)

vated by phorbol esters which are thought to substitute for endogenous diacylglycerol. Phorbol esters inhibit Ang II-induced IP_3 generation and calcium release in rat aortic VSMC,[35] suggesting that endogenous diacylglycerol serves as a feedback inhibitor to terminate agonist-mediated PIP_2 breakdown.

F. Contraction of VSMC in Culture

Primary cultures of enzymatically dissociated rat mesenteric artery VSMC will contract in response to Ang II (Figure 6).[14] Responsiveness usually was maximal (30% of cells responsive) at 3 days in culture, but diminished greatly during subsequent cell proliferation. Contractile responsiveness to hormone was again manifested after confluence was reached in a manner similar to that described previously for other VSMC culture systems.[9]

Subcultured rat mesenteric artery or aortic VSMC have not been observed to contract, except when plated under a layer of collagen, on top of which a monolayer of endothelial cells has been grown (Figure 7). In the absence of endothelium, the VSMC are fibroblast-like in morphology, appear to proliferate extensively, and are unresponsive to Ang II. Within 24 hr after the seeding of an overlying monolayer of endothelial cells, the VSMC change morphologically and develop a distinctly bipolar appearance. Furthermore, a significant number of these cells now contract in response to Ang II.[44]

The data in this and preceeding sections provide evidence that biochemical mechanisms necessary for angiotensin-induced contraction of intact blood vessels, up to and including the phosphorylation of the myosin light chain, are expressed in enzymatically dissociated rat aortic and mesenteric artery VSMC in both primary- and subcultures. In spite of the presence of the functional enzymatic machinery required for contraction, contraction appears to occur only when the cells are not in a proliferative mode, either before they have begun to divide or after they are confluent, or when they have been exposed to the differentiating influence of endothelium (see Volume I, Chapter 4; also, later).[41]

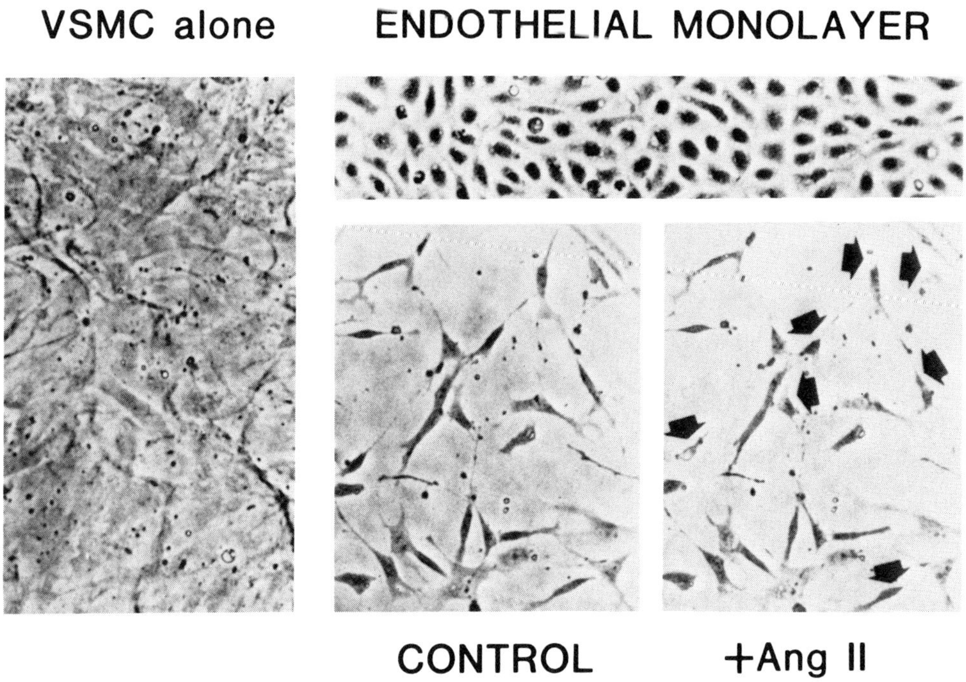

FIGURE 7. Influence of vascular endothelial cells on VSMC morphology and contractile responsiveness to Ang II. (Far left panel) subcultured rat aortic VSMC plated on plastic culture dish with collagen (Vitrogen) gel overlay. Note dense growth of cells with fibroblast-like morphology. (Top panel) monolayer of bovine aortic endothelial cells seeded on top of collagen gel/VSMC culture. (Lower left panel) note bipolar appearance of VSMC when cultured beneath endothelial/collagen gel overlay. (Control = no added Ang II.) (Lower right panel) contractile response of VSMC (arrows), in same field as lower left panel, 5 min after addition of 10 n*M* Ang II to the co-culture.[44]

G. α-Adrenergic Receptors

Although α_1-adrenergic receptors are present in both the rat aorta and mesenteric arteries, neither primary cultures of aortic or mesenteric VSMC nor subcultured aortic VSMC express α_1-receptors. In contrast, subcultured rabbit aortic VSMC express α_1-receptors in moderately high-density ($\sim$100 fmol/mg) protein.[22] These receptors stimulate release of calcium from intracellular storage sites and are down-regulated by α_1-adrenergic catecholamines.[22] These receptors have a nonlinear occupancy response relationship for mediation of Ca^{++} flux.[36] We have not detected α_2-adrenergic receptors in cultured vascular smooth muscle cells (SMC).

H. Muscarinic Cholinergic Receptors

Muscarinic cholinergic receptors are present in relatively high density in primary cultures of rat mesenteric VSMC,[37] but not in subcultured rat aortic VSMC. The mesenteric VSMC cholinergic receptors are coupled to a guanine nucleotide regulatory protein, but do not inhibit adenylate cyclase.[37] These receptors weakly stimulate $^{45}Ca^{++}$ efflux in these cells.

I. Receptors Stimulating Adenylate Cyclase

Rat aortic and mesenteric VSMC have α-adrenergic, prostaglandin E_1, and vasoactive intestinal peptide receptors as evidenced by the ability of these agonists to stimulate cyclic AMP accumulation in these cells.[20,38] These receptors have not been characterized by ligand binding techniques.

IV. PHENOTYPIC MODULATION IN CULTURED VSMC

VSMC in culture appear especially susceptible to phenotypic modulation: a potentially reversible change in differentiated functional status, as defined by various morphological, biochemical, and immunological criteria.[9] This process has a number of implications for in vitro studies of vasoactive hormone responsiveness, as well as VSMC pathobiology.

In cultured VSMC, loss of contractile responsiveness to a given agonist may be the simple consequence of loss of appropriate cell surface receptors. As discussed above and illustrated in Table 1, the pattern of expression of specific vasoactive hormone receptors by SMC cultured from different vessels is extremely variable. A given VSMC culture may continue to express functional receptors for a certain agonist after loosing receptors for another agonist to which it is normally responsive in vivo. For example, subcultured rat aortic VSMC retain coupled Ang II receptors,[21] but lack α_1-adrenergic binding sites. The reasons for this variability in receptor expression in certain cultured VSMC remain incompletely understood but most probably relate to a lack of appropriate trophic stimuli in vitro.

Global contractile unresponsiveness, characteristically seen with explant outgrowth aortic VSMC or subcultured VSMC from many sources, may indicate disruption of more distal, common pathways of stimulus-response coupling or of the contractile apparatus per se. Indeed, alterations in the contractile components of the cytoskeleton of cultured VSMC are a common occurrence and can have various morphological, biochemical, and immunochemical manifestations.[9] For example, primary rat mesenteric artery VSMC cultures typically lack ultrastructurally demonstrable, myosin-containing thick (12 to 18 nm diameter) filaments, and show alterations in smooth-muscle-type and nonmuscle-type myosin immunofluorescent staining, while their total myosin content remains unchanged.[14,39] Despite these alterations, as described above, a significant proportion of these cells continue to respond to physiological concentrations of Ang II with biochemically detectable myosin light chain phosphorylation and microscopically visible, reversible cellular contraction. In contrast, VSMC isolated from other vascular sources and species have been reported to undergo both quantitative and qualitative changes in myosin expression which appear to be related to growth status and population density in culture.[6,9] It is noteworthy that heterogeneity in myosin antigenic expression has been described in vivo in VSMC at different vascular sites in various species.[40] The possible explanations for this observation (e.g., expression of different gene products, myosin *isozymes*, vs. post-translational alterations in a single myosin species) are a matter of ongoing investigation (see Chapter 5). These and related studies should be aided by the development and application of appropriate molecular biological probes to analyze patterns of gene expression in VSMC in culture and *in situ*.

The phenomenon of phenotypic modulation in cultured VSMC, with its various biochemical and morphological manifestations, raises a number of interesting cell biology issues. It has been suggested that this process represents an intrinsic cellular response to an altered environment and, further, that phenotypic status, susceptibility to mitogens, and cell proliferation are causally interrelated.[9,12,41] This working concept has been especially useful in studies of the pathogenesis of atherosclerosis.[41,42] In the context of normal and altered vasoactive hormone responsiveness, the phenotypic modulation observed in cultured VSMC might also be considered a consequence of altered trophic stimuli. Indeed, the act of isolating VSMC from the vessel wall and maintaining them in a petri dish constitutes a form of "neuroendocrine ablation" experiment. Relevant trophic stimuli normally derived in vivo from autonomic innervation or interactions with extracellular matrix components or other vascular cells (e.g., endothe-

Table 1
VASOACTIVE HORMONE RECEPTOR EXPRESSION IN CULTURED VASCULAR SMOOTH MUSCLE CELLS

Receptor type	Rat mesenteric artery (primary)	Rat aortic (subcultured)	Rat aortic (neonatal)	Bovine aortic (enzyme-dissociated)	Bovine aortic (explant)	Rabbit aortic (subcultured)	Comments	Ref.
Angiotensin II	++	+++	ND	–	+	ND	Robust Ca^{++} flux and phosphatidyl inositol response in rat aortic cells	14, 19,21,27,28,30
α_1-Adrenergic	–	–	+	ND	ND	+++	Ca^{++} efflux easily measured in rabbit arotic cells	22,36,45
α_2-Adrenergic	–	–	ND	ND	ND	–		45
Muscarinic cholinergic	+++	+/–	ND	ND	ND	ND	Stimulates Ca^{++} Flux but does not inhibit adenylate cyclase in rat mesenteric cells	37,46
5-HT_2	ND	++	ND	ND	ND	+	Robust Ca^{++} signal in rat aortic cells	45

Note: Receptor density: +++, high; +, low; –, absent; ND, not determined.

lium) are typically lacking under standard in vitro culture conditions. Interestingly, co-cultivation with vascular endothelial cells, as well as treatment with aortic tissue extracts or commercial preparations of heparin, have been reported to inhibit spontaneous modulation of phenotype in cultured aortic VSMC.[42] As discussed above and illustrated in Figure 7, the morphology of subcultured rat aortic VSMC is dramatically altered, and their contractile responsiveness to Ang II is restored following co-culture with vascular endothelial cells. The potential interactions of SMC and endothelial cells in this setting undoubtedly are complex and are worthy of further study.

In conclusion, phenotypic modulation of VSMC in culture poses both practical difficulties and conceptual challenges. As they become better understood, the factors influencing the expression of altered phenotypes may provide new insights into developmental and pathophysiologic mechanisms in vascular smooth muscle.

V. SUMMARY AND FUTURE DIRECTIONS

As the experimental observations summarized in this chapter illustrate, VSMC cultured from different blood vessels and species can be fruitfully employed for the in vitro study of vasoactive hormone responsiveness. In particular, the regulation of expression of specific cell surface receptors and the biochemical processes involved in their activation-response coupling can be readily examined in cultured VSMC. The use of whole, living cells, in which dynamic feedback regulatory mechanisms remain intact, also permits study of the integration of multiple (synergistic or antagonistic) stimuli at the cellular level. The collective properties of mass cultures can be examined biochemically or the responses of individual cells assessed microscopically. Furthermore, through the application of co-culture techniques (see Chapter 15), the reciprocal interactions of the two principal cellular components of blood vessels, endothelium and smooth muscle (and potentially other cell types), can be effectively investigated. Looking to the future, homogenous cultures of VSMC will undoubtedly provide valuable raw materials for development of molecular biological probes to analyze various aspects of gene expression, both in vitro and in vivo.

Although considerable progress has been made relating to the theme of this chapter, several basic questions remain unanswered. What are the necessary trophic stimuli for the in vitro maintenance of *functional differentiation* of VSMC? What are the relative contributions of cell-cell interactions and matrix-cell interactions to this process? Do the altered phenotypes displayed by VSMC in culture bear any relationship to pathophysiologic processes that occur in blood vessels *in vivo*? Indeed, can studies like those described in this chapter provide useful insights into the pathogenesis of disease states such as atherosclerosis and hypertension which primarily involve vascular smooth muscle cells? Hopefully, the answers to these and other important questions in vascular biology and pathobiology will be forthcoming through the application of appropriate in vitro model systems utilizing cultured vascular smooth muscle cells.

ACKNOWLEDGMENTS

The following colleagues and co-workers have contributed over the past 5 years to the original research studies summarized in this chapter: William J. Atkinson, Brad Berk, Tommy A. Brock, Wilson S. Colucci, Laurie S. Ekstein, Keigi Fujiwara, Peter Ganz, Stephen Gunther, David M. Larson, Marc Taubman, and Gregory B. Wright. These studies were supported by grants from the National Institutes of Health (HL-22602, HL-20054/HL-35013, HL-29763, HL-34874) and the American Heart Association and its Massachusetts affiliate. We thank Catherine Curtis and Donna Hickey for their assistance in preparing this manuscript.

REFERENCES

1. Gimbrone, M. A., Jr. and Alexander, R. W., Tissue culture of blood vessel cells, in *Vascular Neuroeffector Mechanisms,* Bevan, J. A. et al., Eds., Raven Press, New York, 1980, 13.
2. Ross, R., The smooth muscle cell. II. Growth of smooth muscle in culture and formation of elastic fibers, *J. Cell Biol.,* 50, 172, 1971.
3. Gimbrone, M. A., Jr., Cotran, R. S., and Folkman, J., Human vascular endothelial cells in culture. Growth and DNA synthesis, *J. Cell Biol.,* 60, 673, 1974.
4. Gimbrone, M. A., Jr. and Cotran, R. S., Human vascular smooth muscle in culture: growth and ultrastructure, *Lab. Invest.,* 33, 16, 1975.
5. Hermsmeyer, K., De Cino, P., and White, R., Spontaneous contractions of dispersed vascular muscle in cell culture, *In Vitro,* 12, 628, 1976.
6. Chamley, J. H., Campbell, G. R., McConnell, J. D., and Gröschel-Stewart, U., Comparison of vascular smooth muscle cells from adult human, monkey, and rabbit in primary culture and in subculture, *Cell Tissue Res.,* 177, 503, 1977.
7. Ives, H. E., Schultz, G. S., Galardy, R. E., and Jamieson, J. D., Preparation of functional smooth muscle cells from the rabbit aorta, *J. Exp. Med.,* 148, 1400, 1978.
8. Gimbrone, M. A., Jr., Culture of vascular endothelium, in *Progress in Hemostasis and Thrombosis,* Vol. 3, Spaet, T., Ed., Grune & Stratton, New York, 1976, 1.
9. Chamley-Campbell, J., Campbell, G. R., and Ross, R., The smooth muscle cell in culture, *Physiol. Rev.,* 59, 1, 1979.
10. Martin, G. M. and Ogburn, C. E., Cell, tissue, and organoid cultures of blood vessels, in *Growth, Nutrition, and Metabolism of Cells in Culture,* Vol. 3, Rothblat, G. H. and Christofalo, V. J., Eds., Academic Press, New York, 1977, 1.
11. Ross, R. and Glomset, J., Atherosclerosis and the arterial smooth muscle cell, *Science,* 180, 1332, 1973.
12. Chamley-Campbell, J. H., Campbell, G. R., and Ross, R., Phenotype-dependent response of cultured aortic smooth muscle to serum mitogens, *J. Cell Biol.,* 89, 379, 1980.
13. Thomas, W. A., Jones, R., Scott, R. F., Morrison, E., Goodale, F., and Imai, H., Production of early atherosclerotic lesions in rats characterized by proliferation of "modified smooth muscle cells", *Exp. Mol. Pathol.,* 1, 40, 1963.
14. Gunther, S., Alexander, R. W., Atkinson, W. J., and Gimbrone, M. A., Jr., Functional angiotensin II receptors in cultured vascular smooth muscle cells, *J. Cell Biol.,* 92, 289, 1982.
15. Gunther, S., Gimbrone, M. A., Jr., and Alexander, R. W., Identification and characterization of the high affinity vascular angiotensin II receptor in rat mesenteric artery, *Circ. Res.,* 47, 278, 1980.
16. Gunther, S., Gimbrone, M. A., Jr., and Alexander, R. W., Regulation by angiotensin II of its receptors in resistance blood vessels, *Nature (London),* 287, 230, 1980.
17. Anderson, J. M., Gimbrone, M. A., Jr., and Alexander, R. W., Angiotensin II stimulates phosphorylation of the myosin light chain in cultured vascular smooth muscle cells, *J. Biol. Chem.,* 256, 4693, 1981.
18. Alexander, R. W., Hyman, S., Atkinson, W., and Gimbrone, M. A., Jr., Regualtion of angiotensin II receptors in cultured vascular smooth muscle cells, *Circulation,* 62, III, 90, 1980.
19. Gunther, S., Alexander, R. W., and Gimbrone, M. A., Jr., Angiotensin II binding, prostaglandin synthesis, and contraction in cultured vascular smooth muscle cells, *Circulation,* 60, II, 225, 1979.
20. Alexander, R. W., Neer, E. J., Dugan, M. E., Atkinson, W., and Gimbrone, M. A., Jr., Prostacyclin stimulation of adenylate cyclase in cultured vascular smooth muscle, *Fed. Proc.,* 39, 3, 742, 1980.
21. Brock, T. A., Alexander, R. W., Ekstein, L. S., Atkinson, W. J., and Gimbrone, M. A., Jr., Angiotensin increases cytosolic free calcium in cultured vascular smooth muscle cells, *Hypertension,* 7(3), Suppl. I, I-105, 1984.
22. Colucci, W. S., Brock, T. A., Gimbrone, M. A., Jr., and Alexander, R. W., Regulation of alpha$_1$-adrenergic receptor-coupled calcium flux in cultured vascular smooth muscle cells, *Hypertension,* 6(2), Suppl. I, I-19, 1983.
23. Hokin, M. R. and Hokin, L. E., Enzyme secretion and the incorporation of ^{32}P phospholipids of pancreas slices, *J. Biol. Chem.,* 203, 967, 1977.
24. Michell, R. H., Inositol phospholipids and cell surface receptor function, *Biochim. Biophys. Acta,* 415, 81, 1975.
25. Berridge, M. J., Inositol trisphosphate and diacylglycerol as second messengers, *Biochim. J.,* 220, 345, 1984.
26. Nishizuka, Y., The role of protein kinase C in cell surface signal transduction and tumor promotion, *Nature (London),* 308, 693, 1984.
27. Alexander, R. W., Brock, T. A., Gimbrone, M. A., Jr., and Rittenhouse, S. E., Angiotensin increases inositol trisphosphate and calcium in vascular smooth muscle, *Hypertension,* 7, 447, 1985.

28. Griendling, K. K., Brock, T. A., Rittenhouse, S. E., Gimbrone, M. A., Jr., and Alexander, R. W., Angiotensin II-induced formation of diacylglycerol in cultured vascular smooth muscle, *Hypertension*, 7, 844, 1985.
29. Morgan, J. P. and Morgan, K. G., Vascular smooth muscle: The first recorded Ca^{2+} transients, *Pfluegers Arch.*, 395, 75, 1982.
30. Brock, T. A., Alexander, R. W., Taubman, M. B., and Gimbrone, M. A., Jr., Angiotensin II receptor expression in cultured rat aortic smooth muscle cells, *Fed. Proc.*, 42, 1348, 1983.
31. Adelstein, R. S., Phosphorylation of muscle contractile proteins, *Fed. Proc.*, 39, 1544, 1980.
32. Morel, N., Wibo, M., and Godfraind, T., A calmodulin-stimulated Ca^{2+} pump in rat aorta plasma membranes, *Biochim. Biophys. Acta*, 644, 82, 1981.
33. Smith, J. B. and Brock, T. A., Analysis of angiotensin-stimulated sodium transport in cultured smooth muscle cells from rat aorta, *J. Cell. Physiol.*, 114, 284, 1983.
34. Moolenaar, W. H., Tertoolen, L. G. J., and de Laat, S. W., Phorbol esters and diacylglycerol mimic growth factors in raising cytoplasmic pH, *Nature (London)*, 312, 371, 1984.
35. Brock, T. A., Rittenhouse, S. E., Powers, C. W., Ekstein, L. S., Gimbrone, M. A., Jr., and Alexander, R. W., Phorbol esters and 1-oleoyl-2-acetyl-glycerol inhibit angiotensin activation of phospholipase C in cultured vascular smooth muscle cells, *J. Biol. Chem.*, 260, 14158, 1985.
36. Colucci, W. S., Brock, T. A., Gimbrone, M. A., Jr., and Alexander, R. W., Nonlinear relationship between α-adrenergic receptor occupancy and norepinephrine-stimulated calcium flux in cultured vascular smooth muscle cells, *Mol. Pharmacol.*, 27, 51[illegible], 1985.
37. Ganz, P., Gimbrone, M. A., Jr., Galper, J. B., Atkinson, W. J., and Alexander, R. W., Expression of muscarinic receptors in cultured vascular smooth muscle cells, *Circulation*, 66(Suppl. 2), II-71, 1982.
38. Ganz, P., Sandrook, A., Landis, S. C., Leopold, J., Gimbrone, M. A., Jr., and Alexander, R. W., Vasodilation and cAMP stimulation by vasoactive intestinal peptide, *Am. J. Physiol.*, 250, H755, 1986.
39. Larson, D. M., Fujiwara, K., Alexander, R. W., and Gimbrone, M. A., Jr., Heterogeneity of myosin antigenic expression in vascular smooth muscle *in vivo*, *Lab. Invest.*, 50(4), 401, 1984.
40. Larson, D. M., Fujiwara, K., Alexander, R. W., and Gimbrone, M. A., Jr., Myosin in cultured vascular smooth muscle cells: immunofluorescence and immunochemical studies of alterations in antigenic expression, *J. Cell Biol.*, 99, 1582, 1984.
41. Chamley-Campbell, J. H. and Campbell, G. R., What controls smooth muscle phenotype? *Atherosclerosis*, 40, 347, 1981.
42. Campbell, G. R. and Campbell, J. H., Smooth muscle phenotype changes in arterial wall homeostasis: implications for the pathogenesis of atherosclerosis, *Exp. Mol. Pathol.*, 42, 139, 1985.
43. Brock, T. A., unpublished observations.
44. Atkinson, W., unpublished observations.
45. Colucci, W., unpublished observations.
46. Ganz, P., unpublished observations.

CONCLUDING REMARKS

Julie H. Campbell and Gordon R. Campbell

From all the chapters it is clear that cell culture has contributed much to our understanding of the biology of vascular smooth muscle cells (SMC). While the properties of smooth muscle in culture may differ considerably from those displayed by their in vivo progenitors, there is good reason to believe that similar phenotypic changes occur in vivo since regenerating smooth muscle and some cells of atherosclerotic plaques are similar morphologically and functionally to synthetic state cells in culture.

Vascular smooth muscle in culture produces a wide range of extracellular matrix molecules, with a reciprocal modulation of SMC function by the extracellular matrix (i.e., growth, migration, and differentiation). Several chapters in this book demonstrate the importance of cell-matrix interactions in the regulation of biology and synthetic activity of SMC and suggest that modulation of extracellular matrix components may alter the structural and/or functional properties of the vessel wall. In particular, the effect of heparin and heparin-like glycosaminoglycans has been described. Heparin-treated SMC synthesize increased amounts of a cell-layer-associated-M_r-60,000-collagen protein and two noncollagenous proteins (M_r 37,000 and 39,000). They also produce decreased amounts of type III procollagen relative to type I procollagen. Heparin is very effective in maintaining smooth muscle morphologically in the contractile phenotype and in suppressing the growth of synthetic state smooth muscle and inhibiting their migration. Confluent, quiscent endothelial cells inhibit smooth muscle phenotypic change and cell division through a heparin-like molecule, and confluent but not exponentially growing SMC synthesize a highly antiproliferative heparin species, raising the possibility of an autocrine regulatory mechanism mediated by heparin operating in SMC. Endothelial cells produce a factor able to stimulate glycosaminoglycan synthesis by SMC.

Matrix-degrading enzymes are produced by SMC in culture, particularly in the presence of low-density lipoprotein, leading to the suggestion that in atherogenesis an elastase-type protease may facilitate migration of SMC in vivo by detaching them from anchorage sites and facilitating their passage through the elastic lamellae. The elastin-derived peptides in turn are chemotactic for monocyte/macrophages, which in turn can excrete an elastase-type protease, liberating more elastin peptides.

Platelet-derived growth factor (PDGF) has been identified as the principal mitogen responsible for smooth muscle growth in vitro. It is also chemokinetic and chemotactic for smooth muscle. Nanogram quantities of PDGF elicit pleiotropic responses resulting in an increase in protein synthesis, stimulation of polysome formation, induction of specific mRNAs, and the induction of synthesis of specific "competence" proteins. PDGF selectively stimulates smooth muscle thrombospondin production, while heparin-treated SMC release increased amounts of thrombospondin. This suggests that thrombospondin may be involved in the smooth muscle growth response.

Cultured vascular SMC undergo differential expression of isoactins in relation to their growth state, suggesting that growth arrest of cells may promote cytodifferentiation. Cell culture has also proven to be an excellent tool for studying the production of prostanoids and eicosanoids by SMC and the regulation of vasoactive hormone expression.

Finally, many of the authors of this book have independently expressed the view that knowledge gained in culture on the biology of vascular smooth muscle may provide explanations for changes in the artery wall following injury or in atherogenesis and hypertension. The testing of the hypotheses expressed will be an exciting addition to vascular smooth muscle research.

INDEX

A

B

C

D

E

F

K

L

M

Q

R

S

T

U

V

W

X

Y

Vascular Smooth Muscle in Culture

Volume I

Editors

Julie H. Campbell, Ph.D.
Head
Cell Biology Laboratory
Baker Medical Research Institute
Senior Research Fellow
National Health and Medical
Research Council of Australia
Melbourne, Victoria, Australia

Gordon R. Campbell, Ph.D.
Reader in Anatomy
Head
Cardiovascular Research Unit
Department of Anatomy
University of Melbourne
Melbourne, Victoria, Australia

CRC Press, Inc.
Boca Raton, Florida

Library of Congress Cataloging-in-Publication Data

Vascular smooth muscle in culture.

Includes bibliographies and index.
1. Vascular smooth muscle. 2. Tissue culture.
I. Campbell, Julie H. II. Campbell, Gordon R.
[DNLM: 1. Muscle, Smooth, Vascular--cytology. 2. Tissue Culture. WE 500 V3308]
QP110.V37V358 1987 591.1'16 86-30953
ISBN 0-8493-4325-9 (set)
ISBN 0-8493-4326-7 (v. 1)
ISBN 0-8493-4327-5 (v. 2)

This book represents information obtained from authentic and highly regarded sources. Reprinted material is quoted with permission, and sources are indicated. A wide variety of references are listed. Every reasonable effort has been made to give reliable data and information, but the author and the publisher cannot assume responsibility for the validity of all materials or for the consequences of their use.

Direct all inquiries to CRC Press, Inc., 2000 Corporate Blvd., N.W., Boca Raton, Florida, 33431.

International Standard Book Number 0-8493-4325-9 (Set)
International Standard Book Number 0-8493-4326-7 (Volume I)
International Standard Book Number 0-8493-4327-5 (Volume II)

Library of Congress Card Number 86-30953
Printed in the United States

PREFACE

Smooth muscle was first grown in culture in 1913/1914 by Champy,[1] Laquer[2] and Lewis and Lewis.[3] For the next 55 years, most of thc reports were descriptive. However, from the late 1960s onwards, there has been an ever-increasing interest and volume of papers on cultured smooth muscle, many concerned with the vascular smooth muscle cell and its role in arterial disease. For example, in 1966, 135 papers were published on smooth muscle in culture, while in 1984, there were 847, of which 416 were specifically on vascular smooth muscle.

For these volumes we invited contributions from several of the major laboratories in the world which use cell culture as a tool to study the biology of vascular smooth muscle. These contributions cover methodology, structural and functional modulation, alterations in contractile and cytoskeletal proteins, differentiation, growth factors, growth inhibitors, collagen, glycosaminoglycan and elastin synthesis and degradation, production of prostaglandins, lipoprotein metabolism, endothelial-smooth muscle interactions, vasoactive hormone receptor expression and regulation, hypertrophy, hyperploidy, and innervation. The books thus provide a near-complete dossier of what is currently known about the vascular smooth muscle cell in culture.

Julie H. Campbell
Gordon R. Campbell
Melbourne, 1985

REFERENCES

1. **Champy, C.,** Quelques resultats de la methode de culture des tissus. I. Generalities. II. Le muscle lisse (note preliminaire), *Arch. Zool. Exp. Gen.*, 53, 42, 1913/1914.
2. **Laqueur, E.,** Zur Uberlebensdauer von Saugetierorganen mit Automatie, *Zentralbl. Physiol.*, 28, 728, 1914.
3. **Lewis, M. R. and Lewis, W. H.,** Mitochondria in tissue culture, *Science*, 39, 330, 1914.

THE EDITORS

Julie H. Campbell, Ph.D., is a Senior Research Fellow with the National Health and Medical Research Council of Australia and Head of the Cell Biology Laboratory, Baker Medical Research Institute, Prahran, Victoria, Australia.

Dr. Campbell received her B.Sc. (Hons) degree from the University of New South Wales, Sydney, Australia in 1968, and her Ph.D. degree in 1973 from the University of Melbourne, Australia. After two postdoctoral fellowships at the University of Melbourne, she was awarded the John H. Halliday Travelling Fellowship of the Life Insurance Medical Research Fund of Australia and New Zealand and further studied at University College, London, England, the University of Iowa, Iowa City and the University of Washington, Seattle, during 1976-1977. In 1978, she assumed her present position at the Baker Medical Research Institute in Melbourne, Australia.

Dr. Campbell is a member of the Australian and New Zealand Society for Cell Biology, and the Australian Society for Experimental Pathology. During 1985, she was Chairman of the Australian Atherosclerosis Group, a Committee Member for the 7th International Conference on Atherosclerosis, in Melbourne, and co-organizer for its satellite symposium "Cell Biology of the Artery Wall" held at Hamilton Island, Australia.

Dr. Campbell is the author of more than 80 papers and is coauthor of a book on cardiac muscle. Her current major research interests relate to the role of smooth muscle cells in the etiology of atherosclerosis.

Gordon R. Campbell, Ph.D., is Reader in Anatomy in the School of Medicine at the University of Melbourne, Australia. He is also Head of the Cardiovascular Research Unit within the Department of Anatomy.

Dr. Campbell received his B.Sc. (Hons) and Ph.D. degrees at the University of Melbourne in 1969 and 1974, respectively. After gaining postdoctoral experience at the University of Melbourne, University College, London, England, the University of Iowa, Iowa City and the University of Washington, Seattle, he was appointed Head, Morphology and Cell Biology Laboratory at the Baker Medical Research Institute, Prahran, Victoria, Australia in 1978. In 1980, he was appointed Senior Lecturer in the Department of Anatomy, University of Melbourne, and Reader in the same department in 1984.

Dr. Campbell is a Fellow of the Royal Society of Medicine, London, England and a member of the American Society for Cell Biology. He is also a member of the Australian and New Zealand Society for Cell Biology, the Australian Atherosclerosis Society, the Australian Society for Experimental Pathology and the Anatomical Society of Australia and New Zealand. In October 1985 he was co-organizer of an international symposium "Cell Biology of the Artery Wall" held at Hamilton Island, Australia.

Dr. Campbell is the author of more than 80 papers and the coauthor of two books on muscle structure and function. His current major research interests relate to the role of smooth muscle cells in the etiology of arteriosclerosis.

CONTRIBUTORS

R. Wayne Alexander, Ph.D., M.D.
Associate Professor of Medicine
Harvard Medical School
Cardiologist
Division of Cardiovascular Medicine
Brigham and Women's Hospital
Boston, Massachusetts

Edwin L. Bierman, M.D.
Professor of Medicine
Department of Medicine
University of Washington
Seattle, Washington

Alex Bobik, Ph.D.
Associate Director
Biochemical Pharmacology Laboratory
Alfred Hospital and Baker Medical Research Institute
Prahran, Victoria, Australia

Jacques Bonnet, M.D.
Chef de Clinique — Assistant
Department of Cardiology
Groupe Hospitalier Haut-Levêque-Xavier Arnozan
Pessac, France

Paul Bornstein, M.D.
Professor of Biochemistry and Medicine
Department of Biochemistry
University of Washington
Seattle, Washington

Daniel Bowen-Pope, Ph.D.
Research Assistant Professor
Department of Pathology
University of Washington
Seattle, Washington

H. Bricaud, M.D.
Professor of Cardiology
Chief
Department of Cardiology
Groupe Hospitalier Haut-Leveque-Xavier Arnozan
Pessac, France

John J. Castellot, Jr., Ph.D.
Assistant Professor
Department of Pathology
Harvard Medical School
Boston, Massachusetts

Alan Chait, M.D.
Professor of Medicine
Department of Medicine
University of Washington
Seattle, Washington

Peter F. Davies, Ph.D.
Associate Professor of Pathology
Department of Pathology
Brigham and Women's Hospital
Harvard Medical School
Boston, Massachusetts

B. Dorian, Ph.D.
Assistant
Unité de Recherches de Cardiologie
INSERM U8
Pessac, France

Michael A. Gimbrone, Jr., M.D.
Professor of Pathology
Brigham and Women's Hospital
Harvard Medical School
Boston, Massachusetts

David Gordon
Department of Pathology
University of Washington
Seattle, Washington

M. Daria Haust
Professor
Department of Pathology
University of Western Ontario
London, Ontario, Canada

William Hornebeck, Ph.D.
Laboratoire de Biochemie du Tissu Conjonctif
Faculte de Medicine
Universite Paris val de Marne
Creteil, France

Olli Jaakkola, M.Sc.
Assistant
Department of Biomedical Sciences
University of Tampere
Tampere, Finland

Olli-Pekka Kallioniemi, M.D.
Department of Biomedical Sciences
University of Tampere
Tampere, Finland

Morris J. Karnovsky
Professor
Department of Pathology
Harvard Medical School
Boston, Massachusetts

J. Larrue, Ph.D.
Directeur de Recherche
Unité de Recherches de Cardiologie
INSERM U8
Pessac, France

James R. A. Leushner
Department of Pathology
University of Western Ontario
London, Ontario, Canada

Richard A. Majack, Ph.D.
Research Scientist
Atherosclerosis and Thrombosis Research
The Upjohn Company
Kalamazoo, Michigan

Mark W. Majesky, Ph.D.
Postdoctoral Fellow
Department of Pathology
School of Medicine
University of Washington
Seattle, Washington

M. J. Merrilees, Ph.D.
Senior Lecturer
Department of Anatomy
University of Auckland
Auckland, New Zealand

Richard A. Murphy, Ph.D.
Professor of Physiology
Department of Physiology
University of Virginia School of Medicine
Charlottesville, Virginia

Seppo Nikkari, M.D.
Department of Biomedical Sciences
University of Tampere
Tampere, Finland

Tapio Nikkari, M.D.
Professor
Department of Biomedical Sciences
University of Tampere
Tampere, Finland

Susan E. O'Connor
Department of Pathology
Brigham and Women's Hospital
Harvard Medical School
Boston, Massachusetts

John F. Oram, Ph.D.
Research Assistant Professor
Department of Medicine
University of Washington
Seattle, Washington

Gary K. Owens, Ph.D.
Assistant Professor
Department of Physiology
University of Virginia School of Medicine
Charlottesville, Virginia

Kari Pietilä, M.D.
Special Lecturer
Department of Biomedical Science
University of Tampere
Tampere, Finland

Leslie Robert, M.D., Ph.D.
Director of Research
Laboratoire de Biochimie du Tissu Conjonctif
Faculte de Medicine
Universite Paris val de Marne
Creteil, France

Russell Ross, Ph.D.
Professor and Chairman
Department of Pathology
University of Washington
Seattle, Washington

Arthur S. Rovner, Ph.D.
Postdoctoral Fellow
Department of Physiology
University of Virginia School of Medicine
Charlottesville, Virginia

Stephen M. Schwartz, Ph.D.
Associate Professor
Department of Pathology
University of Washington
Seattle, Washington

George A. Truskey, Ph.D.
Assistant Professor of Chemical Engineering
Department of Chemical Engineering
Tufts University
Medford, Massachusetts

TABLE OF CONTENTS

Volume I

Volume II

Chapter 1

ARTERIAL SMOOTH MUSCLE DIFFERENTIATION

David Gordon and Stephen M. Schwartz

TABLE OF CONTENTS

I. INTRODUCTION

Abnormalities of vascular smooth muscle differentiation and proliferation are characteristics of both the atherosclerotic plaque and the pathologic changes of hypertensive microvessels.[1,2] Unfortunately, in the case of vascular smooth muscle cells (SMC), phenotypic states have been defined only morphologically, with hardly any biochemical characterization. Additionally, the morphological "criteria" often rest on nonspecific features, such as "numerous microfilament bundles" vs. "large amount of rough endoplasmic reticulum." Given the sampling and fixation dependence of such features, it is not surprising that there is much disagreement from one observer to the next on the state of any given cell. Finally, since these features are not really specific for SMC and since other cell types (e.g., fibroblasts, endothelial cells, and monocytes/macrophages) are known to be in the proximity of (if not within) the vessel wall, it is not always even clear whether a given cell is a "dedifferentiated" SMC or some other cell type. This is true both in vivo and in cultures derived from blood vessels.

This situation is in sharp contrast to the current understanding of the development and differentiation of striated muscle. Here the morphologic distinctions are much more sharply defined, and there has been extensive biochemical characterization of the cytoskeletal and associated proteins in relation to the different stages of proliferation and differentiation. Since the SMC has many similarities in function and cytoskeletal composition to the striated muscle, our approach is to use the knowledge already gained from skeletal muscle as an outline for investigating vascular smooth muscle proliferation and differentiation. Accordingly, this review section is organized with this analogy in mind. We begin by comparing the morphological states of skeletal vs. smooth muscle and then go on to discuss what is known about the specific muscle proteins: actin isotypes, desmin, CPK isozymes, and other cytoskeletal proteins. We end by briefly discussing atherosclerotic carotid disease, the response to endarterectomy, and suggest how a better knowledge of the controls on SMC phenotype may help in understanding this human disease and response to injury.

II. MORPHOLOGY AND CYTOSKELETAL BIOCHEMISTRY

A. Morphology

Presumptive skeletal muscle cells begin as spindle-shaped, mononucleated, diploid cells, with rather nonspecific cytoplasmic features and indeed are morphologically indistinguishable from proliferating fibroblasts.[3,4] At the time of differentiation, these precursor cells cease dividing and fuse into elongated, multinucleated "myotubes". These cells then assemble their cytoplasm into the well-known sarcomeric morphology of adult skeletal muscle.[3-5] Finally, these cells contract spontaneously in culture (in the absence of innervation), and indeed innervation is not required for the establishment of this differentiated state.[4,5]

Other differentiated features include the development of the sarcoplasmic reticulum and the T-tubule system. Each of these cells also possesses a surrounding basement membrane. The nuclei of the differentiated muscle cells are all postmitotic, diploid nuclei, and never again synthesize DNA. All muscle "regeneration" seems attributable to the proliferation and eventual fusion of undifferentiated "satellite" cells located among the well-developed myotubes.[4,6,7] The morphology of satellite cells is quite similar to that of the "presumptive myoblasts". Finally, true hypertrophy of skeletal muscle cells (cytoplasmic enlargement) can occur, for example, as a response to increased work demands. It is unclear whether or not the recruitment of satellite cells to form new myotubes contributes to this process.[8,9]

The vascular (and other) SMC are also mesenchymally derived cells and resemble fibroblasts in early development and postnatal growth.[10,11] In the developing aorta they are proliferating, spindle-shaped cells with initially much rough endoplasmic reticulum, numerous ribosomes, and otherwise nondistinguishing cytoplasmic features. During normal growth and development of the animal, there is a gradual transition to the adult morphology, which is generally a mononucleated, diploid cell whose cytoplasm is packed with actin and myosin filaments. These "myofilaments" appear randomly arranged in contrast to the highly ordered sarcomeric pattern of skeletal muscle.[11] Electron-dense "dense bodies" in the cytoplasm and adjacent to the plasma membrane are felt to be characteristic of SMC. Since actin filaments emanate from these "dense bodies", they are felt by some investigators to be the SMC counterpart to the skeletal muscle Z band.[12] The differentiated SMC also has a surrounding basement membrane and numerous pinocytotic vesicles, the latter possibly serving as an analogue to the T-tubule system of skeletal muscle. These cells can be binucleated, and with aging and hypertension, a high proportion of cells become hypertrophied with tetraploid, octaploid, or hexadecaploid content of DNA.[13-15] In this respect, the vascular SMC is more analogous to the cardiac muscle cell.[16] Finally, although some nonvascular SMC can perform spontaneous contractions in vitro,[17] vascular SMC generally require exogenous stimulation to exhibit significant contraction.[11,18,19]

In contrast to adult skeletal muscle cells, differentiated SMC do have the capacity to reenter the cell cycle in response to certain injurious stimuli,[1] and in the adult mammalian vessel wall, no morphologic subpopulation of undifferentiated "stem" or "satellite" cells have been described.[20] After injury, (e.g., balloon catheter-induced endothelial denudation of the aorta or carotid artery), the proliferating cells become morphologically indistinguishable from their less differentiated developmental precursors described above. After cessation of division, these cells resume the adult differentiated morphology.[21-23] Actually, this view is overly simplistic since one sees a whole spectrum of morphologies among these cells, with nothing approaching the clear-cut morphological changes of the skeletal muscle system. The changes are relative since each morphologic feature (e.g., dense bodies, rough endoplasmic reticulum) can be seen to some degree among the different proposed phenotypic states of adult cells.[21] Similar morphologic features can also occasionally be seen among nonmuscle cells, such as fibroblasts or endothelial cells.[11]

There is a debate over whether or not SMC showing differentiated features can also be actively proliferating at the same time. Many investigators have taken a cue from the skeletal muscle observations and have stated that SMC can be either in a "contractile" state or a proliferative/synthetic state, but not in both. The Campbells have been most vocal in this viewpoint, reporting that in vitro freshly isolated adult vascular SMC change to an undifferentiated morphology before an increase in cell number occurs (see Chapter 4). Also, the "contractile" cells do not appear to be responsive to common mitogens, such as the platelet-derived growth factor, before this morphologic transition has occurred.[21] Additionally, in those few in vitro instances in which the electron microscopic "contractile" state can be reestablished (e.g., plating at high density, co-culture with endothelium, or with heparin[21]), proliferation also ceases. They have termed this transition in phenotype "modulation"[21] as opposed to "dedifferentiation", which might imply the potential to redifferentiate also along nonsmooth muscle cell lines (something never observed). This is not a trivial theory since it implies that this phenotypic change is a requirement for SMC proliferation. Conversely, factors which might hold SMC in a differentiated state would also prevent SMC proliferation according to this theory.

However, the dichotomy between proliferation and differentiation has not been proven. Most studies in support of this theory have been done on bulk, in vitro cultures, without looking for proliferation and differentiation markers within the same individual cells. On the contrary, the Campbells have reported seeing individual SMC from vas deferens contract spontaneously, then pause for several minutes while undergoing mitosis, and then promptly resume spontaneous contractions.[24] Additionally, other investigators have reported obtaining proliferating, contractile mesenteric artery SMC in culture.[19] This suggests caution should be used in trying to predict a smooth muscle cell's functional capabilities simply from its morphological appearance. Thus, the proposed dichotomy is not absolute among SMC and may simply represent an average observation under conditions of extreme wholesale proliferation.

Again the SMC perhaps bears closer similarities to the cardiac myocytes which can possess sarcomeres and undergo mitosis simultaneously.[16,25] Through studying the expression of muscle-related proteins in various states of arterial smooth muscle, we hope to arrive at a biochemical definition of different smooth muscle phenotypic states, as well as of smooth muscle lineage, rather than relying simply on morphology. Therefore, we now turn to a discussion of muscle-specific proteins.

B. Actin Isotypes

Actin is a 42-kdalton protein existing in virtually all cell types. There are at least six distinct mammalian actin isotypes present with varying distributions among the muscle and nonmuscle tissues.[26-30] Nevertheless, amino acid sequencing has shown that this is a highly conserved class of proteins with only a small number of amino acid substitutions — indeed the same tissues from different species have much more similar actins than do different tissues within the same species. Isoelectric focusing separates the actins by isoelectric points into three general classes: α-, β-, and γ-actin.[26,29] Peptide analysis or amino acid sequencing is required to further subdivide these isotypes. Thus, adult skeletal muscle has essentially only "skeletal muscle α-actin", which differs at only four amino acid positions (out of a total of 375 residues) from "cardiac α-actin", which comprises essentially all of the actin in adult cardiac muscle cells.[29,31] These two actin isotypes are not found outside striated muscle systems. Both of these differ from the "smooth muscle α-actin", which together with "smooth muscle γ-actin", are found only in SMC. However, SMC also contain "β-actin" and "nonmuscle γ-actin", these latter two isotypes being present in most nonmuscle cells, with fibroblasts being an example.[30] Thus, as far as actin composition is concerned, the SMC appears to be somewhere between striated and nonmuscle mesenchymal cells. Although these different actin isotypes are useful for marking different tissues, the functional significance of these different isotypes is at present unknown, especially since they all can polymerize into filaments and can all interact with myosin.[31]

Within striated muscle tissues, rather striking actin isotype changes occur during normal development.[32] Thus, in skeletal muscle development, the "presumptive myoblasts" contain only β- and nonmuscle γ-actins. However, with cessation of proliferation, fusion, and during sarcomere formation, the synthesis of these actins is replaced by the production of skeletal muscle α-actin.[32,33] This may not be a simple transition, however, given observations that fetal actin mRNA from mouse skeletal muscle or from a differential skeletal muscle cell line is very similar, if not identical to, adult cardiac muscle mRNA.[35,36] Detailed analyses of proliferation and actin isotype expression in the same cell have not been possible since only recently have actin isotype-specific antibodies been generated.[37-39]

The situation in smooth muscle is even less well characterized. Chicken gizzard actin is composed essentially of only nonmuscle β- and γ-actin (presumably smooth muscle and nonmuscle types) and during its pre- and posthatching development, the γ-actin fraction increases markedly relative to the β-fraction.[40] Adult aortic smooth muscle appears unique in having a relatively high content of smooth muscle α-actin.[30,41] Thus, in adult rat aorta, 68% of the actin is smooth muscle α-actin as opposed to 18% of the total actin in rat taenia coli.[30]

Using a purified preparation of chicken gizzard actin, we have developed a monoclonal antibody which in tissue sections specifically reacts with vascular and nonvascular SMC.[38] Neither skeletal muscle nor cardiac muscle is stained with this antibody. One-dimensional "Western" blots reveal this antibody to bind exclusively to actin from smooth muscle tissues (e.g., monkey ileum) and not to skeletal muscle actin (e.g., human or rabbit skeletal muscle). Two-dimensional "Western" blots with this antibody against the chicken gizzard actin antigen and preparations of adult rat and cultured rat aorta reveal a specificity for a common antigen in α- and γ-actin isotypes. Two-dimensional gels of the immunoprecipitate of this antibody and the purified chicken gizzard actin give the same findings. Given that this monoclonal antibody stains neither striated muscle (rich in skeletal or myocardial α-actins) nor fibroblasts (cells with significant amounts of β- and nonmuscle γ-actin), we conclude that this antibody is specific for an antigen shared between smooth muscle α- and smooth muscle γ-actin. In the rat, this antibody stains all the SMC in the carotid artery and aorta. However, in the chicken thoracic aorta, it stains only alternating layers in a pattern similar to that reported for desmin. This is consistent with the ultrastructural implication that in the chicken the "interlaminar" cells are undifferentiated cells.[42] We have also seen similar heterogeneous reactivity in the bovine aorta. While the nature of the determinant common to the two smooth muscle specific actins remains unknown, this antibody offers a unique opportunity to define the cell's differentiation state in vivo and in vitro in terms of expressions of a unique determinant.

C. Desmin Expression

Desmin is one of a class of proteins called intermediate filament proteins — so named because they have diameters in the range of 100 nm, intermediate between the "thin" actin filaments and the "thick" myosin filaments.[43,44] Monomeric desmin is an approximately 52-kdalton protein present only in differentiated, striated, and smooth muscle tissues. Its function is unknown. However, in skeletal muscle, given its localization to the peri-Z-band areas in the form of a filamentous network seemingly interconnecting the Z-disks of adjacent sarcomeres, it may serve as the essential cytoskeletal framework holding the sarcomeres together in an organized pattern.[43]

More importantly for our purpose, the appearance of this protein during skeletal muscle development coincides with the transition from the proliferating myoblast to the postmitotic muscle cell, together with the switch in actin isotype to α-actin and the early formation of sarcomeres.[34] Thus it is a convenient biochemical marker for the "contractile" state in skeletal muscle development.

Another major intermediate filament protein, vimentin (molecular weight approximately 58 kdalton), is slightly more acidic than desmin on two-dimensional gels.[45-47] Vimentin is the predominant intermediate filament protein in the proliferating myoblasts. After sarcomere formation, desmin comprises the vast bulk, if not all, of the intermediate filament protein. Indeed there is some controversy as to whether or not vimentin is present in mature "contractile" skeletal muscle.[34,48]

Although intermediate filaments are visible in SMC,[11,49] their function is even less clear and the relation, if any, to the dense bodies has not been clarified.[50] The situation differs further in vascular SMC since these cells also contain substantial amounts of vimentin while in the "contractile" state, in contrast to the skeletal muscle situation.[41,51,52] Reports on the time course of appearance of desmin in smooth muscle development are currently lacking.

In the rat thoracic aorta and carotid arteries, only approximately one half of the SMC present in the media appear to react positively with antidesmin antibodies, whereas nearly all the cells react positively with antivimentin antibodies.[51] This suggests that at least for the large elastic arteries, the medial smooth muscle population is heterogeneous despite ultrastructural impression. As one goes through the abdominal aorta and into the small muscular arteries, an increasing proportion of the SMC stain positively for desmin,[53] suggesting that the SMC composition of an artery is dependent upon the size and possibly function of that artery (from elastic conductance vessels to more contractile resistance vessels, for example). Along these lines, it is interesting to note that in avian aortas (e.g., chicken and pigeon) the larger elastic arterial medias have two morphologically distinct cell populations in alternating layers: an ultrastructurally well-differentiated SMC and an "interlaminar" cell which resembles more closely a fibroblast with much less "myofilaments" and more prominent rough endoplasmic reticulum.[42,54] In the chicken, immunofluorescent stains for desmin and vimentin give results consistent with the presence of both desmin and vimentin in the smooth muscle-appearing cells, but only vimentin in the "interlaminar" cells.[52] It is interesting to speculate on the nature of this "interlaminar" cell, given the presence of desmin-negative cells in mammalian aortas. Could "interlaminar" cells be a type of smooth muscle myoblast? One still unresolved question in the rat aorta is whether or not those cells which stain negatively with the antidesmin antibody may still contain desmin, but in a nonfilamentous form.

Finally, using this same antidesmin antibody, Gabbiani et al.[51] have shown that after balloon catheter-induced arterial injury, the proliferating SMC which begin forming the neointima lack desmin. Thus desmin expression could be a cytoskeletal marker for the "contractile" differentiated state of smooth muscle.

D. Creatine Phosphokinase Isotypes

Creatine phosphokinase (CPK) is another muscle-related protein with an important role in the muscle cell's high-energy phosphate storage and delivery system. This enzyme is a dimer whose monomers come in three distinct isotypes separable by gel electrophoresis: a mitochondrial form, an M form, and a B form. Like the α-actin and desmin proteins, the M-type CPK is specific for muscle tissues.[55] The M and the B forms also have characteristic appearances in the course of skeletal muscle development. Thus in vivo, the proliferating myoblasts contain BB-CPK, but at the time of transition to postmitotic, sarcomeric muscle cells, this isotype is totally replaced by MM-CPK.[56] MM-CPK also appears with differentiation in vitro, although the transition is not complete.[56,57] Immunofluorescence studies using antibodies specific for the M form show that the onset of M-CPK synthesis is sharp with regard to the cell cycle since no cells are simultaneously positive for tritiated thymidine labeling and M-CPK labeling.[58] The presence of M-CPK is therefore a useful marker of the differentiated "contractile" state in skeletal muscle.

CPK isozyme patterns have been hardly studied at all in SMC. A few reports suggest that smooth muscle tissue (e.g., chicken gizzard, uterine smooth muscle) contains some M but mostly the B form.[55,59-61] Whether segregation by isotype exists on a cell-by-cell basis is not known. Kimes and Brandt[62] reported on two cell lines derived from rat thoracic aorta that were felt to be smooth muscle by ultrastructural criteria. These lines were reported to synthesize mainly the M form after cessation of cell division. Nevertheless, there is no clear description of the relationship of CPK isozyme expression to vascular SMC phenotype.

E. Other Muscle-Related Protein Changes

Changes in myosin composition have also been reported in the skeletal muscle systems.[32,63] Thus in rat and chicken skeletal muscle, the myosin heavy chain of embryonic muscle is different from that in neonatal muscle, which in turn is different from that in adult muscle. The first heavy chain transition is associated with the transition from proliferation to differentiation.[64] Similar changes among the different light chains have also been described.[32,65] Also of note is that slow and fast skeletal muscles contain different myosin isozymes,[65,66] a difference which appears to be a consequence of innervation by different neuron classes.[107] Although SMC have been reported to contain a distinct smooth muscle myosin as well as a nonmuscle myosin,[67-71] further detailed characterization with regard to phenotypic state is needed. For example, Larson et al.[70] have developed two polyclonal antimyosin heavy chain antibodies, one of which is smooth muscle specific (raised against human uterine myosin) and the other of which reacts with muscle and nonmuscle cells (raised against human platelet myosin). Yet since they precipitate the same myosin heavy chain from vascular smooth muscle, they have suggested that the smooth muscle distinctive feature may be some conformational change, rather than a separate smooth muscle isotype with a distinct amino acid sequence.

Tropomyosin is reported to be essentially absent in prefusion myoblast cultures of skeletal muscle and appears after fusion with differentiation.[33,34,72] Tropomyosin is present in smooth muscle,[73] but, again, there has been no full characterization with regard to development and proliferation.

III. HUMAN CAROTID ARTERY DISEASE AND MODELS OF ARTERIAL INJURY

Endarterectomy, the surgical removal of atheromatous material from an artery, is a common treatment for carotid artery disease. Unfortunately, as might be expected from animal studies, endarterectomy is probably itself a stimulus for smooth muscle proliferation and intimal thickening. A major objective is to correlate changes in animal model systems with observations on human tissue. Strandness has shown that after carotid artery endarterectomy, significant carotid stenosis of 50 to 100% luminal diameter recurs in 19% of patients within a mean postoperative follow-up interval of 16 months.[74] Some of these patients (approximately 4% of the total) will later require further vascular reconstruction at the same site for recurrent symptomatic disease. In contrast to identifiable risk factors for the development of the initial carotid artery disease lesion (diabetes, cigarette smoking, age),[75,76] the relationship between accepted atherosclerosis risk factors and recurrent carotid stenosis remains unclear.[74] Although some studies have reported restenosis rates of less than 5%,[77,78] the indication for repeat studies after surgery in these cases was chiefly neurologic symptoms. When all patients are studied postoperatively (usually by noninvasive means), higher recurrence rates are reported (9% in Turnipseed et al.,[79] 9.8% in Kremen et al.[80]). It is not surprising, therefore, that Zierler et al., using a more sophisticated imaging and flow analysis system, find a 19% recurrent rate.[74]

Other investigators have looked at the morphology of the original atherosclerotic plaque and the hyperplastic lesion recurring after endarterectomy.[77,81-83] These recurrent lesions have been variously likened to diffuse myointimal thickenings or to atherosclerotic plaques. Yet these have been strictly light microscopic studies without quantitation of the proliferative or differentiated state of the involved SMC. In particular, the relationship between the growth state of the SMC in the original plaque and the above-mentioned risk factors has not been studied. Secondly, the growth rate of the SMC remaining in the medial remnant (as represented by the portion of media removed at endarterectomy) and its relationship to the extent of subsequent intimal proliferation after endarterectomy have not been explored.

A. Kinetics of Smooth Muscle Proliferation Following Arterial Injury

Numerous animal studies have been conducted on the proliferative response of SMC to various forms of arterial injury.[1,22] We will focus on studies of a model developed in the adult rat carotid artery.[23,84-86] In this model, the formation of a thickened intima after balloon catheter-induced endothelial denudation is first due to SMC proliferation, causing a four- to fivefold increase in SMC number by 2 weeks. Thereafter, SMC number remains constant, with the further increase in intimal mass occurring by an increase in extracellular matrix. This intimal thickening, and at times also vasospasm, is responsible for luminal narrowing. In normal vessels, the thymidine labeling index of undisturbed arterial SMC is very low (0.06%). However, after arterial injury, the thymidine index rises to 40 to 70% in the media and intima within 2 days. As SMC migrate into the intima and the intima progressively widens, nearly all of the proliferation occurs within the few cell layers adjacent to the vessel lumen and ceases in reendothelialized regions. The surface of persistently denuded areas has the prespective labeling indices of 4 and 1% at 3 and 6 months after injury.

Only a few investigators have attempted to obtain cell growth kinetic data from human arteries. The frequency of polyploidy increases with age in arteries from humans.[15] Experimental studies by Owens and Schwartz[13,14] revealed a similar age dependence of the ploidy in rats. Rats also show a strong positive correlation between ploidy and systemic blood pressure. Studies to ascertain the relative proliferative capacities of diploid vs. polyploid SMC are currently under way. Preliminary results suggest a higher growth fraction among diploid as opposed to tetraploid cells in culture (unpublished results). We do not know as yet the significance of vascular SMC polyploidy. Our hypothesis is that smooth muscle polyploidization, like multinucleation in skeletal muscle or polyploidy in cardiac muscle, is characteristic of an increase in mass in differentiated muscle tissues. Polyploid SMC then might be expected to have a decreased ability to participate in the hyperplastic response required for formation of an atherosclerotic lesion.

The percent of SMC undergoing DNA synthesis was not estimated in any of the above in vivo studies. To this end, Spagnoli et al.,[88] using tritiated thymidine autoradiography on a limited number of human arterial specimens removed at surgery, found a very low labeling index (0.00 to 0.09%) in normal media, similar to that seen in adult experimental animals.[85] However, in segments of media underlying atherosclerotic plaques, there was a trend towards an increased labeling index (0.00 to 0.96%). These same investigators have published a similar preliminary thymidine labeling study on human atherosclerotic plaques and claim to see labeling only in "foam cells" or "monocyte-like cells" and only rarely in recognizable smooth muscle cells.[89] If true, this is surprising since the general view is that the proliferative population of the atherosclerotic plaque is derived from vessel wall SMC.[1] This study, however, was conducted only at the light microscopic level without specific smooth muscle and monocyte/macrophage markers and thus is not convincing. These investigators made no attempt to correlate their findings with the clinical progression of symptomatic disease at the sites examined. Given that monocytes/macrophages can produce factors that are mitogenic for mesenchymal cells,[90,91] the number of such cells in the lesion may be an important determinant of lesion progression.

In summary, there are scant data concerning the growth state and degree of SMC differentiation in adult human arteries. No one has studied the correlation in man between the progression of clinically significant atherosclerotic lesions and intimal SMC growth state or derived smooth muscle subpopulation. Variability in the proliferative and differentiated states of the cells in the lesion or underlying media could well be a valuable predictor of the fate of vessels following endarterectomy. Such studies using smooth muscle-specific and leukocyte-specific antibodies are currently under way in our laboratories.

B. Actin Isotypes of Vascular Smooth Muscle Cells

We have studied the actin isotype composition of adult rat aortic smooth muscle. Two-dimensional gels of both whole homogenized media and isolated cells obtained through enzymatic dissociation reveal that the bulk of the actin is composed of the α-isotype, with the remainder split between β- and γ-forms. This is in agreement with tryptic peptide analysis by Vandekerckhove and Weber[30] and protein electrophoresis.[92] Two-dimensional gels of multiply passaged rat aortic SMC in culture, however, reveal a marked decrease in the percentage of α-actin isotype, with the bulk of the actin now being composed of β- and γ-forms.[92] We have also seen a similar pattern in preparations of neonatal rat aortas. Since both the neonatal aortas and the cultured cells exhibit a substantial amount of proliferation in contrast to the adult rat aorta, it would appear that vascular SMC α-actin content is inversely associated with the proliferative state. In these samples we do not know whether the small amount of α-actin present represents a decrease in all of the cells or possibly an absence in all proliferating cells with full presence in noncycling, more differentiated cells.

C. Replication In Vitro vs. In Vivo

As already noted above, replication of SMC follows two quite distinct pathways in vivo. In hypertension, with the exception of necrotizing malignant hypertension, the major change is an orderly increase in cellular DNA without movement of the replicating cells.[93] At its extreme, this change occurs by endoreplications; that is, cells in the aorta and large vessels of hypertensive animals become polyploid.[94] This is reminiscent of the increase in DNA/cell seen in skeletal muscle, although in that case the change reflects fusion of differentiated cells with residual, undifferentiated stem cells.[3-5,7] In contrast, the characteristic proliferation of diffuse intimal thickening involves migration of SMC from the media into the intima.[95]

The stimuli for these responses remain unknown. For hypertension, at least in large vessels, replication occurs without evidence of platelet interaction either morphologically or by quantitative analysis of platelet adhesion.[96-98] This is important because of the large body of evidence implicating platelet release as the initiating stimulus for smooth muscle replication in atherosclerosis.[99] Even here, however, this answer may be oversimplified. Recently, Reidy and Silver[100] have shown that extensive areas of endothelium can be gently denuded without a smooth muscle proliferative response despite an exuberant thrombotic response. This contrasts with the usual proliferative response seen with the balloon catheter denudation technique.[99] We need to conclude that platelets can stimulate smooth muscle replication since they do so in vitro. The absence of an effect in vivo suggests that the normal SMC in vivo is refractory to the platelet-derived growth factor. Possible auxiliary factors include mitogenic material released from dying cells,[101] mitogens secreted by endothelial cells,[102] or mitogens released by SMC themselves.[103] Perhaps most attractive, however, is the idea that SMC in vivo exist in a state which is initially unresponsive to mitogens. This idea, originally proposed by the Campbells and discussed in Chapter 4 remains central and leaves us with the identity of the stimulus that modulates the SMC into a responsive state as a critical question.

Similarly, the stimulus for endoreplication in hypertension remains unknown. One of the few well-established facts about chronic hypertension is the establishment of a fixed increase in peripheral resistance.[104] The increase in DNA could provide a "memory" for this phenomenon. Moreover, increase within a nondividing cell might be able to explain some of the abnormal physiology associated with "hypertensive" smooth muscle. Here, also, in vitro models may be useful. Goldberg et al.[105] have recently reported that isolated arterial SMC can be separated into ploidy classes by cell sorting. The cells are viable and maintain their ploidy distribution in vitro. In contrast to these results, we have found that cells in the newborn animal are diploid. When placed in culture, however, about 50% of the cultures rapidly and spontaneously develop a high frequency of polyploidy.[106] Thus it is likely that we will be able to use cell culture to study both the effects of polyploidy on cell function and the mechanism of polyploid formation itself.

IV. SUMMARY

SMC are highly differentiated cells characterized by a set of specific contractile proteins similar to those seen in skeletal muscle. In the latter cell type, differentiation is closely linked to loss of ability to divide. This tight linkage is absent in vascular smooth muscle cells since at least most of the SMC in the adult wall are capable of replicating in response to hypertension or atherosclerosis. We do, however, have probes for the specific contractile proteins and both animal cell culture model systems that should allow us to explain the nature of the linkage between differentiation and proliferation in the smooth muscle systems. We plan to apply the knowledge of SMC types and states of differentiation gained from such studies to studies of human arterial disease.

REFERENCES

1. Ross, R., Atherosclerosis: a problem of the biology of arterial wall cells and their interactions with blood components, *Arteriosclerosis,* 1, 293, 1981.
2. Benditt, E. P. and Gown, A. M., Atheroma: the artery wall and the environment, *Int. Rev. Exp. Pathol.,* 21, 55, 1980.
3. Lentz, T. L., Myogenesis: differentiation of skeletal muscle fibers, in *Developmental Regulation: Aspects of Cell Differentiation,* Coward, S. J., Ed., Academic Press, New York, 1973, 169.
4. Dientsman, S. R. and Holtzer, H., Myogenesis: a cell lineage interpretation, in *Cell Cycle and Cell Differentiation,* Reinert, J. and Holtzer, H., Eds., Springer-Verlag, New York, 1975, 1.
5. Konigsberg, I. R., Progression through G_1 and myogenic differentiation *in vitro,* in *Differentiation In Vitro,* Cambridge University Press, New York, 1982, 141.
6. Konigsberg, U. R., Lipton, B. H., and Konigsberg, I. R., The regenerative response of single mature muscle fibers isolated *in vitro, Dev. Biol.,* 45, 260, 1975.
7. Allbrook, D., Skeletal muscle regeneration, *Muscle Nerve,* 4, 234, 1981.
8. Seiden, D., A quantitative analysis of muscle cell changes in compensatory hypertrophy and work-induced hypertrophy, *Am. J. Anat.,* 145, 459, 1976.
9. DeGirolami, U. and Smith, T. W., Pathology of skeletal muscle diseases, *Am. J. Pathol.,* 107, 234, 1982.
10. Gerrity, R. G. and Cliff, W. J., The aortic tunica media of the developing rat. I. Quantitative stereologic and biochemical analysis, *Lab. Invest.,* 32, 585, 1975.
11. Chamley-Campbell, J., Campbell, G. R., and Ross, R., The smooth muscle cell in culture, *Physiol. Rev.,* 59, 1, 1979.
12. Bond, M. and Somlyo, A. V., Dense bodies and actin polarity in vertebrate smooth muscle, *J. Cell Biol.,* 95, 403, 1982.
13. Owens, G. K., Rabinovitch, P. S., and Schwartz, S. M., Smooth muscle cell hypertrophy versus hyperplasia in hypertension, *Proc. Natl. Acad. Sci. U.S.A.,* 78, 7759, 1981.
14. Owens, G. K. and Schwartz, S. M., Alterations in vascular smooth muscle mass in the spontaneously hypertensive rat. Role of cellular hypertrophy, hyperploidy and hyperplasia, *Circ. Res.,* 51, 280, 1982.
15. Barrett, T. B., Benditt, E. P., Owens, G. K., and Schwartz, S. M., Changes in cell ploidy with age in the human arterial smooth muscle cell, *Proc. Natl. Acad. Sci. U.S.A.,* 80, 882, 1982.
16. Manasek, F. J., Some comparative aspects of cardiac and skeletal myogenesis, in *Development Regulation: Aspects of Cell Differentiation,* Coward, S. J., Ed., Academic Press, New York, 1973, 193.
17. Chamley, J. H., Campbell, G. R., and Burnstock, G., Dedifferentiation, redifferentiation and bundle formation of smooth muscle cells in tissue culture: the influence of cell number and nerve fibres, *J. Embryol. Exp. Morphol.,* 32, 297, 1974.

18. Chamley-Campbell, J. H., Campbell, G. R., and Ross, R., Phenotype-dependent response of cultured aortic smooth muscle to serum mitogens, *J. Cell Biol.*, 89, 379, 1981.
19. Gunther, S., Alexander, R. W., Atkinson, W. J., and Gimbrone, M. A., Functional angiotensin II receptors in cultured vascular smooth muscle cells, *J. Cell Biol.*, 92, 289, 1982.
20. Pease, D. C. and Paule, W. J., Electron microscopy of elastic arteries: the thoracic aorta of the rat, *J. Ultrastruct. Res.*, 3, 469, 1960.
21. Chamley-Campbell, J. H. and Campbell, G. R., What controls smooth muscle phenotype? *Atherosclerosis*, 40, 347, 1981.
22. Fishman, J. A., Ryan, G. B., and Karnovsky, M. J., Endothelial regeneration in the rat carotid artery and the significance of endothelial denudation in the pathogenesis of myointimal thickening, *Lab. Invest.*, 32, 339, 1975.
23. Clowes, A. W., Reidy, M. A., and Clowes, M. M., Mechanisms of stenosis after arterial injury, *Lab. Invest.*, 49, 208, 1983.
24. Chamley, J. H. and Campbell, G. R., Mitosis of contractile smooth muscle cells in tissue culture, *Exp. Cell Res.*, 84, 105, 1974.
25. Goode, D., Mitosis of embryonic heart muscle cells *in vitro*. An immunofluorescence and ultrastructural study, *Cytobiologie Z. Exp. Zellforsch.*, 11, 203, 1975.
26. Garrels, J. I. and Gibson, W., Identification and characterization of multiple forms of actin, *Cell*, 9, 793, 1976.
27. Whalen, R. G., Burtler-Browne, G. S., and Gros, F., Protein synthesis and actin heterogeneity in calf muscle cells in culture, *Proc. Natl. Acad. Sci. U.S.A.*, 73, 2018, 1976.
28. Vandekerckhove, J. and Weber, K., At least six different actins are expressed in a higher mammal: an analysis based on the amino acid sequence of the amino-terminal tryptic peptide, *J. Mol. Biol.*, 126, 783, 1978.
29. Vandekerckhove, J. and Weber, K., The complete amino acid sequence of actins from bovine aorta, bovine heart, bovine fast skeletal muscle, and rabbit slow skeletal muscle, *Differentiation*, 14, 123, 1979.
30. Vandekerckhove, J. and Weber, K., Actin typing on total cellular extracts, *Eur. J. Biochem.*, 113, 595, 1981.
31. Korn, E. D., Actin polymerization and its regulation by proteins from nonmuscle cells, *Physiol. Rev.*, 62, 672, 1982.
32. Caplan, A. I., Fiszman, M. Y., and Eppenberger, H. M., Molecular and cell isoforms during development, *Science*, 221, 921, 1983.
33. Devlin, R. B. and Emerson, C. P., Coordinate regulation of contractile protein synthesis during myoblast differentiation, *Cell*, 13, 599, 1978.
34. Gard, D. L. and Lazarides, E., The synthesis and distribution of desmin and vimentin during myogenesis *in vitro*, *Cell*, 19, 263, 1980.
35. Minty, A. J., Alonso, S., Caravatti, M., and Buckingham, M. E., A fetal skeletal muscle actin mRNA in the mouse and its identity with cardiac actin mRNA, *Cell*, 30, 185, 1982.
36. Bains, W., Ponte, P., Blau, H., and Kedes, L., Cardiac actin is the major actin gene product in skeletal muscle cell differentiation *in vitro*, *Mol. Cell Biol.*, 4, 1449, 1984.
37. Bulinski, J. C., Kumar, S., Titani, K., and Hauschka, S. D., Peptide antibody specific for the amino terminus of skeletal muscle α-actin, *Proc. Natl. Acad. Sci. U.S.A.*, 80, 1506, 1983.
38. Gown, A. M., Vogel, A. M., Gordon, D., and Lu, P. L., A smooth muscle-specific monoclonal antibody recognizes smooth muscle actin isozymes, *J. Cell Biol.*, 100, 807, 1985.
39. Herman, I. M. and D'Amore, P. A., Microvascular pericytes contain muscle and nonmuscle actins, *J. Cell Biol.*, 101, 43, 1985.
40. Hirai, S. and Hirabayashi, T., Developmental change of protein constituents in chicken gizzards, *Dev. Biol.*, 97, 483, 1983.
41. Gabbiani, G., Schmid, E., Winter, S., Chaponnier, C., Chastonay, C. D., Vandekerckhove, J., Weber, K., and Franke, W. W., Vascular smooth muscle cells differ from other smooth muscle cells: predominancy of vimentin filaments and a specific α-type actin, *Proc. Natl. Acad. Sci. U.S.A.*, 78, 298, 1981.
42. Moss, N. S. and Benditt, E. P., Spontaneous and experimentally induced arterial lesion. I. An ultrastructural survey of the normal chicken aorta, *Lab. Invest.*, 22, 166, 1970.
43. Lazarides, E., Intermediate filaments as mechanical integrators of cellular space, *Nature (London)*, 283, 249, 1980.
44. Lazarides, E., Intermediate filaments: a chemically heterogeneous, developmentally regulated class of proteins, *Annu. Rev. Biochem.*, 51, 219, 1982.
45. Gard, D. L., Bell, P. B., and Lazarides, E., Coexistence of desmin and the fibroblastic intermediate filaments subunit in muscle and nonmuscle cells: identification and comparative peptide analysis, *Proc. Natl. Acad. Sci. U.S.A.*, 76, 3894, 1979.

46. Bravo, R. and Celis, J. E., Gene expression in normal and virally transformed mouse 3T3B and hamster BHK21 cells, *Exp. Cell Res.*, 127, 249, 1980.
47. Frank, E. D. and Warren, L., Aortic smooth muscle cells contain vimentin instead of desmin, *Proc. Natl. Acad. Sci. U.S.A.*, 78, 3020, 1981.
48. Bennett, G. S., Fellini, S. A., Toyama, Y., and Holtzer, H., Redistribution of intermediate filament subunits during skeletal myogenesis and maturation *in vitro, J. Cell Biol.*, 82, 577, 403, 1979.
49. Somlyo, A. P. and Somlyo, A. V., Ultrastructural aspects of activation and contraction of vascular smooth muscle, *Fed. Proc. Fed. Am. Soc. Exp. Biol.*, 35, 1288, 1976.
50. Cooke, P., A filamentous cytoskeleton in vertebrate smooth muscle fibers, *J. Cell Biol.*, 68, 539, 1976.
51. Gabbiani, G., Rungger-Brändle, E., de Chastonay, C., and Franke, W. W., Vimentin-containing smooth muscle cells in aortic intimal thickening after endothelial injury, *Lab. Invest.*, 47, 265, 1982.
52. Schmid, E., Osborn, M., Rungger-Brändle, E., Gabbiani, G., Weber, K., and Franke, W., Distribution of vimentin and desmin filaments in smooth muscle tissue of mammalian and avian aorta, *Exp. Cell Res.*, 137, 329, 1982.
53. Osborn, M., Caselitz, J., and Weber, K., Heterogeneity of intermediate filament expression in vascular smooth muscle: a gradient in desmin positive cells from the rat aortic arch to the level of the arteria iliaca communis, *Differentiation*, 20, 196, 1981.
54. Lauper, N. T., Unni, K. K., Kottke, B. A., and Titus, J. L., Anatomy and histology of aorta of White Carneau Pigeon, *Lab. Invest.*, 32, 536, 1975.
55. Rosenberg, U. B., Eppenberger, H. M., and Perriard, J., Occurrence of heterogenous forms of the subunits of creatine kinase in various muscle and nonmuscle tissues and their behavior during myogenesis, *Eur. J. Biochem.*, 116, 87, 1981.
56. Perriard, J., Caravatti, M., Perriard, E. R., and Eppenberger, H. M., Quantitation of creatine kinase isoenzyme transitions in differentiating chicken embryonic breast muscle and myogenic cell cultures by immunoadsorption, *Arch. Biochem. Biophys.*, 191, 90, 1978.
57. Caravatti, M., Perriard, J., and Eppenberger, H. M., Developmental regulation of creatine kinase isoenzymes in myogenic cell cultures from chicken, *J. Biol. Chem.*, 254, 1388, 1979.
58. Kligman, D. and Nameroff, M., Analysis of the myogenic lineage in chick embryos. I. Studies on the terminal cell division, *Exp. Cell Res.*, 125, 201, 1980.
59. Jockers-Wretou, E., Giebel, W., and Pfleiderer, G., Immunohistochemical localization of creatinkinase isoenzymes in human tissue, *Histochemistry*, 54, 83, 1977.
60. Hoag, G. N., Franks, C. R., Smith, C., and DeCoteau, W. E., Creatine kinase isoenzyme patterns in normal smooth muscle and smooth muscle neoplasms, *Clin. Biochem.*, 13, 149, 1980.
61. Iyengar, M. R., Fluellen, C. E., and Iyengar, C. W. L., Increased creatine kinase in the hormone-stimulated smooth muscle of the bovine uterus, *Biochem. Biophys. Res. Commun.*, 94, 948, 1980.
62. Kimes, B. W. and Brandt, B. L., Characterization of two putative smooth muscle cell lines from rat thoracic aorta, *Exp. Cell Res.*, 98, 349, 1976.
63. Whalen, R. G., Sell, S. M., Butler-Browne, G. S., Schwartz, K., Bouveret, P., and Pinset-Härström, I., Three myosin heavy-chain isozymes appear sequentially in rat muscle development, *Nature (London)*, 292, 805, 1981.
64. Gorza, L., Sartore, S., Triban, C., and Schiaffino, S., Embryonic-like myosin heavy chains in regenerating chicken muscle, *Exp. Cell Res.*, 143, 395, 1983.
65. Gauthier, G. F., Lowey, S., Benfield, P. A., and Hobbs, A. W., Distribution and properties of myosin isozymes in developing avian and mammalian skeletal muscle fibers, *J. Cell Biol.*, 92, 471, 1982.
66. Schiaffino, S., Askanas, V., Engel, W. K., Vitadello, M., and Sartore, S., Myosin isoenzymes in cultured human muscle, *Arch. Neurol. (Chicago)*, 39, 347, 1982.
67. Burridge, K., A comparison of fibroblast and smooth muscle myosins, *FEBS Lett.*, 45, 14, 1974.
68. Chamley, J. H., Campbell, G. R., McConnell, J. D., and Gröschel-Stewart, U., Comparison of vascular smooth muscle cells from adult human, monkey and rabbit in primary culture, *Cell Tissue Res.*, 177, 503, 1977.
69. Larson, D. M., Fujiwara, K., Alexander, R. W., and Gimbrone, M., Heterogeneity of myosin antigenic expression in vascular smooth muscle *in vivo, Lab. Invest.*, 50, 401, 1984.
70. Larson, D. M., Fujiwara, K., Alexander, R. W., and Gimbrone, M., Myosin in cultured vascular smooth muscle cells: immunofluorescence and immunochemical studies of alterations in antigenic expression, *J. Cell Biol.*, 99, 1582, 1984.
71. Longtine, J. A., Pinkus, G. S., Fujiwara, K., and Corson, J. M., Immunohistochemical localization of smooth muscle myosin in normal human tissues, *J. Histochem. Cytochem.*, 33, 179, 1985.
72. Crisona, N. J. and Strohman, R. C., Inhibition of contraction of cultured muscle fibers results in increased turnover of myofibrillar proteins but not of intermediate-filament proteins, *J. Cell Biol.*, 96, 684, 1983.

73. Joyce, N. C., Haire, M. F., and Palade, G. E., Contractile proteins in pericytes. I. Immunoperoxidase localization of tropomyosin, *J. Cell Biol.*, 100, 1379, 1985.
74. Zierler, R. E., Bandyk, D. F., Thiele, B. L., and Strandness, D. E., Carotid artery stenosis following endarterectomy, *Arch. Surg. (Chicago)*, 117, 1408, 1982.
75. Roederer, G. O., Langlois, Y. E., Lusiani, L., Jager, K. A., Primozich, J. F., Lawrence, R. J., Phillips, D. J., and Strandness, D. E., Natural history of carotid artery disease on the side contralateral to endarterectomy, *J. Vasc. Surg.*, 1, 62, 1984.
76. Roederer, G. O., Langlois, Y. E., Jager, K. A., Primozich, J. F., Lawrence, R. J., Beach, K. W., Phillips, D. J., and Strandness, D. E., The natural history of carotid arterial disease in asymptomatic patients with cervical bruits, *Stroke*, 15, 605, 1984.
77. Stoney, R. J. and String, S. T., Recurrent carotid stenosis, *Surgery*, 80, 705, 1976.
78. Hertzer, N. R., Martinez, B. D., and Beven, E. G., Recurrent stenosis after carotid endarterectomy, *Surg. Gynecol. Obstet.*, 149, 360, 1979.
79. Turnipseed, W. D., Berkoff, H. A., and Crummy, A., Postoperative occlusion after carotid endarterectomy, *Arch. Surg. (Chicago)*, 115, 573, 1980.
80. Kremen, J. E., Gee, W., Kaupp, H. A., and McDonald, K. M., Restenosis or occlusion after carotid endarterectomy, *Arch. Surg. (Chicago)*, 114, 608, 1979.
81. Imparato, A. M., Bracco, A., Kim, G. E., and Zeff, R., Intimal and neointimal fibrous proliferation causing failure of arterial reconstructions, *Surgery*, 72, 1007, 1972.
82. French, B. N. and Rewcastle, N. B., Sequential morphological changes at the site of carotid endarterectomy, *J. Neurosurg.*, 41, 745, 1974.
83. Cossman, D., Callow, A. D., Stein, A., and Matsumoto, G., Early restenosis after carotid endarterectomy, *Arch. Surg. (Chicago)*, 113, 275, 1978.
84. Clowes, A. W. and Clowes, M. M., The influence of chronic hypertension on injured and uninjured arteries in spontaneously hypertensive rats, *Lab. Invest.*, 43, 535, 1980.
85. Clowes, A. W., Reidy, M. A., and Clowes, M. M., Kinetics of cellular proliferation after arterial injury. I. Smooth muscle growth in the absence of endothelium, *Lab. Invest.*, 49, 327, 1983.
86. Reidy, M. A., Clowes, A. W., and Schwartz, S. M., Endothelial regeneration. V. Inhibition of endothelium in arteries of rat and rabbit, *Lab. Invest.*, 49, 569, 1983.
87. Orekhov, A. N., Kosykh, V. A., Repin, V. S., and Smirnov, V. N., Cell proliferation in normal and atherosclerotic human aorta. I. Flow cytofluorometric determination of cellular DNA content, *Lab. Invest.*, 48, 395, 1983.
88. Spagnoli, L. G., Villaschi, S., Neri, L., Palmieri, G., Taurino, M., Faraglia, V., and Fiorani, P., Autoradiographic studies of the smooth muscle cells in human arteries, *Paroi Arterielle/Arterial Wall*, 7, 107, 1981.
89. Villaschi, S. and Spagnoli, L. G., Autoradiographic and ultrastructural studies on the human fibro-atheromatous plaque, *Atherosclerosis*, 48, 95, 1983.
90. Glenn, K. C. and Ross, R., Human monocyte-derived growth factor(s) for mesenchymal cells: activation of secretion by endotoxin and concanavalin A, *Cell*, 24, 603, 1981.
91. Martin, B. M., Gimbrone, M. A., Jr., Unanue, E. R., and Cotran, R. S., Stimulation of nonlymphoid mesenchymal cell proliferation by a macrophage-derived growth factor, *J. Immunol.*, 126, 1510, 1981.
92. Gabbiani, G., Kocher, O., Bloom, W. S., Vandekerckhove, J., and Weber, K., Actin expression in smooth muscle cells of rat aortic intimal thickening, human atheromatous plaque, and cultured rat aortic media, *J. Clin. Invest.*, 73, 148, 1984.
93. Wiener, J., Loud, A. V., Giacomelli, F., and Anversa, P., Morphometric analysis of hypertension-induced hypertrophy of rat thoracic aorta, *Am. J. Pathol.*, 88, 619, 1977.
94. Owens, G. K. and Schwartz, S. M., Vascular smooth muscle cell hypertrophy and hyperploidy in the Goldblatt hypertensive rat, *Circ. Res*, 53, 491, 1983.
95. Clowes, A. W. and Schwartz, S. M., Significance of quiescent smooth muscle migration in the injured rat carotid artery, *Circ. Res.*, 56, 139, 1985.
96. Reidy, M. A., personal communication, 1985.
97. Limas, C., Westrum, B., and Limas, C. J., The evolution of vascular changes in the spontaneously hypertensive rat, *Am. J. Pathol.*, 98, 357, 1980.
98. Chobanian, A. V., Prescott, M. F., and Haudenschild, C. C., Recent advances in molecular pathology. The effects of hypertension on the arterial wall, *Exp. Mol. Pathol.*, 41, 153, 1984.
99. Schwartz, S. M. and Ross, R., Cellular proliferation in atherosclerosis and hypertension, *Prog. Cardiovasc. Dis.*, 26, 355, 1984.
100. Reidy, M. A. and Silver, M., Endothelial regeneration. VII. Lack of intimal proliferation after defined injury to rat aorta, *Am. J. Pathol.*, 118, 173, 1985.
101. Gajdusek, C. M. and Schwartz, S. M., Comparison of intracellular and extracellular mitogen activity, *J. Cell Physiol.*, 121, 316, 1984.

102. Barrett, T. B., Gajdusek, C. M., Schwartz, S. M., McDougall, J. K., and Benditt, E. P., Expression of the *sis* gene by endothelial cells in culture and *in vitro, Proc. Natl. Acad. Sci. U.S.A.*, 81, 6772, 1984.
103. Seifert, R. A., Schwartz, S. M., and Bowen-Pope, D. F., Developmentally regulated production of platelet-derived growth factor-like molecules, *Nature (London)*, 311, 669, 1984.
104. Folkow, B., Physiological aspects of primary hypertension, *Physiol. Rev.*, 62, 347, 1982.
105. Goldberg, I. D., Rosen, E. M., Shapiro, H. M., Zoller, L. C., Myrick, K., Levenson, S. E., and Christenson, L., Isolation and culture of a tetraploid subpopulation of smooth muscle cells from the normal rat aorta, *Science*, 226, 559, 1984.
106. Gordon, D., Mohai, L. G., and Schwartz, S. M., Induction of polyploidy in cultures of neonatal rat aortic smooth muscle cells, in preparation.
107. Salmons, A. and Sreter, F. A., Significance of impulse activity in the transformation of skeletal muscle type, *Nature (London)*, 263, 30, 1976.

Chapter 2

METHODS OF GROWING VASCULAR SMOOTH MUSCLE IN CULTURE

Julie H. Campbell and Gordon R. Campbell

TABLE OF CONTENTS

I. INTRODUCTION

The methodology, enzymes, culture medium, substrate, and chambers used for growing smooth muscle in culture vary with the type and purpose of the experiment, the age and species of the donor, and the personal preference of the investigators. In this chapter, the systems used by some of the established laboratories will be described. Most researchers use similar methods, modified slightly to suit their particular requirements.

II. CULTURE PROCEDURES

A. Enzyme-Dispersed Cells in Primary Culture

The methods developed in our laboratories will be described in detail. The enzymes used are collagenase (Worthington CLS III, approximately 105 units/mg) at 3 mg/mℓ in Medium 199 minus serum (M199-S) and elastase (Sigma E-0127, 60 units/mg) at 1 mg/mℓ in M199-S. Six hundred milligrams of collagenase is placed in 200 mℓ M199-S and dissolved by stirring over ice for 1 hr. In order to remove residual particulate material and sterilize the solution, it is filtered by negative pressure successively through 5 μm, 0.8 μm, 0.45 μm, and 0.2 μm Millipore® filters. It is then aliquoted into 20 × 10 mℓ sterile plastic tubes, frozen immediately at −20°C, and used within 1 month. 10 Milligram elastase is dissolved in 10 mℓ M199-S, and the pH is adjusted to 7 with sterile NaOH. The solution is sterilized by negative pressure through 0.2-μm Millipore® filters and used the same day.

1. Elastic Arteries (Pig, Rabbit, Rat Aortas)

Freshly dissected aortas from adult animals are placed in cold Hank's Balanced Salt Solution (HBSS) plus 5% fetal calf serum (FCS). The vessels are cleaned by removing the fat and connective tissue under a dissecting microscope, cut longitudinally; and, using watchmaker forceps, the intima plus the inner two thirds of the media is removed in 1-mm-wide horizontal strips from the adventitia. This procedure is carried out in a 90-mm glass petri dish containing HBSS-S and a scintered glass plate to prevent sliding of the tissue. The muscle strips are then transferred to collagenase in a 50-mℓ Erlenmeyer flask. The methodology can then proceed in either of two ways depending on the available time:

Method 1. The tissue plus collagenase is gently stirred on an orbital shaker for 1 hr at 37°C. The pH is regularly adjusted with 1 *M* NaOH. The collagenase is removed from the tissue with a Pasteur pipette and discarded, elastase added and the tissue pipetted up and down in a wide-bore pipette then stirred at 37°C for a further hour. Finally, more collagenase is added and the tissue stirred and regularly pipetted until all tissue has dispersed into single cells (about $1^1/_2$ hr).

Method 2. If there is lack of time, an equal volume of M199-S is added to the tissue/collagenase and the flask placed in a 37°C incubator overnight. (The extra volume prevents an undesirable change in pH.) The following morning, fresh collagenase is added on top of the M199/collagenase/tissue, gently pipetted, and left for 30 min to 1 hr at 37°C with stirring until the tissue has completely dispersed into single cells.

2. Muscular Arteries (Rat Caudal Artery, Rabbit Ear Artery)

The vessels are cleaned of fat and connective tissue and placed in collagenase in a 60-mm petri dish. The vessels are stirred gently on an orbital shaker at 37°C. At regular 10-min intervals, the adventitia is very gently pipetted away from the underlying muscle. When the vessel becomes translucent, only the muscle layer is present. The vessels are placed in fresh collagenase, cut into 3-mm lengths, transferred to an Erlenmeyer flask with an equal volume of M199, and placed in a 37°C incubator overnight. The following morning the tissue suspension is centrifuged at 900 rpm for 5 min and the supernatant discarded. The tissue is resuspended in 0.125% trypsin-versene solution, gently stirred, and pipetted at 37°C until the cells are completely dissociated ($^1/_2$ to $^3/_4$ hr). FCS is added to inactivate the trypsin, and the suspension is again spun at 900 rpm for 5 min.

3. Arterioles (Rat Mesenteric Vessels)

Mesenteric vessels are embedded in a large amount of fat. To make the adipose tissue firm for ease of removal, the tissue is placed in HBSS on ice. It is then placed in collagenase at 37°C for 10 min, transferred back into cold HBSS, and the fat and connective tissue is stripped away. The cold HBSS is replaced frequently so that fat globules are removed. The mesenteric vein with its anastomosing branches are separated from the artery and arterioles and discarded. The mesenteric arterioles are now separated from the mesenteric artery and placed in 60-mm petri dishes with collagenase for 10 min so that the adventitia disperses away with gentle pipetting. The muscle layer is transferred to fresh collagenase, cut into small pieces, and dispersed into single cells the same as for muscular arteries.

4. Embryonic Blood Vessels (Chick Aorta)

Embryonic and neonatal blood vessels disperse very easily and require only a 30-min incubation in collagenase (discarded), followed by successive 10-min incubations in 0.1% trypsin (1:250; Nutritional Biochemicals) in Ca^{2+} and Mg^{2+}-free HBSS.

5. Plating of Dispersed Cells

The enzyme-cell suspensions are transferred to 10-mℓ centrifuge tubes containing 1 mℓ of FCS and spun at 900 rpm for 5 min. A drop of the supernatant is placed on a microscope slide to check that all cells have pelleted. If some cells remain in suspension, the supernatant is transferred to fresh tubes and respun at 1200 rpm. The cell pellets are gently resuspended in nutrient medium, a cell count performed, then the cell concentration adjusted to the required amount and the cells plated out.

References 1 to 13 provide variations of all of the above methods.

B. Reaggregrates of Enzyme-Dispersed Cells

The methodology described is from Sperelakis' laboratory.[3-5]

The blood vessels are dispersed into single cells, pelleted, and resuspended in nutrient medium to a concentration of about 10^6 cells per milliliter. Spherical reaggregates of the separated cells are obtained by two methods:

Method 1 — One milliliter of cell suspension is placed in a well-chamber made from a glass ring attached to boiled cellophane dialysis tubing (2 cm diameter) by high-vacuum silicone grease, enclosed within a Carrel flask. After 2 mℓ of culture medium is placed around the glass rings in the Carrel flask, the culture is incubated at 37°C. The cells do not adhere to the dialysis tubing, and reaggregates of dispersed cells begin to form within 36 hr. After 3 to 5 days, the reaggregates (50 to 200 μm diameter) become round, translucent, and firmly packed.

Method 2 — In this method, which is based on that of Moscona,[14] 2 to 3 mℓ of cell suspension is placed in 25-mℓ Erlenmeyer flasks, sealed with rubber stoppers, and covered with parafilm. The flasks are rotated in a gyratory shaker bath at 37°C for 48 hr at a speed of 70 rpm.

C. Free-Floating Explants

The methodology is from Jarmolych and colleagues[15-17] (see also Reference 18).

Medial tissue is cut into segments (1 × 1 mm to 1 × 5 mm) and placed in 30-mℓ plastic culture bottles containing 5 mℓ of nutrient medium. The explants do not attach to the substrate, and there is no cell outgrowth beyond the periphery of the explant itself.

D. Substrate-Attached Explants

The methodology is from Wissler and colleagues.[19,20]

Round explants, 2 mm in diameter, are punched out from cleaned medial tissue with a sterile skin biopsy punch. These explants are placed in 30-mℓ plastic flasks, usually one in each flask, and incubated in 2.5 mℓ medium plus serum at 37°C. To facilitate adherence of the explants to the substrate, the flasks are turned upside down for 2 hr each day. Initial outgrowth occurs within 1 to 2 weeks.

E. Subcultured Cells

The methodology is from Ross.[21,22]

Intimal-medial strips are placed in a petri dish containing nutrient medium and cut into 1-mm^3 pieces using a scissoring action with two Number 11 Bard-Parker surgical blades. Explants are cut cleanly without tearing as cells do not appear to migrate readily from torn edges of tissue. The explants are washed several times in nutrient medium and dispensed into pregassed, 75-cm^2 plastic flasks with 3 mℓ of medium containing 100 to 150 explants per flask. The flasks are swirled to disperse the explants evenly. When the explants have attached to the bottom of the flask (about 1 week), a greater volume of medium is added. Alternatively, the flask can be maintained upright for 2 to 3 hr to encourage attachment of explants.[23] A coverslip[24] or dialysis membrane[25] is placed over the explants to hold them in place, or each explant is immobilized into the plastic surface of the flask with a platinum-Teflon®-steel wire positioner.[26] Outgrowth from the explants reaches confluency in 2 to 3 weeks. They are then washed in Tris-versene buffer (0.54 m*M* versene and 0.02 *M* Tris-HCl pH 7.4 at 37°C) and detached from the substrate with 0.05% trypsin (Difco® 1:250 trypsin) in Tris-versene buffer by incubation for 10 min at 37°C. The trypsin is inactivated with medium containing 10% FCS, and the suspension is centrifuged at 1000 rpm for 7 min. The cell pellet is resuspended in medium plus serum and dispensed into culture dishes at a known concentration. When confluency is reached, the cells are subcultured, using the trypsinization procedure described above.

III. CULTURE MEDIUM

A. Composition

The most commonly used medium for growth of vascular smooth muscle in culture is the Dulbecco-Vogt modification of Eagle's minimal essential medium[27] plus 5 or 10% serum. Frequent additions are 2 to 4 m*M* glutamine, 0.28 *M* bicarbonate, and 100 m*M* nonessential amino acids;[28] sometimes, 1 m*M* sodium pyruvate is also added.[21] Eagle's minimal essential medium, either with[23] or without[10,19] supplements, is also popular. Several laboratories, including our own, use Medium 199 with Hank's salts,[1,15-18] while in other laboratories Ham's F10[29] and Ham's F12[26,30] media are used. Antibiotics are used universally, generally 100 Iu/mℓ penicillin plus 100 μg/mℓ streptomycin. Some laboratories use 50 Iu/mℓ penicillin plus 50 μg/mℓ streptomycin plus 100 μg/mℓ kanamycin, while others use 50 μg/mℓ gentamycin alone. In our laboratories, 100 Iu/mℓ penicillin alone is used.

B. Serum

For convenience and good growth characteristics, most laboratories use either 5 or

10% FCS (whole blood serum) in nutrient medium for vascular smooth muscle cultures. However, because of the escalating cost of this product, many laboratories are making their own serums. This is not difficult and has the advantage that serum from the same species from which the cells are derived can be used. Additionally, as pointed out by Ross et al.[31] (see also Chapter 6, this volume), vascular smooth muscle cells (SMC) in vivo come into contact only with whole blood serum when platelet aggregation and release has occurred in a vessel with an injured endothelium. Under normal circumstances, SMC are bathed by a filtrate of plasma. For vascular smooth muscle cultures, Ross has pioneered the use of homologous plasma-derived serum, which does not contain platelet-releaseate products, and in which the cells remain quiescent as in vivo.

The methodology for preparation of whole blood serum and plasma-derived serum comes from Ross and Kariya.[21]

1. Whole Blood Serum for Stock Cultures

Blood from several animals is pooled and allowed to clot for at least 24 hr at 4°C. The resulting serum is separated from the clots, pooled, and centrifuged at 22,000 × g for 15 min at 4°C. The centrifuged serum is filtered through a 0.22-μm Millipore filter using positive pressure and heat inactivated at 56°C for 30 min; it is then stored at −70°C.

2. Whole Blood Serum

Using plastic or siliconized glass syringes, the blood is drawn from at least four animals into 3.8% sodium citrate, one volume citrate to ten volumes blood. Each donor's blood is separately calcified with 1.0 *M* $CaCl_2$ to a final concentration of 14 μ mol/mℓ allowed to clot at 37°C for 2 hr, and then centrifuged at 1085 × g for 15 minutes at 4°C. The serums are respun at 22,000 × g for 30 min at 4°C, pooled, and dialyzed (Dialya Por, 6000 to 8000 mol wt cutoff) against Ringers at 4°C for 24 hr. It is then heat inactivated at 56°C for 30 min, filtered through 0.22-μm Millipore®, and stored at −70°C.

3. Plasma-Derived Serum

The blood is drawn into prechilled (4°C) citrated plastic or siliconized glass syringes. The blood from each donor is spun separately in plastic or siliconized glass tubes at 1085 × g for 15 min at 4°C and the resulting plasma respun at 22,000 × g for 30 minutes at 4°C. The platelet-poor plasma is pooled and kept on ice for 3 hr; 1.0 *M* $CaCl_2$ to a final concentration of 20 μ mol/mℓ and one volume of Ringers for six volumes plasma are added; then the plasma is incubated at 37°C for 2 hr. The plasma is spun at 22,000 × g for 30 min to remove the fibrin clot and dialyzed against 0.1 *M* Tris pH 7.4 overnight. The plasma-derived serum is applied to a CM-Sephadex C-50 column and eluted with 0.1 *M* Tris pH 7.4. The eluate is concentrated back to its original volume by ultrafiltration using an Amicon Diaflo PM-10 membrane, dialyzed for 24 hr against Ringers at 4°C, heat inactivated, and stored at −70°C.

IV. CULTURE CHAMBERS AND SUBSTRATES

Vascular SMC are generally grown in plastic culture dishes or flasks; however, they also attach well to very clean glass coverslips placed either in plastic dishes or in specialized chambers, such as the Rose chamber. They grow well on collagen membranes,[32] elastic membranes,[33] smooth silicone rubber substrata,[34] polyacrylonitrile (orlon) fabrics, dacron velour, and Parylene-C coated polypropylene microfabric,[35] and microcarrier beads (see Chapter 3).

ACKNOWLEDGMENTS

The expert assistance of Janet Rogers, Lucy Popadynec, Liana Butera, Bridget Southwell, and Mary Jane Black is gratefully acknowledged.

REFERENCES

1. Chamley, J. H., Campbell, G. R., McConnell, J. D., and Gröschel-Stewart, U., Comparison of vascular smooth muscle cells from adult human, monkey and rabbit in primary culture and in subculture, *Cell Tissue Res.*, 177, 503, 1977.
2. Chamley-Campbell, J. H., Campbell, G. R., and Ross, R., The smooth muscle cell in culture, *Physiol. Rev.*, 59, 1, 1979.
3. Harder, D. R. and Sperelakis, N., Action potential generation in reaggregates of rat aortic smooth muscle cells in primary culture, *Blood Vessels*, 16, 186, 1979.
4. Ives, H. E., Schultz, G. S., Galardy, R. E., and Jamieson, J. D., Preparation of functional smooth muscle cells from the rabbit aorta, *J. Exp. Med.*, 148, 1400, 1978.
5. McLean, M. J. and Sperelakis, N., Electrophysiological recordings from spontaneously contracting reaggregates of cultured vascular smooth muscle cells from chick embryos, *Exp. Cell Res.*, 104, 309, 1977.
6. Martin, G. M., Ogburn, C. E., and Wight, T. N., Comparative rates of decline in the primary cloning efficiencies of smooth muscle cells from the aging thoracic aorta of two murine species of contrasting maximum life span potentials, *Am. J. Pathol.*, 110, 236, 1983.
7. Hermsmeyer, K., De Cino, P., and White, R., Spontaneous contractions of dispersed vascular muscle in cell culture, *In Vitro*, 12, 628, 1976.
8. Gimbrone, M. A. and Cotran, R. S., Human vascular smooth muscle in culture. Growth and ultrastructure, *Lab. Invest.*, 33, 16, 1975.
9. Nilsson, J., Ksiazek, T., Heldin, C.-H., and Thyberg, J., Demonstration of stimulatory effects of platelet-derived growth factor on cultivated rat arterial smooth muscle cells. Differences between cells from young and adult animals, *Exp. Cell Res.*, 145, 231, 1983.
10. May, J. F., Paule, W. J., Rounds, D. E., Blankenhorn, D. H., and Zemplenyi, T., The induction of atherosclerotic plaque-like mounds in cultures of aortic smooth muscle cells, *Virchows Arch. B*, 18, 205, 1975.
11. Garay, R. P., Moura, A. M., Osborne-Pellegrin, M. J., Papadimitriou, A., and Worcel, M., Identification of different sodium compartments from smooth muscle cells, fibroblasts and endothelial cells, in arteries and tissue culture, *J. Physiol. (London)*, 287, 213, 1979.
12. Yau-Young, A. O., Shio, H., and Fowler, S., Growth, biochemistry, and morphology of isolated rabbit aortic smooth muscle cells maintained in the presence or absence of serum, *J. Cell. Physiol.*, 108, 461, 1981.
13. Martin, W. and Gordon, J. L., Spontaneous and agonist-induced ^{86}Rb efflux from rabbit aortic smooth muscle cells in culture: a comparison with fresh tissue, *J. Cell. Physiol.*, 115, 53, 1983.
14. Moscona, A., Rotation-mediated histogenic aggregation of dissociated cells. A quantifiable approach to cell interactions in vitro, *Exp. Cell Res.*, 22, 455, 1961.
15. Jarmolych, J., Daoud, A. S., Landau, J., Fritz, K. E., and McElvene, E., Aortic media explants. Cell proliferation and production of mucopolysaccharides, collagen, and elastic tissue, *Exp. Mol. Pathol.*, 9, 171, 1968.
16. Daoud, A. S., Fritz, K. E., and Jarmolych, J., Increased DNA synthesis in aortic explants from swine fed a high-cholesterol diet, *Exp. Mol. Pathol.*, 13, 377, 1970.
17. Fritz, K. E., Jarmolych, J., and Daoud, A. S., Association of DNA synthesis and apparent dedifferentiation of aortic smooth muscle cells *in vitro*, *Exp. Mol. Pathol.*, 12, 354, 1970.
18. Rossi, G. L., Alroy, J., and Röthenmund, S., Morphological studies of cultured swine aorta media explants, *Virchows Arch. B*, 12, 133, 1973.
19. Fisher-Dzoga, K., Jones, R. M., Vesselinovitch, D., and Wissler, R. W., Ultrastructural and immunohistochemical studies of primary cultures of aortic media cells, *Exp. Mol. Pathol.*, 18, 162, 1973.
20. Fisher-Dzoga, K., Chen, R., and Wissler, R. W., Effects of serum lipoproteins on the morphology, growth, and metabolism of arterial smooth muscle cells, in *Arterial Mesenchyme and Arteriosclerosis*, Wagner, W. D. and Clarkson, T. B., Eds., Plenum Press, New York, 1974, 299.

21. Ross, R. and Kariya, B., Morphogenesis of vascular smooth muscle in atherosclerosis and cell culture, in *Handbook of Physiology,* Section 2: The Cardiovascular System, *Vascular Smooth Muscle,* Vol. 2, Bohr, D., Somlyo, A. P., and Sparks, H. V., Jr., Eds., American Physiological Society, Washington, D.C., 1980, 69.
22. Ross, R., The smooth muscle cell. II. Growth of smooth muscle in culture and formation of elastic fibers, *J. Cell Biol.,* 50, 172, 1971.
23. St. Clair, R. W., Smith, B. P., and Wood, L. L., Stimulation of cholesterol esterification in Rhesus monkey arterial smooth muscle cells, *Circ. Res.,* 40, 166, 1977.
24. Brown, B. G., Mahley, R., and Assman, G., Swine aortic smooth muscle in tissue culture. Some effects of purified swine lipoproteins on cell growth and morphology, *Circ. Res.,* 39, 415, 1976.
25. Chamley, J. H., Goller, I., and Burnstock, G., Selective growth of sympathetic nerve fibers to explants of normally densely innervated autonomic effector organs in tissue culture, *Dev. Biol.,* 31, 362, 1973.
26. Björkerud, S. and Ekroth, R., The growth of human atherosclerotic and non-atherosclerotic aortic intima and media in vitro, *Artery,* 8, 329, 1980.
27. Vogt, M. and Dulbecco, R., Steps in the neoplastic transformation of hamster embryo cells by polyoma virus, *Proc. Natl. Acad. Sci. U.S.A.,* 49, 171, 1963.
28. Pietilä, K. and Nikkari, T., Effect of phase of growth and hyperlipidemic serum on the synthesis of collagen in rabbit aortic smooth muscle cells in culture, *Med. Biol.,* 56, 111, 1978.
29. Larrue, J., Daret, D., Demond-Henri, J., Allières, C., and Bricaud, H., Prostacyclin synthesis by proliferative aortic smooth muscle cells. A kinetic in vivo and in vitro study, *Atherosclerosis,* 50, 63, 1984.
30. Thyberg, J., Nilsson, J., Palmberg, L., and Sjölund, M., Adult human arterial smooth muscle cells in primary culture. Modulation from contractile to synthetic phenotype, *Cell Tissue Res.,* 239, 69, 1985.
31. Ross, R., Nist, C., Kariya, B., Rivest, M.-J., Raines, E., and Callis, J., Physiological quiescence in plasma-derived serum: influence of platelet-derived growth factor on cell growth in culture, *J. Cell. Physiol.,* 97 (Suppl.1), 497, 1978.
32. Csonka, E., Szemenyei, K., Miskulin, M., and Robert, A. M., Morphological examination of aortic endothelial and smooth muscle cells grown *in vitro* on collagen membranes, *Artery,* 8, 253, 1980.
33. Leung, D. Y. M., Glagov, S., and Mathews, M. B., Cyclic stretching stimulates synthesis of matrix components by arterial smooth muscle cells *in vitro, Science,* 191, 475, 1976.
34. Buck, R. C., Behaviour of vascular smooth muscle cells during repeated stretching of the substratum *in vitro, Atherosclerosis,* 46, 217, 1983.
35. Eskin, S. G., Armeniades, C. D., Lie, J. T., Trevino, L., and Kennedy, J. H., Growth of cultured calf aortic smooth muscle cells on cardiovascular prosthetic materials, *J. Biomed. Mater. Res.,* 10, 113, 1976.

Chapter 3

MICROCARRIER CULTURE OF VASCULAR SMOOTH MUSCLE CELLS

Susan E. O'Connor and Peter F. Davies

TABLE OF CONTENTS

I. INTRODUCTION

The in vitro culture of vascular smooth muscle cells (SMC) is an integral component of cardiovascular research in relation to both normal vascular physiology and the pathogenesis of atherosclerosis. Any procedures which offer new and potentially valuable methods for propagating vascular cells are therefore of significant interest. Microcarrier systems, in addition to providing scaled-up culture of vascular cells, enable a variety of innovative approaches to vascular cell research. In this chapter we present straightforward techniques for the propagation on microcarriers of anchorage-dependent cells in general and vascular SMC in particular, using methods in routine use in this laboratory.

II. CONCEPT

Anchorage-dependent cells die quickly without attachment to a substratum and therefore cannot be maintained in suspension culture. In an attempt to overcome this limitation, the use of small beads to propagate anchorage-dependent cells in suspension culture was first introduced by van Wezel[1] in 1967. Significant advances in the development of microcarrier technology, particularly since the mid-1970s, have resulted in the culture of many different kinds of cells on beads in suspension. Development was stimulated primarily by a need to scale up cultures of anchorage-dependent animal cell lines for the efficient production of biological products. Examples include the production of vaccines,[2-5] interferon,[6] and other commercially valuable cell products.[7-11] The advantages of scale-up have also been utilized to obtain large numbers of cells synchronized in mitosis[12] and high yields of purified membrane fractions.[13]

Very recently, novel manipulations of relatively small quantities of cells have been used for research purposes. Cardiovascular research, in particular, has made use of a number of microcarrier types to address questions relevant to vascular cell function that were previously difficult to investigate. For example, Ryan et al.[14] have used a microcarrier system to monitor cell-surface events in pulmonary artery endothelium. Previous studies were hindered by the need for proteolytic enzyme digestion during isolation and subculture procedures. Furthermore, the ease of transfer of anchorage-dependent cells has been effectively utilized — first, to prepare microcarrier beds in glass columns for biochemical studies in endothelial cells using flow-through systems[15,16] and, second, in studies of vascular cell interactions[17,18,34,35] (see also Davies, Volume II, Chapter 15).

III. MICROCARRIERS

A. General Characteristics

The earliest microcarriers developed from DEAE Sephadex[1] possessed high positive charges distributed throughout a porous matrix. The adsorption of nutrients and cofactors from the culture medium onto a large internal surface area and the restriction by high electrostatic interactions of normal cell movements led to poor plating efficiencies and low replication rates. It has since been shown that the lowest possible positive charge or low negative charge is optimal for cell attachment and spreading.[19] When the charge is limited to the surface of the microcarrier, adsorption of serum proteins by the large internal surface area of a porous bead is markedly reduced.[20] The introduction of solid beads minimized these problems and also reduced the volume of culture medium required to bathe the cells by eliminating diffusion of medium into the bead. The smooth surface of solid microcarriers also promotes efficient cell attachment and spreading.

The composition of the bead matrix determines the ease of preparation of microcarriers prior to cell culture. Hydration procedures involving multiple washings are inconvenient features of some microcarriers. If prepared swollen beads are stored, bactericidal agents must be removed before their use with cultured cells. The most convenient forms of microcarriers are solid matrices supplied in a sterilized, dry form.

Because microcarriers are best suited for suspension culture, the specific density of the beads must allow them to be easily mixed at low stirring speeds. Most fall in the density range of 1.03 to 1.045 g/mℓ. Those at the higher end of the range rapidly settle upon cessation of stirring; although this can be a useful feature for the separation of medium and beads, such microcarriers often require higher stirring speeds. The density of the microcarrier changes with the addition of cells and their subsequent proliferation. With increasing cell numbers, it is sometimes necessary to increase the stirring speed to maintain the microcarriers in suspension.

For visualizing cells on microcarriers either by phase-contrast microscopy of living cells or after staining, a transparent microcarrier is useful. Under microscopic observation, two planes of focus are possible, giving visual access to both the "front" and "rear" of the microcarrier and enabling a simple estimate to be made of the extent of colonization.

B. Commercially Available Microcarriers

The different types of commercially available microcarriers are listed in Table 1 along with their major properties. While all of the microcarriers listed will support the attachment and growth of anchorage-dependent cells, some are more suited for use with either epithelial or fibroblast-like cells. Biocarrier, Cytodex 1, Superbeads, and Cytodex 2 are reported to be more useful with cells having a fibroblast-like morphology, while Cytodex 3, Biosilon, and Cytosphere are suggested for cells with epithelial morphology.[21,22] The choice of microcarrier, however, is best made with the type of experiment in mind since all will, with appropriate handling, provide viable cultures. For example, is an intrabead porous volume important for the experiments? Are morphological studies (including scanning and transmission electron microscopy) important, and will bead shrinkage compromise their interpretation?

For vascular cell culture, our laboratory has had experience primarily with Biosilon (Nunc, Denmark; Vangard International, Inc., Neptune, N.J.). This choice arose simply because these microcarriers, which we use extensively for studies of cellular biochemistry, have the closest composition to tissue culture plastic and, in the system described below, reproducibly propagate vascular endothelial and SMC, skin fibroblasts, and 3T3 cells with identical characteristics (as far as we can determine) to the same cells grown in dishes and flasks. They also maintain suspension cultures of adherent human blood monocytes and mouse peritoneal macrophages for short periods of time. Properties which render this microcarrier particularly suitable for biochemical experiments with cultured cells are

1. Nonporous solid polystyrene (Figure 1) of similar composition to standard tissue culture dishes and flasks (the nonporous nature eliminates high adsorption of radiolabeled tracers and metabolic products; cells are readily removed from the plastic surface by trypsin:EDTA for cell counts and for the measurement of cell-to-cell bead ratios)
2. Transparent, nonshrinking upon air-drying, and extractable into organic solvents thereby allowing cells to be fixed and stained for observation and processed for electron microscopy without shrinkage

Table 1
COMMERCIAL MICROCARRIERS

Name	Manufacturer	Type[a]
Biosilon	Nunc, Denmark	Polystyrene, NP
Biocarriers	Biorad, U.S.	Polyacrylamide, P
Cytodex 1, 2, 3	Pharmacia, Sweden	Dextran, P
Cytospheres	Lux, U.S.	Polystyrene, NP
DE-52, DE-53	Whatman, U.K.	Microgranular cellulose, P
Gelibeads	KC Biological, U.S.	Cross-linked gelatin, P
Superbeads	Flow Labs, U.S.	Dextran, P

[a] P, porous matrix; NP, non-porous matrix.

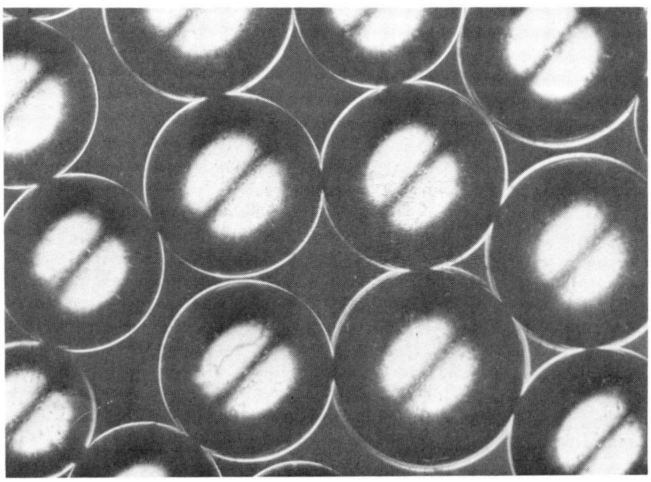

FIGURE 1. Solid polystyrene microcarriers (Biosilon; Nunc, Denmark) suitable for SMC culture. Average diameter, 208 μm. Photographed by dark-field microscopy. (Magnification × 125.)

A reported disadvantage of these microcarriers is the sensitivity of anchored cells to shear forces developed during stirring.[20] This may lead to cell loss and cell injury resulting from collisions of the rigid spheres. In practice, however, we have found that an appropriate choice of stirring system eliminates these failings.

IV. STIRRER SYSTEMS

Microcarriers are routinely maintained in suspension culture (rather than in perfused columns or stationary cultures) because conditions for efficient nutrient and metabolite diffusion are met by the constant movement of the stirred medium. The relatively large numbers of cells grown require uniform exposure to fresh medium throughout the culture flask. For laboratory-scale cultures which can be operated in standard incubators, the primary method for maintaining a suspended microcarrier culture is the stirrer system.

The requirements of a stirrer system for this purpose are numerous. First and foremost, it must keep all of the microcarriers in suspension at stirring speeds consistent with good cell growth and replication. The microcarriers should be in a homogeneous solution with no pockets of beads left stagnant or trapped in a limited area. This ensures that the cells are all maintained in the same environment experiencing similar low-shear forces. The stirrer flask itself must allow for gas exchange and be able to maintain a suitable pH. Accessible sample ports and ease of cleaning and sterilization are also important.

Available systems range from simple paddle stirrers to sophisticated designs which impose more gentle conditions of culture. The earliest microcarrier cultures were grown in spinner flasks designed for use with transformed cells normally grown in suspension. Hirtenstein et al.,[23] however, have observed that optimal conditions for the suspension of single cells are probably different from those required for microcarriers. For example, simple paddle stirrers often have too high a stirring speed for microcarriers and the presence of an immersed spinner-bearing that tends to crush circulating beads. For these reasons a modified spinner vessel was introduced (Bellco Glass, Inc.). These flasks made use of a paddle attached to the impeller, which allowed the microcarriers to be suspended at a lower stirring speed. This change resulted in an increase in the yield of several cell types. Unfortunately, the paddles produced uneven flow patterns that created different local environments within the flask.[23] To address this problem, Techne Ltd. (Cambridge, U.K.) introduced a rod-stirred culture system with an indented base. As Figure 2 indicates, the rod is attached by a rubber gasket to a screw cap. The bulb at the end of the rod contains a magnet that is drawn around by another magnet placed in the stand on which the flask is mounted. The indented base creates a trough which conforms to the shape of the bulb. This combination of rod and trough forces the medium to circulate in a manner which uniformly suspends the microcarriers. Figure 3 illustrates the pattern of flow of an ink drop placed on the surface of a stirred 0.4% polyacrylamide solution. The motion of the rod and bulb forces the liquid to flow in a peripheral downward helical path and then up to the surface in a spiral with ever-increasing radius.[24] Horizontal and vertical circulation creates a constantly moving solution with no static area beneath the stirrer, as is common with flat-bottomed flasks. The Techne system includes a "softstart" facility that gently pushes the microcarriers into suspension, avoiding excessive turbulence. The entire Techne MCS-104 system is engineered for use in an incubator; the magnetic stirrer produces very little heat or noise and accommodates four flasks. We have found this particular system to be well-suited to the growth and maintenance of vascular SMC and endothelial cells.[18]

Our microcarrier cultures are routinely grown in 1 ℓ Techne stirrer flasks that have a working volume of 500 mℓ. Before use, the interior of each flask is treated with a silicon solution (Prosil®-28, SCM Corporation, Gainesville, Fla.; 1% in distilled water) and rinsed with distilled water. This procedure is repeated when necessary to prevent cell attachment to the walls of the stirrer flask.

V. ROLLER BOTTLES

Roller bottles may also be used with microcarrier cultures, although cell yields are less than those reported for spinner and rod-stirred cultures,[21] and special incubators are usually required. The microcarriers can be used to increase the surface area of the roller bottle by the simple addition of empty beads, along with the medium or initial cell inoculum. The microcarriers will adhere to the walls of the bottle, and the rolling speed is maintained optimal for each individual cell type. Siliconized roller bottles may be used for traditional suspension cultures; however, this requires that the bottles be completely filled with medium.

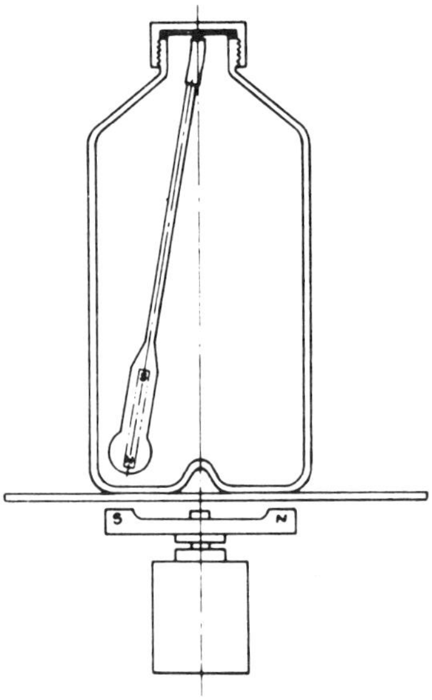

FIGURE 2. Outline of Techne MCS-104 microcarrier stirring system. A bulbous rod is attached to the inside of the cap by a length of silicon rubber. A magnet in the bulb induces pendulous rotation by attraction for another magnet in the base turned by an electric motor. (From De Bruyne, N. A. and Morgan, B. J., *Am. Lab.*, June 1981. With permission.)

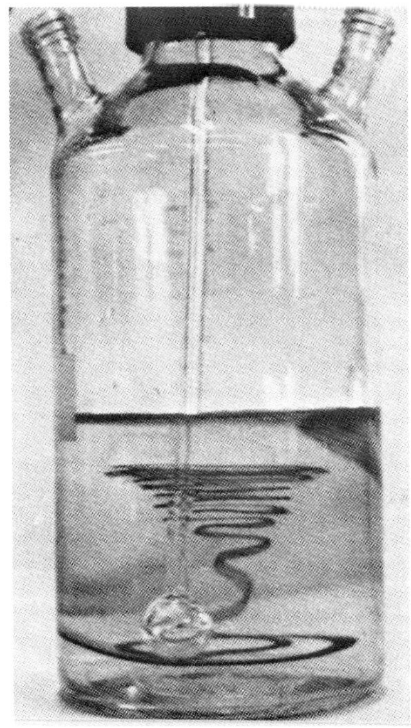

FIGURE 3. Helical path followed by an ink drop placed on the surface of a stirred 0.4% polyacrylamide solution in the MCS-104 stirrer. A combination of primary horizontal rotation and secondary motion at the start of the upward climb results in outward movement towards the surface. (From De Bruyne, N. A. and Morgan, B. J., *Am. Lab.*, June 1981. With permission.)

VI. SHORT-TERM STATIC CULTURES

For pilot studies, it is often useful to initiate small microcarrier cultures in static conditions. Microcarrier cultures of this type are plated and grown in tissue culture dishes that have been treated with an inert polymer, hydroxyethyl methacrylate (Hydron Laboratories, New Brunswick, N.J.; 1.2% solution in ethanol) to prevent the cells from attaching to the bottom of the dish.[16] Bacteriological plastic is also suitable to prevent adhesion to petri dish surfaces. Under static conditions, many more cells than usual grow in the petri dish. Therefore, the medium must be changed frequently to maintain the proper pH and adequate diffusion of nutrients and metabolites.

VII. CULTURES OF VASCULAR SMOOTH MUSCLE CELLS ON MICROCARRIERS

A. Smooth Muscle Cell Propagation

SMC obtained by nonenzymatic explant culture[25] and primary culture through enzymatic digestion[26] are suitable for use on microcarriers. The techniques described below are standard in our laboratory and are appropriate for enzymatically digested primary cells in suspension or cells which have been removed from standard tissue culture dishes by trypsinization.

All procedures are carried out in a laminar flow hood. Microcarriers (Biosilon), which are supplied dry and sterile, are simply transferred to a Techne stirrer flask (capacity 1ℓ) containing 250 mℓ of culture medium with 10% serum several hours before use. The serum concentration should be increased to 20% for primary cells or for other cells with low plating efficiency. Presoaking in a growth medium enhances attachment by coating the beads with plasma cold-insoluble globulins. These amphoteric bridging proteins link the negatively charged bead surface to the net negatively charged cell surface. In the absence of linking protein (either from serum or pretreatment of the beads with purified fibronectin), plating efficiency is very poor.[16]

A suspension of SMC (obtained through the methods described above) is added to the stirrer flask containing the soaked microcarriers, and the cell/bead suspension may be left static or, if automation is available, stirred intermittently (3 min on, 2 min off) for up to 24 hr. The flask is then filled to a final volume of 500 mℓ and left stirring. Hirtenstein et al.[23] have emphasized the importance of maintaining a head space above the culture medium that is at least as great in volume as the culture medium below it. Our experience has shown that a speed of 40 to 50 rpm in the Techne stirrer system is optimal to maintain all the beads in suspension while minimizing shear effects. Recently, a stirring speed of 18 rpm has been reported optimal for endothelial cells grown on Cytodex 3 microcarriers.[27]

The microcarriers should be inoculated with between 2×10^6 and 7×10^6 cells per gram of beads to achieve confluence within 5 to 10 days. This initial plating density of between 5 and 20 cells per bead will yield a confluent culture of about 150 to 200 cells per bead. An example of a growth curve for aortic SMC is shown in Figure 4. The number varies with the size distribution of the beads, the age of the culture, and the extent of bead clumping (see later). One gram of dry Biosilon microcarriers contains approximately 3.7×10^5 beads, giving a total surface area of 490 cm^2.

SMC are readily maintained in a growing state in Dulbecco's Modified Eagle's Medium containing 10% calf serum (M.A. Bioproducts, Watersville, Md.), 2 μmol/mℓ glutamine and 100 units each of penicillin and streptomycin. If a quiescent (nongrowing) culture of SMC is desired, the microcarriers are washed with Hank's Balanced Salt Solution (HBSS) to remove most serum growth factors and kept in 5% Plasma-derived serum prepared according to the methods of Vogel et al.[28]

B. Stain for Light Microscopy

Limited observation of the microcarriers under phase microscopy is possible. The perimeter of the sphere is visible, and the cells are seen as "bumps" along this edge (Figure 5). The orientation of the edge is random; therefore, some impression of the extent of colonization of the beads is possible. To visualize the cells in more detail, it is necessary to fix and stain them. A sample of microcarriers is rinsed several times with HBSS to remove the culture medium. The microcarriers are then fixed for 2 to 3 min in 95% ethanol and stained for 3 to 4 min in hematoxylin.* These procedures can be readily carried out in a conical centrifuge tube; the beads settle rapidly allowing removal of unwanted supernatant. After rinsing off the excess hematoxylin with distilled water, the stained beads are placed on a microscope slide and observed under

* With the aid of heat, dissolve 50 g of hematoxylin crystals in 50 mℓ of 100% alcohol and 100 g of alum in 1000 mℓ distilled water. Remove from heat and mix the two solutions together. Bring solution to a rapid boil (less than 1 min with stirring) and remove from heat. Add 2.5 g mercuric oxide (red) slowly and reheat to a simmer until it becomes a dark purple. Immediately plunge beaker in ice water. Stain is ready for use when cool. Addition of 3 mℓ glacial acetic acid per 100 mℓ of solution increases the precision of nuclear stain.[25]

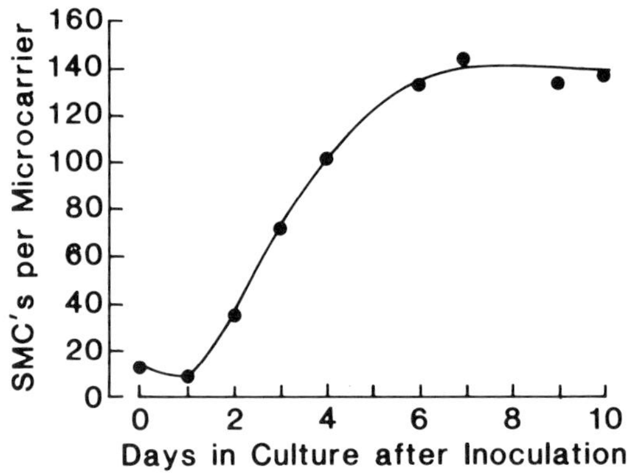

FIGURE 4. Growth curve of bovine aortic SMC isolated by the explant technique (25) and plated on Biosilon microcarriers. Initial plating density was ten cells per bead. Confluence (120 cells per bead) occurred after 6 days of suspension culture.

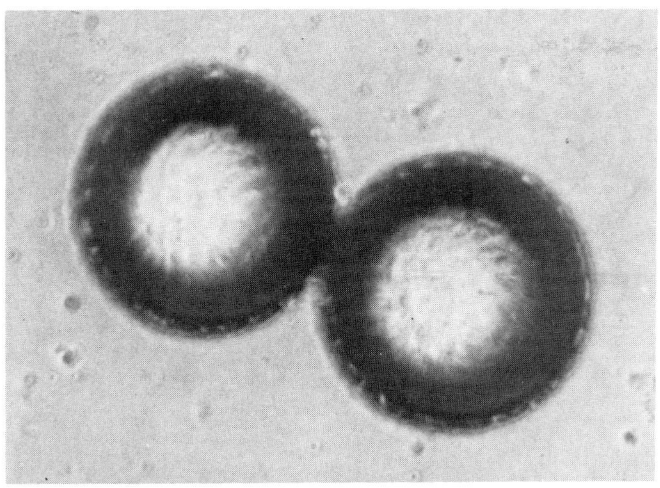

FIGURE 5. Phase-contrast microscopic appearance of vascular SMC at subconfluent density (90 cells per Biosilon bead). Although cells occupying the front and rear faces of each microcarrier are not clearly seen, an estimate of the extent of colonization can be made from the bead periphery. (Magnification unstained × 175.)

10X power with a standard light microscope. If a permanent record is desired, the beads can be covered with a thin layer of mounting medium (e.g., per mount).

Measurement of cell numbers following trypsinization is similar to that used with standard tissue culture flasks because the microcarriers are also made of polystyrene. A sample of microcarriers is placed in a conical tube, the microcarrier-bound cells are removed with trypsin: EDTA, gently vortexed, and the beads are allowed to settle to the bottom of the tube. The released cells remain in suspension much longer than the beads. The cell number in the supernatant is then determined using a hemocytometer or Coulter Counter (Coulter Electronics, Hialeah, Fla.). The bead number in the same sample can be determined by counting a diluted aliquot of resuspended beads (vortex) in the light microscope. The cell-to-bead ratio can then be calculated.

Total cell protein is determined by dissolving microcarrier-bound cells in 0.1% sodium dodecyl sulfate (30 min at room temperature) with occasional vortexing. The insoluble beads settle, and the supernatant is assayed by the Lowry procedure.[29]

C. Descriptive Morphology of Smooth Muscle Cells on Microcarriers

At a plating density of 5 to 20 cells per bead, individual SMC assume a fusiform morphology with random orientation (Figures 6a and 6b). As the beads become more heavily colonized (Figures 6c and 6d), the fusiform shape becomes less apparent. A characteristic feature of vascular SMC in culture is the formation of a ''hill and valley'' conformation after reaching confluence. We have never observed multilayers of SMC on single microcarriers although multilayers will form on occasion between beads if ''bridging'' is extensive. One may speculate that the inhibition of multilayer formation is associated with significant shear forces generated in stirred suspension. Once a confluent density is achieved, it is common for two or more microcarriers to become ''bridged'' by migrating SMC. These cells have an elongated morphology and are often clearly aligned (Figures 7a and 7b). Large, multibead clumps may develop if the culture is left static for any length of time or is stirred at too slow a speed (Figure 7c). Maintaining the stirring speed at 40 to 50 rpm will minimize bead clumping. If the vessel wall is improperly treated with silicon or if any area of silicon has worn thin, the bridged microcarriers will become attached to the wall and can form long strands of cells, beads, and matrix. Two- and three-bead clumps are found in almost all cultures regardless of their age but do not present a significant problem.

The ''bridging'' noted with SMC is in contrast to vascular endothelial cells, a highly contact inhibited cell with marked polarity of apical and basal surfaces. These cells, for example, are easily grown in completely static conditions, with little evidence of bead clumping (Figure 7d).

Older cultures which have laid down a large amount of extracellular matrix will sometimes shear off in sheets if the stirring speed is too great. The effect can be identified by the appearance of matrix or cells which can be seen dangling from partially or completely denuded beads. Pipetting the microcarriers through too small an opening will also produce shearing of cells. To avoid this, we routinely use wide-bore pipettes to dispense the colonized microcarriers. Any microcarrier culture will contain a few unpopulated beads even at their most mature state. These represent a tiny fraction of the commercial microcarriers that remain unattractive to cells, probably because of incomplete treatment of the bead surface during manufacture.

D. Scanning Electron Microscopy

Microcarriers can readily be processed for scanning electron microscopy (SEM). The use of solid beads minimizes shrinkage artifact, whereas porous beads are less suitable. After fixation in 2% glutaraldehyde in buffered salt solution, pH 7.4, for 1 hr at 4°C, the cells are washed twice with deionized water. All manipulations can be performed in a plastic conical centrifuge tube, with gentle inversion of the tube between each step. After the beads settle, the supernatant is removed and replaced with the next solution. Cell water is gradually exchanged with alcohol by replacement with ethanol solutions of increasing concentrations (10 to 100% at 10% increments for 10 min each step at room temperature). Microcarriers are then either critical-point dried from ethanol/CO_2 or air-dried from 100% ethanol, transferred to sticky copper tape mounted on an SEM stub, and coated with a thin layer (approximately 200 Å) of gold-palladium (Hummer IV sputter coater, Technics Instruments, Alexandria, Va.). An example of endothelial cells prepared by this procedure and viewed in an AMR 1000 scanning electron microscope is shown in Figure 8a.

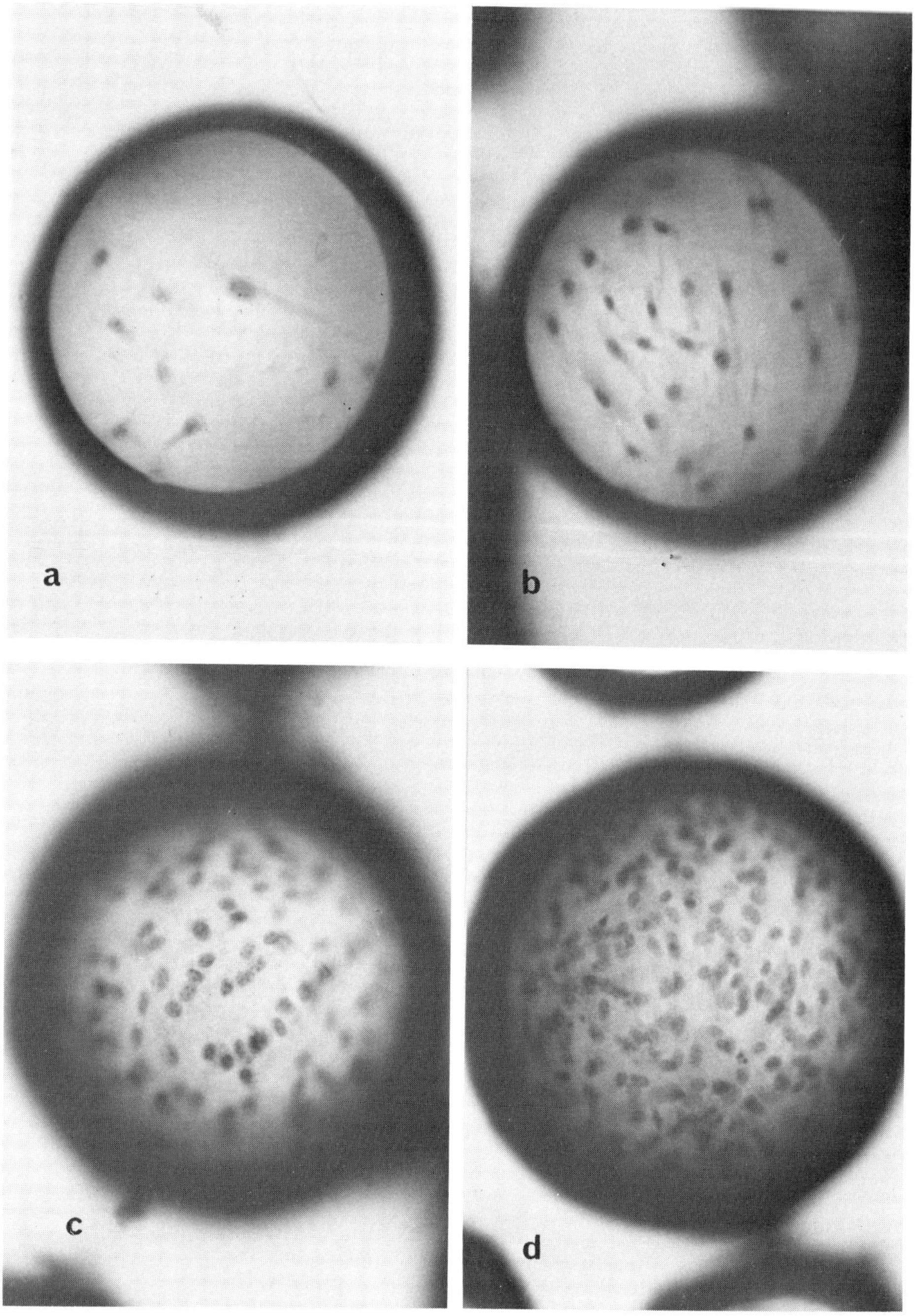

FIGURE 6. Vascular SMC stained with hemotoxylin at various cell densities on solid polystyrene microcarriers. Average cell-to-bead ratios in the cultures from which these examples were taken were (a) 30, (b) 60, (c) 110, (d) 155. (Magnification × 280.)

E. Transmission Electron Microscopy

The following procedure is a modification of that published by Sargent et al.[30] It was developed by Netland and Damm of the Department of Physiology and Biophysics, Harvard Medical School, and was kindly provided for this chapter by them.

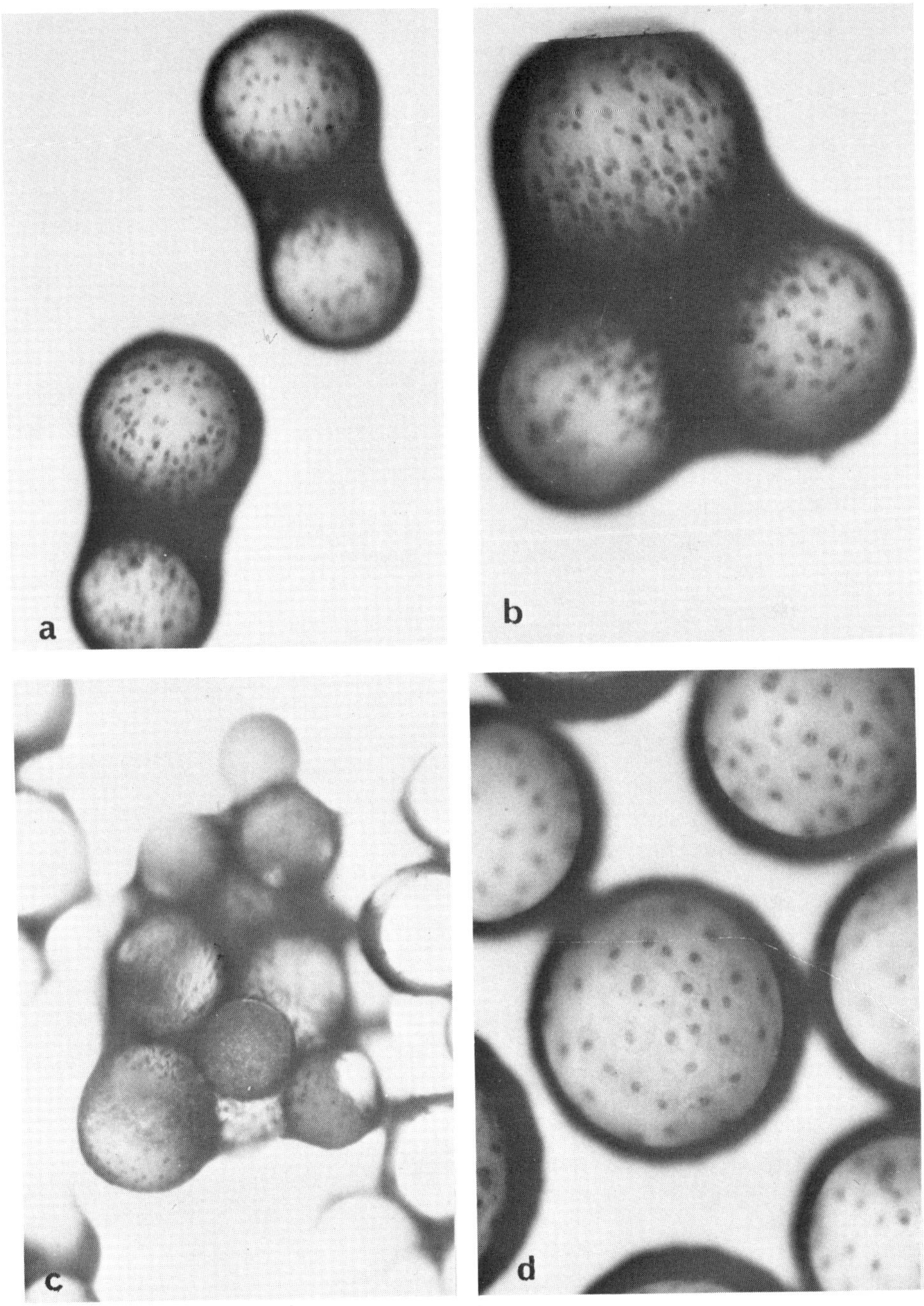

FIGURE 7. Examples of microcarrier aggregates which often occur in cultures of vascular SMC and fibroblasts. (a) Doublets, common in most SMC cultures even under optimal stirring conditions; magnification × 120. (b) Triplets, occasionally observed in normal SMC cultures; magnification × 155. (c) Extensive aggregation and clumping of SMC microcarriers in an insufficiently stirred culture. Cells in the interior of such aggregates will become necrotic; magnification × 90. (d) In contrast to SMC and fibroblasts, microcarrier cultures of vascular endothelial cells do not readily form aggregates; magnification × 185. Biosilon microcarriers. Hematoxylin stain.

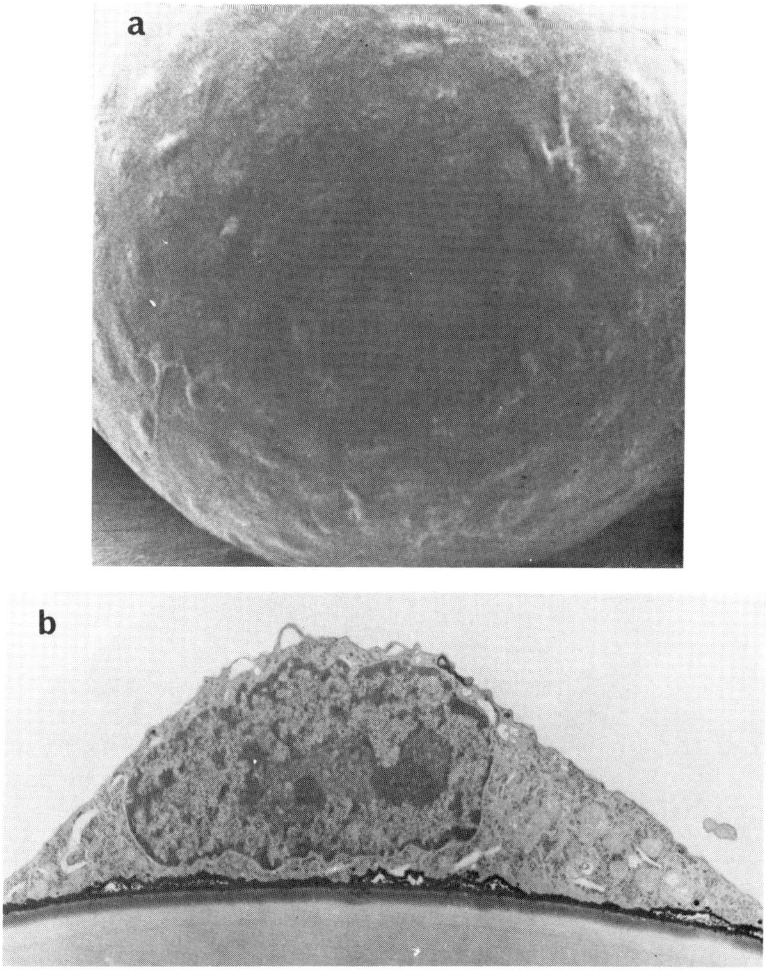

FIGURE 8. Electron microscopy of microcarrier culture (Biosilon) demonstrated for vascular endothelial cells. (a) Scanning electron microscopy of confluent bovine aortic endothelial cells; magnification × 500. (b) Transmission electron microscopy of same culture as in (a). Tannic acid was used postfixation to emphasize the interface between cell and bead surface; magnification × 20,000.

Following fixation and washing as described above for SEM, the microcarriers in buffered salt solution are warmed to 45°C in a water bath; 2% agar in PBS is prepared and also warmed to 45°C. A few drops of 1% eosin are added to make the agar visible during processing; 1 to 2 mℓ of the agar solution is added to the sample. The sample and agar solution are then gently mixed, using a wooden stick. The sample is centrifuged at 1000 rpm for 2 min. After the agar block is formed, the sample is removed by cutting the centrifuge tube and flooding with PBS. The excess agar is cut off the agar block. The block of agar containing the sample is diced into 1 mm cubes which are then transferred to a glass vial. Following postfixation for 1 hr in 0.2 *M* cacodylate buffer containing 1% osmium tetroxide, the cubes are washed in three changes (10 min each) of 0.2 *M* cacodylate buffer. The samples are then washed three times (5 min each) with distilled water and gently shaken in 0.2 *M* cacodylate buffer containing 1% (w/v) uranyl acetate. After 1 hr of staining, cubes are washed in three changes of distilled water and processed through graded ethanol solutions (50%, 10 min; 70%, 10 min; 95%, 10 min; 100%, 10 min; 100%, 15 min). The samples are then processed through three changes of 1,2 epoxypropane and finally embedded in resin.[31] The changeover from dehydration fluid to embedding fluid is made in three stages: 1/1 dehydrating/embedding fluid for a half hour; 1/3 dehydrating/embedding fluid for a half hour; 100% embedding fluid for 1 hr; 100% embedding fluid overnight. Samples are cured for at least 10 hr in a 70°C oven. Semithin sections are cut and stained with 0.1% toluidine blue in 1% sodium borate and examined with the light microscope. Ultrathin sections are prepared from selected areas, picked up on copper grids, and stained with 7.5% uranylacetate in 50% ethanol followed by lead citrate stain.[32] The sections can then be examined in the transmission electron microscope, usually at 60 KV. An example of Biosilon-bound endothelial cells prepared for transmission electron microscopy (TEM) is shown in Figure 8b.

F. Applications in Vascular Research

The most useful properties of microcarriers as substrata for anchorage dependent cells are the high surface area to volume ratio and the ease with which the cells can be transferred between different locations without enzymatic removal from the substratum. The latter property, in particular, has proved useful for studies of the biochemistry of cell surface receptors and other surface proteins whose integrity is destroyed by proteolytic enzymes such as trypsin. The introduction of naked beads to a stirring microcarrier culture of SMC results in their colonization and hence an effective increase in the cell population. Such a phenomenon may be useful for the continuous culture of cells, avoiding the use of trypsin.[33] The property of cell migration onto and off beads has been used to selectively isolate microvessel endothelial cells[34] and to "plate" cells into petri dishes without using trypsin, the cells simply migrating onto the dish surface. Busch et al.[15] and this laboratory[16,33] have set up perfusion beds of microcarrier-borne cells to collect, in concentrated form, metabolites secreted by the cells, thus using the high surface area to volume ratio of microcarriers to create a very small interstitial volume of medium.

Each bead is essentially a microculture of up to 200 anchorage-dependent vascular cells. This fact provides great versatility in moving different numbers of cells into and out of selected environments. We have used such an approach to study vascular cell interactions in co-culture.[17,18,35,36] There are subtle but important differences between studies of intercellular metabolism in co-culture compared with the use of conditioned medium. Co-culture allows the potential for multiple interactions between the cell populations whereas there is an inherent restriction of interactions when conditioned medium is used. First, there is no provision for signals or messages from the target cell to reach the cell that is conditioning the medium. Second, there is the possibility that short-lived potent factors produced by the conditioning cell may be inactive either because of short half-life or by dilution when applied as conditioned medium to the target cell. Third, the separation of cell populations for the production of conditioned medium removes the normal checks and balances which presumably exist between cell types such as endothelium and SMC residing so close together in vivo. Co-culture minimizes these restrictions. Two examples of the usefulness of this approach have recently been reported.[18,35,36,37] We show in Figures 9a and 9b the two major co-culture systems used in this laboratory for vascular cells, one involving humoral interactions only and the other which allows both contact between the cell populations and humoral interactions to occur simultaneously.

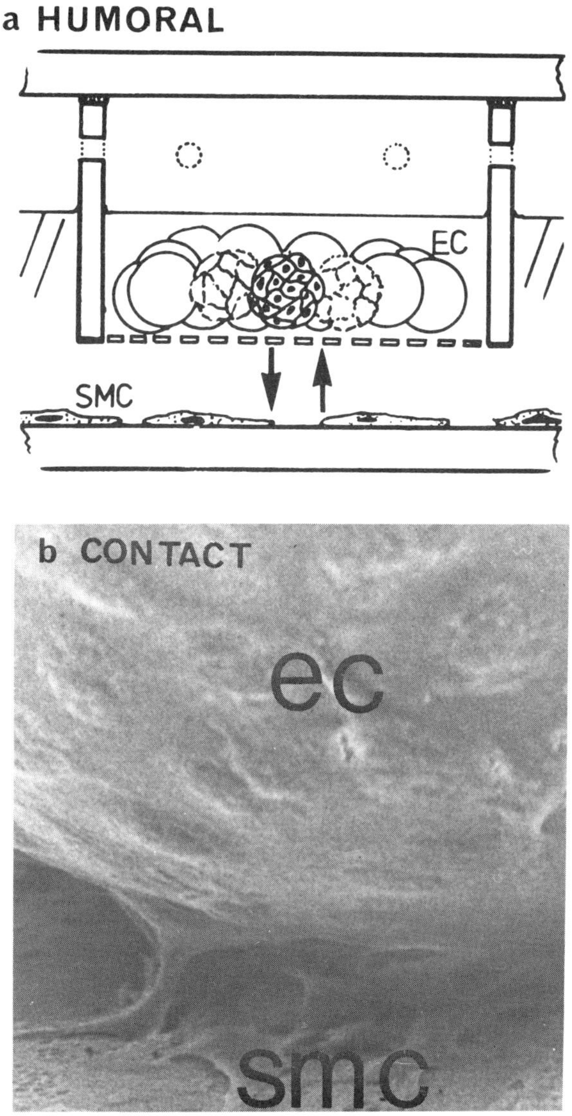

FIGURE 9. Two systems for the study of vascular cell interactions utilizing microcarrier cultures. (a) Humoral interactions between confluent endothelial cells on microcarriers and SMC grown in conventional petri dish culture. See References 17 and 18. (b) Contact co-culture between endothelial (ec) and smooth muscle cells (smc). In such a configuration, intercellular communication by both humoral diffusion and junctional transfer has been demonstrated. See References 35, 36, and 37.

VIII. CONCLUDING REMARKS

Microcarriers have now become a useful and highly versatile tool for small-scale (nonindustrial scale) cell research. Many innovative applications, in addition to those cited above, are ripe for investigation, including the possible use of microcarriers in the seeding of vascular grafts, the isolation of endothelial cells in poorly accessible regions of the microcirculation, and the assay of cellular metabolism in living cells in a cuvette by fluorescence spectrophotometry. Such approaches should provide insight into the role of SMC, endothelial cells, and monocyte-derived macrophages in vascular biology and pathology.

ACKNOWLEDGMENTS

This work is funded by grants to Dr. Davies from the National Heart Lung and Blood Institutes at the National Institutes of Health (HL24612 and HL22602). We gratefully acknowledge the following members of the group and collaborators involved in microcarrier technology and related biochemical studies during the past 5 years: Catherine Kerr, Lesley Kuczera, Barbara Eisenhaure, Debbie Sandstrom, Pip Diehl and Drs. Henry Warren, George Truskey, and Peter Ganz.

REFERENCES

1. van Wezel, A. L., Growth of cell strains and primary cells on microcarriers in homogeneous culture, *Nature (London),* 216, 64, 1967.
2. Montagnon, B. J., Vincent-Falquet, J. C., and Fanget, B., Thousand liters scale microcarrier culture of vero cells for killed polio virus vaccine; promising results, *Dev. Biol. Stand.,* 55, 37, 1984.
3. van Wezel, A. L., van der Velden de Groot, C. A. M., and van Herwaarden, J. A. M., The production of inactivated polio vaccine on serially cultivated kidney cells from captive-bred monkeys, *Dev. Biol. Stand.,* 46, 151, 1980.
4. Meignier, B., Mougeot, H., and Favre, H., Foot and mouth disease virus production on microcarrier-grown cells, *Dev. Biol. Stand.,* 46, 249, 1980.
5. van Hemert, P., Kilburn, D. G., and van Wezel, A. L., Homogenous cultivation of animal cells for the production of virus and virus products, *Biotechnol. Bioeng.,* 11, 875, 1969.
6. Edy, V. G., Augenstein, D. C., Edwards, C. R., Cruttenden, V. F., and Lubiniecki, A. S., Large-scale tissue culture for human IFN-production, *Tex. Rep. Biol. Med.,* 41, 169, 1982.
7. Page, M. and Dufour, C., Growth of human colon carcinoma cells on beaded microcarriers, *J. Cell Biol.,* 83, 302a, 1979.
8. Griffiths, B., Atkinson, T., Electricwala, A., Latter, A., McEntree, I., Riley, P. A., and Sutton, P. M., Production of a fibrinolytic enzyme from cultures of guinea pig keratocytes grown on microcarriers, *Dev. Biol. Stand.,* 55, 31, 1984.
9. Prestidge, R. L., Sandlin, G. M., Koopman, W. J., and Bennett, J. C., Interleukin 1: production by P388D cells attached to microcarrier beads, *J. Immunol. Methods,* 46, 197, 1981.
10. Scott, R. W., Eaton, D. L., and Baker, J. B., Rapid purification of protease nexin and plasminogen activator released by human fibroblasts in microcarrier culture, *J. Cell Biol.,* 95, 121a, 1982.
11. Norrgren, G., Ebendal, T., Gelb, C., and Wikstrom, H., The use of Cytodex 3 microcarriers and reduced serum media for the production of nerve growth promoters from chicken heart cells, *Dev. Biol. Stand.,* 55, 43, 1984.
12. Thilly, W. G. and Levine, D. W., Microcarrier culture: a homogeneous environment for studies of cellular biochemistry, *Methods Enzymol.,* 58, 184, 1979.
13. Gotlib, L. J., Isolation of cell plasma membranes on microcarrier culture beads, *Biochim. Biophys. Acta,* 602, 207, 1980.
14. Ryan, U. S., Mortara, M., and Whitaker, C., Methods for microcarrier culture of bovine pulmonary artery endothelial cells avoiding the use of enzymes, *Tissue Cell,* 12, 619, 1980.
15. Busch, C., Cancilla, P. A., DeBault, L. E., Goldsmith, J. C., and Owen, W. G., Use of endothelium cultured on microcarriers as a model for the microcirculation, *Lab. Invest.,* 47, 498, 1982.
16. Davies, P. F., Microcarrier culture of vascular endothelium, *Exp. Cell Res.,* 134, 365, 1981.
17. Davies, P. F. and Kerr, C., Co-cultivation of vascular endothelial and smooth muscle cells using microcarrier techniques, *Exp. Cell Res.,* 141, 455, 1982.
18. Davies, P. F., Truskey, G. A., Warren, H. B., O'Connor, S. E., and Eisenhaure, B. H., Metabolic cooperation between vascular endothelial cells and smooth muscle cells in coculture, *J. Cell Biol.,* 101, 871, 1985.

19. Gebb, C., Clark, J. H., Hirtenstein, M. D., Lindgren, G., Lindskog, V., Lindgren, B., and Uretblad, P., Alternative surface for microcarrier culture of animal cells, *Dev. Biol. Stand.*, 50, 93, 1982.
20. Reuveny, S., Microcarriers for culturing mammalian cells and their applications, *Adv. Biotechnol. Processes*, 2, 1, 1983.
21. Pharmacia Fine Chemicals: *Microcarrier Cell Culture: Principle and Methods*, Trade Publication, 1982.
22. Johansson, A. and Nielsen, V., Biosilon, a new microcarrier, *Dev. Biol. Stand.*, 46, 125, 1980.
23. Hirtenstein, M. D., Clark, J. M., and Gebb, C., A comparison of various laboratory scale culture configurations for microcarrier culture of animal cells, *Dev. Biol. Stand.*, 50, 73, 1982.
24. DeBruyne, N. A. and Morgan, B. J., Stirrer for suspension cell cultures, *Am. Lab.*, June 1981.
25. Ross, R., The smooth muscle cell. II. Growth of smooth muscle in culture and formation of elastin fibers, *J. Cell Biol.*, 50, 172, 1971.
26. Chamley-Campbell, J. H., Campbell, G. R., and Ross, R., Phenotype-dependent response of cultured aortic smooth muscle to serum mitogens, *J. Cell Biol.*, 89, 378, 1981.
27. Cocks, T. M., Angus, J. A., Campbell, J. H., and Campbell, G. R., Release and properties of endothelium-derived relaxing factor (EDRF) from endothelial cells in culture, *J. Cell. Physiol.*, 123, 310, 1985.
28. Vogel, A. Raines, E., Kariya, B., Rivest, M.-J., and Ross, R., Coordinate control of 3T3 cell proliferation by platelet-derived growth factor and plasma components, *Proc. Natl. Acad. Sci. U.S.A.*, 75, 2810, 1978.
29. Lowry, D. H., Rosebrough, N. J., Farr, A. L., and Randall, R. J., Protein measurement with the folin phenol reagent, *J. Biol. Chem.*, 193, 265, 1951.
30. Sargent, G. F., Sims, T. A., and McNeish, A. S., The use of polystyrene microcarriers to prepare cell monolayers for transmission electron microscopy, *J. Microsc. (Oxford)*, 122, 204, 1980.
31. Spurr, A. R., A low-viscosity epoxy embedding medium for electron microscopy, *J. Ultrastruct. Res.*, 26, 31, 1969.
32. Sato, J., Lead citrate stain in electron microscopy, *Electron Microsc.*, 17, 158, 1968.
33. Davies, P. F., Microcarrier cultures in vascular endothelial research, *Dev. Biol. Stand.*, 50, 125, 1982.
34. Folkman, J., Capillary endothelial cells — the use of microcarrier beads for isolation and long-term culture, *J. Cell Biol.*, 95, 485 A, 1982.
35. Davies, P. F., Ganz, P., and Diehl, T. S., Reversible microcarrier-mediated junctional communication between endothelial and smooth muscle cell monolayer: an in vitro model of vascular cell interactions, *Lab. Invest.*, 85, 710, 1985.
36. Ganz, P., Davies, P. F., Leopold, J., Gimbrone, M. A., and Alexander, R. W., Short and longterm interactions of endothelium and vascular smooth muscle in coculture: effects on cyclic GMP production, *Proc. Natl. Acad. Sci. U.S.A.*, 83, 3552, 1986.
37. Davies, P. F., Biology of disease — vascular cell interactions with special reference to the pathogenesis of atherosclerosis, *Lab. Invest.*, 55, 5, 1986.

Chapter 4

PHENOTYPIC MODULATION OF SMOOTH MUSCLE CELLS IN PRIMARY CULTURE

Gordon R. Campbell and Julie H. Campbell

TABLE OF CONTENTS

I. INTRODUCTION

Various cell types can alter their character when the environment changes. These alterations in character are called modulations of the differentiated state and involve reversible interconversions between phenotypes. Modulations in cell phenotype may occur as a result of a number of factors, such as cell interactions, alterations of extracellular matrix, or in response to other signals such as hormones.

Smooth muscle cells (SMC) are capable of expressing a range of phenotypes. At one end of this spectrum of phenotypes are the SMC whose function is almost exclusively that of contraction ("contractile state"). This function is reflected structurally with 80 to 90% of the cell cytoplasmic volume occupied with contractile apparatus. Organelles such as rough endoplasmic reticulum (ER), Golgi, and free ribosomes are few in number and located in the perinuclear region (Figure 1). Cells of the taenia coli, vas deferens, circular muscle of the ileum, and smaller muscular arteries express this phenotype. These muscles contain relatively little connective tissue (e.g., the volume of extracellular space is about 30% in taenia coli and 10 to 15% in the circular muscle of the ileum),[1] and in visceral muscle much of this connective tissue is synthesized by constituent fibroblasts. Therefore, SMC need to express minimal synthetic function. At the opposite end of the spectrum of phenotypic expression is the muscle cell, whose function is almost exclusively that of synthesis ("synthetic state") (Figure 2). As with other cell types actively engaged in the production of extracellular matrix (such as fibroblasts), the cytoplasm contains few filament bundles but large amounts of rough ER, Golgi, and free ribosomes. Cells in the synthetic state are seen in development, repair, and pathological conditions.[2]

It must be emphasized that the contractile and synthetic states as described above represent the extreme ends of a continuous spectrum of phenotypes, with most smooth muscle expressing intermediate morphology. For example, in large mammalian elastic arteries, smooth muscle is the only cell type present,[3-5] and 60 to 70% of the cell volume is occupied with myofilaments.[6,7] The volume of the connective tissue is 50 to 60%; therefore, this muscle cell has a dual function, being responsible for contraction/relaxation and the normal replacement of extracellular matrix components.

II. STRUCTURAL AND FUNCTIONAL CHANGES OF ARTERIAL MEDIAL SMOOTH MUSCLE IN PRIMARY CULTURE

A. Explant Cultures

Kasai and Pollak in 1964[8] were the first to describe phenotypic changes of SMC in culture. They examined the cellular outgrowth from rabbit arterial wall explants and suggested that "fibroblasts" appeared within 3 to 5 days and "smooth muscle cells" within 8 to 10 days. Similar observations were made on explants of human aorta in culture.[9] However, even special light microscope stains (such as Pollak's trichrome), are inadequate to distinguish the spectrum of phenotypes that SMC express. The electron microscope is far more appropriate for this task, and Dauod, Fritz, Jarmolych, and colleagues[10,11] described the presence of four "cell types" in outgrowth from pig aortic media explants. These were termed "primitive cells", "fibroblast-like cells", "modified smooth muscle cells", and "mature smooth muscle cells", according to the number of filaments and the concomitant increase or decrease in the number of synthetic organelles present. They suggested that mature SMC "dedifferentiated" in the first few days in culture to modified SMC, then to fibroblast-like cells, then finally to primitive cells, where they rapidly proliferated. Peak proliferation (as determined by ^{3}H-thymidine incorporation into DNA) occurred between 9 to 14 days in culture, whereas production of extracellular matrix (collagen, elastin, and glycosaminoglycans)

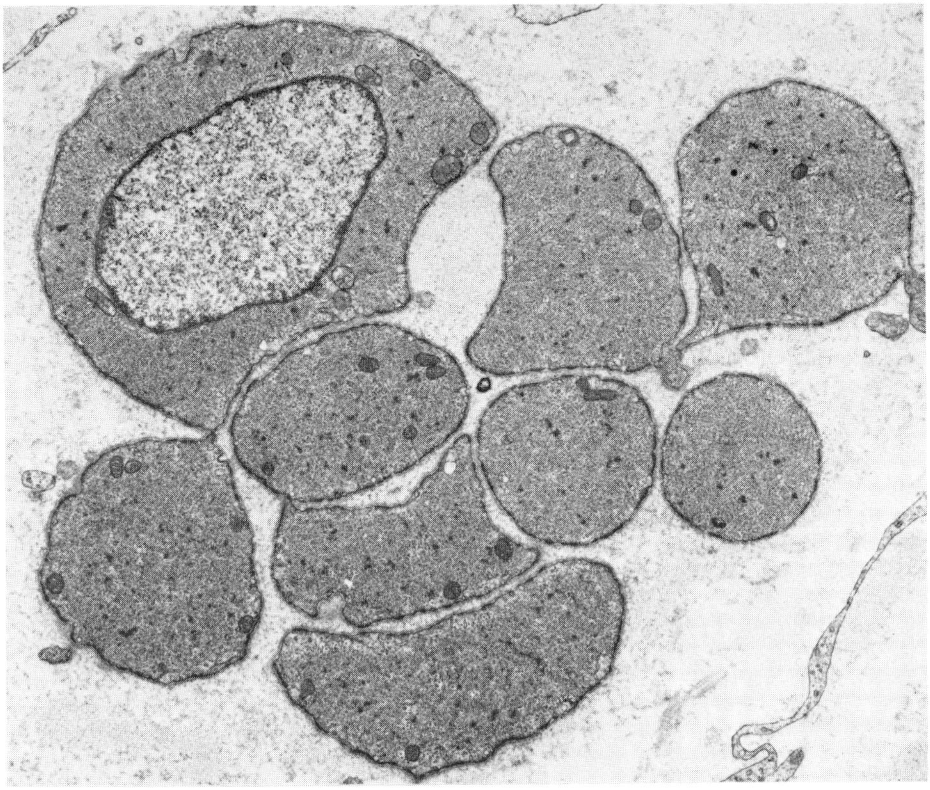

FIGURE 1. SMC from the mouse vas deferens. Most of the cytoplasm is filled with myofilaments. These cells could be considered to be in the "contractile state". (Magnification × 4500.)

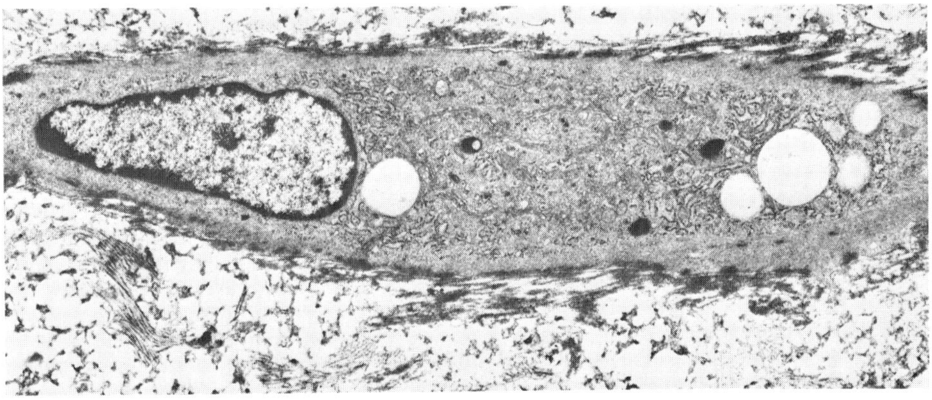

FIGURE 2. SMC from the intima of a hypercholesterolemic rabbit. Most of the cytoplasm is filled with organelles generally associated with synthesis. Myofilament bundles are small and located towards the periphery of the cell. This cell is towards the "synthetic state". (Magnification × 3000.)

was minimal at 7 to 9 days, but then increased up to 21 days. The primitive cells subsequently "redifferentiated" back to smooth muscle. These findings have more recently been substantiated by Rossi et al.[12] and Wight et al.[13]

B. Enzyme-Dispersed Cells

1. Terminology

When SMC from the guinea pig vas deferens and taenia coli are enzymatically dispersed and placed in primary culture, they undergo similar morphological changes to those described in Section A. These changes have been described as dedifferentiation and redifferentiation,[14-19] but it has since been recognized that this terminology is not strictly correct since there is no evidence that the more "primitive"-looking SMC return to a multipotential state (true dedifferentiation). The word "modulation" has subsequently been used to describe the changes which occur in smooth muscle phenotype in response to an altered environment.[2,20-23]

2. Changes in Morphology

Vascular and visceral smooth muscle enzyme-dispersed into single cells and plated in primary culture attach and flatten on the culture substratum within 1 to 2 days. They then closely resemble the same cells in vivo[20,21] (Figure 3). That is, their cytoplasm contains substantial bundles of myofilaments. They are therefore described as being in the contractile phenotype. If they are seeded below a critical cell concentration, the cells undergo a series of spontaneous changes in phenotype with time to what is termed the synthetic state.[16,19,21,22] In the synthetic state, SMC contain few filaments but increased numbers of organelles involved with synthesis (Figure 4). At the same time, there is a decrease or loss in staining reaction with FITC-labeled antibodies to the heavy meromyosin end of smooth muscle myosin.[19] The number of lysosomes also increases.[21] With phase-contrast microscopy, the cells change from being phase-dense and ribbon or fusiform in shape, to phase-lucent, broad, and flat (Figures 5 and 6). The time of phenotypic change is dependent on the donor species, age, and organ.[20,24] While phenotypic modulation from the contractile state to the synthetic state occurs in plasma-derived serum as well as in whole blood serum,[21,25] platelet factors can affect this process since platelet-derived-growth-factor (PDGF) antibodies delay the onset of phenotypic change in 10% whole blood serum, and purified PDGF speeds up the process in 10% plasma-derived serum.[21] Prostaglandin E1 also stimulates the transition of SMC from the contractile to the synthetic state during their first few days in culture. However, at a later time, when the majority of cells are in the synthetic state and have undergone one or more cell divisions, prostaglandin E1 slows down the rate of initiation of DNA synthesis.[26]

Thyberg et al.[21] have examined the cytoplasmic volume density of organelles in rat aortic smooth muscle with time in culture after enzyme dispersal and found that the volume percentage of filaments decreases from 60.32 on day 0 to 5.34 on day 4, while the volume percentage of rough endoplasmic reticulum increases from 5.33 on day 0 to 23.77 on day 4. Golgi cisternae also increases from 1.79 to 5.5 over the same time period, while lysosomal volume percent increases from 3.8 at day 0 to 6.53 on day 10.

3. Factors Affecting the Reversibility of Smooth Muscle Phenotypic Changes In Vitro

Smooth muscle phenotypic change is reversible or irreversible, depending on the initial cell seeding density.[24,27] If the cells are seeded at 10^6 cells per milliliter or greater, they form a confluent monolayer from the first day in culture. These cells do not undergo a spontaneous phenotypic change but remain in the contractile phenotype. If they are seeded sparser (i.e., at $5 \times 10^4 \rightarrow 1 \times 10^5$ cells per milliliter), they undergo the spontaneous phenotypic change on days 6 to 8, then proliferate until they form a confluent monolayer. If the cells undergo fewer than five cell doublings in forming this confluent monolayer, they will revert back to the contractile state within 1 to 2 days of confluency being reached. If, however, they have been seeded very sparsely (i.e., 1 ×

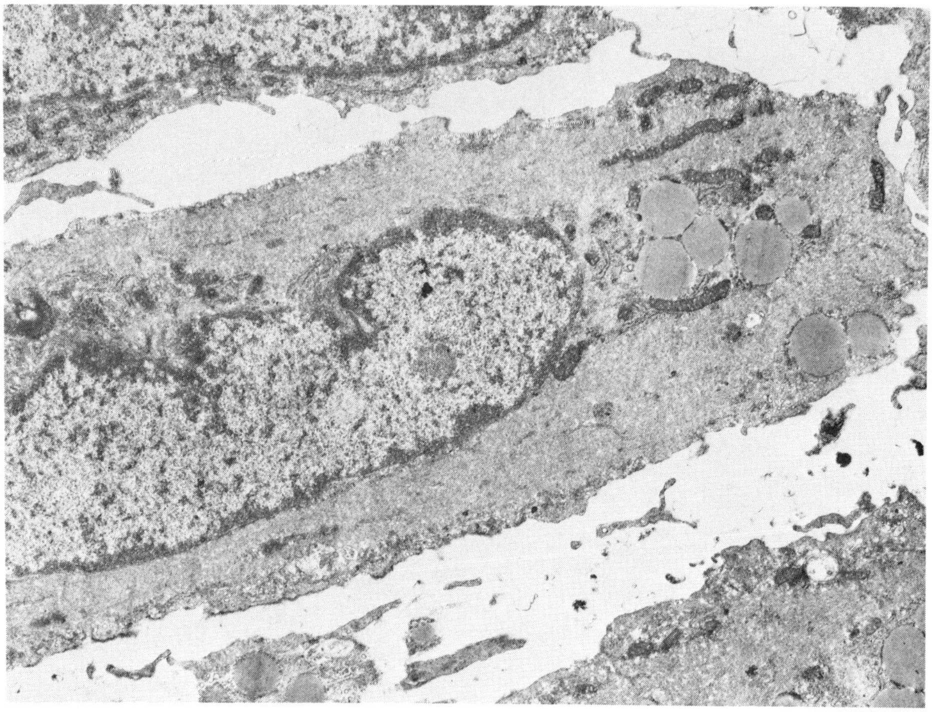

FIGURE 3. Seven-week-old rabbit aorta 4 days in primary culture. SMC have a similar appearance to those of the intact media, with much of their cytoplasm filled with myofilaments. (Magnification × 3000.) (From Schwartz, S. M., Campbell, G. R., and Campbell, J. H., *Circ. Res.*, 58, 427, 1986. With permission.)

$10^3 \rightarrow 5 \times 10^3/m\ell$), the cells will undergo the phenotypic change on days 6 to 8, but then need considerably greater than five cell doublings to achieve confluency. These cells do not return to the contractile phenotype, but remain permanently in the synthetic phenotype. SMC that are in the synthetic state but capable of returning to the contractile state have been termed "reversible synthetic". Cells which are incapable of returning to the contractile state have been termed "irreversible synthetic".[23] This loss of reversion of phenotype is not related to "senescence" demonstrated by Ross and Kariya[28] in late passage smooth muscle, since the primary cultured cells have undergone many fewer cell doublings and are still capable of intense proliferation. However, "irreversible synthetic" SMC after further cell doublings eventually become senescent and do not proliferate in response to serum mitogens.

4. Contraction

In the first few days in primary culture while the cells morphologically express a contractile phenotype, spontaneous contractions at a rate of one to eight per minute have been reported in single SMC from the guinea pig vas deferens,[14,16,17,29-31] taenia coli,[31-33] ureter,[18,31] and chicken gizzard.[15,31,34,35] There are a few reports of spontaneous contractions in single vascular SMC in culture[19,36] and of their stimulation to contract by vasoactive agents.[19,37]

Concomitant with the change in phenotype to a synthetic state, the muscle cells lose their ability for spontaneous or induced contraction.[20]

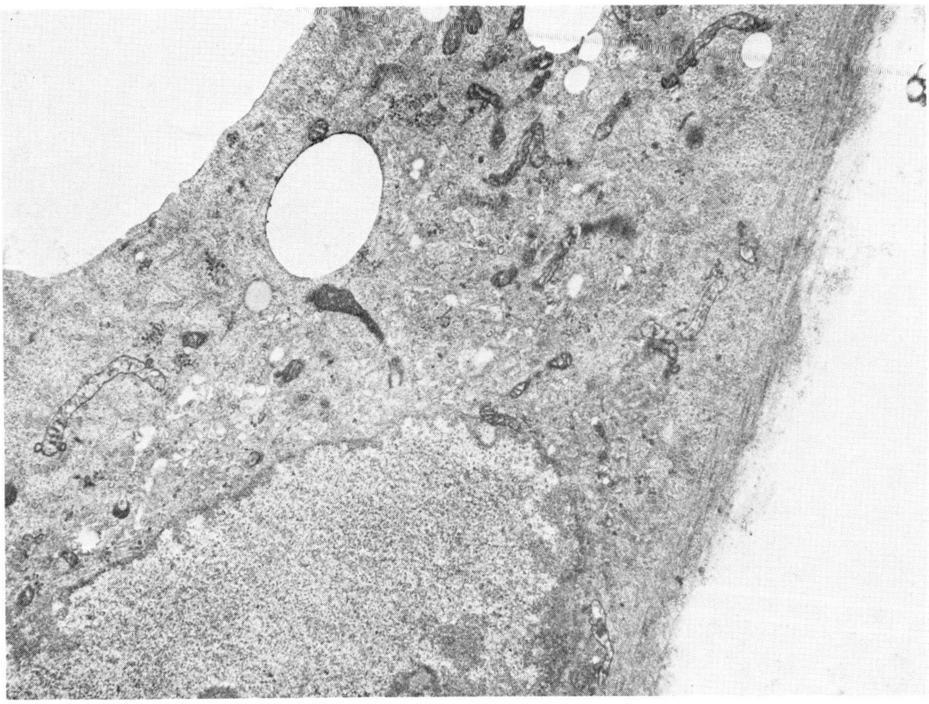

FIGURE 4. Seven-week-old rabbit aorta 11 days in culture (first subculture). Although a filament bundle extends along the right-hand side of the cell (note plasmalemmal vesicles of cell membrane), most of the cytoplasm is filled with organelles associated with synthesis. (Magnification × 3500.) (From Schwartz, S. M., Campbell, J. H., and Campbell, G. R., *Circ. Res.*, 58, 427, 1986. With permission.)

5. Division

Only 3 to 5% of aortic SMC from the adult pig and monkey in the first 6 or 7 days of primary culture incorporate ^{3}H-thymidine into their nuclei during a 4-hr, pulse-labeling period in the presence of 5% whole blood serum.[25,38] However, on day 7, 8, or 9 (i.e., the day after phenotypic modulation to the synthetic state is first evident morphologically), the number of labeled nuclei increases to 10 to 20% (see also Chapter 13). The percentage of cells incorporating ^{3}H-thymidine into DNA then increases linearly with time until on day 14, 40 to 60% of cell nuclei are labeled during the 4-hr, pulse-labeling period. The cells begin to proliferate logarithmically in 5% whole blood serum about 24 hr after they show an increased incorporation of ^{3}H-thymidine. There is no significant increase in cell number while the cells are in the contractile state; however, some contractile SMC are capable of division.[29]

The time of phenotypic change and subsequent proliferation is dependent upon the donor species, age, and organ. Thyberg et al.[21] studied isolated SMC from 8-month-old rat aorta arteries and found that by day 3 structural modification had occurred and cells began to proliferate logarithmically on day 5.

Phenotypic modulation occurs in the absence of the PDGF[21,25] and in the presence of mitomycin C[21] but in these cases is not followed by cell division. This demonstrates that while modulation is an essential but not sufficient prerequisite for SMC proliferation, the PDGF and/or other serum factors are necessary for mitosis to occur.

Recent observations by Nilsson et al.[39] show that, at least in the rat, modulation of SMC from the contractile to the synthetic phenotype is accompanied by the production of a PDGF-like protein and autocrine initiation of DNA synthesis. Serum-free condi-

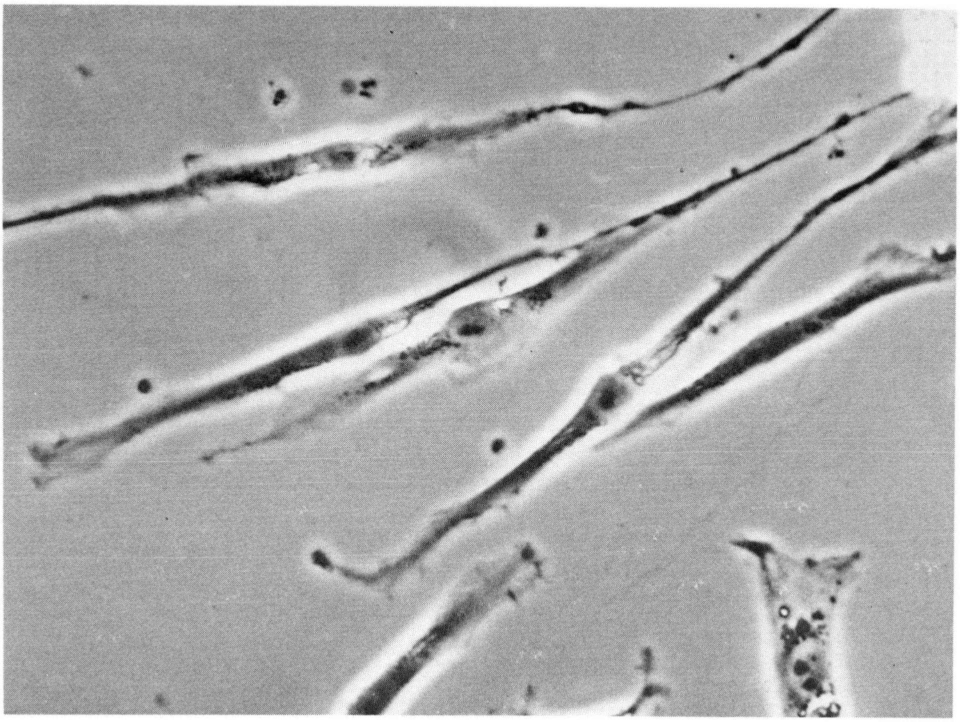

FIGURE 5. Enzyme-dispersed SMC from the adult pig aortic media, 3 days in primary culture. (Magnification × 800.)

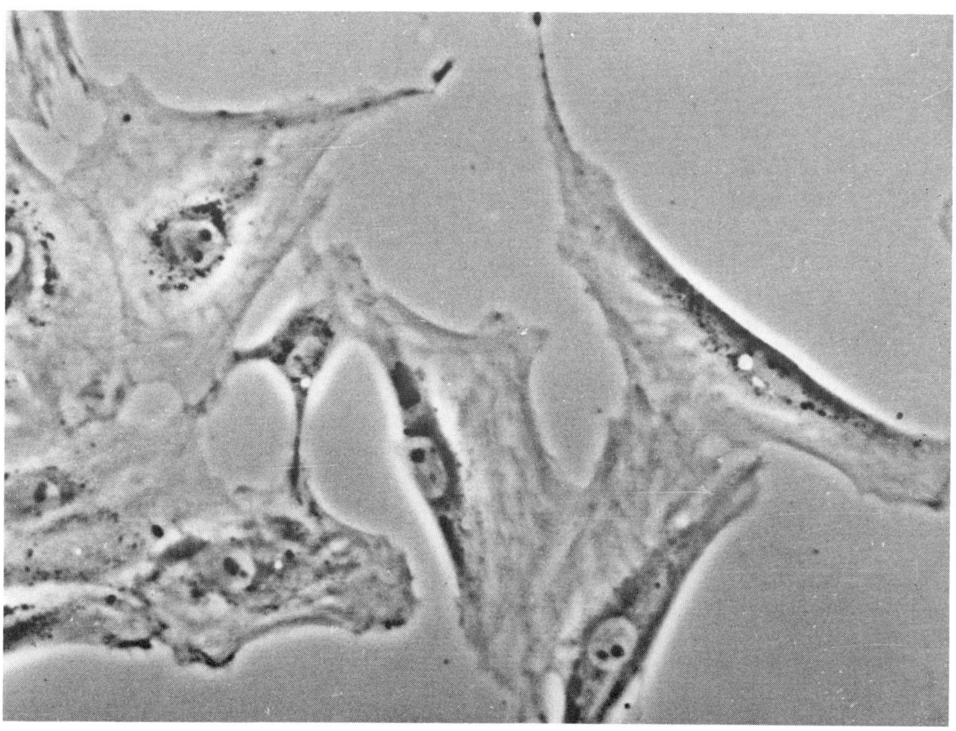

FIGURE 6. Enzyme-dispersed SMC from the adult pig aortic media, 9 days in primary culture. (Magnification × 800.)

tioned medium from primary cultures of adult rat arterial SMC contains a factor that initiates DNA synthesis in growth-arrested subcultures of SMC. The mitogenic activity can be neutralized by antibodies to PDGF, and no mitogenic activity occurs in conditioned medium from cultures pretreated with actinomycin D, excluding release into the medium of PDGF adsorbed to the plastic vessels during the initial culture in serum-containing medium. Exposure of human fibroblasts to samples of the conditioned media at 4°C inhibits subsequent binding of ^{125}I-labeled PDGF. Furthermore, SMC in primary cultures are able to initiate DNA synthesis in a chemically defined medium lacking PDGF and other growth factors.[39]

6. Synthesis of Extracellular Matrix

Synthetic state aortic SMC under basal conditions synthesize fourfold the amount of collagen as contractile state cells, as measured by the incorporation of ^{3}H-proline into hydroxyproline (see Reference 23). The amount of noncollagen protein synthesized doubles under the same conditions. Synthetic state cells also synthesize fivefold the contractile state level of sulfated glycosaminoglycans, as measured by uptake of inorganic sulfur-35.[23] These increases are not related to cell proliferation since in these experiments the synthetic state cells were maintained in a quiescent growth state.

7. Enzyme Alterations

Concomitant with the increased amount of synthetic organelles in the synthetic state SMC,[21] the specific activities of enzymes associated with mitochondria and rough endoplasmic reticulum increase.[40] Cytochrome C oxidase and NADPH-dependent cytochrome C reductase increase 2.3 and 1.8-fold, respectively. Increases of three- to fourfold in activity of the lysosomal enzymes acid phosphatase and *N*-acetyl-β-glucosaminidase occur,[40] consistent with the larger numbers of lysosomes present in synthetic state cells.[21] However, acid cholesteryl esterase, which is also found in lysosomes and is responsible for the hydrolysis of cholesteryl esters, decreases slightly but not significantly upon alteration to the synthetic state.[40]

8. Lipoprotein Metabolism

Cultured SMC in the synthetic state have an altered ability to metabolize lipoproteins.[38,40,41] Morphological examination of rabbit aortic SMC, incubated for 24 hr in 75 μg/mℓ β-very-low-density lipoprotein (β-VLDL) from the serum of cholesterol-fed rabbits, shows few lipid droplets, as demonstrated by Fettrot staining in "contractile"-state cells, with some increase in "reversible synthetic"-state cells, but with substantial numbers of lipid droplets in "irreversible synthetic"-state cells (Figures 7, 8, 9). This pattern of differential cholesteryl ester accumulation was confirmed by gas chromatography and by incorporation of [^{3}H] sodium oleate into cholesteryl oleate. "Irreversible synthetic"-state cells have a considerably greater capacity to bind and degrade β-VLDL than "reversible synthetic" cells, which in turn have a greater capacity than "contractile"-state cells (Figure 10). With all phenotypes the binding is receptor-mediated, of high affinity, and saturable. Similar results were found with normal VLDL, but the extent of the binding, degradation, and cholesteryl ester accumulation was lower than with β-VLDL. In contrast, cells of all three phenotypes bind and degrade considerably less low-density lipoprotein (LDL) under identical conditions, and the cells do not accumulate appreciable cholesteryl ester. Thus at least in the rabbit, lipoproteins of the triglyceride-rich spectrum (β-VLDL and VLDL) are more atherogenic than those of the cholesterol-rich spectrum (LDL), with "irreversible synthetic"-state cells more susceptible to lipid accumulation than "reversible synthetic"-state cells, which in turn are more susceptible than "contractile"-state cells.[41]

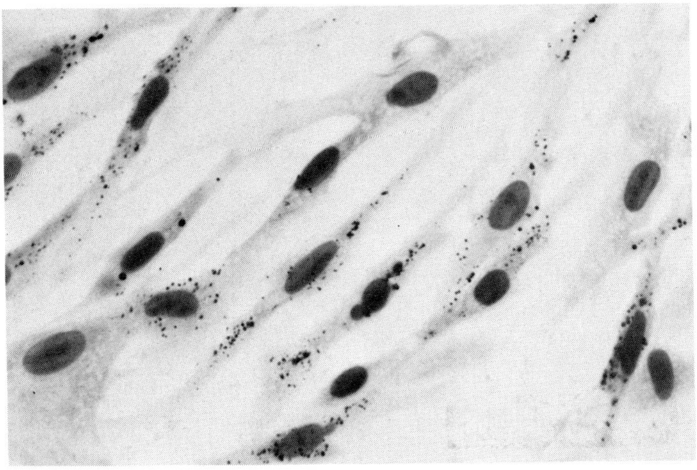

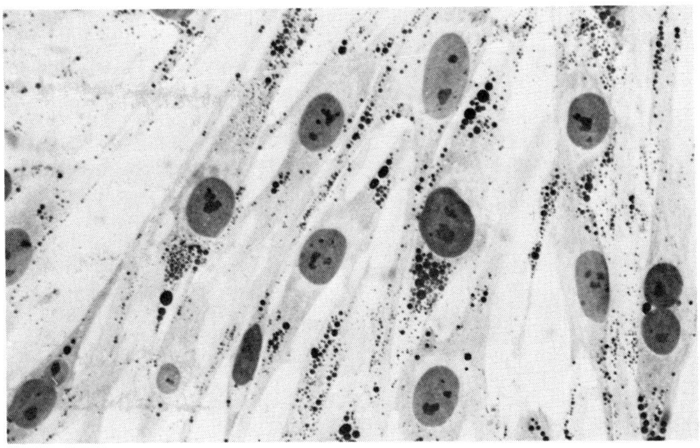

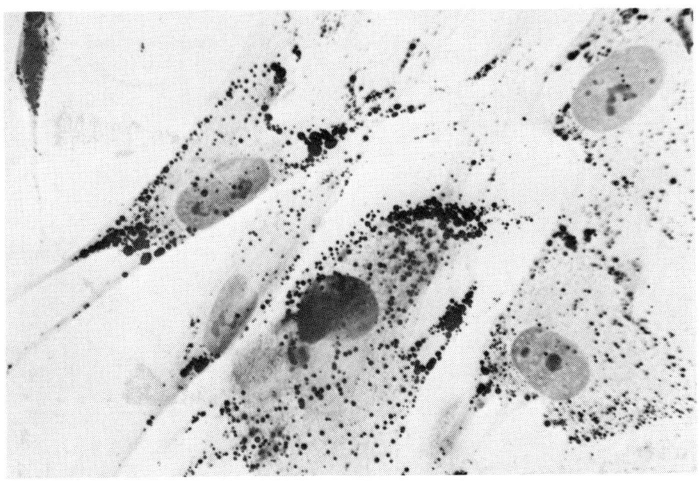

FIGURES 7, 8, and 9. Contractile (top, 7), reversible synthetic (middle, 8), and irreversible synthetic (bottom, 9) state cells stained with Fettrot solution for lipid droplets and counterstained with Meyer's Haemalum following 17-hr incubation in 5% LDS, then 24-hr incubation with 75 μg/mℓ β-VLDL in 5% LDS. (Magnification × 600.) (From Campbell, J. H., Reardon, M. F., Campbell, G. R., and Nestel, P. J., *Arteriosclerosis*, 5, 318, 1985. With permission.)

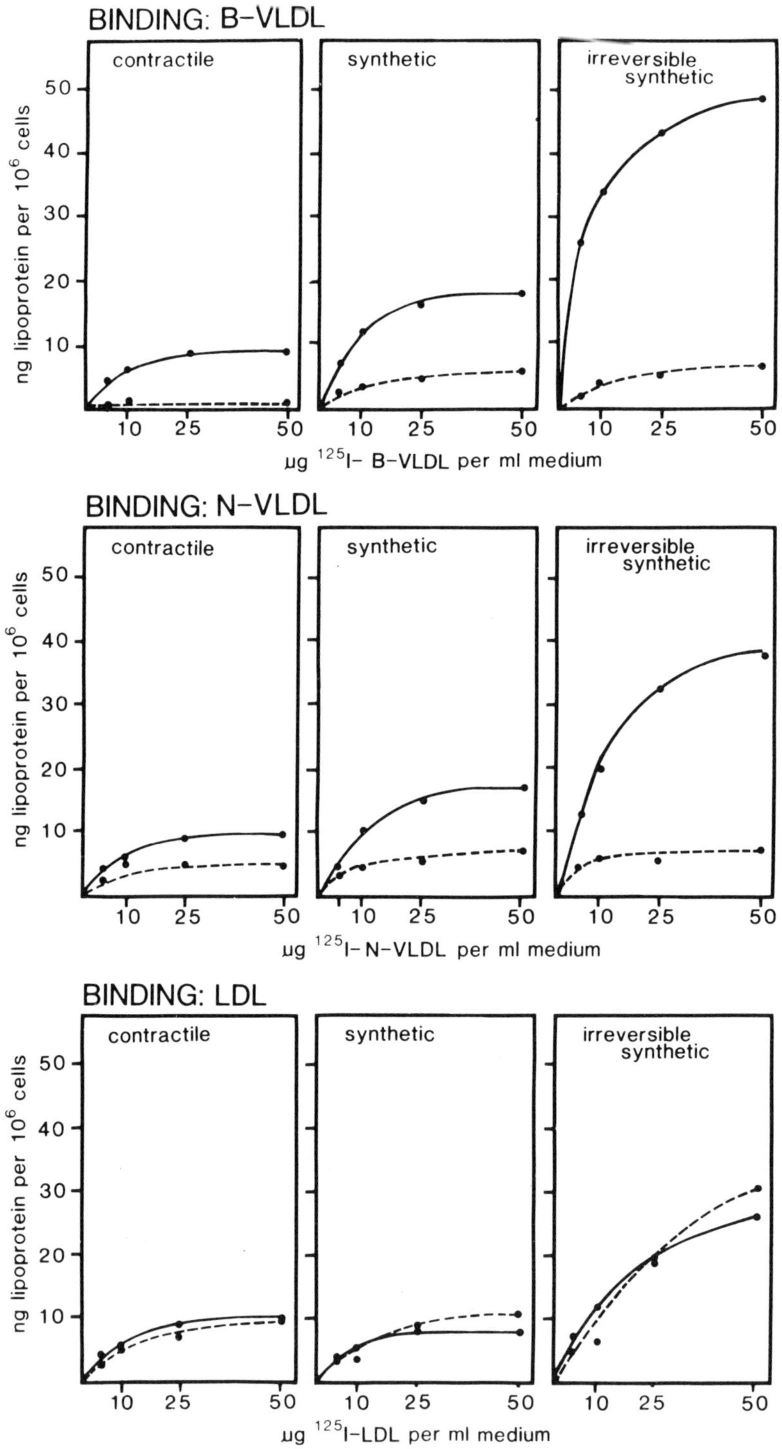

FIGURE 10. Specific (• — •) and nonspecific (O — O) binding of ^{125}I-labeled lipoproteins to rabbit aortic SMC in culture. (From Campbell, J. H., Reardon, M. F., Campbell, G. R., and Nestel, P. J., *Arteriosclerosis*, 5, 318, 1985. With permission.)

III. INFLUENCES OF ENDOTHELIUM ON SMOOTH MUSCLE PHENOTYPIC MODULATION AND PROLIFERATION

A. Influences on Smooth Muscle Phenotype

Spontaneous phenotypic modulation of enzymatically isolated smooth muscle in primary cell culture is prevented if the cells are grown in co-culture with a confluent monolayer of endothelial cells.[2,16,24,17] For this effect to occur, the two cell layers do not have to be in contact, but bathed by the same nutrient medium. The system used for these experiments comprises the modified Rose chamber, where the test and feeder cell layers are grown on opposite coverslips.[27] A feeder layer of confluent, contractile SMC (which is above the critical initial cell seeding density of $10^6/m\ell$ and does not undergo the spontaneous phenotypic change) also prevents the test, sparsely-seeded, contractile SMC from undergoing a spontaneous change in phenotype. In contrast, coculture with confluent adventitial fibroblasts, confluent and quiescent subcultured synthetic state SMC or subconfluent proliferating endothelial cells does not prevent the phenotypic modulation of the test contractile smooth muscle.[24]

The insertion of Spectrapor wet cellulose dialysis membranes of different molecular-weight cutoff between the feeder and test layers has demonstrated that the approximate molecular weight of the inhibitory substance or substances produced by confluent endothelial cells and contractile SMC is 10,000 to 15,000.[27] This is in agreement with our earlier studies which demonstrated that a glycosaminoglycan extract of about 12,000 daltons from the artery wall inhibits smooth muscle phenotypic change.[24] Treatment of this aortic glycosaminoglycan extract with four units per milliliter heparinase from *Flavobacterium heparinum* for 6 hr at 37°C destroys the active factor, suggesting that it is heparin or a related glycosaminoglycan. Addition of sodium heparin to culture medium also inhibits smooth muscle phenotypic change and subsequent proliferation.[24,27,42,43]

Cultured endothelial cells secrete about 50% of their glycosaminoglycan as a highly sulfated (heparin-like) heparan sulfate[44-47] and also produce a factor or factors able to stimulate glycosaminoglycan synthesis by SMC.[48] Heparan sulfate is the predominant glycosaminoglycan in the pericellular coat immediately adjacent to the plasma membrane of cultured SMC,[43,49,50] but by the seventh subculture, this is replaced by dermatan sulfate as the predominant species.[50]

B. Influences on Smooth Muscle Proliferation

Simms and Stillman in 1936[51] first discovered that the aorta contains growth inhibitory substances. Florentin et al.[52] showed that intraperitoneal injections of alcohol-precipitable components of an aqueous extract of pig aorta into 8-week-old living swine, in quantities as low as 500 μg of protein, drastically reduces the rate of entry of arterial SMC into mitosis, with no demonstrable effect on epidermal mitosis. Alcohol precipitates from aqueous extracts of pig aorta can be fractionated to produce both stimulators and inhibitors of synthetic state smooth muscle in culture.[53]

In culture, endothelial cells produce both stimulators and inhibitors of smooth muscle proliferation. The growth stimulator is called the endothelial-derived growth factor (EDGF),[54] and is mitogenic for many mesenchymally derived cells but not for endothelial cells themselves.[54-58] EDGF is a polypeptide which is not homogeneous and contains one factor that is similar to PDGF. This PDGF-like factor accounts for about 25% of the mitogenic effect, at least with 3T3 cells as the target.[59-61] The proliferative state of the endothelial cell determines whether a stimulator or inhibitor is released or which one predominates. When synthetic state smooth muscle is the test tissue and proliferating endothelium the feeder layer in a co-culture situation, the rate of proliferation of the test smooth muscle is stimulated. But when the feeder layer consists of confluent, quiescent endothelium, the normal growth of the test synthetic state smooth muscle is totally inhibited. A feeder layer of confluent contractile smooth muscle inhibits the proliferation of synthetic state cells, while a feeder layer of proliferating synthetic state cells sometimes stimulates, and other times inhibits, smooth muscle growth[24,27] (Table 1).

Similarly, conditioned medium containing 20% whole blood serum from confluent endothelial cells inhibits the proliferation of subcultured SMC, while conditioned medium from proliferating endothelial cells and from proliferating or confluent subcultured SMC and fibroblasts do not inhibit SMC growth.[55] The inhibitory activity has been amply demonstrated to be due to production of heparin-like glycosaminoglycans[43,55,62-64] (see also Chapter 7 for full discussion). Furthermore, heparan sulfate isolated from the surface of postconfluent SMC has recently been shown to exhibit a specific antiproliferative activity on cultured SMC 13 times greater than mucopolysaccharide obtained from the surface of exponentially growing SMC and more than 40 times greater than commercially available heparin.[65]

C. Possible Effects In Vivo

In the normal arterial wall, the SMC and abluminal surface of the endothelium are surrounded by a basal lamina consisting of (among other substances) laminin, heparan sulfate proteoglycan, and type IV collagen.[66,67] The basal lamina is, in turn, closely associated with the continuum of collagen, elastin, and proteoglycans of the intercellular matrix. Their association not only establishes the spatial arrangements of components within the vessel wall,[68] but may be responsible for maintaining SMC in the contractile phenotype, thereby inhibiting cell division (see Reference 69). Following endothelial denudation, platelets are deposited on the subendothelium, releasing PDGF from their alpha granules and platelet heparitinase (endoglycosidase) from their lysosomes. The endoglycosidase may cleave the heparin-like substance from the basal lamina proteoglycans of the SMC closest to the damaged lumen and from remaining endothelial cells and then be removed[62,70] (see Chapter 7). If a heparin-like glycosaminoglycan is the low-molecular-weight substance in the artery wall that maintains smooth muscle in the contractile phenotype, then the loss of this substance would result in SMC modulating to the synthetic phenotype (in primary cell culture it is due to dilution of the factor with decreasing cell seeding concentration). The synthetic-state muscle cells are responsive to substances from the blood and/or regenerating endothelium and/or macrophages, and the cells migrate into the intima and proliferate. Upon restitution of the endothelial lining, the confluent, quiescent endothelium and surrounding contractile-state SMC release the growth inhibitor for synthetic-state cells, which soon builds to a critical level, and development of the myointimal thickening is halted. The SMC then return to the contractile state (see also Chapter 7).

The notion that the extracellular matrix components can control the phenotype a cell expresses is not new. For instance, recent studies have shown that collagen type II and certain proteoglycans are influential in chondrogenic differentiation and in the regulation of chondrocyte phenotype.[71-73]

IV. SIGNIFICANCE OF SMOOTH MUSCLE PHENOTYPIC MODULATION IN PRIMARY CULTURE TO THE PATHOGENESIS OF ATHEROSCLEROSIS

Diffuse intimal thickenings of humans, like the fibromusculo-elastic intimal thickenings formed in experimental animals as a result of endothelial injury, are sites of predilection for atheromatous plaque formation but do not invariably develop into

Table 1
INFLUENCE ON SYNTHETIC STATE SMC PROLIFERATION OF CELL FEEDER LAYERS AFTER 5 DAYS IN CO-CULTURE

Feeder layer[a]	No. SMC/chamber × 10^5 ± S.D.
None (control)	20.6 ± 2.4
Confluent EC	0.9 ± 0.1 ($p < 0.001$)
Proliferating EC	25.2 ± 0.3 ($0.01 < p < 0.05$)
Confluent contractile SMC	1.7 ± 0.2 ($p < 0.001$)
Proliferating synthetic SMC	19.5 ± 6.5 ($p < 0.05$)

Note: Number of cells per chamber on day 0 is 0.8 ± 0.1 × 10^5.

[a] EC, endothelial cells; SMC, smooth muscle cells.

plaques.[74-77] Two mechanisms have been suggested by which diffuse intimal thickenings develop: (1) a response of the vessels wall to repeated injury and (2) a response of the vessel wall to postnatal growth and increase in blood pressure.[78] The nodular proliferation of SMC and accumulation of foam cells and extracellular lipid results in a reorganization of these thickenings in atherogenesis.

The vast majority of cells in human diffuse intimal thickenings are smooth muscle. These, like the SMC in lesions, vary in size and shape.[76,79-81] The volume fraction of synthetic organelles in SMC from human carotid endarterectomy and autopsy material has been measured by morphometric techniques,[82,83] and while intimal SMC from unaffected regions approximate those of the media, there is a 100% increase in volume fraction of synthetic organelles in SMC of diffuse intimal thickenings near lesions, as compared with those of the media. That is, the cells morphologically express the synthetic phenotype. Consistent with an altered phenotypic expression are the recent observations of Gabbiani et al.[84] that, unlike the aortic media which shows a predominance of actin in the α-isoform, human atheromatous plaques and surrounding adjacent diffuse intimal thickenings show a predominance of β-actin with some γ-isoform. Some of the SMC present in the diffuse intimal thickenings near lesions may be senescent, having exhausted their proliferative capacity during the formation of the thickening,[28,85] but others may actively express the same characteristics as the morphologically equivalent synthetic state SMC in culture. These cells respond rapidly to mitogens (whether they are from the serum, proliferating endothelium, or macrophages), synthesize substantial amounts of collagen, and exhibit enhanced binding and degradation of atherogenic lipoproteins, resulting in a substantial lipid accumulation,[38,40,41,69,76] all of which are features essential to the process of atherogenesis.

REFERENCES

1. Gabella, G., Structural apparatus for force transmission in smooth muscles, *Physiol. Rev.*, 64, 455, 1984.
2. Campbell, G. R., Chamley-Campbell, J. H., and Burnstock, G., Differentiation and phenotypic modulation of arterial smooth muscle cells, in *Structure and Function of the Circulation*, Vol. 3, Schwartz, C. J., Werthessen, N. T., and Wolf, S., Eds., Plenum Press, New York, 1981, 357.
3. Pease, D. C. and Paule, W. J., Electron microscopy of elastic arteries. The thoracic aorta of the rat, *J. Ultrastruct. Res.*, 3, 469, 1960.

4. Karrer, H. E., An electron microscope study of the aorta in young and in aging mice, *J. Ultrastruct. Res.,* 5, 1, 1961.
5. Paule, W. J., Electron microscopy of the newborn rat aorta, *J. Ultrastruct. Res.,* 8, 219, 1963.
6. Gerrity, R. G. and Cliff, W. J., The aortic tunica media of the developing rat. I. Quantitative stereologic and biochemical analysis, *Lab. Invest.,* 32, 585, 1975.
7. Olivetti, G., Anversa, P., Melissari, M., and Loud, A. V., Morphometry of medial hypertrophy in the rat thoracic aorta, *Lab. Invest.,* 42, 559, 1980.
8. Kasai, T. and Pollak, O. J., Smooth muscle cells in aortic cultures of untreated and cholesterol-fed rabbits, *Z. Zellforsch. Mikrosk. Anat.,* 62, 743, 1964.
9. Pollak, O. J. and Adachi, M., Human and rabbit arterial cells compared in tissue cultures, *Prog. Biochem. Pharmacol.,* 4, 294, 1968.
10. Jarmolych, J., Daoud, A. S., Landau, J., Fritz, K. E., and McElvene, E., Aortic media explants. Cell proliferation and production of mucopolysaccharides, collagen, and elastic tissue, *Exp. Mol. Pathol.,* 9, 171, 1968.
11. Fritz, K. E., Jarmolych, J., and Daoud, A. S., Association of DNA synthesis and apparent dedifferentiation of aortic smooth muscle cells *in vitro, Exp. Mol. Pathol.,* 12, 354, 1970.
12. Rossi, G. L., Alroy, J., and Röthenmund, S., Morphological studies of cultured swine aorta media explants, *Virchows Arch. B,* 12, 133, 1973.
13. Wight, T. N., Cooke, P. H., and Smith, S. C., An electron microscopic study of pigeon aorta cell cultures. Cytodifferentiation and intracellular lipid accumulation, *Exp. Mol. Pathol.,* 21, 1, 1977.
14. Chamley, J. H., Campbell, G. R., and Burnstock, G., An analysis of the interactions between sympathetic nerve fibres and smooth muscle cells in tissue culture, *Dev. Biol.,* 33, 344, 1973.
15. Campbell, G. R., Chamley, J. H., and Burnstock, G., Development of smooth muscle cells in tissue culture, *J. Anat.,* 117, 295, 1974.
16. Chamley, J. H., Campbell, G. R., and Burnstock, G., Dedifferentiation, redifferentiation and bundle formation of smooth muscle cells in tissue culture: the influence of cell number and nerve fibres, *J. Embryol. Exp. Morphol.,* 32, 297, 1974.
17. Chamley, J. H. and Campbell, G. R., Trophic influences of sympathetic nerves and cyclic AMP on differentiation and proliferation of isolated smooth muscle cells in culture, *Cell Tissue Res.,* 161, 497, 1975.
18. Chamley, J. H. and Campbell, G. R., Isolated ureteral smooth muscle cells in culture. Including their interaction with intrinsic and extrinsic nerves, *Cytobiologie Z. Exp. Zellforsch.,* 11, 358, 1975.
19. Chamley, J. H., Campbell, G. R., McConnell, J. D., and Groschel-Stewart, U., Comparison of vascular smooth muscle cells from adult human, monkey and rabbit in primary culture and in subculture, *Cell Tissue Res.,* 177, 503, 1977.
20. Chamley-Campbell, J., Campbell, G. R., and Ross, R., The smooth muscle cell in culture, *Physiol. Rev.,* 59, 1, 1979.
21. Thyberg, J., Palmberg, L., Nilsson, J., Ksiazek, T., and Sjolund, M., Phenotype modulation in primary cultures of arterial smooth muscle cells. On the role of platelet-derived growth factor, *Differentiation,* 25, 156, 1983.
22. Thyberg, J., Nilsson, J., Palmberg, L., and Sjolund, M., Adult human arterial smooth muscle cells in primary culture. Modulation from contractile to synthetic phenotype, *Cell Tissue Res.,* 239, 69, 1985.
23. Campbell, J. H. and Campbell, G. R., Chemical stimuli of the hypertrophic response to smooth muscle, in *Hypertrophic Response of Smooth Muscle,* Seidel, C. L., Ed., CRC Press, Boca Raton, Fla., 1987, in press.
24. Chamley-Campbell, J. H. and Campbell, G. R., What controls smooth muscle phenotype? *Atherosclerosis,* 40, 347, 1981.
25. Chamley-Campbell, J. H., Campbell, G. R., and Ross, R., Phenotype-dependent response of cultured aortic smooth muscle to serum mitogens, *J. Cell Biol.,* 89, 379, 1981.
26. Sjölund, M., Nilsson, J., Palmberg, L., and Thyberg, J., Phenotype modulation in primary cultures of arterial smooth-muscle cells. Dual effect of prostaglandin E1, *Differentiation,* 27, 158, 1984.
27. Campbell, J. H. and Campbell, G. R., Cellular interactions in the artery wall, in *The Peripheral Circulation,* Hunyor, S., Ludbrook, J., Shaw, J., and McGrath, M., Eds., Elsevier, New York, 1984, 33.
28. Ross, R. and Kariya, B., Morphogenesis of vascular smooth muscle in atherosclerosis and cell culture, in *Handbook of Physiology - Section 2, The Cardiovascular System, Vol. 2, Vascular Smooth Muscle,* Bohr, D., Somlyo, A. P., and Sparks, H. V., Eds., American Physiological Society, Bethesda, Md., 1980, 69.
29. Chamley, J. H. and Campbell, G. R., Mitosis of contractile smooth muscle cells in tissue culture, *Exp. Cell Res.,* 84, 105, 1974.
30. Mark, G. E., Chamley, J. H., and Burnstock, G., Interactions between autonomic nerves and smooth and cardiac muscle cells in tissue culture, *Dev. Biol.,* 32, 194, 1973.

31. Gröschel-Stewart, U., Chamley, J. H., Campbell, G. R., and Burnstock, G., Changes in myosin distribution in dedifferentiating and redifferentiating smooth muscle cells in tissue culture, *Cell Tissue Res.*, 165, 13, 1975.
32. Purves, R. D., Mark, G. E., and Burnstock, G., The electrical activity of single isolated smooth muscle cells, *Pfluegers Arch.*, 341, 325, 1973.
33. Purves, R. D., Hill, C. E., Chamley, J. H., Mark, G. E., Fry, D. M., and Burnstock, G., Functional autonomic neuromuscular junctions in tissue culture, *Pfluegers Arch.*, 350, 1, 1974.
34. Campbell, G. R., Uehara, Y., Mark, G., and Burnstock, G., Fine structure of smooth muscle cells grown in tissue culture, *J. Cell Biol.*, 49, 21, 1971.
35. Chamley-Campbell, J. H. and Campbell, G. R., Development of smooth muscle and autonomic nerves in culture, in *Somatic and Autonomic Nerve-Muscle Interactions*, Burnstock, G., O'Brien, R., and Vrbova, G., Eds., Elsevier, Amsterdam, 1983, 35.
36. Hermsmeyer, K., De Cino, P., and White, R., Spontaneous contractions of dispersed vascular muscle in cell culture, *In Vitro*, 12, 628, 1976.
37. Mauger, J. P., Worcel, M., Tassin, J., and Courtois, Y., Contractility of smooth muscle cells of rabbit aorta in tissue culture, *Nature (London)*, 255, 337, 1975.
38. Chamley-Campbell, J. H., Nestel, P., and Campbell, G. R., Smooth muscle metabolic reactivity in atherogenesis: LDL metabolism and response to serum mitogens differ according to phenotype, in *Factors in Formation and Regression of the Atherosclerotic Plaque*, Born, G. R. V., Catapano, A. L., and Paoletti, R., Eds., Plenum Press, New York, 1982, 115.
39. Nilsson, J., Sjölund, M., Palmberg, L., Thyberg, J., and Heldin, C.-H., Arterial smooth muscle cells in primary culture produce a platelet-derived growth factor-like protein, *Proc. Natl. Acad. Sci. U.S.A.*, 82, 000, 1985.
40. Campbell, J. H., Popadynec, L., Nestel, P. J., and Campbell, G. R., Lipid accumulation in arterial smooth muscle cells. Influence of phenotype, *Atherosclerosis*, 47, 279, 1983.
41. Campbell, J. H., Reardon, M. F., Campbell, G. R., and Nestel, P. J., Metabolism of atherogenic lipoproteins by smooth muscle cells of different phenotype in culture, *Arteriosclerosis*, 5, 318, 1985.
42. Melzig, von M. and Teuscher, E., The influence of blood factors on the myosin content of vascular smooth muscle cells in culture, *Acta Histochem.*, 73, 289, 1983 (in German).
43. Nilsson, J., Ksiazek, T., Thyberg, J., and Wasteson, A., Cell surface components and growth regulation in cultivated arterial smooth muscle cells, *J. Cell Sci.*, 64, 107, 1983.
44. Busch, C., Ljungman, C., Heldin, C.-M., Waskson, E., and Obrink, B., Surface properties of cultured endothelial cells, *Haemostasis*, 8, 142, 1979.
45. Gamse, G., Fromme, H. G., and Kresse, H., Metabolism of sulfated glycosaminoglycans in cultured endothelial cells and smooth muscle cells from bovine aorta, *Biochim. Biophys. Acta*, 544, 514, 1978.
46. Oohira, A., Wight, T. N., and Bornstein, P., Sulfated proteoglycans synthesized by vascular endothelial cells in culture, *J. Biol. Chem.*, 258, 2014, 1983.
47. Wasteson, Å., Glimelius, B., Busch, C., Westermark, H., Heldin, C.-H., and Norling, B., Effects of a platelet endoglycosidase on cell surface associated heparan sulphate of human cultured endothelial and glial cells, *Thromb. Res.*, 11, 309, 1977.
48. Merrilees, M. J. and Scott, J., Interaction of aortic endothelial and smooth muscle cells in culture. Effect of glycosaminoglycan levels, *Atherosclerosis*, 39, 147, 1981.
49. Heickendorff, L. and Ledet, T., Glycosaminoglycans of arterial basement membrane-like material from cultured rabbit aortic myomedial cells, *Biochim. Biophys. Acta*, 798, 276, 1984.
50. Yamamoto, H., Kanaide, H., and Nakamura, M., Metabolism of glycosaminoglycans of cultured rat aortic smooth muscle cells altered during subculture, *Br. J. Exp. Pathol.*, 64, 156, 1983.
51. Simms, H. S. and Stillman, N. P., Substances affecting adult tissue in vitro. II. A growth inhibitor in adult tissue, *J. Gen. Physiol.*, 20, 621, 1937.
52. Florentin, R. A., Nam, S. C., Janakidevi, K., Lee, K. T., Reiner, J. M., and Thomas, W. A., Population dynamics of arterial smooth-muscle cells. II. In vivo inhibition of entry into mitosis of swine arterial smooth-muscle cells by aortic tissue extracts, *Arch. Pathol.*, 95, 317, 1973.
53. Eisenstein, R., Harper, E., Kuettner, K. E., Schumacher, B., and Matijevitch, B., Growth regulators in connective tissues. II. Evidence for the presence of several growth inhibitors in aortic extracts, *Paroi Arterielle*, 5, 163, 1979.
54. Gajdusek, C., DiCorleto, P., Ross, R., and Schwartz, S. M., An endothelial cell-derived growth factor, *J. Cell Biol.*, 85, 467, 1980.
55. Castellot, J. J., Jr., Addonizio, M. L., Rosenberg, R., and Karnovksy, M. J., Cultured endothelial cells produce a heparinlike inhibitor of smooth muscle cell growth, *J. Cell Biol.*, 90, 372, 1981.
56. Fass, D. N., Downing, M. R., Meyers, P., Bowie, E. J. W., and Witte, L. D., Cell growth stimulation by normal and von Willebrand porcine platelets and endothelial cells, *Blood*, 52 (Suppl. 1), 181, 1978.
57. Wang, C.-H., Largis, E. E., and Schaffer, S. A., The effects of endothelial cell-conditioned media on the proliferation of aortic smooth muscle cells and 3T3 cells in culture, *Artery*, 9, 358, 1981.

58. Witte, L. D., Cornicelli, J. A., Miller, R. W., and Goodman, D. S., Effects of platelet-derived and endothelial cell-derived growth factors on the low density lipoprotein receptor pathway in cultured human fibroblasts, *J. Biol. Chem.*, 257, 5392, 1982.
59. Bowen-Pope, D. F., Vogel, A., and Ross, R., Production of platelet-derived growth factor-like molecules and reduced expression of platelet-derived growth factor receptors accompany transformation by a wide spectrum of agents, *Proc. Natl. Acad. Sci. U.S.A.*, 81, 2396, 1984.
60. DiCorleto, P. E., Cultured endothelial cells produce multiple growth factors for connective tissue cells, *Exp. Cell Res.*, 153, 167, 1984.
61. DiCorleto, P. E. and Bowen-Pope, D. F., Cultured endothelial cells produce a platelet-derived growth factor-like protein, *Proc. Natl. Acad. Sci. U.S.A.*, 80, 1919, 1983.
62. Castellot, J. J., Jr., Favreau, L. V., Karnovsky, M. J., and Rosenberg, R. D., Inhibition of vascular smooth muscle cell growth by endothelial cell-derived heparin. Possible role of a platelet endoglycosidase, *J. Biol. Chem.*, 257, 11256, 1982.
63. Hatcher, V. B., Tsien, G., Oberman, M. S., and Burk, P. G., Inhibition of cell proliferation and protease activity by cartilage factors and heparin, *J. Supramol. Struct.*, 14, 33, 1980.
64. Hoover, R. L., Rosenberg, R., Haering, W., and Karnovsky, M. J., Inhibition of rat arterial smooth muscle cell proliferation by heparin. II. In vitro studies, *Circ. Res.*, 47, 578, 1980.
65. Fritze, M. S., Reilly, C. F., and Rosenberg, R. D., An antiproliferative heparan sulfate species produced by postconfluent smooth muscle cells, *J. Cell Biol.*, 100, 1041, 1985.
66. Kjellén, L., Pettersson, I., and Höök, M., Cell-surface heparan sulfate: an intercalated membrane proteoglycan, *Proc. Natl. Acad. Sci. U.S.A.*, 78, 5371, 1981.
67. Palotie, A., Tryggvason, K., Peltonen, L., and Seppä, H., Components of subendothelial aorta basement membrane. Immunohistochemical localization and role in cell attachment, *Lab. Invest.*, 49, 362, 1983.
68. Wight, T. N., Vessel proteoglycans and thrombogenesis, in *Progress in Hemostasis and Thrombosis*, Spaet, T., Ed., Grune & Stratton, New York, 1980, 1.
69. Campbell, G. R. and Campbell, J. H., Smooth muscle phenotypic changes in arterial wall homeostasis: implications for the pathogenesis of atherosclerosis, *Exp. Mol. Pathol.*, 42, 139, 1985.
70. Rosenberg, R. D., Castellot, J. J., Jr., and Karnovsky, M. J., Role of heparin-like molecules in atherogenesis, in *Heparin: New Biochemical and Medical Aspects*, Witte, I., Ed., Walter de Gruyter, Berlin, 1982, 261.
71. Lash, J. W. and Vasan, N. S., Somite chondrogenesis in vitro. Stimulation by exogenous extracellular matrix components, *Dev. Biol.*, 66, 151, 1978.
72. Hay, E. D., Collagen and embryonic development, in *Cell Biology of Extracellular Matrix*, Hay, E. D., Ed., Plenum Press, 1981, 379.
73. Archer, C. W., Rooney, P., and Wolpert, L., Cell shape and cartilage differentiation of early chick limb bud cells in culture, *Cell Differ.*, 11, 245, 1982.
74. Geer, J. C. and Haust, M. D., Smooth muscle cells in atherosclerosis, in *Monographs on Atherosclerosis*, Vol. 2, Pollak, O. J., Simms, H. S., and Kirk, S. E., Eds., S. Karger, Basel, 1972.
75. McGill, H. C., Jr., The lesion, in *Atherosclerosis. III. Proc. 3rd Int. Symp. Atherosclerosis*, Schettler, G. and Weizel, A., Eds., Springer-Verlag, Berlin, 1974, 27.
76. Campbell, G. R. and Chamley-Campbell, J. H., The cellular pathobiology of atherosclerosis, *Pathology*, 13, 423, 1981.
77. Velican, C. and Velican, D., Intimal thickening in developing coronary arteries and its relevance to atherosclerotic involvement, *Atherosclerosis*, 23, 345, 1976.
78. Velican, C. and Velican, D., The precursors of coronary atherosclerotic plaques in subjects up to 40 years old, *Atherosclerosis*, 37, 33, 1980.
79. Haust, M. D., Atherosclerosis and smooth muscle cells, in *Biochemistry of Smooth Muscle*, Stephens, N. L., Ed., CRC Press, Boca Raton, Fla., 1983, 189.
80. Orekhov, A. N., Karpova, I. I., Tertov, V. V., Rudchenko, S. A., Andreeva, E. R., Krushinsky, A. V., and Smirnov, V. N., Cellular composition of atherosclerotic and uninvolved human aortic subendothelial intima. Light-microscopic study of dissociated aortic cells, *Am. J. Pathol.*, 115, 17, 1984.
81. Campbell, G. R. and Campbell, J. H., Smooth muscle cells, in *The Biology and Clinical Science of Atherosclerosis*, European Atherosclerosis Group, Churchill Livingstone, Edinburgh, 1986, in press.
82. Mosse, P. R. L., Campbell, G. R., Wang, T. L., and Campbell, J. H., Smooth muscle phenotypic expression in human carotid arteries. I. Comparison of cells from diffuse intimal thickenings adjacent to atheromatous plaques with those of the media, *Lab. Invest.*, 53, 556, 1985.
83. Mosse, P. R. L., Campbell, G. R., and Campbell, J. H., Smooth muscle phenotypic expression in human carotid arteries. II. Comparison of cells from areas of atherosclerosis-free intimal thickenings with those of the media, *Arteriosclerosis*, 6(6), 1986.
84. Gabbiani, G., Kocher, O., Bloom, W. S., Vandekerckhove, J., and Weber, K., Actin expression in smooth muscle cells of rat aortic intimal thickening, human atheromatous plaque, and cultured rat aortic media, *J. Clin. Invest.*, 73, 148, 1984.

85. Ross, R., Wight, T. N., Strandness, E., and Thiele, B., Human atherosclerosis. I. Cell constitution and characteristics of advanced lesions of the superficial femoral artery, *Am. J. Pathol.*, 114, 79, 1984.

Chapter 5

CONTRACTILE PROTEIN EXPRESSION AND CYTODIFFERENTIATION IN CULTURED VASCULAR SMOOTH MUSCLE CELLS

Gary K. Owens, Arthur S. Rovner, and Richard A. Murphy

TABLE OF CONTENTS

I. INTRODUCTION

There is much interest in the development of cultured vascular smooth muscle (VSM) cells for use in studying receptor or contractile function in vitro. Isolated cells have unique advantages for studying mechanisms of action of vasoactive substances without the complicating influences of other cell types, diffusional limitations, innervation, as well as technical limitations in the types of measurements that can be performed on a whole tissue (e.g., optical measurements of Ca^{2+} concentrations using fluorescent indicators). However, Chamley-Campbell et al.[1] and others[2] presented electron microscopic and immunocytochemical evidence suggesting that VSM cells do not proliferate in cell culture until they have lost much of their contractile apparatus. The Campbells suggested that VSM cells normally exist in a nondividing "contractile state" and phenotypically modulate to a "synthetic state" in cell culture. Other studies, however, have demonstrated that established cultures of VSM cells express muscle-specific contractile proteins[3-8] and exhibit some contractile properties[9-12] characteristic of differentiated smooth muscle.

In this chapter we will

1. Review the composition, structure, and function of the contractile apparatus in smooth muscle cells
2. Present evidence showing that VSM cells continue to express smooth muscle-specific contractile proteins in culture and that this expression is related to the cell's growth state
3. Examine whether additional factors characterizing VSM differentiation are also promoted by conditions that increase expression of smooth muscle cell-specific contractile proteins
4. Review known factors that promote cytodifferentiation in cultured VSM cells

II. CONTRACTILE SYSTEM OF SMOOTH MUSCLE CELLS IN VIVO

Smooth muscle, like striated muscle, is a specialized cell type with an organized myofilament lattice for the expression of external force or shortening. There is a generally shared consensus, based primarily on mechanical and biochemical analysis, that contraction is due to a sliding filament/crossbridge mechanism. Interdigitation of thin filaments, consisting of actin and tropomyosin, into a myosin-containing thick filament lattice appears to reflect crossbridge cycling powered by ATP hydrolysis.[13-15] However, the assumption that smooth and striated muscles differ significantly only in the structural organization of the contractile proteins is incorrect. This section summarizes recent information showing that the contractile system of smooth muscle has unique properties underlying the ability to perform a variety of functions.

A. Characteristics of the Contractile System

The ultrastructural appearance of smooth muscles, typified by a densely packed array of axially oriented thin filaments with scattered thick filaments, is paralleled by a correspondingly high content of thin filament proteins and low myosin content compared to mammalian skeletal muscles (Table 1). Within the precision of the estimates, all mammalian smooth muscles have a comparable myosin content, but arteries differ from veins and a wide variety of other tissues in having cells with higher thin filament protein contents.

The estimated mechanical output of smooth muscle cells also contrasts with striated muscle (Table 1). These figures are based on data obtained from the few preparations

Table 1
CONTRACTILE PROTEIN COMPOSITION AND MECHANICAL OUTPUT

	Content[a] (mg/g cell wet weight)			Mechanical output	
	Myosin	Actin	Tropomyosin	Isometric stress[b] (× 10^5 N/m^2)	V_0[c] (L_0/sec)
Skeletal muscle	62	22	5	2—3.5	4—24
Arterial smooth muscle	18	50	13	Up to 6.7	0.1
Veins and smooth muscles of airway, gastrointestinal, and other organs	18	29	8	Up to 7.3	0.4

[a] Summary from Murphy et al.[16]
[b] Maximum reported estimates for cells (may be underestimates for smooth muscles due to tissue damage, incomplete activation): swine carotid media,[17] guinea pig taenia coli.[18]
[c] Values for mammalian skeletal muscles depend on myosin isoenzyme.[19] Values for smooth muscle also depend on level of crossbridge phosphorylation. Values for maximal unloaded shortening velocities were extrapolated for 100% phosphorylation: swine carotid media,[16] feline esophageal,[20] bovine trachealis.[21]

in which tissue measurements can be corrected to provide data on cellular output and in which efforts have been made to achieve maximal activation. Two striking differences distinguish smooth and striated muscles. The latter have very high estimated unloaded shortening velocities (V_0). Differences in V_0 among striated muscle cells reflect synthesis of different myosin isoenzymes. The velocity of a given striated muscle cell also depends on load, but V_0 is not directly determined by cell [Ca^{2+}]. In contrast, smooth muscles are slow, and the V_0 for a given cell can vary over a wide range.[22] In smooth muscle, crossbridge cycling rates appear to be a regulated parameter reflecting cell [Ca^{2+}] and the level of crossbridge phosphorylation. Thus, smooth muscles have properties that are absent in striated muscles.

Smooth muscles also differ from striated muscles by generating higher levels of isometric stress (force/cross-sectional area of cells). This difference represents a major puzzle because the myosin and crossbridge content of smooth muscles is only 30% of that in striated muscles (Table 1). Stresses and velocities in muscles depend not only on the nature of the contractile proteins, but also on their organization into the filament lattice. The latter is not known in smooth muscles, and the relative contributions of protein differences and filament lattice structure to estimated cellular contractile outputs is uncertain.

B. Contractile Function in Smooth Muscle

Skeletal muscle cells extend from one tendon to another. The skeleton bears most gravitational loads, and the cells are normally relaxed, contracting when needed to produce work. Furthermore, each cell (or motor unit) is recruited and functions independently. These conditions do not apply to smooth muscle cells in the walls of hollow organs. The connection of the small cells in series around the organ requires that such cells must generate and bear equal stresses. Furthermore, contraction in part of a tissue produces changes in pressure that are transmitted to all other cells, so the elements are not independent. A final point is that smooth muscles function not only to produce work, but must be capable of tonic contractions to maintain the circumference or volume of the organ (e.g., vascular resistance). Smooth muscles exhibit a wide variety of activity patterns ranging from normal tonic contractions (i.e., sphincters) to intermittent phasic contractions comparable to skeletal muscle twitches. The available evidence is consistent with the hypothesis that all smooth muscles have a similar contractile apparatus and that unique Ca^{2+}-dependent regulatory mechanisms allow very different types of contractions.[22] Physiological diversity appears to arise from differences in the ways tissues control myoplasmic [Ca^{2+}].

The flexibility of the smooth muscle contractile apparatus, at least in part, arises from properties which allow two types of crossbridge interactions with the thin filaments.[22-25] Contraction of a relaxed cell is initiated by a rapid increase in myoplasmic [Ca^{2+}] to levels that activate myosin kinase. This leads to phosphorylation of the crossbridges at a site on the regulatory light chains of myosin. Phosphorylated crossbridges cycle rapidly and produce fast responses, with correspondingly high rates of energy consumption. However, activation is characteristically associated with a transient increase in myoplasmic [Ca^{2+}], which falls to an intermediate sustained level.[26] Mechanical studies indicate that reductions in cell [Ca^{2+}] to intermediate levels leading to dephosphorylation by myosin phosphatase are associated with the formation of a non- or very slowly cycling attachment of the crossbridges with the thin filament.[23,24] In this state, the contractile system can maintain a stress against an imposed load (such as blood pressure) with greatly reduced cycling and a very high economy. This state has been termed "latch" and appears to characterize tonic contractions in sphincters[20] or arterial smooth muscle.[23,24] The latch state is very sensitive to Ca^{2+}, but reductions in Ca^{2+} lead to relaxation.[27] In summary, any analysis of the contractile protein variants expressed in smooth muscle must consider their role in the function of the tissue, which has elements not exhibited by striated muscle.

C. Molecular Diversity of the Contractile Proteins and Functional Significance

Striated muscles express a single actin variant. The functional differences between skeletal muscle cell types are associated with isoenzymes of myosin and the metabolic adaptations necessary to match ATP production with consumption in cells with widely differing shortening velocities. There is no compelling evidence for the expression of myosin variants in vertebrate smooth muscle[16] except for an avian embryonic form.[28] Several laboratories have reported preliminary evidence that smooth muscles have two or more myosin heavy chains differing in their molecular weights.[29-31] However, proteolytic cleavage during tissue processing readily occurs, leading to possible artifacts. Our studies[31] show equal amounts of two heavy chains in several types of smooth muscle. However, only a single myosin type was detected on nondenaturing pyrophosphate gels. These observations are consistent with an interpretation that mature smooth muscle contains a single myosin form that is a heterodimer consisting of two different heavy chains (plus two 20,000- and two 17,000-dalton light chains). If this hypothesis is correct, the two heads of the crossbridge in smooth muscle may differ, with possible functional significance with respect to crossbridge interactions with the thin filament discussed above.

Smooth muscle myosin is immunologically and electrophoretically distinct from the isomyosins of striated muscles and that present in nonmuscle cells (Figure 1).[32-35] Although myosin variants have not been shown to contribute to functional diversity, the expression of the smooth muscle-specific myosin or its denatured heavy chains is a readily measured and potentially useful marker for assessing cytodifferentiation in cultured or developing smooth muscle.

In contrast to striated muscle, the molecular diversity in the contractile proteins of smooth muscle is found in the thin filament proteins. Vandekerckhove and Weber[38] demonstrated that four forms of actin are expressed in smooth muscles. These include two smooth muscle-specific actins (α-SM and γ-SM) and two variants expressed in nonmuscle cells (β-NM and γ-NM), where the α, β, and γ designate variants distinguish-

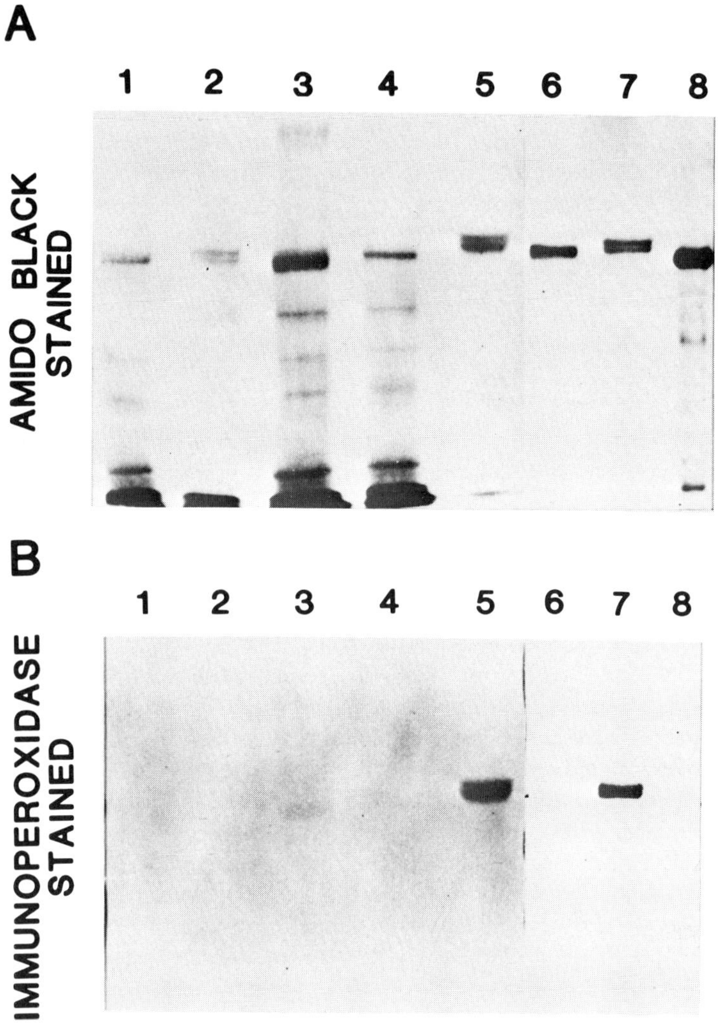

FIGURE 1. Immunological characterization of myosins from a variety of cells and tissues, using the smooth muscle myosin-specific antibody of Groschel-Stewart et al.[37] Myosins were resolved by sodium dodecyl sulfate (SDS) gel electrophoresis (3 to 4% gradient gel) and blotted onto nitrocellulose paper.[36] Panel A shows an amido black stain illustrating the proteins present on the nitrocellulose. Panel B shows results of immunoperoxidase staining of these same gels with the Groschel-Stewart et al.[37] anti-myosin antibody. Lanes: (1) Swiss 3T3 cells; (2) cultured rat coronary artery endothelial cells; (3) cultured rat aortic smooth muscle cells at confluency; (4) cultured rat aortic smooth muscle cells during log phase growth; (5) purified myosin from swine stomach; (6) purified rabbit skeletal muscle myosin: (7) purified myosin from the media of swine carotid artery; and (8) rat left ventricle tissue homogenate. Note that myosin was present in all lanes (Panel A), but only those from swine stomach (Lane 5) and carotid artery (Lane 7) reacted with the Groschel-Stewart antimyosin antibody. In contrast, the myosins from all cultured cells reacted with an antiplatelet myosin antibody provided by D. Larsen (data not shown). Controls were done using nonimmune serum (data not shown).

able on the basis of their isoelectric points. Only three variants are found in two-dimensional gels of smooth muscle proteins because the γ-SM and γ-NM actin variants comigrate. Despite this limitation, two-dimensional gel electrophoresis provides a relatively simple method to estimate actin variant contents in smooth muscle tissue samples lacking significant amounts of other cell types.[39] Our results[6,7,39] and those of others[40,41] clearly show that the actin variants are highly tissue-specific. All arteries, for example, exhibit comparable actin variant distributions irrespective of species. Measurements of the isoactin distribution and content has proven to be a useful and readily determined marker for studies of cytodifferentiation in smooth muscle.

Expression of muscle (i.e., α-SM and γ-SM) and nonmuscle (β-NM and γ-NM) actins appears to be developmentally regulated in smooth muscle. Saborio et al.[42] found a continuous increase in γ-SM actin and a decrease in nonmuscle actins in the chicken gizzard during embryonic development and showed that the differential expression of actins was controlled at the transcription level. We demonstrated that similar changes occur during developmental growth of VSM cells.[6] β-NM actin comprised about 60% of the total actin in VSM cells from newborn rats. The amount of β-NM actin decreased, whereas the α-SM actin increased with age, comprising 70% of the actin in VSM cells from adult rats.

The functional significance of changes in isoactin expression during developmental growth of VSM is unclear, but may reflect the physiological requirements for specific actin variants for specialized cellular functions. There is considerable evidence supporting this idea in skeletal muscle. Whereas prefusion skeletal myoblasts contain principally nonmuscle isoactins, a dramatic change in isoactin expression occurs after fusion, with α-actin (the skeletal muscle type) becoming the only significant actin variant present in differentiated skeletal muscle.[43,44] Concurrent with these changes in actin expression, extensive changes in the structure and function (i.e., sarcomeres form and cells become contractile) of actin occur in these cells. Recent immunocytological studies by Pardo et al.,[45] demonstrating differential subcellular localization of muscle and nonmuscle actins in skeletal muscle cells, also support the idea that isoactins have specialized roles within the cell. However, all actins are similar in their primary structure,[38] physical properties,[45] and actin binding sites.[47] Therefore, the precise nature of purported functional differences between isoactins is unclear. Despite these uncertainties, measurements of changes in isoactin expression appear to be a very useful marker for studying cytodifferentiation of smooth muscle during development or culture.

III. CONTRACTILE PROTEIN EXPRESSION IN CULTURED VASCULAR SMOOTH MUSCLE CELLS

A. Actin Expression in Cultured Vascular Smooth Muscle Cells

Our laboratory has been engaged in developing a functional culture model for studying VSM contractile responsiveness in vitro. However, assessment of contractile responsiveness is difficult to measure quantitatively in cultured cells. Therefore, our research strategy is to study factors that promote cytodifferentiation in cultured smooth muscle cells, utilizing expression of the smooth muscle-specific forms of actin (i.e., α-SM and γ-SM isoactins) as a marker for differentiation in these cells. Changes in isoactin expression in relation to growth state were evaluated in both primary and subpassaged rat aortic smooth muscle cells obtained by enzyme dispersion techniques.[1,48] Isoactin expression was evaluated by (1) measurements of relative isoactin content and rates of synthesis (^{35}S-methionine incorporation) by densitometric evaluation[49] of two-dimensional isoelectric focusing (IEF)-sodium dodecyl sulfate (SDS) gels[50] and (2) by immunocytological examination of individual smooth muscle cells utilizing a smooth muscle-specific isoactin antibody (designated "CGA7"),[51] provided by Gown and Gordon (University of Washington, Seattle). These studies[6,7] yielded the following results:

1. Gel electrophoretic analysis showed no detectable decreases in α-smooth muscle isoactin content or myosin content (heavy chain) in primary cultures of VSM cells prior to the onset of cellular proliferation. In addition, cells identified as undergoing DNA synthesis by ^{3}H-thymidine autoradiography simultaneously stained with the smooth muscle-specific isoactin antibody. Thus, loss of smooth muscle-specific isoactins and myosin was not a prerequisite for initiation of cellular proliferation. Significant levels of α-SM actin were present at the onset of proliferation, although the fractional synthesis of this actin had virtually ceased (Figure 2).
2. Expression of smooth muscle-specific isoactins (synthesis and content) was drastically reduced in log phase growth cells and then increased in association with density-induced decreases in cellular growth rates as cells reached confluency (Figure 2). Conversely, β-NM actin synthesis and content were increased in rapidly dividing smooth muscle cells, but decreased in density-arrested cells. Significantly, these changes were observed in both primary and subpassaged VSM cultures.
3. There was a dramatic decrease (Figure 3a) in the relative synthesis of α-smooth muscle isoactin when saturation density cells were passaged and plated at low densities in serum-containing medium, which persisted until cells reached confluency (Figure 3d). However, this decrease could be almost totally prevented by plating cells in serum-free medium[52] (data not shown), plasma derived serum (Figure 3c),[53] or by plating cells in serum at a density exceeding saturation density (Figure 3b). If cells were initially plated at a sparse density in the presence of serum and then switched to serum-free conditions, only moderate increases in the relative synthesis of α-SM isoactin occurred within the first 24 hr.
4. Serum stimulation of cells that had been growth-arrested in either plasma-derived serum[53] or serum-free medium[52] resulted in a dramatic decrease in α-SM actin expression and an increase in β-NM expression that preceded the onset of cellular proliferation.[7]

These findings demonstrate that cultured VSM cells undergo differential expression of isoactins in relation to their growth state, and suggest that growth arrest of cells promotes cytodifferentiation in cultured VSM cells. Strauch and Rubenstein[5] reported similar findings in studies of BC_3H_1 cells, a smooth muscle-like cell line derived from a mouse brain tumor. Similarly, Franke et al.[3] demonstrated continued expression of the m-RNA for α-SM actin in an established smooth muscle cell line derived from the rat inferior vena cava. Larsen et al.[8] described continued myosin expression in primary and established cultures of rat mesenteric VSM cells. Thus, loss of cell-specific contractile proteins does not appear to be prerequisite for cellular proliferation in cultures of VSM cells. However, our studies[6,7] and those of Strauch and Rubenstein[5] do show that smooth muscle cells in both primary and subpassage undergo differential expression of isoactins in relation to their growth state. We want to emphasize that these results provide evidence that expression of cell-specific characteristics and cellular growth are coupled, rather than evidence that phenotypic modulation is a prerequisite for smooth muscle cell proliferation.

It is important to note that these studies also suggest that cell-cell contact has an important permissive effect on induction of α-SM actin synthesis. Strauch and Rubenstein[5] found that α-SM actin synthesis could be induced much sooner in BC_3H_1 cells by growth-arresting confluent cells by withdrawal of serum, but no changes were ob-

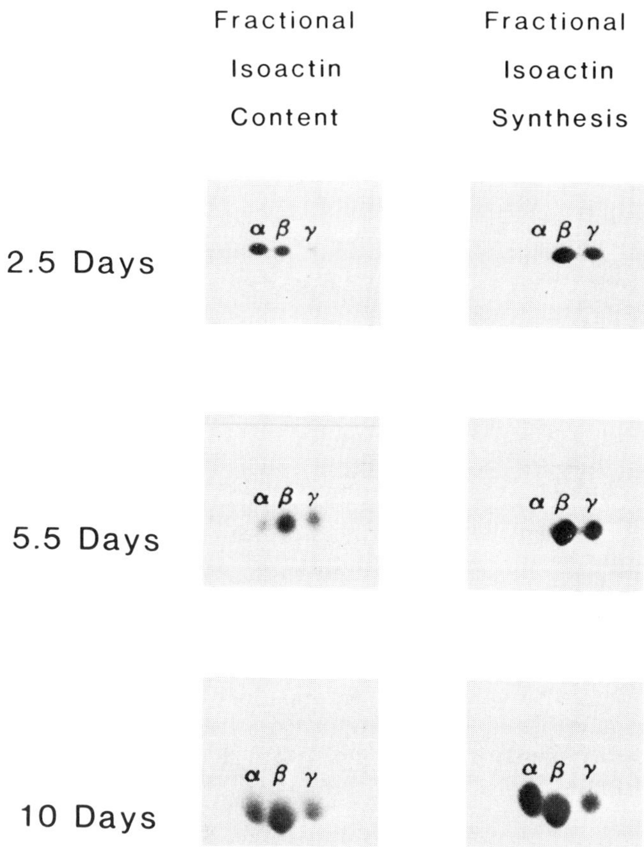

FIGURE 2. Two-dimensional isoelectric focusing — SDS gels showing the fractional content (silver-stained gel) and synthesis (^{35}S-methionine autoradiographs) of isoactins in rat aortic smooth muscle cells at 2.5 days, 5.5 days, and 10.0 days in primary culture. For measurements of isoactin synthesis, duplicate culture dishes were pulsed with ^{35}S-methionine (4 hr, 80 μCi/mℓ, 986 to 1103 Ci/mmol). Samples were harvested, pooled, solubilized, and isoactins resolved by two-dimensional gel electrophoresis.[50] Replicate dishes were pulsed with ^{3}H-thymidine (1 μCi/mℓ, 1 hr) for determination of the frequency of replicating cells (data not shown). At 2.5 days a large fraction of cells were labeled with ^{3}H-thymidine, and α-SM actin content was high, although α-SM actin synthesis was very low. Cells were undergoing logarithmic growth at 5.5 days, and both α-SM actin content and synthesis were extremely low. Cells were postconfluent at 10.0 days; growth rates had decreased dramatically, and both α-SM actin content and synthesis had increased substantially. α = α-SM actin; β = β-NM actin; γ = γ-SM + γ-NM actin. (Reproduced from *The Journal of Cell Biology*, 1986, Vol. 102, pp. 343-352 by copyright permission of the Rockefeller University Press.)

served if cells were serum-deprived when subconfluent. In our studies, induction of α-SM isoactin coincided with attainment of cell confluency, although maximal α-SM isoactin expression did not occur until cells were several days postconfluent. Whereas high levels of isoactin synthesis could be maintained in sparse cultures in serum-free medium or plasma-derived serum, we found that growth arrest of sparse density cells that were not already induced was not very effective in increasing α-SM actin expression unless serum withdrawal was for extended time periods. Furthermore, the fact that cells continue to express high levels of nonmuscle actins even when growth-ar-

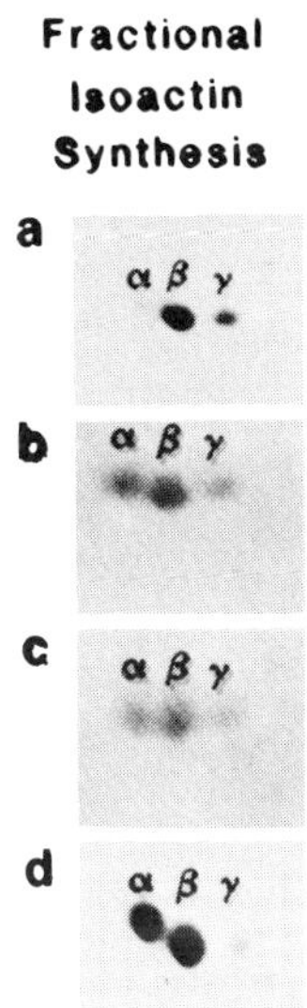

FIGURE 3. ^{35}S-methionine autoradiographs of two-dimensional IEF/SDS gels illustrating the effects of cellular growth state on the fractional synthesis (i.e., ^{35}S-methionine autoradiographs) of isoactins in subpassaged rat aortic smooth muscle cells. Cells at saturation density were harvested with a trypsin-EDTA solution and plated in the medium indicated. All cells other than those illustrated in (b) were plated at 10^4 per square centimeter. Replicate dishes of each group were pulsed for 1 hr with ^{3}H-thymidine for determination of the frequency of cells undergoing DNA replication (data not shown). (a) 2.5 days after plating in 10% fetal calf serum (FCS) (cells were growing logarithmically); (b) 2.5 days after plating in 10% FCS at a density (i.e., 5.0×10^5 cm^{-2}) exceeding saturation density for these cells (replication rates were <1%); (c) 2.5 days following plating in plasma-derived serum[53] (the frequency of replicating cells was <5%); (d) 10 days after plating in 10% FCS (cells were postconfluent, and the frequency of replicating cells was <2%). Note that the fractional synthesis of α-SM actin is markedly increased in growth-arrested cells (b to d) as compared to rapidly dividing cells (a). α = α-SM actin; β = β-NM actin; γ = γ-smooth muscle actin + γ-NM actin.

rested indicates that additional criteria other than cessation of an initiation of cellular proliferation must be important in inducing cytodifferentiation in these cells.

B. Myosin Expression in Cultured Smooth Muscle Cells

Using electron microscopy and a smooth muscle cell-specific myosin antibody,[37] Chamley-Campbell and co-workers[1,55] reported that VSM cells characteristically lose myosin prior to the onset of cellular proliferation and only variably regain it at confluency, depending on culture conditions and initial plating densities. However, SDS-polyacrylamide gel electrophoresis shows that smooth muscle myosin is present at all times in primary and passaged smooth muscle cell cultures (see Figure 1).[7,8] Larsen et al.[8] found changes in VSM myosin antigenic expression in culture, but presented convincing evidence that the changes reflected conformational alterations rather than synthesis of a new myosin variant. Recent studies by Rovner et al.[56] confirm the results of Owens et al.[7] and Larsen et al.[8] and appear to resolve the apparent discrepancies between the findings of these workers and those of Chamley-Campbell. Based on Western blot analysis, Rovner et al.[56] found that the antisera utilized by Chamley-Campbell et al.[1] is specific for smooth muscle myosin and does not stain myosin isolated from a variety of nonmuscle cells or tissues or from skeletal and cardiac muscles (Figure 1). In agreement with observations of Larsen et al.[8] and Owens et al.,[7] some form of myosin was present in cultured smooth muscle cells at all times by SDS-PAGE. However, the myosin antibody utilized by Chamley-Campbell did not react with the myosin derived from cultured VSM cells in Western blot experiments, but the antiplatelet myosin (APM) and antismooth muscle myosin (ASMM) (both provided by Larsen) did react (data not shown). Our interpretation of these results is that VSM cells synthesize a myosin in vitro that is distinct from the variant found in vivo, and that the conformational changes observed by Larsen et al.[8] are not necessarily related to this phenomenon. The studies of Rovner et al.[56] also demonstrated that the myosin heavy chain present in cultured cells consisted of a single molecular weight variant of approximately 205,000 daltons, while the myosin expressed in vivo appears to be a heterodimer consisting of two heavy chains of approximately 207,000 and 211,000 daltons.[31] The molecular weight of the myosin heavy chain derived from cultured VSM cells was identical to that found in several nonmuscle cells. Studies are in progress to determine under what conditions the in vivo myosin variants might be expressed in cultured VSM cells. It is interesting that Chamley-Campbell et al.[1,55] observed that cultured VSM cells characteristically lose smooth muscle-specific myosin staining at the onset of cell proliferation, but regain it at confluency if plated at a high initial density.[55] In contrast, neither cells plated at low densities nor subpassaged cells showed positive staining with this antibody under their culture conditions.

C. Contractile Responsiveness of Cultured Vascular Smooth Muscle Cells

Cultured VSM cells do not generally appear to be capable of force generation. However, there is now good evidence showing that several elements of excitation-contraction coupling are functional in cultured cells. Established cultures of rat mesenteric smooth muscle cells retain high affinity receptors to angiotensin II and undergo dose-dependent A-II-induced phosphorylation of the 20,000-dalton myosin light chain.[57] Furthermore, a variable but significant proportion of these cells contracted (reversible, agonist-specific cell shortening) in response to angiotensin II.[9] Martin and Gordon[10] observed changes in ^{86}Rb efflux in cultured rabbit aortic smooth muscle cells in response to stimulation with norepinephrine or histamine. In addition, Colucci et al.[12] recently demonstrated α_1-adrenergic receptor-coupled calcium flux in cultured smooth muscle cells derived from rabbit aorta. Thus, it appears that important steps in receptor activation-contraction coupling continue to be expressed in vitro.

Cultured VSM cells are, however, "phenotypically modulated"* according to many criteria.[1,2,58] For example, they have a decreased actin thin filament content, increased synthetic cellular organelles, and lack ultrastructurally demonstrable myosin-containing thick filaments, although cultured cells do have prominent cytoplasmic stress fibers. Consistent with the morphological data, cultured cells have a decreased absolute content of actin and myosin,[7,8] exhibit increased proliferative and biosynthetic activities,[1,48] and with few exceptions, do not appear to be capable of stress development. However, observations that subpassaged smooth muscle cells continue to express a number of cell-specific contractile proteins (e.g., smooth muscle-specific isoactins, myosin light chain kinase) and that cells continue to show a variety of characteristics indicative of contractile responsiveness, indicate that the concept of a "synthetic state" vs. "contractile state" is somewhat misleading and overly simplistic in describing the differentiated state of VSM cells in culture.**

* Chamley-Campbell et al.[1] have utilized the term "modulated" to refer to changes in phenotype from a predominantly contractile state to a predominantly synthetic state. This term is more appropriate than the often-used term "dedifferentiated", which is clearly incorrect since there is no evidence that VSM cells return to a multipotent state.

** While the usage of the terms "synthetic state" and "contractile state" are not technically incorrect, they imply absolute rather than relative changes in cell phenotype. The usage of these terms in the literature has often not been that originally intended by Chamley-Campbell et al.[1]

IV. FACTORS CONTROLLING VSM CELL CYTODIFFERENTIATION IN CULTURE

Our understanding of the factors influencing the expression of cytodifferentiated characteristics in cultured VSM cells is extremely limited. As noted previously, our studies[6,7] and those of Strauch and Rubenstein[5] demonstrated the importance of cell density and growth state in controlling expression of smooth muscle cell-specific isoactins. Furthermore, there is substantial evidence suggesting that other differentiated properties of smooth muscle cells are also promoted in association with growth arrest. Schubert et al.[59] demonstrated an increase in the specific activity of creatine phosphokinase and myokinase associated with increased cell density and the cessation of cell division in BC_3H_1 cells. Subsequently, Olson et al.[60] demonstrated that the induction of creatine phosphokinase in these cells occurred at the transcriptional level. Chamley-Campbell and Campbell[55] presented morphological evidence suggesting that the loss of contractile myofilaments in primary smooth muscle cell culture could be inhibited by plating cells at high density, by growth in medium containing heparin or by growth in co-culture with endothelium (see Chapter 4). Martin and Gordon[10] found that the responsiveness of primary cultures of rabbit aortic smooth muscle cells to agonist-induced changes in membrane conductance could be promoted with heparin. Observations with heparin and endothelium are relevant to this discussion, since Karnovsky and co-workers[61] reported that heparin inhibits smooth muscle cell proliferation in vivo and in vitro, and that endothelial cells produce a heparin-like inhibitor of smooth muscle cell growth (see Chapter 7). However, it is not clear from these cited studies whether the effects of heparin on smooth muscle cell differentiation were in fact related to growth inhibition. Furthermore, the nature of the endothelial-derived differentiation-promoting factor is unclear.

Chamley-Campbell et al.[1] presented evidence suggesting that "phenotypic modulation" in primary smooth muscle cell cultures can be delayed in sparse VSM cell cultures by factors produced by confluent smooth muscle cell cultures, by growth in the presence of sympathetic neurons or nerve extracts, and by growth in medium containing dibutyryl cyclic AMP or theophylline (see Chapter 17). However, these studies were based on morphological evaluations, and the relationship of morphologic changes to smooth muscle cell contractile responsiveness is uncertain. Nevertheless, these results are intriguing, and suggest a number of approaches that should be further examined using more definitive criteria for assessing the differentiated state of VSM cells. Our studies suggest that the expression of smooth muscle cell-specific isoactins and myosin heavy chains will be useful in this regard. However, we want to emphasize that it is important to obtain measures of contractile responsiveness as well.

V. SUMMARY AND CONCLUSIONS

VSM cells undergo marked changes in phenotype when grown in cell culture. However, cells continue to express a variety of cell-specific characteristics that distinguish them as smooth muscle cells. Whereas cultured cells appear to have a much greater synthetic capability than their in vivo counterparts, the concept of a "contractile" vs. a "synthetic" state fails to adequately describe the differentiated state of VSM cells in culture.

There is now good evidence that the expression of cytodifferentiated characteristics in cultured VSM cells is closely related to their growth state and can be promoted by modification of their growth medium. Furthermore, there are now a variety of definitive, quantitative markers of VSM cytodifferentiation that can be systematically applied to studies of VSM cytodifferentiation. In particular, we can now begin to explore the molecular controls of VSM differentiation in a manner similar to that done in skeletal muscle. These studies may result in more useful cultured smooth muscle cells for studying contractile function in vitro. More importantly, such studies will contribute substantially to our understanding of the interrelationship between growth and cytodifferentiation in VSM cells, which, at present, is a poorly understood area of smooth muscle cell biology.

REFERENCES

1. Chamley-Campbell, J., Campbell, G. R., and Ross, R., The smooth muscle cell in culture, *Physiol. Rev.*, 59, 1, 1979.
2. Thyberg, J., Palmberg, L., Nilsson, J., Ksiazek, T., and Sjolund, M., Phenotype modulation in primary cultures of arterial smooth muscle cells on the role of platelet-derived growth factor, *Differentiation*, 25, 156, 1983.
3. Franke, W. W., Schmid, E., Vandekerckhove, J., and Weber, K., A permanently proliferating rat vascular smooth muscle cell with maintained expression of smooth muscle characteristics, including actin of the vascular smooth muscle type, *J. Cell Biol.*, 87, 594, 1980.
4. Gabbiani, G., Kocher, O., Bloom, W. S., Vandekerckhove, J., and Weber, K., Actin expression in smooth muscle cells of rat aortic intimal thickening, human atheromatous plaque, and cultured rat aortic media, *J. Clin. Invest.*, 73, 148, 1984.
5. Strauch, A. R. and Rubenstein, P. A., Induction of vascular smooth muscle α-isoactin expression in BC_3H_1 cells, *J. Biol. Chem.*, 259, 3152, 1984.
6. Owens, G. K. and Thompson, M. M., Developmental changes in isoactin expression in rat aortic smooth muscle cells *in vivo:* relationship between growth and cytodifferentiation, *J. Biol. Chem.*, in press, 1986.
7. Owens, G. K., Gordon, D., Loeb, A., and Thompson, M., Expression of smooth muscle specific isoactins in cultured vascular smooth muscle cells: relationship between growth and cytodifferentiation, *J. Cell Biol.*, 102, 343, 1986.
8. Larsen, D. M., Fujiwara, K., Alexander, R. W., and Gimbrone, M. A., Myosin in cultured vascular smooth muscle cells: immunofluorescence and immunochemical studies of alterations in antigenic expression, *J. Cell Biol.*, 99, 1582, 1984.
9. Gunther, S., Alexander, W., Atkinson, W. J., and Gimbrone, M. A., Functional angiotensin II receptors in cultured vascular smooth muscle cells, *J. Cell Biol.*, 92, 289, 1982.
10. Martin, W. and Gordon, J. L., Spontaneous and agonist induced Rb efflux from rabbit aortic smooth muscle cells in culture: a comparison with fresh tissue, *J. Cell. Physiol.*, 115, 53, 1983.
11. Smith, J. B. and Brock, T. A., Analysis of angiotensin-stimulated sodium transport in cultured smooth muscle cells from rat aorta, *J. Cell. Physiol.*, 114, 284, 1983.
12. Colucci, W. S., Brock, T. A., Gimbrone, M. A., and Alexander, R. W., Regulation of $alpha_1$-adrenergic receptor coupled calcium flux in cultured vascular smooth muscle cells, *Hypertension*, 6, I19, 1984.
13. Hartshorne, D. J. and Gorecka, A., Biochemistry of the contractile proteins of smooth muscle, in *Handbook of Physiology, Section 2, The Cardiovascular System*, Vol. 2, *Vascular Smooth Muscle*, Bohr, D. F., Somlyo, A. P., and Sparks, H. V., Jr., Eds., American Physiological Society, Bethesda, Md., 1980, 93.
14. Murphy, R. A., Mechanics of vascular smooth muscle, in *Handbook of Physiology, Section 2, The Cardiovascular System, Vol. 2, Vascular Smooth Muscle*, Bohr, D. F., Somlyo, A. P., and Sparks, H. V., Jr., Eds., American Physiological Society, Bethesda, Md., 1980, 325.
15. Somlyo, A. V., Bond, M., Berner, P. F., Ashton, F. T., Holtzer, H., and Somlyo, A. P., The contractile apparatus of smooth muscle: an update, in *Smooth Muscle Contraction*, Stephens, N. L., Ed., Marcel Dekker, New York, 1984, 1.
16. Murphy, R. A., Aksoy, M. O., Cohen, D. M., Fatigati, V., and Gerthoffer, W. T., Contractile apparatus and functional diversity in vertebrate smooth muscle, in *Vascular Neuroeffector Mechanisms: 4th Int. Symp.*, Bevan, J. A., Maxwell, R. A., Shibata, S., Fujiwara, M., Mohri, K., and Toda, N., Eds., Raven Press, New York, 1983, 37.
17. Dillon, P. F. and Murphy, R. A., High force development and crossbridge attachment in smooth muscle from swine carotid arteries, *Circ. Res.*, 50, 799, 1982.
18. Gabella, G., The force generated by a visceral smooth muscle, *J. Physiol. (London)*, 263, 199, 1976.

19. Barany, M., ATPase activity of myosin correlated with speed of muscle shortening, *J. Gen. Physiol.*, 50, 197, 1967.
20. Weisbrodt, N. W. and Murphy, R. A., Myosin phosphorylation and contraction of feline esophageal smooth muscle, *Am. J. Physiol.*, in press, 1985.
21. Kamm, K. E. and Stull, J. T., Myosin phosphorylation, force and V_0 in neurally stimulated tracheal smooth muscle, *Am. J. Physiol.*, in press, 1985.
22. Murphy, R. A., Gerthoffer, W. T., Trevethick, M. A., and Singer, H. A., Ca^{2+}-Dependent regulatory mechanisms in smooth muscle, in *Vasodilator Mechanisms*, Vanhoutte, P. M. and Vatner, S. F., Eds., S. Karger, Basel, 1984, 99.
23. Aksoy, M. O., Mras, S., Kamm, K. E., and Murphy, R. A., Ca^{2+}, cAMP, and changes in myosin phosphorylation during contraction of smooth muscle, *Am. J. Physiol.*, 245(14), C255, 1983.
24. Chatterjee, M. and Murphy, R. A., Calcium-dependent stress maintenance without myosin phosphorylation in skinned smooth muscle, *Science*, 221, 464, 1983.
25. Siegman, M. J., Butler, T. M., Mooers, S. U., and Davies, R. E., Calcium-dependent resistance to stretch and stress relaxation in resting smooth muscles, *Am. J. Physiol.*, 231, 1501, 1976.
26. Morgan, J. P. and Morgan, K. G., Calcium and cardiovascular function. Intracellular calcium levels during contraction and relaxation of mammalian cardiac and vascular smooth muscle as detected with aequorin, *Am. J. Med.*, 77, 33, 1984.
27. Gerthoffer, W. T. and Murphy, R. A., Ca^{2+}, myosin phosphorylation, and relaxation of arterial smooth muscle, *Am. J. Physiol.*, 245(14), C271, 1983.
28. Takano-Ohmuro, H., Obinata, T., Mikawa, T., and Masaki, T., Changes in myosin isoenzymes during development of chicken gizzard muscle, *J. Biochem. (Tokyo)*, 93, 903, 1983.
29. Burridge, K. and Bray, D., Purification and structural analysis of myosin from brain and other non-muscle tissues, *J. Mol. Biol.*, 99, 1, 1975.
30. Seidel, C. L., White, V., and Schildmeyer, L., Intervessel differences in smooth muscle myosin heavy chains, *Physiologist*, 26, A-12, 1983.
31. Rovner, A. S., Thompson, M. M., and Murphy, R. A., Detection of myosin heavy chain variants in smooth muscle by SDS polyacrylamide gel electrophoresis, *Fed. Proc.*, 43, 427, 1984.
32. Groschel-Stewart, U., Comparative studies of human smooth and striated muscle myosins, *Biochim. Biophys. Acta*, 229, 322, 1971.
33. Groschel-Stewart, U., Chamley, J. H., Campbell, G. R., and Burnstock, G., Changes in myosin distribution in dedifferentiating and redifferentiating smooth muscle cells in tissue culture, *Cell Tissue Res.*, 165, 13, 1975.
34. Larsen, D. M., Fujiwara, K., Alexander, R. W., and Gimbrone, M. A., Jr., Heterogeneity of myosin antigenic expression in vascular smooth muscle in vivo, *Lab. Invest.*, 50, 401, 1984.
35. Burridge, K., A comparison of fibroblast and smooth muscle myosins, *FEBS Lett.*, 45, 14, 1974.
36. Towbin, H., Staehelin, T., and Gordon, J., Electrophoretic transfer of proteins from polyacrylamide gels to nitrocellulose sheets: procedure and some applications, *Proc. Natl. Acad. Sci. U.S.A.*, 76, 4350, 1979.
37. Groschel-Stewart, U., Schreiber, J., Mahlmeister, C., and Weber, K., Production of specific antibodies to contractile proteins, and their use in immunofluorescence microscopy. I. Antibodies to smooth and striated chicken muscle myosins, *Histochemie*, 46, 229, 1976.
38. Vandekerckhove, J. and Weber, K., The complete amino acid sequence of actins from bovine aorta, bovine heart, bovine fast skeletal muscle, and rabbit slow skeletal muscle, *Differentiation*, 14, 123, 1979.
39. Fatigati, V. and Murphy, R. A., Actin and tropomyosin variants in smooth muscles. Dependence on tissue type, *J. Biol. Chem.*, 259, 14383, 1984.
40. Vandekerckhove, J. and Weber, K., At least six different actins are expressed in a higher mammal: an analysis based on the amino acid sequence of the amino-terminal tryptic peptide, *J. Mol. Biol.*, 126, 783, 1978.
41. Gabbiani, G., Schmid, E., Winter, S., Chaponnier, C., DeChastonay, C., Vandekerckhove, J., Weber, K., and Franke, W. W., Vascular smooth muscle cells differ from other smooth muscle cells: predominance of vimentin filaments and a specific α-type actin, *Proc. Natl. Acad. Sci. U.S.A.*, 78, 298, 1981.
42. Saborio, J. L., Segura, M., Flores, M., Garcia, R., and Palmer, E., Differential expression of gizzard actin genes during chick embryogenesis, *J. Biol. Chem.*, 254, 11119, 1979.
43. Devlin, R. B. and Emerson, C. P., Jr., Coordinate regulation of contractile protein synthesis during myoblast differentiation, *Cell*, 13, 599, 1978.
44. Bulinski, J. C., Kumar, S., Titani, K., and Hauschka, S. D., Peptide antibody specific for the amino terminus of skeletal muscle α-actin, *Proc. Natl. Acad. Sci. U.S.A.*, 50, 1506, 1983.
45. Pardo, J. V., Pittenger, M. F., and Craig, S. W., Subcellular sorting of isoactins: selective association of γ-actin with skeletal muscle mitochondria, *Cell*, 32, 1093, 1983.

46. Pollard, T. D., Cytoplasmic contractile proteins, *J. Cell Biol.*, 91, 1565, 1981.
47. McKenna, N., Meigs, J. B., and Wang, Y. L., Identical distribution of fluorescently labeled brain and muscle actins in living cardiac fibroblasts and myocytes, *J. Cell Biol.*, 100, 292, 1985.
48. Chamley-Campbell, J. H., Campbell, G. R., and Ross, R., Phenotype-dependent response of cultured aortic smooth muscle to serum mitogens, *J. Cell Biol.*, 89, 379, 1981.
49. Garrison, J. C. and Johnson, M. L., A simplified method for computer analysis of autoradiograms from two-dimensional gels, *J. Biol. Chem.*, 257, 13144, 1982.
50. O'Farrell, P. H., High resolution two-dimensional electrophoresis of proteins, *J. Biol. Chem.*, 250, 4007, 1975.
51. Gown, A. M., Vogel, A. M., Gordon, D., and Lu, P. L., A smooth muscle cell specific monoclonal antibody that recognizes smooth muscle actin isozymes, *J. Cell Biol.*, in press, 1985.
52. Libby, P. and O'Brien, K. V., Culture of quiescent arterial smooth muscle cells in a defined serum-free medium, *J. Cell. Physiol.*, 115, 217, 1983.
53. Ross, R., Nist, C., Kariya, B., Rivest, M. J., Raines, E., and Callis, J., Physiological quiescence in plasma-derived serum: influence of platelet-derived growth factor on cell growth in culture, *J. Cell. Physiol.*, 97, 497, 1978.
54. Baserga, R., *Multiplication and Division in Mammalian Cells*, Marcel Dekker, New York, 1976.
55. Chamley-Campbell, J. H. and Campbell, G. R., What controls smooth muscle phenotype? *Atherosclerosis*, 40, 347, 1981.
56. Rovner, A. S., Murphy, R. A., and Owens, G. K., Expression of smooth muscle and nonmuscle myosin heavy chains in cultured vascular smooth muscle cells, *J. Biol. Chem.* 1986, in press.
57. Anderson, J. M., Gimbrone, M. A., Jr., and Alexander, R. W., Angiotensin II stimulates phosphorylation of the myosin light chain in cultured vascular smooth muscle cells, *J. Biol. Chem.*, 256, 4693, 1981.
58. Yau-Young, A. O., Shio, H., and Fowler, S., Growth, biochemistry, and morphology of isolated rabbit aortic smooth muscle cells maintained in the presence or absence of serum, *J. Cell. Physiol.*, 108, 461, 1981.
59. Schubert, D., Harris, A. J., Devine, C. E., and Heinemann, S., Characterization of a unique muscle cell line, *J. Cell Biol.*, 61, 398, 1974.
60. Olson, E. N., Caldwell, K. L., Gordon, J. I., and Glaser, L., Regulation of creatine phosphokinase expression during differentiation of BC_3H_1 cells, *J. Biol. Chem.*, 258, 2644, 1983.
61. Karnovsky, M. J., Endothelial-vascular smooth muscle cell interactions, *Am. J. Pathol.*, 105, 200, 1981.

Chapter 6

GROWTH FACTORS FOR VASCULAR SMOOTH MUSCLE CELLS

Daniel F. Bowen-Pope, Mark W. Majesky, and Russell Ross

TABLE OF CONTENTS

I. INTRODUCTION

The size, elasticity, and strength of the large arteries is largely determined by the smooth muscle cells (SMC) of the tunica media and by the macromolecules (especially collagen and elastin) synthesized and deposited by these cells. Weakness of, or damage to, this layer can result in the formation of aneurysms or hemorrhages. Conversely, excessive growth of SMC in the tunica intima can impede the flow of blood, as in atherosclerosis[1,2] and hypertension.[3] How is the architecture and mass of the vessel wall regulated? This chapter will discuss some of the information which has been gained from studying vascular SMC in culture. The information should be evaluated with the following considerations in mind.

A. The In Vivo vs. Cell Culture Environments

The environment of an SMC in culture may be very different from that of an SMC in vivo. Some of these differences may affect the way an SMC would respond to a given stimulus. The culture environment itself can vary tremendously between different experimental protocols. Certain protocols may predispose the cells to respond to specific variables. When stimulation of cell proliferation is studied, a low basal (control) rate of proliferation must first be established. This has been variously accomplished by allowing the cultures to proliferate until growth is slowed by some combination of cell density and growth factor limitations, by reducing the concentrations of serum added to the nutrient medium, or by replacing the whole blood serum with plasma-derived serum or by a defined mixture of supplementary nutrients and factors. Each different protocol could predispose the test cells to respond to a different "growth factor". For example, single amino acids can become growth stimulatory when assayed using SMC cultured in medium depleted specifically of that amino acid. Studies using cultured cells can thus indicate which factors *could* stimulate SMC proliferation, but do not in themselves indicate that changes in levels of these factors occur, or are important, in vivo. Indeed, none of the factors studied using cultured SMC have yet been unambiguously demonstrated to function as growth factors for SMC in vivo. As an aid to evaluating the significance of results obtained with different putative growth factors in culture, we will briefly describe the specific culture system used to obtain the result and will mention the arguments adduced for a physiological role for the factor.

B. Phenotypic Modulation and Heterogeneity

The properties of SMC in culture may differ considerably from those displayed by their in-vivo progenitors. Such differences could arise through phenotypic "modulation" and/or through selection of subpopulations. SMC in the arteries of normal adults (and during the first days in culture) are characteristically well filled with thick and thin myofilaments and dense bodies and contain a poorly developed Golgi apparatus and rough endoplasmic reticulum.[4-6] When SMC are isolated from the tunica media by enzymatic digestion and put into culture, they lose most of their observable myofilaments and develop an extensive Golgi and rough endoplasmic reticulum.[4,7] This process will be discussed extensively in other chapters of this book (see Chapters 4 and 13). Observations in several systems suggest that these morphological changes are accompanied by changes in responsiveness to mitogens. Jarmolych et al.[5] and Fritz et al.[6] observed that during the first 2 days after explanting, very few (0 and 0.4%) of the SMC in explants of pig and rabbit thoracic aortas incorporated ^{3}H-thymidine during a 2-hr labeling period. During the next 2 days, increasing numbers of labeled cells (11% on day 4) were observed. During the same period, many of the cells were undergoing the morphological changes described above, and electron microscope autoradiography indicated that *only* modulated (synthetic phenotype) cells incorporated ^{3}H-thymidine.[6] A comparable phenomenon has been observed using enzymatically isolated SMC. The percentage of pig and monkey SMC incorporating ^{3}H-thymidine increases rapidly at about 7 days after plating.[4] This correlates with the appearance of cells with a well-developed synthetic phenotype. Enzymatically isolated rat SMC undergo a similar modulation at 2 to 4 days after isolation.[7] Only cells in the synthetic phenotype were observed by electron microscopic autoradiography to be incorporating ^{3}H-thymidine.

Chamley-Campbell et al.[4] reported conditions under which enzymatically isolated SMC could be kept in the contractile phenotype. However, the culture procedures routinely used by virtually all investigators yield cells in the synthetic phenotype, and the observations reported in this chapter may be applicable only to SMC with this phenotype. If the "synthetic phenotype" was expressed only in the tissue culture environment, this could compromise the utility of studying SMC in culture. There is reason to speculate, however, that transitions between contractile and synthetic phenotypes occur in vivo as well. SMC in the aortas of immature rats[8-10] and after experimental injury[11] have been described as having the morphological characteristics of the synthetic phenotype. Explants cultured from rabbit[12] and rat[13] aortas, which were injured by balloon catheter deendothelialization 4 to 7 days before sacrifice, showed more rapid outgrowth of cells, possibly as a result of prior modulation to the synthetic phenotype. It seems possible that proliferation of SMC in vivo, as well as in culture, is controlled at two levels: (1) by a transition into (or out of) a mitogenically competent synthetic phenotype and (2) by the presence (or absence) of "growth factors" active on the synthetic phenotype cells. Each level of control may be exerted by a different set of factors. Thus, the growth factors in platelets, which are so active on synthetic phenotype SMC, do not seem to influence the transition of pig and monkey SMC from contractile to synthetic phenotype.[14] Thyberg et al.,[7] however, reported that modulation of rat SMC is more rapid in whole blood serum (WBS) than in plasma-derived serum (PDS) and that treatment of WBS with antibodies against the platelet-derived growth factor (PDGF) delays modulation.

A second consideration which complicates analysis of SMC responses both in vivo and in culture is the possibility that the cells in the tunica media are phenotypically heterogeneous. The tunica media of the large arteries of many species is usually considered to consist entirely of a single cell type so that cells obtained from this source are all considered to be SMC.[15] However, in some species the tunica media contains more than one morphologically[16] or histochemically[17] distinguishable cell type. If subsets of SMC with different growth properties existed within the artery wall, this would cause problems for cell culture analysis of growth in cell culture. On one hand, the cells studied in culture could represent a subset of the SMC in the vessel wall that have been selected for their ability to proliferate well in culture. The information obtained in culture would then be applicable to only a subset of the SMC in the vessel wall. On the other hand, if one subtype is *not* preferentially obtained in culture, then analysis of response of cultured cells to growth factors will be complicated by the possibility that the different growth factors are stimulating different subpopulations. This particularly complicates analysis of the effects of simultaneous addition of more than one factor, since each factor could be acting on either the same or different subtypes. The cloning of SMC offers a possible approach toward investigating the possibility, and consequences, of cell heterogeneity in the vessel wall.

C. Use of the Term "Growth"

The final caveat is that the term "growth" in "growth factor" will be considered here to include all processes which would contribute toward an increase in the mass of cells in the tunica media. As measured in cell culture, these processes include an increase in the number of cells synthesizing DNA (determined by ^{3}H-thymidine incorporation and flow microfluorometry), an increase in the number of cells, an increase in the amount of protein or DNA per culture, or an increase in colony size. These processes are not necessarily equivalent mechanistically; e.g., an increased rate of entry of cells into the DNA synthetic phase of the cell cycle would not lead to an increase in cell number if karyokinesis did not occur (Owens et al.[3] have shown that vascular SMC can become polyploid) or if cell survival declined. Conversely, a change in cell survival could lead to a change in cell number even if the rate of entry into S was not affected.

II. GROWTH FACTORS IN BLOOD

A. Analysis of Blood Constituents

Whole blood serum (WBS usually ambiguously referred to simply as "serum") is the archetypal "growth factor" for most cultured mesenchymal cells, including vascular SMC. It has been used to supplement nutrient medium since the earliest days of cell culture. It was well recognized that the serum could be supplying "growth factors", as well as the essential nutrients and vitamins that were not included in the chemically defined portion of culture medium. The problem was to determine the identity of these factors. Two approaches have been especially fruitful:

1. Serum has been obtained from animals in different nutritional, hormonal, or metabolic states and tested for differential ability to stimulate the test cells. If a difference is found, knowledge about the state of the animals is then used to suggest a candidate for the key variable from among the spectrum of factors known to be present in serum. Ideally, this choice is confirmed by verifying that specific neutralization of the factor eliminates the difference and that specific addition of the factor reproduces the difference. This approach is obviously particularly well suited to evaluate the role of already well-characterized growth factors (e.g., insulin — see later).
2. A second approach has been to start with serum from normal animals and attempt to isolate the active components by biochemical techniques, using growth-promoting activity as an assay to identify the active fractions. This approach is necessary for characterizing growth factors that have not been previously identified or purified and has resulted in the discovery of several new factors (e.g., Somatomedin, PDGF). One specific form of analysis of blood into components has both biochemical utility and physiological significance — the division into plasma and cell-derived constituents.

B. Growth Factors in Platelets

1. Plasma-Derived Serum vs. Whole Blood Serum

Although blood derivatives have long been used to supplement nutrient medium, whole blood is very rarely, if ever, used. The relationships between some of the commonly used blood derivatives are diagramed in Figure 1. Carrell and Burrows[18] placed tissue explants in plasma, which rapidly coagulated around the tissue and provided a semisolid environment into which cells migrated and proliferated. Current cell culture techniques are hindered by the presence of the clot, so the coagulation cascade is activated in vitro prior to exposure of the plasma to cells, and only the supernatant "serum" is used. If the cellular elements of blood are removed (usually by centrifugation) before coagulation, the fluid is designated "plasma-derived serum" (PDS). If not, it is properly designated "whole blood serum" (WBS) but is usually referred to

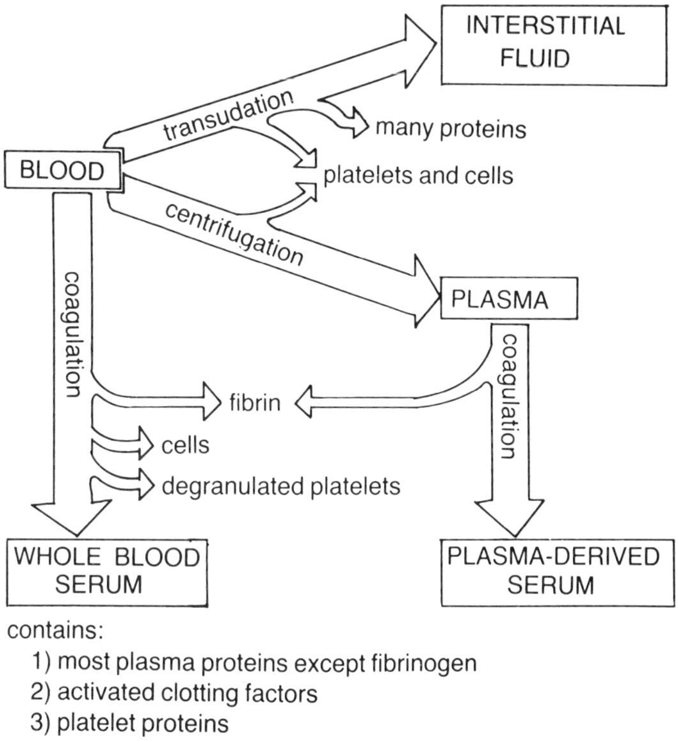

FIGURE 1. Derivation of different fluids from blood. (From Bowen-Pope, D. F., in *The Cell Surface in Development and Cancer,* Browder, L., Ed., Plenum Press, New York, in press. With permission.)

simply as "serum". As will be described below for SMC, WBS was found to support more rapid cell proliferation than did PDS.[19-21] This difference was found to be due to the release of platelet components into serum as a consequence of the activation of platelet degranulation during coagulation.[20-23] Several growth factors are now known to be released from platelets: PDGF, type-beta transforming growth factor (β-TGF), and a factor related to epidermal growth factor (EGF). The effects of individual factors on SMC growth will be described later. Although such studies provide more information as to which platelet factors might be capable of stimulating SMC, and to what extent, the use of WBS is still informative. Since WBS contains plasma and all of the platelet growth factors in the proportions in which they are released from platelets, it may provide the closest available approximation to the mixture of the growth factors to which SMC are actually exposed in vivo at sites of vascular injury.

The greater potency of WBS than of PDS in stimulating SMC growth has been demonstrated for SMC from many species using both homologous and heterologous sera. Ross et al.,[21] Rutherford and Ross,[24] and Burke and Ross[25] showed that monkey (*Macaca nemestrina*) thoracic SMC responded to 5% monkey WBS with greater rates of proliferation and percent labeled nuclei, and that the potency of PDS could be increased to that of WBS by adding material released by platelets in response to thrombin.[21] Similar reports of differential response to homologous PDS and WBS have been made for human arterial SMC[21,26,27] and rabbit thoracic SMC.[28] PDS and WBS retain their differential stimulatory capacity when tested on heterologous SMC, e.g., human sera tested on rat aortic SMC[7,29] or monkey aortic SMC.[30]

Although this chapter focuses on growth factors, the relative lack of potency of PDS as a growth factor is equally important for understanding growth control. SMC in the artery wall of normal adult animals are healthy but not rapidly proliferating.[31] These cells are exposed to the subset of blood components ("interstitial fluid") which pass through the vascular endothelium. As is diagramed in Figure 1, interstitial fluid differs from both PDS and WBS in that it does not contain activated clotting factors. It shares with PDS the absence of growth factors from platelets. Given the relative ease with which PDS can be prepared (e.g., see Ross et al.[21]), it has been proposed as a useful substitute for interstitial fluid in bringing SMC into a state of healthy quiescence in culture.[30] In some cases, PDS has been further processed by incubation with carboxymethyl sephadex to remove cationic factors, including any PDGF which might have been released from the platelets before their removal.[30,32] Now that specific assays for PDGF are available, it has been found[33-35] that carefully prepared PDS does not contain detectable PDGF. Since treatment with carboxymethyl sephadex removes many cationic proteins from serum and the accompanying dialysis and ultrafiltration steps can cause loss of soluble nutrients, this procedure is no longer routinely performed. As an alternative to the use of PDS, Libby and O'Brien[36] have developed a chemically defined culture medium which maintains bovine arterial SMC in a stable quiescent state (stable DNA content per culture). This medium is based on a 1:1 mixture of Dulbecco's modified Eagle's medium and Ham's medium F-12 supplemented with 10^{-6} M insulin, 5 μg/mℓ transferrin, and 0.2 mM ascorbate.

Use of chemically defined and complex (e.g., PDS) supplements can each contribute toward an analysis of SMC response to different growth factors. Use of a simple defined medium might not permit cells to respond to certain factors since required "cofactors" which may normally be present in blood or in interstitial fluid are not present. A striking example of this which has been observed using fibroblastoid cells, but not yet using SMC, is the synergism between PDGF, EGF, and β-TGF in stimulating the proliferation of cells suspended in soft agar (see later). Alone, none of these factors stimulates efficient growth in suspension. In combination, they are very potent.[37,38] The original observations of soft agar growth-promoting activity were possible because the assay was performed in nutrient medium supplemented with subthreshold concentrations of WBS that contributed the necessary cofactors.[39,40] Now that the synergism between these three factors has been recognized, the mechanism(s) of their interactions can be investigated using defined medium without serum. In general, it seems that chemically defined medium may be very useful for studying mechanisms, but that it is susceptible to generating both false negatives (due to absence of a "cofactor" present in vivo) and false positives (due to presence of a factor not present in blood or present at much lower concentrations) when used to investigate which factors may actually function in vivo.

2. Platelet-Derived Growth Factor

The original observations of the differences between PDS and WBS in stimulating proliferation of cultured chicken embryo cells,[19] monkey SMC,[21] mouse "fibroblastoid" 3T3 cells,[20] and a glial cell line[22] and the observation that the difference could be accounted for by growth factors released from platelets[20-22] led eventually to the purification from human platelets[41,42] and from human platelet-rich plasma[43,44] of a mitogenic 30,000-dalton, polypeptide factor designated PDGF. The fact that four laboratories, using different growth assays and biochemical procedures, independently purified a single growth factor from human blood by-products is consistent with the proposal that PDGF is one of the major growth-promoting factors in human blood. The amount of PDGF in human WBS has now been determined by specific radioreceptor assay (15 ng/mℓ,[33] 17.5 ng/mℓ[34]) and by radioimmunoassay (50 ng/mℓ,[45] 50 ng/mℓ,[34] 15.5 ng/mℓ[46]). Since the ED_{50} for stimulation of thymidine incorporation by several connective tissue cell types, including SMC, is about 1 to 3 × 10^{-11} M (0.3 to 1 ng/mℓ[47] and see later), the PDGF content of 5 to 10% human WBS would make a very substantial contribution to the growth-promoting activity of WBS. The preparation of monospecific antisera against human PDGF has allowed the relative contribution of PDGF to the total mitogenicity of human WBS to be determined by specific neutralization. Our own (unpublished) studies and those of Heldin et al.[48] indicate that PDGF accounts for approximately 50% of the stimulatory activity of human WBS for 3T3 and glial cells, respectively. Nilsson et al.[49] confirmed that antiserum against PDGF removed a majority of the ability of human WBS to stimulate proliferation of aortic SMC from 5-day-old rats, but reported that this was not true for adult SMC.

PDGF-like molecules have been found by radioreceptor assay in WBS obtained from all chordates tested,[33] but the concentration of PDGF present can vary considerably from species to species. In our own studies, we have found that mouse WBS also contains high levels of PDGF (≃10 ng/mℓ) but that baboon WBS contains only 2.7 ng/mℓ,[35] and commercial calf serum contains even less (≃0.75 ng/mℓ, our unpublished data). Since the growth-promoting capacity of human and calf WBS are comparable, it would seem that PDGF contributes less to the growth-promoting activity of calf serum than it does to that of human WBS. The relative paucity of PDGF in calf serum could help to explain why PDGF was not obtained in the early attempts to fractionate serum (bovine) into its mitogenically active components (reviewed by Temin et al.[50]).

Purified PDGF has been shown to stimulate the growth of many mesenchymal cell types, including vascular SMC from several species. Incorporation of ^{3}H-thymidine by monkey (*Macaca nemestrina*) and human arterial SMC is stimulated with an ED_{50} of approximately 10^{-11} *M*.[47] Mitogenic response was paralleled by specific high-affinity binding of ^{125}I-PDGF.[47] Parallel stimulation of ^{3}H-thymidine incorporation and specific binding of ^{125}I-PDGF were also reported for bovine aortic SMC,[51] in that case with a somewhat higher ED_{50}. PDGF stimulates proliferation and increases ^{3}H-thymidine labeling indices of adult rat aortic SMC in a base of 0.5 to 1% fetal bovine serum[52] and in serum-free medium.[49,53] The latter authors speculate that previous reports of the need for plasma components for stimulation of certain cell types by PDGF may have resulted from the use of nutritionally inadequate basal medium (i.e., DMEM rather than MCDB 104). Alternatively, the cultured rat SMC could themselves be synthesizing the key factors normally provided by plasma (see Atkinson et al.[54] and Clemmons[55] for evidence that cultured fibroblasts synthesize Somatomedin C). The stimulation of rat SMC by PDGF was inhibited by prostaglandin PGE_1 at 10 ng/mℓ and by PGF_2 and PGD_2 at higher concentrations,[53] confirming previous observations that these prostaglandins inhibited ^{3}H-thymidine incorporation by rabbit aortic SMC cultured in 10% fetal bovine serum[56] and reduced the cloning efficiency of guinea pig aortic SMC in 10% fetal bovine serum.[57] Thyberg et al.[7] found that adult rat aortic SMCs respond to the anionic growth factors in human platelets as well as to PDGF so that the effects of WBS on SMC growth should not all be attributed to PDGF.

The responsiveness of cells to PDGF seems to be mediated through expression of cell-surface receptors for PDGF[47,51,58,59] (reviewed in Bowen-Pope et al.[60]). PDGF receptors have been measured on SMC from human aorta,[47] monkey aorta,[47,61] porcine aorta,[58] rat aorta,[62] and bovine aorta.[51,60,63] PDS contains a high-molecular-weight proteins(s) which prevents binding of PDGF to this cell-surface receptor.[34,35,64,65] We calculate that if a small amount of PDGF was released into plasma, about 75% of this would be present as an inactive complex with the binding protein. The biological effects of complex formation in culture or in vivo are still speculative. In culture, the combination of very high affinity receptors and very low working concentrations of PDGF contributes toward a situation in which the added PDGF can be depleted during the course of a mitogenesis experiment. By preventing the cultures from squandering their PDGF during the first few hours, the binding protein could increase the mitogenic efficacy of PDGF. In vivo, a similar situation could exist or, alternatively, the binding protein could function entirely as a negative mediator by inactivating PDGF, which doesn't very quickly bind to PDGF receptors and/or by affecting the way PDGF is cleared from the plasma compartment by degradation systems.[35]

3. Epidermal Growth Factor

Despite its name, EGF is a potent mitogen for many connective tissue cell types, including SMC (reviewed in Adamson and Rees[66]). EGF was first discovered because of its presence in huge quantities within the mouse salivary glands.[67] Although EGF is now one of the best characterized growth factors and has served as a model for many of the biochemical and cell biological studies performed with PDGF, its source and physiological roles in humans are far from clear. It is not, for example, present in high concentrations in the human salivary gland. Even in the mouse, the relationship between the high concentrations in salivary glands and the concentrations seen in other tissues is far from clear, since surgical removal of the salivary gland does not alter levels of EGF in other tissues or in blood.[68] While investigating interactions between the receptors for PDGF and for EGF, we made measurements of EGF levels in blood, distinguishing what was in platelets from what was in plasma. We found that all EGF detectable in blood appeared to be present within the platelets.[69] Oka and Orth[70] made a similar observation and concluded that platelets are the major repository of EGF in man. It is likely that EGF-like molecules constitute some of the anionic growth factor activity found in WBS.

EGF can stimulate growth of SMC under certain conditions. At 100 ng/mℓ, EGF increases the apparent saturation density of adult bovine aortic SMC in a base of either 2.5% PDS or 2.5% WBS.[71] In serum-free medium supplemented with 250 μg/mℓ of high-density lipoprotein (HDL), EGF stimulates proliferation with an ED_{50} of 5 ng/mℓ and an optimum at 50 ng/mℓ.[72] ^{3}H-thymidine incorporation by confluent cultures of calf aortic SMC is increased tenfold by the addition of 10 ng/mℓ EGF to serum-free medium.[73] Rat abdominal aortic SMCs in a base of 0.5 to 1% FBS were reported to show increased proliferation in response to 10 ng/mℓ EGF only if partially purified Somatomedin A (10 μg/mℓ) was also added.[52]

4. Class β-Transforming Growth Factor

Transforming growth factors (TGF) are operationally defined as substances which promote the growth in suspension of cultured cells that otherwise require attachment to a substratum.[74] Ability to grow in soft agar is one of the characteristics of oncogenically transformed cells which most reliably distinguishes them from their nontransformed counterparts.[75] Class α-TGF were first found to be secreted by cultured transformed cells. These TGF resemble EGF in that they bind to the EGF receptor[76] and are related to EGF in amino acid sequence.[77] Class β-TGF do not bind to the EGF receptor and depend on the presence of EGF in order to display optimal ability to promote growth in soft agar.[37] Surprisingly, the normal tissue richest in class β-TGF seems to be the blood platelets.[39,40] Assoian et al.[38] have provided evidence that the β-TGF in platelets may be strongly supported in its activity by EGF and PDGF together, so that a platelet contains a complete set of three growth factors needed to support optimal growth in soft agar: PDGF, EGF, β-TGF.

To date, β-TGF has been studied almost exclusively using cultured cell lines. Nevertheless, β-TGF receptors seem to be expressed by almost every cell type and may play a role in regulating SMC growth in vivo. The environment of a smooth muscle cell in a damaged artery, and possibly in a normal artery as well, is not identical to that of an attached cell in monolayer culture and may share some characteristics with suspension in soft agar. A "transforming growth factor" would then be necessary to promote optimal cell proliferation. The name "transforming growth factor" should probably be viewed as reflecting the historical circumstances of its initial discovery rather than as implying a unique involvement in oncogenic transformation. This possibility is supported by the fact that β-TGF is encoded by a cellular gene. It thus seems that oncogenic transformation can activate cellular genes encoding for growth factors related to three of the growth factors found in platelets: PDGF (e.g., Bowen-Pope et al.[78]), EGF (e.g., Todaro et al.[76]), and β-TGF,[79] thereby, presumably, making the tumor cells independent of exogenous mitogens.

5. Platelet Factors In Vivo

Since most of the experimental work with the above-mentioned platelet factors has been done in culture, the exact role(s) of these factors in vivo has not been established. Nevertheless, several pieces of evidence favor the hypothesis that factors released from platelets stimulate the proliferation of connective tissue cells at sites of tissue damage:

1. Growth factors from platelets have been localized to the α-granules by studying platelets from patients with α-granule-specific defects,[80] by fractionating subcellular organelles[23] and by studying the differential release of granule components by different platelet-activating agents.[26] Release of granule proteins from the platelet is exquisitely sensitive to environmental stimuli, including contact with exposed subendothelial connective tissue.[81,82] This provides a mechanism for the topical application of growth factors to sites at which a proliferative response would be useful. Delivery of platelet factors in this fashion has been confirmed by Goldberg et al.,[83] who reported that large amounts of PF4, another α-granule protein, have penetrated into the vessel wall within 10 min after balloon catheter injury.
2. Inhibition of platelet function reduces the proliferative response of SMC to experimental injury, presumably by preventing the local release of growth factors.[84-87]

C. Growth Factors in Plasma

1. Insulin and Insulin-like Growth Factors

Insulin and insulin-like growth factors (IGF) constitute a family of evolutionarily related polypeptide factors which can stimulate both growth and insulin-like metabolic effects in several mesenchymal cell types.[88,89] It seems likely that the mitogenic activity of insulin is mediated via the IGF receptors, which can be occupied by insulin, albeit with a much lower affinity than by IGF. This may explain why the mitogenic effects of insulin on cultured cells are often seen only when very high concentrations of insulin are used.

Bovine SMC are not stimulated by 5 μg/mℓ insulin in a base of medium 199 + 0.1% human serum albumin.[90] In a 1:1 mixture of media DV plus F12, 10^{-6} *M* insulin does diminish loss of cell protein and DNA from cultures of bovine SMC previously grown in serum-containing medium. When 5 μg/mℓ transferrin and 0.2 m*M* ascorbate were included, the cultures showed a positive protein balance and did not lose DNA.[36] Gospodarowicz et al.[72] reported that proliferation of bovine SMC in serum-free DME medium supplemented with HDL was stimulated by insulin with an apparent ED_{50} of 150 ng/mℓ and maximally at 2.5 ng/mℓ and was also stimulated by 10 ng/mℓ of Somatomedin-C (IGF-I).

In serum-free medium, insulin at 1 mU/mℓ stimulated a small increase in ^{3}H-thymidine incorporation by rat aortic SMC.[91] In a base of 0.5 to 1% fetal bovine serum, insulin stimulated proliferation and ^{3}H-thymidine incorporation by rat aortic SMC.[52,92] Maximal stimulation was achieved at 500 μU/mℓ, but was only about 20% as great as was achieved with 10% calf serum.[92] Insulin at 100 ng/mℓ was less effective than other members of the "insulin family", including partially purified Somatomedins A and C (10 μg/mℓ), multiplication stimulating activity (0.5 μg/mℓ), and IGF-I (50 ng/mℓ).[52] Proliferation of human arterial SMC in a base of 6% fetal calf serum is also stimulated by insulin, with significant stimulation seen at 10 μU/mℓ and a maximum effect seen at 10,000 μU/mℓ.[93] The maximum effect of insulin was again considerably less than that of 10% fetal bovine serum.

Koschinsky et al.[94] reported that serum from diabetic patients promoted better proliferation of human SMC than did serum from normal or treated diabetics. This confirms the observation by Ledet[95] that diabetic serum promotes more rapid growth of colonies from explants of rabbit aorta. However, increased levels of insulin in diabetic serum did not seem to account for the increased efficacy of the diabetic serum since addition of up to 2000 μU/mℓ of insulin to the normal serum did not stimulate growth.[95]

2. Growth Hormone

Ledet[95] has reported that diabetic serum stimulates more rapid growth of colonies of rabbit aortic SMC than does normal serum. Normal serum can be made more potent by the addition of growth hormone,[95,96] but not by the addition of insulin[95] or glucose.[96] Antiserum against growth hormone reduces the potency of diabetic serum to that of normal serum. The amount of growth hormone required to reproduce the extra stimulation by diabetic serum is in the same concentration range (0.2 ng/mℓ) as could be found in diabetic serum since growth hormone levels in diabetics are elevated three- to fourfold, from 0.4 to 1.4 ng/mℓ.[97] In vivo, considerably less aortic SMC proliferation occurs in response to balloon catheter de-endothelialization in rats that have been hypophysectomized than in control rats.[98,99] This does not seem to be due to deprivation of growth hormone, however, since replacement therapy with growth hormone alone (or together with glucocorticoids, mineralocorticoids, and thyroxine) did not restore the SMC proliferative response.[99]

3. Lipids and Lipoproteins

Several key observations demonstrating that lipoproteins can stimulate growth under certain circumstances have been made using the following culture system.[100-102] Explants of rabbit or Rhesus monkey thoracic aorta are cultured for 5 to 6 months in medium containing 10% normal serum. During this period, SMC migrate out from the explants and from colonies. Test sera are then substituted for 50% of the normal serum or test lipoproteins are added, and the growth response is measured as an increase in colony size. Stimulation was obtained with low-density lipoprotein (LDL) from hyperlipemic serum, but not with LDL from normolipemic serum or with HDL from either serum.[100] The differences remain even when the LDL from the two sera are used at a comparable cholesterol content.[101] Fless et al.[102] used this system to analyze LDL subfractionated by density gradient ultracentrifugation. The "larger LDL species" (molecular weight greater than 3.0×10^{-6}, density greater than 1.030 g/mℓ) from both normal or hyperlipemic monkeys or from some normal human donors was mitogenic. The "smaller LDL" (molecular weight = 2.6 to 2.7×10^{-6}) from normal monkeys or from some normal human donors was not mitogenic. "LDL-III", the Rhesus monkey equivalent of human Lp(a), was also mitogenic, but only after removal of most of its sialic acid moieties.

Using a culture system in which initial rates of proliferation of porcine aortic SMC were measured in a base of 1.5% porcine serum, Brown et al.[103] determined the dose response to several species of lipoproteins: HDL_c, HDL_2, LDL, and VLDL, listed in order of increasing maximum potency. Maximum effects of each were achieved at 10 mg/dℓ of lipoprotein cholesterol, with all responses being less than that produced by 10% porcine serum. The source of the lipoproteins (normal vs. hyperlipemic serum) did not make a difference. At triglyceride levels above 15 mg/dℓ, VLDL was reported to lead to foam cell formation. Whole hyperlipemic serum has been reported to be more stimulatory than normolipemic serum for rat,[91] rabbit,[104] and pig and monkey[14] SMC. Extraction of lipids from normolipemic serum with acetone/ethanol/ether reduced its ability to stimulate ^{3}H-thymidine incorporation by rat aortic SMC.[91] However, the extraction procedure could be affecting serum components in addition to lipoproteins, and certain fatty acids are essential nutrients for cultured mammalian cells. Specific removal of LDL and most HDL from normolipemic monkey WBS permitted proliferation of monkey SMC, though to a lesser extent than did reconstituted serum.[105]

In some culture systems, LDL seems to be toxic for SMC. Hessler et al.[106] reported that LDL from normolipemic human serum caused a decrease in the number of human SMC per culture, as well as in ^{3}H-thymidine labeling index, over a period of 3 days. By contrast, HDL was never toxic and prevented the toxicity of LDL. Gospodarowicz et al.[72] confirmed that LDL was toxic for cultured bovine aortic SMC and found that HDL was stimulatory at 250 μg/mℓ and used it to supplement DME medium in preparing a serum-free culture medium.

4. Other Factors in Plasma

Among the other factors present in plasma which have been tested for ability to stimulate growth of cultured SMC are the following: Thrombin (1 μg/mℓ), hydrocortisone (5×10^{-5} *M*) and transferrin (10 μg/mℓ) were reported to stimulate proliferation of rat abdominal aortic SMC in a base of 0.5 to 1% fetal bovine serum.[52] Ascorbate (50 μg/mℓ) in a base of 10% fetal bovine serum increased growth rate and plating efficiency, but did not alter the saturation density of bovine aortic SMC.[107] Libby and O'Brien[36] found that ascorbate (0.2 m*M*) in combination with insulin and transferrin could prevent the cell protein and DNA loss, which occurs when cultures of calf aortic SMC are transferred from medium supplement with serum to serum-free medium. The steroid hormones ethinylesteradol, estrone, and estriol at 10^{-8} *M* did not affect ^{3}H-thymidine incorporation by rat aortic SMC,[91] nor did thyroxine or several steroids or vasoactive hormones affect the survival of bovine aortic SMC in serum-free medium.[36]

III. GROWTH FACTORS FROM CULTURED CELLS

A. Growth Factors from Endothelial Cells

Cultured endothelial cells from several species (human, pig, bovine) have been shown to produce a growth factor(s), endothelial cell-derived growth factor (ECDGF), which can stimulate several connective tissue cell types.[108-110] ECDGF produced by bovine aortic endothelial cells cultured in serum-free medium stimulated a large increase in the ^{3}H-thymidine labeling index of bovine aortic SMC in serum-free medium.[108] ECDGF collected in 5% PDS supported proliferation of bovine aortic SMC as well as did 5% WBS.[108] ECDGF produced by bovine aortic endothelial cells cultured in serum-free medium or in 1% PDS also stimulated proliferation of human aortic SMC.[109] Serum-free medium conditioned for 1 day was found to be about two thirds as effective as 5% bovine serum.[109]

ECDGF is probably a mixture of several different factors. One of these factors can bind to the PDGF receptor and is recognized by antiserum prepared against pure

PDGF.[63] This PDGF-like factor accounts for approximately 25% of the mitogenic capacity of human umbilical vein ECDGF when tested by ability to stimulate ^{3}H-thymidine incorporation by 3T3 cells.[63,78] DiCorleto[111] has recently separated the PDGF-like and PDGF-unlike factors in bovine aortic ECDGF by cation exchange chromatography and confirmed that at least two biochemically distinct growth factors are present. Growth factor production by vascular endothelial cells thus resembles growth factor release by platelets in that both sources yield multiple factors. Since PDGF is a potent mitogen for SMC (see earlier), it is likely that the PDGF-like component of ECDGF will be active on SMC. The relative contribution of the PDGF-like component to the overall potency of ECDGF will depend on the susceptibility of the test cells to the other components of ECDGF and will not necessarily be comparable to the 25% value obtained, using 3T3 cells as the test cells. Endothelial cells from different vessels or from different species may also make different proportions of the PDGF-like and other components and may alter the proportion of PDGF-like components under different circumstances. Although we are not discussing growth inhibitors in this chapter, it should be noted that cultured vascular endothelial cells have also been reported to produce substances which inhibit the proliferation of SMC[110] (see also Chapters 4 and 7). Castellot et al.[110] have presented evidence that this inhibitory factor is a heparin-like molecule. Heparin from other sources has been demonstrated to inhibit the proliferation of SMC that occurs in response to vascular injury.[112]

It is not known whether endothelial cells in vivo release PDGFc. However, it has been reported that 3.7-kb mRNA hybridizing with a *sis* cDNA probe can be detected in endothelial cells scraped from human umbilical veins and from bovine aortas.[113] The *sis* gene encodes a protein homologous to one of the two related polypeptides found in preparations of pure PDGF and is probably the cellular gene for this PDGF peptide. The presence of *sis*-hybridizing mRNA in endothelial cells scraped directly from tissues is consistent with some expression of this PDGF gene in vivo. The bovine aortic and human umbilical vein endothelial cells scraped from vessels yielded approximately 1.3 and 10%, respectively, as much *sis*-hybridizing RNA as did the same cell types in culture, suggesting that endothelial cells in undamaged vessels in vivo produce less PDGFc than do their cultured counterparts. PDGFc production by cultured endothelial cells can be stimulated further by several agents. Fox and DiCorleto[114] have reported that tumor promoters and endotoxin can increase the rate of secretion by about twofold. Physiological concentrations of thrombin (1 to 10 units/mℓ) can increase rates of PDGFc secretion by HUVE by at least threefold.[115] The thrombin stimulation is not associated with decreases in the intracellular levels of PDGFc, suggesting that thrombin is not stimulating release of preformed, active PDGF. The effect of thrombin may thus be on the rate of synthesis of PDGFc by endothelial cells or on the rate of processing of an inactive PDGF processor to a secreted active PDGFc. These results suggest that thrombin that is generated from prothrombin as one of the end results of the activation of the clotting cascade (e.g., at sites of vascular damage) might participate in stimulating SMC proliferation both directly, as a mitogen,[116,117] and indirectly, by stimulating nearly endothelial cells to release PDGFc.

B. Growth Factors from Vascular Smooth Muscle Cells

A second vascular cell that can make a PDGFc under certain conditions is the smooth muscle cell itself. We have recently reported[62] that aortic SMC cultured from the aortas of 2-week-old rats secrete substantial amounts of PDGFc, whereas SMC from adult rats do not. Rates of secretion of PDGFc by the pup rat SMC are comparable to the rates of secretion by vascular endothelial cells. Goat anti-PDGF IgG can abolish the binding of pup SMC PDGFc to test cells and totally eliminates the ability of pup SMC-conditioned medium to stimulate ^{3}H-thymidine incorporation by 3T3 cells. Thus, in contrast to growth factor release from platelets and endothelial cells, PDGFc appears to be the only mitogen secreted by pup rat SMC, at least when assayed on 3T3 test cells.

Since SMC express PDGF receptors and respond mitogenically to PDGF, the PDGFc produced by pup rat SMC may be an example of what Sporn and Todaro[118] have called an "autocrine hormone": a hormone that stimulates the cells that produce it. Two observations support this possibility:

1. Pup rat SMC express fewer cell-surface PDGF receptors than do adult rat SMC.[62] We have shown that the number of PDGF receptors on adult rat SMC after preincubation with pup rat SMC-conditioned medium is reduced toward the level of PDGF receptors expressed by pup rat SMC. This suggests that PDGFc production by pup rat SMC may be sufficient to explain their low levels of PDGF receptors through a mechanism of receptor occupation and downregulation. If this is the case, it is reasonable to propose that the pup rat SMC would be mitogenically stimulated by this PDGFc in an autocrine fashion.
2. If the pup rat SMC were producing a self-mitogen that was not produced by adult rat SMC, we would expect to see a difference in the mitogen requirements of these cells. Indeed, we have found that pup rat SMC do have a higher ^{3}H-thymidine labeling index in low concentrations of PDS than do adult rat SMC.[119]

We have recently reported that adult rat SMC might be activated to secrete PDGFc by conditions associated with wounding in vivo.[120] In these studies, the carotid artery was injured by scraping away the endothelium with an inflated balloon catheter. Two weeks after this injury, extensive proliferation of SMC in the intima of the artery had occurred, and the ^{3}H-thymidine labeling index of the intimal SMC was still high.[31] At this point, the intima was dissected away from the media and cultured. When the PDGF-related phenotype of the intimal SMC was compared with that of SMC from uninjured media, it was found that the number of PDGF receptors expressed by the intimal SMC was only 50% as high as the level of PDGF receptors expressed by cells from the uninjured media. In addition, cells from intima produced up to tenfold higher levels of PDGF than did SMC from the uninjured media. The differences between intimal and medial SMC seem to be at least partially stable in culture since the differences between medial and neointimal smooth cells were observed using cells that had been cultured in vitro for at least 3 weeks. These findings suggest that production of PDGFc by SMC might be activated in response to wounding and might supplement the PDGF derived from attached, degranulated platelets and from activated endothelial cells in contributing to the extensive and prolonged proliferation of SMC in the intima of the wounded vessel (Figure 2). The relative importance of these three sources of PDGF in stimulating SMC proliferation is not yet known and may depend on the type of injury and on the time after injury.

C. Growth Factors from Leukocytes

Interleukin-1 (Il-1) is a member of a group of polypeptide factors which mediate some of the complex series of interactions that occur between the cells of the immune system[121] and which may also affect connective tissue cell types. However, recent data from Libby et al.[90] suggest that whereas Il-1 stimulates proliferation of human fibroblasts, it does not significantly stimulate human, bovine, or rabbit SMC.

Leibovich and Ross[122] observed delayed healing of skin wounds in monocytopenic guinea pigs and reported that culture medium conditioned by macrophages can stimulate growth of cultured guinea pig wound fibroblasts. Liebovich[123] later reported that

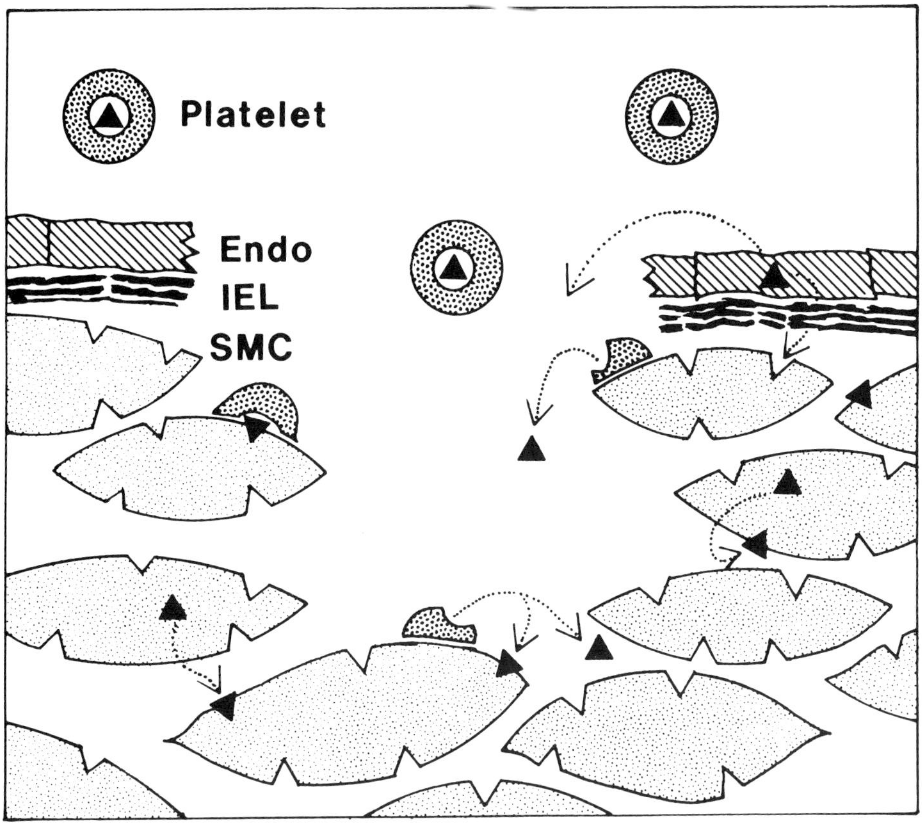

FIGURE 2. Sources of PDGFc for vascular SMC in an injured artery. A small injury to a musculoelastic artery is cartooned as a break in the endothelial cell monolayer (diagonal hatching) and in the internal elastic lamina (IEL, shown as rough parallel bundles) and with some loss of SMC (light stipples). Platelets are dark stippled disks containing PDGF (triangles) within alpha-granules (open circles). The illustration depicts release of PDGFc from adherent platelets, and adjacent endothelial cells and SMC, and its binding to receptors (triangular notches) on SMC. (From Bowen-Pope, D. F. and Seifert, R. A., *Cancer Cells*, Vol. 3, Ferramisco, J., Ozanne, B., and Stiles, C., Eds., Cold Spring Harbor Press, Cold Spring Harbor, N.Y., 1985, 183. With permission.)

the presence of PDS was required for production of growth factor and suggested that the growth factor was produced by modification of a plasma constituent. Subsequent experiments, however, indicate that macrophages can release growth factor activity even in serum-free medium.[124-127] In the case of macrophages derived from peripheral blood monocytes, it seems that serum plays a role in the maturation of the monocytes into macrophages capable of producing growth factor but that, once mature, the serum is not longer necessary.[127] Growth factor production by macrophages is stimulated by attachment to the substratum[128] and further stimulated by several agents, including endotoxin, concanavalin A, opsinized zymosan, and phorbol myristate acetate.[124-127]

The growth factors released by macrophages have not yet been purified or completely characterized. Martin et al.[126] reported that the growth-promoting activity produced by mouse peritoneal macrophages was not adsorbed by carboxymethyl sephadex under conditions which removed PDGF. Shimokado et al.[129] found that human peritoneal and lung macrophages do produce a PDGF-like factor but that most of this factor is present in the form of a complex which does not bind to PDGF receptors in a radioreceptor assay. Complexes may be in equilibrium with some free PDGF since the conditioned medium does contain mitogenic activity which is neutralized by antiserum to PDGF. Molecular seive chromatography under acidic conditions allows the PDGF-like activity to be separated from a PDGF-binding activity. This concomitant production of growth factor and growth factor-binding activities is reminiscent of production of IGF-II and its binding protein by cultured rat liver cells.[130]

Medium conditioned by cultured macrophages obtained from Schilling stainless steel wound chambers implanted subcutaneously in rabbits has been reported to stimulate proliferation of adult bovine aortic SMC.[131] When such macrophages were co-cultured with SMC, the growth rate of the SMC was increased. "Wound fluid" obtained from the Schilling chambers was also stimulatory, possibly due to the presence of growth factors produced by macrophages within the chambers.[131] Mouse peritoneal macrophages produce growth factor activity promoting proliferation and ^{3}H-thymidine in corporation by bovine aortic SMC. The amount of growth factor released was increased by incubation of the macrophages with latex, lipopolysaccharide, or phorbol myristate acetate.[126] Human peripheral monocytes, which have been cultured 5 days in homologous serum to permit maturation into macrophage-like cells, produced considerable growth-promoting activity (^{3}H-thymidine incorporation) for human SMC.[125] Endotoxin and concanavalin A stimulated increased rates of growth factor production.

Given the many pathological conditions in which macrophages are observed in association with proliferating SMC (e.g., Faggiotto et al.[132]) and the evidence mentioned above that cultured macrophages can produce a growth factor(s) active on SMC, it seems likely that growth factors from macrophages play a role in stimulating SMC in the artery wall.

IV. SYMPATHETIC NERVES AND VASOACTIVE PEPTIDES

Recognition of the roles of arterial SMC hypertrophy[3,133] and hyperplasia[134,135] in hypertension provides a rational basis for examining the effects of vasoactive agents on SMC growth. A variety of studies have implicated sympathetic nerves and endogenous catecholamines in both normal growth and development of SMC and in the growth response in hypertension. They suggest that the sympathetic nervous system may exert a chronic form of control of artery wall structure and/or function in addition to its well-known short-term control of vascular tone.[136] Bevan[137] and Bevan and Tsuru[138] found that denervation of the central ear artery of growing rabbits produced decreases in medial thickness and ^{3}H-thymidine-labeled SMC nuclei and increased the sensitivity of the vessels to norepinephrine when compared to contralateral innervated vessels. Rusterholz and Mueller[139] reported a decreased resistance to flow in the maximally dilated rabbit ear vascular bed following unilateral superior cervical ganglionectomy. Cavallero et al.[140] reported that epinephrine injections stimulated DNA synthesis in the aorta and pulmonary artery of the rabbit. Thadani and Schanberg[141] found that alpha adrenergic stimulation induced rat aortic ornithine decarboxylase activity and suggested a possible role for sympathetic nerves in regulation of protein synthesis by vascular SMC. Autonomic nerves may, therefore, exert a trophic influence on artery wall growth and metabolism in a manner resembling that of motor nerves on skeletal muscle.[142] However, for issues relevant to the artery wall, it is difficult to distinguish between direct effects of adrenoceptor stimulation on cell growth and indirect effects due to changes in pressure and wall tension in the intact vasculature. This is particularly true for hypertension. Judy et al.[143] reported that sympathetic nerve activity is significantly greater in spontaneously hypertensive rats (SHR) than in normotensive controls. Antiadrenergic drugs[144] or sympathectomy[145] arrested the onset of hypertension in young SHR and prevented the development of medial hypertrophy and enhanced lysine incorporation into noncollagen protein in medium-sized muscular arteries. Similarly, Rorive et al.[146] found that inhibition of aortic DNA replication in renal hypertensive rats by antihypertensive drugs depended on inhibition of the sympathetic nervous system.

While these studies point to a role for catecholamines in ASMC growth in hypertension, the mechanisms for this effect are unknown. Addition of norepinephrine or epinephrine directly to ASMC in culture results in relatively minor effects on cell growth. Blaes and Boissel[147] reported that epinephrine augments the growth of cultured rat ASMC in a serum-dependent fashion, but the increment in cell numbers was slight (20 to 30%). Similar results were reported for human aortic SMC growth in the presence and absence of the vasoactive peptides angiotensin II and vasopressin.[148] Augmentation of proliferation by these peptides was abolished by passage of the homologous serum employed over CM-Sephadex. While these results do not support a role for catecholamines or vasoactive peptides as complete mitogens for ASMC, they suggest that these agents may act synergistically with serum-derived mitogens to augment rates of cell growth. Whether this augmentation reflects an anabolic effect of cellular metabolism and protein syntheis or represents a more specific action in cell cycle progression is not clear at this time. Nevertheless, if such an effect occurs in vivo, it might suggest at least one way that factors associated with stress and hypertension function as risk factors for atherosclerosis.

V. FIBROBLAST GROWTH FACTOR

Fibroblast growth factor (FGF) is a polypeptide factor, or family of factors, first observed in extracts of bovine brain and pituitary.[149] The molecular identity of all factors with FGF activity is not yet clear. Lemmon et al.[150] have reported that that major activity in pituitary extracts is a basic polypeptide, while brain extracts contain a basic polypeptide (which may be identical to that from the pituitary) and also an acidic polypeptide.

FGF at 100 ng/mℓ has been reported to increase the saturation density of bovine aortic SMC in a base of either 2.5% PDS or WBS.[151] In this system, FGF was considerably more potent than 100 ng/mℓ EGF. When grown in 10% serum, the initial rate of proliferation and final saturation density of first or second passage bovine aortic SMC was less in PDS than in WBS, and growth in PDS could be increased to that in WBS by the addition of 100 ng/mℓ FGF.[71] In serum-free medium supplemented with HDL, FGF stimulated SMC proliferation with an ED_{50} of 5 ng/mℓ and a maximum effect at 100 ng/mℓ.[72] Stimulation by FGF was synergistic with HDL, Somatomedin C, or insulin. Tiell et al.[98] speculated that the absence of FGF might account for the suppressive effect of hypophysectomy on the SMC proliferation seen in response to balloon catheter deendothelialization. To date, however, there is not data as to whether FGF is present in blood or in tissue outside the brain and pituitary.

REFERENCES

1. Thomas, W. A. and Kim, D. N., Atherosclerosis as a hyperplastic and/or neoplastic disease, *Lab. Invest.*, 48, 245, 1983.
2. Ross, R., Wight, T. N., Strandness, E., and Thiele, B., Human atherosclerosis. I. Cell constitution and characteristics of advanced lesions of the superficial femoral artery, *Am. J. Pathol.*, 114, 79, 1984.

3. Owens, G. K., Rabinovitch, P. S., and Schwartz, S. M., Smooth muscle cell hypertrophy versus hyperplasia in hypertension, *Proc. Natl. Acad. Sci. U.S.A.*, 78, 7759, 1981.
4. Chamley-Campbell, J., Campbell, G. R., and Ross, R., The smooth muscle cell in culture, *Physiol. Rev.*, 59, 1, 1979.
5. Jarmolych, J., Dauod, A. S., Landau, J., Fritz, E., and McElvene, E., Aortic media explants. Cell proliferation and production of mucopolysaccharides, collagen, and elastic tissue, *Exp. Mol. Pathol.*, 9, 171, 1968.
6. Fritz, K. E., Jarmolych, J., and Daoud, A. S., Association of DNA synthesis and apparent dedifferentiation of aortic smooth muscle cells *in vitro*, *Exp. Mol. Pathol.*, 12, 354, 1970.
7. Thyberg, J., Palmberg, L., Nilsson, J., Ksiazek, T., and Sjolund, M., Phenotype modulation in primary cultures of arterial smooth muscle cells. On the role of platelet-derived growth factor, *Differentiation*, 25, 156, 1983.
8. Paule, W. J., Electron microscopy of the newborn rat aorta, *J. Ultrastruct. Res.*, 8, 219, 1963.
9. Cliff, W. J., The aortic tunica media in growing rats studied with the electron microscope, *Lab. Invest.*, 17, 599, 1967.
10. Gerrity, R. G. and Cliff, W. J., The aortic tunica media of the developing rat. I. Quantitative stereologic and biochemical analysis, *Lab. Invest.*, 32, 585, 1975.
11. Poole, J. C. F., Cromwell, S. B., and Benditt, E. P., Behavior of smooth muscle cells and formation of extracellular structure in the reaction of arterial walls to injury, *Am. J. Pathol.*, 62, 391, 1971.
12. Rhee, C. Y., Herz, F., and Spaet, T. H., Accelerated culture of aortic smooth muscle cells, *Thromb. Res.*, 11, 90, 1977.
13. Grunwald, J. and Haudenschild, C. C., Intimal injury *in vivo* activates vascular smooth muscle cell migration and explant outgrowth *in vitro*, *Arteriosclerosis*, 4, 183, 1984.
14. Chamley-Campbell, J. H., Campbell, G. R., and Ross, R., Phenotype-dependent response of cultured aortic smooth muscle to serum mitogens, *J. Cell Biol.*, 89, 379, 1981.
15. Wissler, R. W., The arterial medial cell: smooth muscle or multifunctional mesenchyme, *Circulation*, 36, 1, 1967.
16. Moss, N. S. and Benditt, E. P., Spontaneous and experimentally induced arterial lesions. I. An ultrastructural survey of the normal chicken aorta, *Lab. Invest.*, 22, 166, 1970.
17. Schmid, E., Osborn, M., Rungger-Brandle, E., Gabbiani, G., Weber, K., and Franke, W. W., Distribution of vimentin and desmin filaments in smooth muscle tissue of mammalian and avian aorta, *Exp. Cell Res.*, 137, 329, 1982.
18. Carrell, A. and Burrows, M. T., Cultivation of tissues *in vitro* and its technique, *J. Exp. Med.*, 13, 387, 1911.
19. Balk, S. D., Calcium as a regulator of the proliferation of normal, but not of transformed, chicken fibroblasts in a plasma-containing medium, *Proc. Natl. Acad. Sci. U.S.A.*, 68, 271, 1971.
20. Kohler, N. and Lipton, A., Platelets as a source of fibroblast growth-promoting activity, *Exp. Cell Res.*, 87, 297, 1974.
21. Ross, R., Glomset, J., Kariya, B., and Harker, L., Platelet-dependent serum factor that stimulates the proliferation of arterial smooth muscle cells in vitro, *Proc. Natl. Acad. Sci. U.S.A.*, 71, 1207, 1974.
22. Westermark, B. and Wasteson, Å., A platelet factor stimulating human normal glial cells, *Exp. Cell Res.*, 98, 170, 1976.
23. Kaplan, D. R., Chao, F. C., Stiles, C. D., Antoniades, H. N., and Scher, C. D., Platelet alpha granules contain a growth factor for fibroblasts, *Blood*, 53, 1043, 1979.
24. Rutherford, R. B. and Ross, R., Platelet factors stimulate fibroblasts and smooth muscle cells quiescent in plasma serum to proliferate, *J. Cell Biol.*, 69, 196, 1976.
25. Burke, J. M. and Ross, R., Collagen synthesis by monkey arterial smooth muscle cells during proliferation and quiescence in culture, *Exp. Cell Res.*, 107, 387, 1977.
26. Witte, L. D., Kaplan, K. L., Nossel, H. L., Lages, B. A., Weiss, H. J., and Goodman, D. S., Studies of the release from human platelets of the growth factor for cultured human arterial smooth muscle cells, *Circ. Res.*, 42, 402, 1978.
27. Thorgeirsson, G. and Robertson, A. L., Platelet factors and the vascular wall. Variations in growth response between endothelial and medial smooth muscle cells, *Atherosclerosis*, 30, 67, 1978.
28. Ihnatowycz, I. O., Cazenave, J. P., Mustard, J. F., and Moore, S., The effect of a platelet-derived growth factor on the proliferation of rabbit arterial smooth muscle cells in tissue culture, *Thromb. Res.*, 14, 477, 1979.
29. Nilsson, J. and Thyberg, J., Fine structure of arterial smooth muscle cells cultured in the presence of whole blood serum or plasma-derived serum, *Cell Tissue Res.*, 223, 87, 1982.
30. Ross, R., Nist, C., Kariya, B., Rivest, M. J., Raines, E., and Callis, J., Physiological quiescence in plasma-derived serum: influence of platelet-derived growth factor on cell growth in culture, *J. Cell. Physiol.*, 97, 497, 1978.

31. Clowes, A. W., Reidy, M. A., and Clowes, M. M., Kinetics of cellular proliferation after arterial injury. I. Smooth muscle growth in the absence of endothelium, *Lab. Invest.*, 59, 327, 1983.
32. Vogel, A., Raines, E., Kariya, B., Rivest, M. J., and Ross, R., Coordinate control of 3T3 cell proliferation by platelet-derived growth factor and plasma components, *Proc. Natl. Acad. Sci. U.S.A.*, 75, 2810, 1978.
33. Singh, J. P., Chaikin, M. A., and Stiles, C. D., Phylogenetic analysis of platelet-derived growth factor by radioreceptor assay, *J. Cell Biol.*, 95, 667, 1982.
34. Huang, J. S., Huang, S. S., and Deuel, T. F., Human platelet-derived growth factor: radioimmunoassay and discovery of a specific plasma-binding protein, *J. Cell Biol.*, 97, 383, 1983.
35. Bowen-Pope, D. F., Malpass, T. W., Foster, D. M., and Ross, R., Platelet-derived growth factor *in vivo*: levels, activity, and rate of clearance, *Blood*, 64, 458, 1984.
36. Libby, P. and O'Brien, K. V., Culture of quiescent arterial smooth muscle cells in a defined serum-free medium, *J. Cell. Physiol.*, 115, 217, 1983.
37. Roberts, A. B., Anzano, M. A., Lamb, L. C., Smith, J. M., and Sporn, M. B., New class of transforming growth factors potentiated by epidermal growth factor: isolation from non-neoplastic tissues, *Proc. Natl. Acad. Sci. U.S.A.*, 78, 5339, 1981.
38. Assoian, R. K., Grotendorst, G. R., Miller, D. M., and Sporn, M. B., Cellular transformation by coordinated action of three peptide growth factors from human platelets, *Nature (London)*, 309, 804, 1984.
39. Childs, C. B., Proper, J. A., Tucker, R. F., and Moses, H. L., Serum contains a platelet-derived transforming growth factor, *Proc. Natl. Acad. Sci. U.S.A.*, 79, 5312, 1982.
40. Assoian, R. K., Komoriya, A., Meyers, C. A., Miller, D. M., and Sporn, M. B., Transforming growth factor-β in human platelets. Identification of a major storage site, purification, and characterization, *J. Biol. Chem.*, 258, 7155, 1983.
41. Antoniades, H. N., Scher, C. D., and Stiles, C. D., Purification of human platelet-derived growth factor, *Proc. Natl. Acad. Sci. U.S.A.*, 76, 1809, 1979.
42. Heldin, C.-H., Westermark, B., and Wasteson, Å., Platelet-derived growth factor: purification and partial characterization, *Proc. Natl. Acad. Sci. U.S.A.*, 76, 3722, 1979.
43. Deuel, T. F., Huang, J. S., Proffitt, R. T., Baenziger, J. U., Chang, D., and Kennedy, B. B., Human platelet-derived growth factor — purification and resolution into two active protein fractions, *J. Biol. Chem.*, 256, 8896, 1981.
44. Raines, E. and Ross, R., Platelet-derived growth factor. I. High yield purification and evidence for multiple forms, *J. Biol. Chem.*, 257, 5154, 1982.
45. Antoniades, H. N. and Scher, C. D., Radioimmunoassay of a human serum growth factor for Balb/c 3T3 cells: derivation from platelets, *Proc. Natl. Acad. Sci. U.S.A.*, 74, 1973, 1977.
46. Raines, E. W., unpublished data, 1985.
47. Bowen-Pope, D. F. and Ross, R., Platelet-derived growth factor. II. Specific binding to cultured cells, *J. Biol. Chem.*, 257, 5161, 1982.
48. Heldin, C.-H., Westermark, B., and Wasteson, Å., Demonstration of an antibody against platelet-derived growth factor, *Exp. Cell Res.*, 136, 255, 1981a.
49. Nilsson, J., Ksiazek, T., Heldin, C.-H., and Thyberg, J., Demonstration of stimulatory effects of platelet-derived growth factor on cultivated rat arterial smooth muscle cells, *Exp. Cell Res.*, 145, 231, 1983b.
50. Temin, H. M., Pierson, R. W., Jr., and Dulak, N. C., The role of serum in the control of multiplication of avian and mammalian cells in culture, in *Growth, Nutrition and Metabolism of Cells in Culture*, Vol. 5, Rothblat, G. H. and Cristofalo, V. J., Eds., Academic Press, New York, 1972, 50.
51. Williams, L. T., Tremble, P., and Antoniades, H. N., Platelet-derived growth factor binds specifically to receptors on vascular smooth muscle cells and the binding becomes nondissociable, *Proc. Natl. Acad. Sci. U.S.A.*, 79, 5867, 1982.
52. Weinstein, R., Stemerman, M. B., and Maciag, T., Hormonal requirement for growth of arterial smooth muscle cells in vitro: an endocrine approach to atherosclerosis, *Science*, 818, 1981.
53. Nilsson, J. and Olsson, A. G., Prostaglandin E_1 inhibits DNA synthesis in arterial smooth muscle cells stimulated with platelet-derived growth factor, *Atherosclerosis*, 53, 77, 1984.
54. Atkinson, P. R., Weidman, E. R., Bhaumick, B., and Bala, R. M., Release of somatomedin-like activity by cultured WI-38 human fibroblasts, *Endocrinology*, 106, 2006, 1980.
55. Clemmons, D. R., Multiple hormones stimulate the production of somatomedin by cultured human fibroblasts, *J. Clin. Endocrinol. Metab.*, 58, 850, 1984.
56. Pietila, K., Moilanen, T., and Nikkari, T., Prostaglandins enhance the synthesis and inhibit the growth of rabbit aortic smooth muscle cells in culture, *Artery*, 7, 509, 1980.
57. Huttner, J. J., Gwebu, E. T., Panganamala, R. V., Milo, G. E., and Cornwell, D. G., Fatty acids and their prostaglandin derivatives — inhibitors of proliferation in aortic smooth muscle cells, *Science*, 197, 289, 1977.

58. Heldin, C.-H., Westermark, B., and Wasteson, Å., Specific receptors for platelet-derived growth factor on cells derived from connective tissue and glia, *Proc. Natl. Acad. Sci. U.S.A.*, 78, 3664, 1981b.
59. Huang, J. S., Huang, S. S., Kennedy, B., and Deuel, T. F., Platelet-derived growth factor: specific binding to target cells, *J. Biol. Chem.*, 257, 8130, 1982.
60. Bowen-Pope, D. F., Seifert, R. A., and Ross, R., The platelet-derived growth factor receptor, in *Cell Proliferation: Recent Advances*, Boynton, A. L. and Leffert, H., Eds., Academic Press, New York, 1985, 287.
61. Glenn, K. C., Bowen-Pope, D. F., and Ross, R., Platelet-derived growth factor. III. Identification of a platelet-derived growth factor receptor by affinity labeling, *J. Biol. Chem.*, 257, 5172, 1982.
62. Seifert, R. A., Schwartz, S. M., and Bowen-Pope, D. F., Developmentally regulated production of platelet-derived growth factor-like molecules, *Nature (London)*, 311, 1984.
63. DiCorleto, P. E. and Bowen-Pope, D. F., Cultured endothelial cells produce a platelet-derived growth factor-like protein, *Proc. Natl. Acad. Sci. U.S.A.*, 80, 1919, 1983.
64. Huang, J. S., Huang, S. S., and Deuel, T. F., Specific covalent binding of platelet-derived growth factor to human plasma alpha$_2$-macroglobulin, *Proc. Natl. Acad. Sci. U.S.A.*, 81, 342, 1984.
65. Raines, E. W., Bowen-Pope, D. F., and Ross, R., Plasma binding proteins for platelet-derived growth factor that inhibit its binding to cell-surface receptors, *Proc. Natl. Acad. Sci. U.S.A.*, 81, 3424, 1984.
66. Adamson, E. D. and Rees, A. R., Epidermal growth factor receptors, *Mol. Cell. Biochem.*, 34, 129, 1981.
67. Savage, C. R. and Cohen, S. J., Epidermal growth factor and a new derivative. Rapid isolation procedures and biological and chemical characterization, *J. Biol. Chem.*, 247, 7609, 1972.
68. Byyny, R. L., Orth, D. N., Cohen, S., and Doyne, E. S., Epidermal growth factor: effects of androgens and andrenergic agents, *Endocrinology*, 95, 776, 1974.
69. Bowen-Pope, D. F. and Ross, R., Is epidermal growth factor present in human blood? Alteration of EGF binding specificity in the radioreceptor assay, *Biochem. Biophys. Res. Commun.*, 114, 1036, 1983.
70. Oka, Y. and Orth, D. N., Human plasma epidermal growth factor/Beta-urogastrone is associated with blood platelets, *J. Clin. Invest.*, 72, 249, 1983.
71. Gospodarowicz, D. and Ill, C. R., Do plasma and serum have different abilities to promote cell growth? *Proc. Natl. Acad. Sci. U.S.A.*, 77, 2726, 1980.
72. Gospodarowicz, D., Hirabayashi, K., Giguere, L., and Tauber, J. P., Factors controlling the proliferative rate, final cell density, and life span of bovine vascular smooth cells in culture, *J. Cell Biol.*, 89, 568, 1981.
73. Bhargava, G., Rifas, L., and Makman, M. H., Presence of epidermal growth factor receptors and influence of epidermal growth factor on proliferation and aging in cultured smooth muscle cells, *J. Cell. Physiol.*, 100, 365, 1979.
74. Sporn, M. B., Newton, D. L., Roberts, A. B., DeLarco, J. E., and Todaro, G. J., Retinoids and suppression of the effects of polypeptide transforming factors — a new molecular approach to chemoprevention of cancer, in *Molecular Actions and Targets for Cancer Chemotherapeutic Agents*, Sartorelli, A. C., Lazo, J. S., and Bertino, J. R., Eds., Academic Press, New York, 1981, 541.
75. Macpherson, I. and Montagnier, L., Agar suspension culture for the selective assay of cells transformed by polyoma virus, *Virology*, 23, 291, 1968.
76. Todaro, G. J., DeLarco, J. E., and Cohen, S., Transformation by murine and feline sarcoma viruses specifically blocks binding of epidermal growth factor to cells, *Nature (London)*, 264, 26, 1976.
77. Marquardt, H., Hunkapiller, M. W., Hood, L. E., Twardzik, D. R., DeLarco, J. E., Stephenson, J. R., and Todaro, G. J., Transforming growth factors produced by retrovirus-transformed rodent fibroblasts and human melanoma cells: amino acid sequence homology with epidermal growth factor, *Proc. Natl. Acad. Sci. U.S.A.*, 80, 4684, 1983.
78. Bowen-Pope, D. F., Vogel, A., and Ross, R., Production of platelet-derived growth factor-like molecules and reduced expression of platelet-derived growth factor receptors accompanies transformation by a wide spectrum of agents, *Proc. Natl. Acad. Sci. U.S.A.*, 81, 2396, 1984.
79. Anzano, M. A., Roberts, A. B., DeLarco, J. E., Wakefield, L. M., Assoian, R. K., Roche, N. S., Smith, J. M., Lazarus, J. E., and Sporn, M. B., Increased secretion of type B transforming growth factor accompanies viral transformation of cells, *Mol. Cell. Biol.*, 5, in press.
80. Gerrard, J. M., Phillips, D. R., Rao, G. H. R., Plow, E. F., Walz, D. A., Ross, R., Harker, L. A., and White, J. G., Biochemical studies of two patients with the gray platelet syndrome, *J. Clin. Invest.*, 66, 102, 1980.
81. Weiss, H. J., Platelet physiology and abnormalities of platelet function, *N. Engl. J. Med.*, 293, 531, 1975.

82. Baumgartner, H. R. and Muggli, R., Adhesion and aggregation: morphological demonstration and quantitation in vivo and in vitro, in *Platelets in Biology and Pathology*, Gordon, J. I., Ed., Elsevier North-Holland Biomedical Press, New York, 1976, 23.
83. Goldberg, I. D., Stemerman, M. B., and Handin, R. I., Vascular permeation of platelet factor 4 after endothelial injury, *Science*, 209, 611, 1980.
84. Harker, L. A., Ross, R., Slichter, S. J., and Scott, C. R., Homocystine-induced arteriosclerosis: the role of endothelial cell injury and platelet response in its genesis, *J. Clin. Invest.*, 58, 731, 1976.
85. Moore, S., Friedman, R. J., Singal, D. P., Gauldie, J., Blajchman, M. A., and Roberts, R. S., Inhibition of injury induced thromboatherosclerotic lesions by antiplatelet serum in rabbits, *Thromb. Haemost.*, 35, 70, 1976.
86. Fuster, V. and Bowie, E. J. W., The von Willebrand pig as a model for atherosclerotic research, *Thromb. Haemost.*, 39, 322, 1978.
87. Friedman, R. J., Stemerman, M. B., Wenz, B., Moore, S., Gauldie, J., Gent, M., Tiell, M. L., and Spaet, T. H., The effect of thrombocytopenia on experimental atherosclerotic lesion formation in rabbits. Smooth muscle cell proliferation and reendothelialization, *J. Clin. Invest.*, 60, 1191, 1977.
88. Blundell, T. L. and Humbel, R. E., Hormone families: pancreatic hormones and homologous growth factors, *Nature (London)*, 287, 781, 1980.
89. Zapf, J., Froesch, E. R., and Humbel, R. E., The insulin-like growth factors (IGF) of human serum: chemical and biological characterization and aspects of their possible physiological role, *Curr. Top. Cell. Regul.*, 19, 257, 1981.
90. Libby, P., Wyler, D. J., Janicka, M. W., and Dinarello, C. A., Differential effects of human interleukin-1 on growth of human fibroblasts and vascular smooth muscle and endothelial cells, ms. submitted.
91. Taggart, H. and Stout, R. W., Control of DNA synthesis in cultured vascular endothelial and smooth muscle cells, *Atherosclerosis*, 37, 549, 1980.
92. Pfeifle, B., Ditschuneit, H. H., and Ditschuneit, H., Insulin as a cellular growth regulator of rat arterial smooth muscle cells in vito, *Horm. Metab. Res.*, 12, 381, 1980.
93. Pfeile, B. and Ditschuneit, H., Effect of insulin on growth of cultured human arterial smooth muscle cells, *Diabetologia*, 20, 155, 1981.
94. Koschinsky, T., Bunting, C. E., Schwippert, B., and Gries, A., Regulation of diabetic serum growth factors for human muscular cells by the metabolic control of diabetes mellitus, *Atherosclerosis*, 39, 313, 1981.
95. Ledet, T., Growth hormone stimulating the growth of arterial medial cells in vitro. Absence of effect of insulin, *Diabetes*, 25, 1011, 1976.
96. Ledet, T., Fischer-Dzoga, K., and Wissler, R. W., Growth of rabbit aortic smooth muscle cells cultured in media containing diabetic and hyperlipemic serum, *Diabetes*, 25, 207, 1976.
97. Ledet, T., Growth hormone antiserum suppresses the growth effect of diabetic serum. Studies on rabbit aortic medial cell cultures, *Diabetes*, 26, 798, 1977.
98. Tiell, M. L., Stemmerman, M. B., and Spaet, T. H., The influence of the pituitary on arterial intimal proliferation in the rat, *Circ. Res.*, 42, 644, 1978.
99. Bettmann, M. A., Stemerman, M. B., and Ransil, B. J., The effect of hypophysectomy on experimental endothelial cell regrowth and intimal thickening in the rat, *Circ. Res.*, 48, 907, 1981.
100. Fischer-Dzoga, K., Fraser, R., and Wissler, R. W., Stimulation of proliferation in stationary primary cultures of monkey and rabbit aortic smooth muscle cells. I. Effect of lipoprotein fractions of hyperlipemic serum and lymph, *Exp. Mol. Pathol.*, 24, 346, 1975.
101. Fischer-Dzoga, K. and Wissler, R. W., Stimulation of proliferation in stationary primary cultures of monkey aortic smooth muscle cells. II. Effect of varying concentrations of hyperlipemic serum and low density lipoproteins of varying dietary fat origins, *Atherosclerosis*, 24, 515, 1976.
102. Fless, G. M., Kirchhausen, T., Fischer-Dzoga, K., Wissler, R. W., and Scanu, A. M., Serum low density lipoproteins with mitogenic effect on cultured aortic smooth muscle cells, *Atherosclerosis*, 41, 171, 1982.
103. Brown, B. G., Mahley, R., and Assmann, G., Swine aortic smooth muscle in tissue culture. Some effects of purified swine lipoproteins on cell growth and morphology, *Circ. Res.*, 39, 415, 1976.
104. Pietila, K., Long-term effect of hyperlipidemic serm on the synthesis of glycosaminoglycans and on the rate of growth of rabbit aortic smooth muscle cells in culture, *Atherosclerosis*, 42, 67, 1982.
105. Ross, R. and Glomset, J. A., Atherosclerosis and the arterial smooth muscle cells, *Science*, 180, 1332, 1973.
106. Hessler, J. R., Robertson, A. L., and Chisolm, G. M., LDL-induced cytoxicity and its inhibition by HDL in human vascular smooth muscle and endothelial cells in culture, *Atherosclerosis*, 32, 213, 1979.
107. Schwartz, E., Bienkowski, R. S., Coltoff-Schiller, B., Goldfischer, S., and Blumenfeld, O. O., Changes in the components of extracellular matrix and in growth properties of cultured aortic smooth muscle cells upon ascorbate feeding, *J. Cell Biol.*, 462, 1982.

108. Gajdusek, C., DiCorleto, P., Ross, R., and Schwartz, S. M., An endothelial cell-derived growth factor, *J. Cell Biol.*, 85, 467, 1980.
109. Wang, C.-H., Largis, E. E., and Schaffer, S. A., The effects of endothelial cell-conditioned media on the proliferation of aortic smooth muscle cells and 3T3 cells in culture, *Artery*, 9, 358, 1981.
110. Castellot, J. J., Addonizio, M. L., Rosenberg, R., and Karnovsky, M. J., Cultured endothelial cells produce a heparin-like inhibitor of smooth muscle cell growth, *J. Cell Biol.*, 90, 372, 1981.
111. DiCorleto, P. E., Cultured endothelial cells produce multiple growth factors for connective tissue cells, *Exp. Cell Res.*, 153, 167, 1984.
112. Clowes, A. W. and Karnovsky, M. J., Suppression by heparin of smooth muscle cell proliferation in injured arteries, *Nature (London)*, 265, 625, 1977.
113. Barrett, T. B., Gajdusek, C. M., Schwartz, S. M., McDougall, J. K., and Benditt, E. P., Expression of the *sis* gene by endothelial cells in culture and *in vivo*, *Proc. Natl. Acad. Sci. U.S.A.*, 81, 6772, 1984.
114. Fox, P. L. and DiCorleto, P. E., Regulation of production of a platelet-derived growth factor-like protein by cultured bovine aortic endothelial cells, *J. Cell. Physiol.*, 121, 298, 1984.
115. Harlan, J., Thompson, P., Ross, R., and Bowen-Pope, D. F., Alpha-thrombin induces release of PDGF-like molecules by cultured human umbilical endothelial cells, *J. Cell Biol.*, in press.
116. Chen, L. B. and Buchanan, J. M., Mitogenic activity of blood components. I. Thrombin and prothrombin, *Proc. Natl. Acad. Sci. U.S.A.*, 72, 131, 1975.
117. Carney, D. H., Glenn, K. C., and Cunningham, D. D., Conditions which affect initiation of animal cell division by trypsin and thrombin, *J. Cell. Physiol.*, 95, 13, 1978.
118. Sporn, M. B. and Todaro, G. J., Autocrine secretion and malignant transformation of cells, *N. Engl. J. Med.*, 303, 878, 1980.
119. Bowen-Pope, D. F. and Seifert, R. A., Exogenous and endogenous sources of PDGF-like molecules and their potential roles in vascular biology, in *Cancer Cells*, Vol. 3, Ferramisco, J., Ozanne, B., and Stiles, C., Eds., Cold Spring Harbor Press, Cold Spring Harbor, N.Y., 1985, 185.
120. Walker, L. N., Bowen-Pope, D. F., and Reidy, M. A., Secretion of platelet-derived growth factor (PDGF)-like activity by arterial smooth muscle cells in induced as a response to injury, *J. Cell Biol.*, 99 (Abstr.), 416a, 1984.
121. Dinarello, C. A., Interleukin-1, *Rev. Infect. Dis.*, 6, 51, 1984.
122. Leibovich, S. J. and Ross, R., A macrophage-dependent factor that stimulates the prevention of fibroblasts *in vitro*, *Am. J. Pathol.*, 84, 501, 1976.
123. Leibovich, S. J., Production of macrophage-dependent fibroblast stimulating activity (M-FSA) by murine macrophages. Effects of BALB/c 3T3 fibroblasts, *Exp. Cell Res.*, 113, 47, 1978.
124. Wahl, S. M., Wahl, L. M., McCarthy, J. B., Chedid, L., and Mergenhagen, S. E., Macrophage activation by mycobacterial water soluble compounds and synthetic muramyl dipeptide, *J. Immunol.*, 122, 2226, 1979.
125. Glenn, K. C. and Ross, R., Human monocyte-derived growth factor(s) for mesenchymal cells: activation of secretion by endotoxin and con A, *Cell*, 25, 603, 1981.
126. Martin, B. M., Gimbrone, M. A., Unanue, E. R., and Cotran, R. S., Stimulation of non-lymphoid mesenchymal cell proliferation by a macrophage-derived growth factor, *J. Immunol.*, 126, 1510, 1981.
127. Leslie, C. C., Musson, R. A., and Henson, P. M., Production of growth factor activity for fibroblasts by human monocyte-derived macrophages, *J. Leuk. Biol.*, 36, 143, 1984.
128. Bitterman, P. B., Rennard, S. I., Hunninghake, G. W., and Crystal, R. G., Human alveolar macrophage growth factor for fibroblasts, *J. Clin. Invest.*, 70, 806, 1982.
129. Shimokado, K., Raines, E. W., Madtes, D. K., Barrett, T. B., Benditt, E. P., and Ross, R., A significant part of macrophage-derived growth factor consists of at least two forms of PDGF, *Cell*, 43, 277, 1986.
130. Moses, A. C., Nissley, S. P., Passamini, J., and White, R. M., Further characterization of growth hormone-dependent somatomedin binding proteins in rat serum and demonstration of somatomedin-binding proteins produced by rat liver cells in culture, *Endocrinology*, 104, 536, 1979.
131. Greenburg, G. and Hunt, T., The proliferative response *in vivo* of vascular endothelial and smooth muscle cells exposed to wound fluids and macrophages, *J. Cell. Physiol.*, 97, 353, 1978.
132. Faggiotto, A., Ross, R., and Harker, L., Studies of hypercholesterolemia in the nonhuman primate. I. Changes that lead to fatty streak formation, *Arteriosclerosis*, 4, 323, 1984.
133. Olivetti, G., Melissari, M., Marchetti, G., and Anversa, P., Quantitative structural changes of the rat thoracic aorta in early spontaneous hypertension: tissue composition, and hypertrophy and hyperplasia of smooth muscle cells, *Circ. Res.*, 51, 19, 1982.
134. Fernandez, D. and Crane, W. A. J., New cell formation in rats with accelerated hypertension due to partial aortic constriction, *J. Pathol.*, 100, 307, 1970.
135. Bevan, R. D., An autoradiographic and pathological study of cellular proliferation in rabbit arteries correlated with an increase in arterial pressure, *Blood Vessels*, 13, 100, 1976.

136. Bevan, R. D. and Tsuru, H., Long-term denervation of vascular smooth muscle causes not only functional but structural changes, *Blood Vessels,* 16, 109, 1979.
137. Bevan, R. D., Effect of sympathetic denervation on smooth muscle cell proliferation in growing rabbit ear artery, *Circ. Res.,* 37, 14, 1975.
138. Bevan, R. D. and Tsuru, H., Functional and structural changes in the rabbit ear artery after sympathetic denervation, *Circ. Res.,* 49, 478, 1981.
139. Rusterholz, D. B. and Mueller, S. M., Sympathetic nerves exert a chronic influence on the intact vasculature that is age related, *Ann. Neurol.,* 11, 365, 1982.
140. Cavallero, C., DiTondo, U., Mingazzini, P. L., Pesando, P. C., and Spagnoli, L. G., Cell proliferation in the atherosclerotic lesions of cholesterol-fed rabbits. II. Histological, ultrastructural, and radioautographic observations on epinephrine-treated rabbits, *Atherosclerosis,* 17, 49, 1973.
141. Thadani, P. V. and Schanberg, S. M., Effect of stress and sympathetic activity on rat cardiac and aortic ornithine decarboxylase activity, *Life Sci.,* 25, 1009, 1979.
142. Gutmann, E., Neutrophic relations, *Annu. Rev. Physiol.,* 38, 177, 1976.
143. Judy, W. V., Watanabe, A. M., Henry, D. P., Besch, H. R., Murphy, W. R., and Hockel, G. M., Sympathetic nerve activity. Role in regulation of blood pressure in the spontaneously hypertensive rat, *Circ. Res.,* 38 (Suppl. 2), 21, 1976.
144. Nakada, T. and Lovenberg, W., Lysine incorporation in vessels of spontaneously hypertensive rats: effects of adrenergic drugs, *Eur. J. Pharmacol.,* 48, 87, 1978.
145. Yamori, Y., Nakada, T., and Lovenberg, W., Effect of antihypertensive therapy on lysine incorporation into vascular protein of the spontaneously hypertensive rat, *Eur. J. Pharmacol.,* 38, 349, 1976.
146. Rorive, G. L., Carlier, P. J., and Foidart, J. M., Hyperplasia of rat arteries smooth muscle cells associated with development and reversal of renal hypertension, *Clin. Sci.,* 59, 335S, 1980.
147. Blaes, N. and Boissel, J. P., Growth-stimulating effect of catecholamines on rat aortic smooth muscle cells in culture, *J. Cell. Physiol.,* 116, 167, 1983.
148. Campbell-Boswell, M. and Robertson, A. L., Jr., Effects of angiotensin II and vasopressin on human smooth muscle cells *in vitro, Exp. Mol. Pathol.,* 35, 265, 1981.
149. Gospodarowicz, D., Localization of a fibroblast growth factor and its effect alone and with hydrocortisone on 3T3 cell growth, *Nature (London),* 249, 123, 1974.
150. Lemmon, S. K., Riley, M. C., Thomas, K. A., Hoover, G. A., Maciag, T., and Bradshaw, R., Bovine fibroblast growth factor: comparison of brain and pituitary preparations, *J. Cell Biol.,* 95, 162, 1982.
151. Gospodarowicz, D., Moran, J., and Braun, D., Control of proliferation of bovine vascular cells, *J. Cell. Physiol.,* 91, 377, 1977.
152. Bowen-Pope, D. F., The growth factor-platelet-transformation connection, in *The Cell Surface in Development and Cancer,* a volume of *Developmental Biology,* Browder, L., Ed., Plenum Press, New York, in press.

Chapter 7

HEPARIN AND THE REGULATION OF GROWTH IN THE VASCULAR WALL

John J. Castellot, Jr. and Morris J. Karnovsky

TABLE OF CONTENTS

I. INTRODUCTION

A salient characteristic of the normal arterial wall is that the component cells are in a quiescent growth state.[1] The importance of the intimal endothelial cells (EC) which line the lumen in maintaining this state has been recognized for nearly a decade, but the precise molecular mechanisms underlying this phenomenon are only beginning to be clarified.

When EC are damaged, a series of events ensues which leads to the migration and proliferation of the medial smooth muscle cells (SMC). First, platelets adhere to the injured area and release their granular contents. One of the α-granule products to which the SMC are exposed is the platelet-derived growth factor (PDGF), which is both chemotactic and mitogenic for SMC.[2,3] Although the vast majority of platelets are present only transiently at the injured site, there are several other sources of SMC mitogens which are present. These include macrophages[4,5] and the regenerating EC.[6] One of the currently intriguing hypotheses of the pathogenesis of arteriosclerosis — the response to injury theory — holds that SMC respond to the presence of the platelet, macrophage, and EC products by migrating into the intima and proliferating, thus giving rise to a hyperplastic mass.[7-11] Uninjured EC at the periphery of the injury migrate and proliferate until the damaged area is re-endothelialized, at which time SMC growth ceases.[7] Repeated cycles of injury and proliferation may then lead to full-blown lesions with their potentially serious consequences.

Many laboratories have provided experimental support for the response to injury hypothesis, including our own. Much of this work has been directed at understanding the proliferative response of SMC to various mitogenic substances and is detailed elsewhere in this volume. Our work has focused on the growth regulatory mechanisms within the vascular wall in both physiological and pathological conditions. In particular, we have studied the potential role of endogenous heparin-like species as regulators of SMC growth.

II. HISTORICAL PERSPECTIVE

A. In Vivo Models for EC Injury Link SMC Proliferation to EC Regeneration

In the mid-1970s, we and others began to examine histologically the response of arteries to an EC injury. The air-dry injury method developed in this laboratory involved ligating a 1.5-cm segment of the rat carotid artery, evacuating the contents, and passing a gentle stream of air through the lumen under carefully controlled pressure, humidity, and time.[7] The endothelium is desiccated and begins to peel off within minutes after restoring blood flow to the carotid. Platelets then carpet the exposed intima, and a dramatic proliferation of SMC is observed within the next 7 to 14 days. The advantages to the air-dry procedure is that the injury to the vessel wall is well controlled, destroying all of the EC without significant injury to the media. The rat carotid artery eliminates complications in studying endothelial regeneration, since there were no ostia in the segment used, and EC regeneration occurs solely from the uninjured proximal and distal portions of the vessel. SMC proliferation, myointimal thickening, and EC regeneration can be quantitated by morphometric and autoradiographic means.

When this type of injury was produced (Figure 1), we observed little myointimal proliferation at the proximal and distal regions of the injury in which re-endothelialization was rapid. In the middle of the segment, however, where endothelial regeneration occurred last, there was massive SMC hyperplasia. The proliferation reached a peak at 10 to 14 days after injury, at which time re-endothelialization was complete.

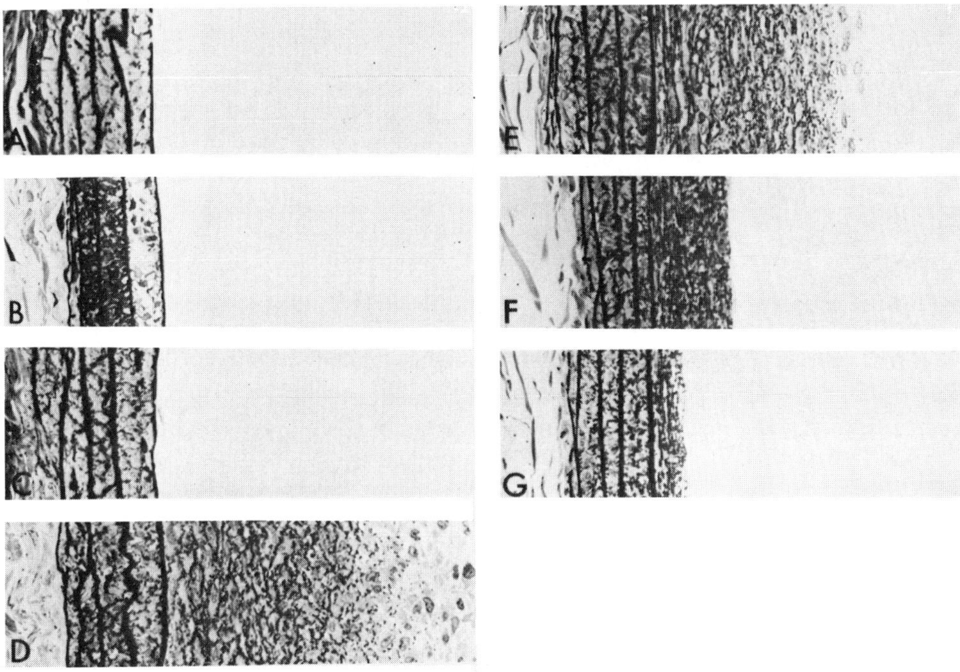

FIGURE 1. Histology of the arterial wall in response to EC injury. Composite histologic figure illustrating the changes occurring in the wall of the carotid artery after endothelial denudation. To aid comparison of intimal thickness at each stage, the elastic laminae of the media are aligned. The vessel lumen is at the right of each picture. This procedure stains EC rather lightly; thus they show up only faintly when photographed. (A) Normal vessel with flat endothelium; (B) central area of the segment 4 days after denudation, with loss of endothelium and showing prominent edema of the innermost zone of the media; (C) newly covered area 7 days after denudation, with plump EC and showing resolution of the medial edema; (D) central area of the segment 14 days after denudation, showing the massive extent of myointimal thickening; (E) central area at 17 days, showing a slight decrease in the thickness of the myointimal layer; (F) and (G) central area at 1 and 3 months, respectively, showing progressive regression of the thickened zone.

In many cases, considerable regression of the hyperplastic lesion had occurred by 1 to 3 months after the injury. Similar results have been obtained by others[11,12] in the aorta, using a balloon catheter-induced injury. This was the first clue we had that EC and/or other cells might produce growth effectors for SMC.

B. Heparin Blocks the Proliferative Response of SMC In Vivo

At about the time that the air-dry injury model was developed, Chen and Buchanan[13] reported that thrombin was mitogenic for certain cell types. Because the clotting sequence is activated in vascular injury, we tested the effect of heparin on the SMC hyperplasia in the rat carotid after the air-dry injury.[14] Heparin was continuously infused into control and injured animals via a catheter placed in the left jugular vein, with the tip lying in the superior vena cava. With this treatment, the SMC proliferation usually seen after EC injury was almost completely abolished (Figure 2). We found no effects of heparin on the number of circulating or deposited platelets or on their structure and degranulation. Neither the rate nor the extent of re-endothelialization was affected by heparin.

Although heparin had markedly suppressed myointimal proliferation, the original rationale — that the antiproliferative effect would be mediated by the antithrombin, anticoagulant activity of heparin — remained an unanswered question. With the sep-

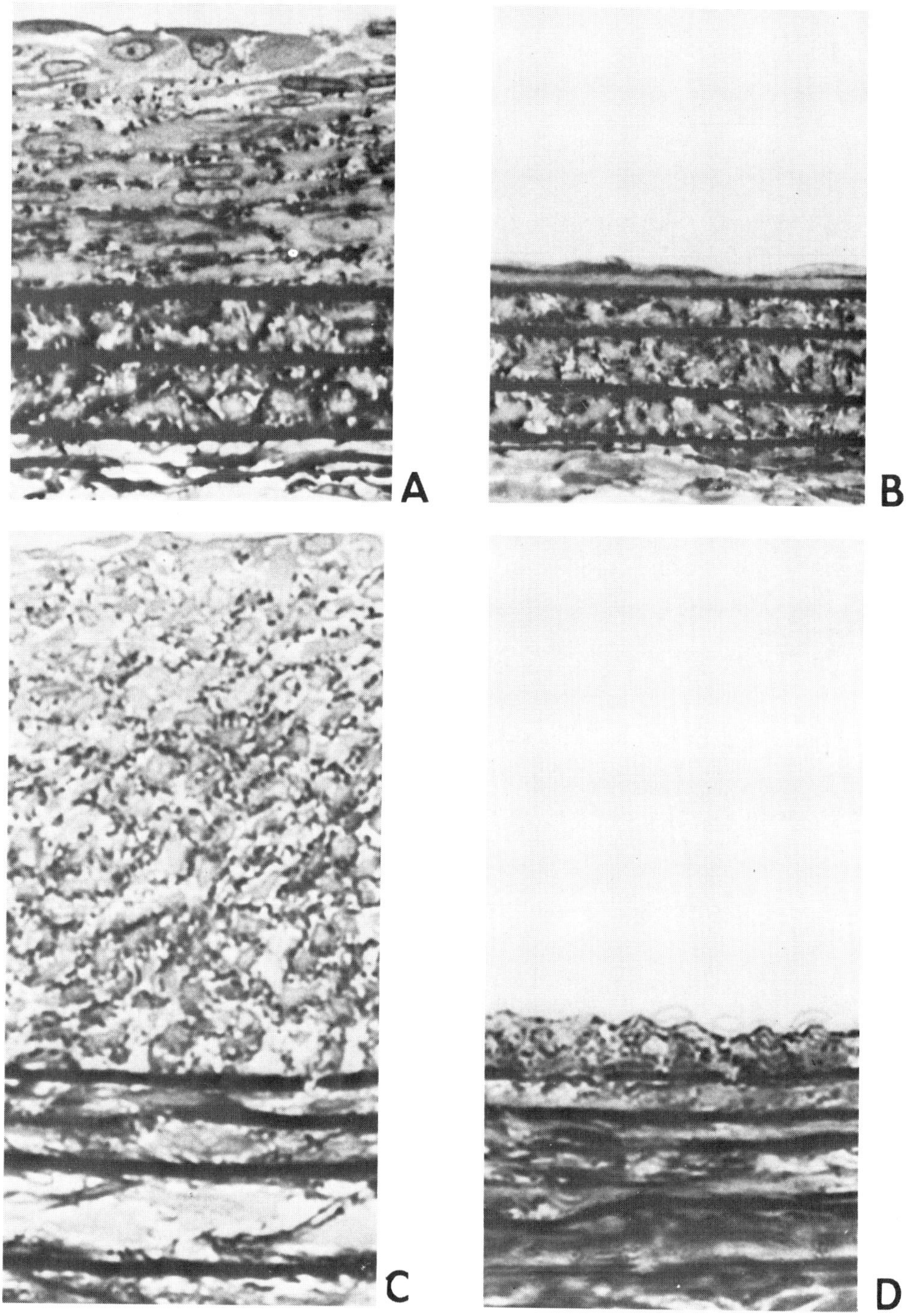

FIGURE 2. Effect of AC and NAC heparin on SMC proliferation following EC injury in vivo. Histological sections are shown of the central segments of air-dried rat carotid arteries 14 days after injury. (A) and (C) Control rats not treated with heparin — note the substantial myointimal proliferation in these animals; (B) rat treated with AC heparin (approximately 0.5 mg/kg/hr) in the same experiment as the rat in panel A — note the greatly reduced degree of myointimal thickening; (D) rat treated with NAC heparin (approximately 0.5 mg/kg/hr) in the same experiment as the rat in panel C — again, note the greatly reduced degree of myointimal thickening.

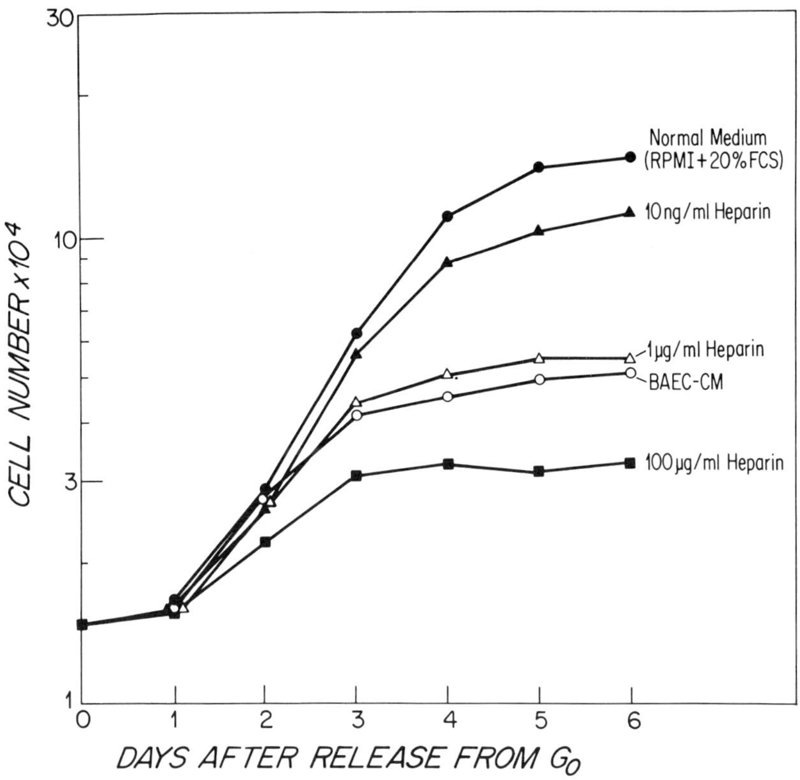

FIGURE 3. Effect of heparin and EC-conditioned medium on SMC growth. Sparsely plated rat aortic SMC were growth-arrested by serum deprivation in G_0. Control cultures were released from the G_0 block by placing them in their normal growth medium (RPMI + 20% fetal calf serum). These cells proliferate until they are confluent. Other cultures were placed in a 1:1 mixture of bovine aortic EC-conditioned medium and RPMI + fetal calf serum (final concentration, 20% fetal calf serum; BAEC-CM) or in RPMI + 20% fetal calf serum containing the indicated concentrations of heparin. Cell numbers were measured at daily intervals. The cells were not fed during the experiment. (From Castellot, J. J., Rosenberg, R. D., and Karnovsky, M. J., *Biology of Endothelial Cells*, Jaffe, E. A., Ed., Martinus Nijhoff, Boston, 1984, 118. With permission.)

aration of heparin into purified anticoagulant (AC) and nonanticoagulant (NAC) fractions by Rosenberg's group[15] and by Lindahl and his colleagues,[16] it now became possible to answer this question directly. In collaboration with Dr. Rosenberg and using his NAC heparin fraction, we repeated the infusion experiments.[17] It was clear that on a mass basis, NAC heparin was as effective as AC material in blocking SMC proliferation (Figure 2). Thus, the original rationale for trying heparin was wrong, and the discovery of the antiproliferative activity of heparin was quite serendipitous. We switched our attention to cultured SMC to characterize the antiproliferative activity of heparin.

C. Cultured SMC Are More Responsive to Heparin than Other Cell Types

To test the ability of heparin to inhibit the growth of cultured SMC, we first growth-arrested the cells at subconfluent densities by serum deprivation. This was done to more closely mimic the in vivo situation in which SMC normally exist in a quiescent growth state. The SMC were released from the growth-arrested (i.e., G_0) state by replacing the serum-poor medium with normal growth medium (containing 20% serum)

Table 1
SENSITIVITY OF VARIOUS CELL TYPES TO HEPARIN

Cell type	ED_{50} (μg/mℓ)
Rat aortic SMC	2
Rat mesenteric artery SMC	7
Calf aortic SMC	4
Cebus monkey aorta SMC	3
Human umbilical vein SMC	4
Canine tracheal SMC	80
Rat kidney glomerular mesangial cells	5
Baby hamster kidney fibroblasts (BHK)	500
Polyoma virus-transformed BHK	>800[a]
Swiss 3T3	>600[a]
BALB/c 3T3	500
Chinese hamster embryo fibroblasts (normal)	500
Chinese hamster embryo fibroblasts (transformed)	>600[a]
Madin-Darby canine kidney epithelial cells	200
Rat kidney epithelial cells	200
Bovine aortic endothelial cells	400
Rat epididymal endothelial cells	300
Mouse epididymal endothelial cells	200
Human umbilical vein endothelial cells	500

Note: The above cell types were growth-arrested and then exposed to a wide range of heparin concentrations (10 ng/mℓ to 1 mg/mℓ). Growth inhibition was determined by cell counts.

[a] An accurate ED_{50} could not be determined because cytotoxicity occurred above that concentration.

in the presence or absence of heparin. The antiproliferative effect was determined by counting cell number at various intervals after release from growth arrest. Heparin was very effective in suppressing the growth of cultured SMC[18,19] (Figure 3). The ED_{50} for the antiproliferative activity is in the 1- to 10-μg/mℓ range.

Many other cell types were examined for their responsiveness to heparin[20] (Table 1). Under these assay conditions, only SMC and related cell types (e.g., mesangial cells) were sensitive to heparin. NAC and AC heparins were found to be equally antiproliferative. There are numerous reports in the literature on the antiproliferative effect of heparin on various nonvascular cells, mostly fibroblasts (cf. Lippman and Mathews[21]). The dose required for 50% inhibition was very high, usually in the 1-mg/mℓ range, compared with 1- to 10-μg/mℓ doses needed for SMC. It should be pointed out that in these experiments, heparin was added to exponentially growing cultures. An interesting characteristic of our system is that SMC which are quiescent (i.e., in G_0) before their exposure to growth medium containing heparin are 50 to 100 times more sensitive to heparin than SMC which are exponentially growing at the time they are exposed. The possible explanations for this will be discussed later.

D. Other Glycosaminoglycans Do Not Inhibit SMC Growth

We used our inhibition assay to compare the effects of heparin and other classes of glycosaminoglycans as SMC antiproliferative agents.[19] Whereas AC and NAC heparins were highly potent and effective (50% inhibition at 1 to 10 μg/mℓ), other glycosaminoglycans such as dermatan sulfate, chondroitin sulfates A and C, and hyaluronic acid required at least 500 μg/mℓ doses to inhibit SMC growth by 50%.

E. EC Secrete a Heparin-Like Inhibitor of SMC Proliferation

In the air-dry model, the cessation of SMC hyperplasia in a particular region of the damaged segment was correlated with the re-endothelialization of that area, as discussed above. We therefore thought it possible that there was a regulatory influence of EC on SMC proliferation and undertook to examine this using cultured cells. Conditioned medium from confluent cultures of EC exerted a strong inhibitory effect on SMC released from G_0 (Figure 3).[19] Interestingly, exponentially growing EC produced a stimulatory effect on SMC growth, thus suggesting that cessation of EC growth after regeneration in vivo may be an important step in the regulation and inhibition of SMC proliferation. The mitogenic factor elaborated by EC has been explored in detail by others.[6]

Biochemical characterization[19] (Table 2) showed that the antiproliferative activity from EC was unaffected by heating and was also insensitive to proteases, hyaluronidases, and chondroitin sulfate ABC lyase. However, a highly purified Flavobacterium heparinase almost completely abolished the activity. This enzyme, which has no detectable activity against proteins or other glycosaminoglycans, degrades heparin into disaccharide and smaller fragments that lack inhibitory activity, as discussed later. In addition, a trichloroacetic acid-soluble, ethanol-insoluble glycosaminoglycan fraction prepared from EC-conditioned medium was highly antiproliferative. When this material was treated with the bacterial heparinase, the activity was abolished. Therefore, we concluded[19] that the inhibitory activity produced by EC under certain requisite conditions was a heparin-like molecule. The possibility that mast cell contamination of the primary cultures was contributing to the presence of antiproliferative heparin in the conditioned medium was ruled out by exhaustive cytochemical examination of the cultures.

We found that only SMC were sensitive to the inhibitory activity of EC-conditioned medium. In addition, media conditioned by a variety of other cell types had no effect on SMC proliferation. Thus, there appeared to be both target and producer cell specificity for the antiproliferative effect. Although we originally reported that conditioned medium from SMC did not affect SMC growth, recent work by Rosenberg and colleagues suggests that confluent, but not exponentially growing, SMC synthesize a highly antiproliferative heparin species.[22] This raises the interesting possibility of an autocrine regulatory mechanism operating in SMC that is mediated by heparin. The roles of EC- and SMC-derived heparin is an open question; one possibility is that there is an EC-SMC interaction in which EC-derived heparin acts as a "trigger" for SMC to begin synthesizing their own heparin.

The combination of in vivo and in vitro experiments described above provided a potential explanation for the findings of Rosenberg and Lindahl that more than half of the heparin molecules present in a typical preparation from beef lung or porcine intestine were devoid of anticoagulant activity and also suggested a new biological role for heparin as a growth regulator in the vascular wall. These studies also indicate a pharmacological rationale for the use of heparin that is discussed later.

III. STRUCTURE-FUNCTION STUDIES

A. The Minimum Effective Size of Antiproliferative Heparin is a Pentasaccharide

In collaboration with Rosenberg, we carried out experiments to establish what size molecule of heparin was effective in inhibiting SMC growth. Fragments of heparin were prepared by limit digest with nitrous acid, and discrete oligosaccharide fragments were separated by gel filtration chromatography.[23] The smallest heparin fragment with antiproliferative activity was a hexamer, whereas di- and tetrasaccharide fractions were inactive (Table 3). The maximum antiproliferative activity was obtained with dodeca-

Table 2
BIOCHEMICAL CHARACTERIZATION OF THE EC-DERIVED ANTIPROLIFERATIVE ACTIVITY

Treatment	Percent inhibition
None	68 ± 12
60°C, 30 min	63 ± 10
90°C, 5 min	62 ± 5
Trypsin (30 μg/mℓ, 2 h, 37°C)	60 ± 10
Chymotrypsin (30 μg/mℓ, 2 h, 37°C)	64 ± 8
Subtilisin (30 μg/mℓ, 60 min, 37°C)	57 ± 7
Hyaluronidase (15 U/mℓ, 90 min, 37°C)	60 ± 12
Chondroitin 80 ABC lyase (1 U/mℓ, 90 min, 37°C)	65 ± 6
Flavobacterium heparinase (10 U/mℓ, 90 min, 37°C)	15 ± 7

Note: Conditioned medium from confluent, primary bovine aortic EC was subjected to the indicated treatments and then assayed for its ability to inhibit rat SMC. The data is expressed as "percent inhibition". This number is obtained by first subtracting the starting cell from the cell number at the endpoint of the experiment (usually 5 to 7 days), when growth has essentially ceased in both control and conditioned medium-exposed cultures. The net growth is set at 100%, and the net growth in conditioned medium-treated cells is expressed as a percentage of the control. The difference is the percent inhibition.

mer and larger fragments — activities equivalent to native (i.e., commercial) heparin at equimolar doses.

The above experiments were very useful in defining the basic size parameters for the antiproliferative effect. However, the limitation of this approach is that the size fractions obtained by gel filtration, while relatively homogeneous with respect to the size and degree of sulfation, are quite heterogeneous with respect to the specific chemical structures within a size class. This problem has been successfully eliminated by Choay and colleagues, who undertook a massive project to synthesize heparin oligosaccharides from precisely defined monosaccharide units, thus yielding molecules of unambiguous structure.[24] After a 200-step process, Choay's laboratory had synthesized pentasaccharide heparin chains. In collaboration with this group, we tested several of these synthetic heparins in our SMC inhibition assay. A pentasaccharide molecule was found to have approximately the same antiproliferative activity as the hexasaccharide fraction obtained from gel filtration (Table 3). All the tetrasaccharides tested were almost completely inactive.[71]

Heparin interacts with several hemostatic enzymes. It appears that to maximally accelerate the inactivation of thrombin, factor IXa, and factor XIa by antithrombin III, a heparin molecule of at least 16 residues is required, although smaller fragments did have some ability to accelerate the factor Xa-antithrombin III reaction.[25] Thus it

Table 3
COMPARISON OF THE ANTIPROLIFERATIVE CAPACITY, ANTICOAGULANT ACTIVITY, AND DEGREE OF SULFATION OF HEPARIN DERIVATIVES

	Antiproliferative activity[a]		Anticoagulant activity[b]	Total sulfates[c]
	1 μg/mℓ	100 μg/mℓ		
Heparin (60 saccharides)	36	75	205	2.7
Disaccharide	0	4	0	1.8
Tetrasaccharide	2	12	0	2.3
Hexasaccharide	21	46	0	2.7
Octasaccharide	29	65	0	2.7
Decasaccharide	40	71	0	2.7
Dodecasaccharide	43	82	30	2.7
Choay pentasaccharide (with 3-O-sulfate)	18	47	0	3.2
Choay pentasaccharide (without 3-O-sulfate)	9	22	0	2.8
N-desulfated	10	18	0	1.4
N-desulfated; N-resulfated	41	82	62	2.3
N-desulfated; N-reacetylated	24	64	0	1.0
Totally desulfated	7	10	0	0
Totally desulfated; N-resulfated	15	26	0	1.0
Totally desulfated; N-reacetylated	3	12	0	0

[a] Percent inhibition of rat aortic SMC.
[b] USP units of thrombin inhibitory activity per milligram.
[c] Moles SO_4/moles glucosamine.

seems that for complete anticoagulant activity, heparin fragments of 16 residues or greater are needed, whereas maximum antiproliferative activity requires only a 12-saccharide heparin molecule.

B. Both N- and O-Sulfates Are Required for Antiproliferative Activity

To examine which chemical moieties were necessary for the antiproliferative effect, native heparin was chemically modified[26] (Table 3). Totally desulfated heparin lost all its inhibitory activity. The N-desulfated heparin lost most of its antiproliferative activity, as well as all its anticoagulant activity. Acetylation of the N-positions of the N-desulfated molecule restored much of the inhibitory potency, but did not restore the anticoagulant capacity. Because it is not possible chemically to directly O-desulfate heparin, this modification was approximated by first totally desulfating and then re-N-sulfating heparin. This derivative also lost most of its inhibitory potential.

These experiments indicated that O-sulfation, or at least a negative charge at the O-position, is necessary for the antiproliferative activity. The situation at the N-position is somewhat different. When the N-sulfates were removed, the N-position is positively charged, and the growth of SMC is not suppressed. Acetylation results in a neutral charge at the N-positions and restored the antiproliferative activity, suggesting that a negative charge at these positions is not required.

To more critically determine the precise molecular determinants of the antiproliferative effect, we have examined the ability of several synthetic heparins provided by

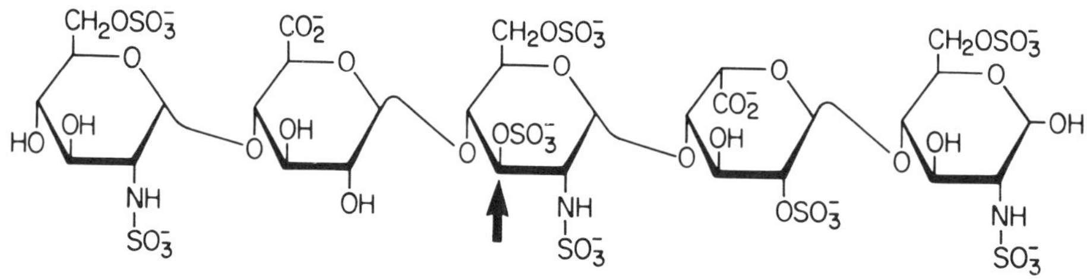

FIGURE 4. Structure of the Choay heparin pentasaccharide. Removal of the 3-O-sulfate denoted by the arrow results in almost complete loss of the antiproliferative activity (Table 3).

Choay to inhibit SMC proliferation. As discussed above, a pentasaccharide species was found to retain significant antiproliferative activity. When a pentasaccharide was synthesized lacking the 3-*O*-sulfate from the internal glucosamine residue, essentially all the antiproliferative activity was lost (Table 3; Figure 4), thus suggesting a critical role for this moiety.

The structure-function studies have a dual purpose: (1) to determine the molecular determinants of the capacity of heparin to inhibit SMC proliferation and (2) to provide molecules which have lost their anticoagulant ability but retain their antiproliferative effect. Such molecules may be potentially useful, as discussed later. Ideally, one would like to isolate heparin from EC or from EC-conditioned medium and chemically analyze it. However, the mass of heparin which can be obtained from either cultured or in vivo endothelium is quite small, and thus this approach has proven to be technically rather difficult. When the endogenous heparin species have been characterized, we speculate that the antiproliferative material from EC and SMC will be rich in the pentasaccharide sequences containing the 3-*O*-sulfate described above.

IV. BINDING AND INTERNALIZATION OF HEPARIN

A. Heparin Binds to Specific Sites on the SMC Surface

To begin to understand how heparin exerts its antiproliferative effect, we carried out studies on the binding and mode of internalization of heparin in heparin-sensitive cell types.[27] The binding of heparin to SMC, utilizing ^{125}I- and ^{3}H-heparin probes, is characterized by specific, saturable binding sites on the cell surface. The affinity ($K_d = 10^{-9}$ *M*) and number of binding sites (100,000 per cell) are typical of regulatory molecules with specific cell surface receptors.

Growth-arrested SMC bound eight times more heparin than exponentially growing cells. We had previously found that growth-arrested SMC were 50 to 100 times more sensitive to the growth inhibitory effect of heparin than exponential cultures;[19] part of this sensitivity may be due to the increased amount of heparin bound. One difference between proliferating and quiescent cells is that quiescent cells have much more cell surface fibronectin, a molecule which has heparin binding sites.[28] We cannot biochemically rule out the possibility of a heparin-fibronectin binding interaction as the reason for the increased heparin binding to quiescent SMC. However, fibronectin is present on the growth-arrested SMC surface in linear arrays, as revealed by indirect immunofluorescence (not shown), whereas heparin displays a diffuse binding pattern (Figure 5), thus making the possibility of a heparin-fibronectin interaction less likely as the explanation for the increased binding of heparin to quiescent SMC. In addition, the reduction in binding was due to the presence of fewer binding sites rather than to a

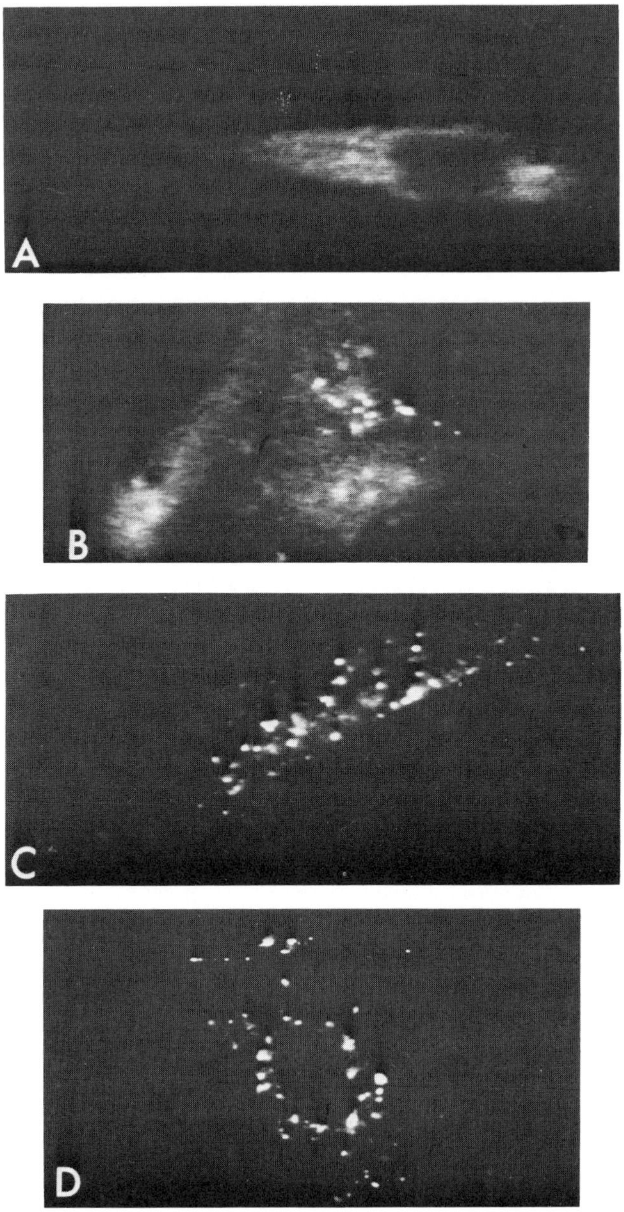

FIGURE 5. Binding and uptake of FITC-heparin. Growth-arrested SMC were exposed to 2 μg/mℓ FITC-heparin for 15 min at 4°C. The FITC-heparin was removed and the cells were placed in normal growth medium at 37°C for the times indicated below. They were then fixed and examined immediately using video image intensification fluorescence microscopy. (A) SMC fixed immediately at 4°C; (B) 2 min at 37°C; (C) 15 min at 37°C; (D) 2 hr at 37°C.

decreased affinity for the ligand, suggesting that a change in receptor number rather than the addition of a new component of binding (such as fibronectin) is responsible.

B. Heparin is Internalized by a Receptor-Mediated Endocytic Mechanism

Work from many laboratories has suggested that cells retrieve biologically important molecules from their environment by characteristic endocytic mechanisms. One of these modes of uptake which recently has been intensely studied is receptor-mediated endocytosis. Several types of ligands including α-2-macroglobulin,[29] low-density lipoprotein,[30] epidermal growth factor,[31] transferrin,[32] Semliki Forest virus,[33] and immunoglobulins[34] appear to follow this pathway, which functions in the delivery of ligands to the endosomal compartment.

We have used two approaches to study the mechanism of heparin uptake and its distribution in SMC. Utilizing FITC-heparin in conjunction with video image intensification fluorescence microscopy (Figure 5), we observed that FITC-heparin was bound to the cell surface at 4°C. Upon warming the cells to 37°C, the FITC-heparin formed surface clusters and was rapidly internalized in endocytic vesicles. These vesicles eventually became localized to the perinuclear region.

Analysis of radiolabeled heparin uptake revealed two distinct rates of uptake (Figure 6). There was an initial rapid entry of labeled heparin into SMC followed by a slow rate of uptake that occurred over several days. The $t_{1/2}$ for the initial rapid uptake phase was approximately 15 min. This is slower than the $t_{1/2}$ of 7 min observed for some receptor-mediated uptake systems,[30] but is comparable to the uptake rate for epidermal growth factor by hepatocytes in the perfused rat liver[35] and faster than the uptake of human chorionic gonadotropin in cultured granulosa cells.[36] The slow phase of uptake could be due to one or more of the following mechanisms: (1) nonfluid phase, nonreceptor-mediated (adsorptive) endocytosis; (2) fluid phase endocytosis, which would require that some of the bound heparin be slowly shed into the medium where it could be internalized by pinocytosis; and (3) receptor-mediated uptake which occurs by more than one rate-limiting mechanism. With regard to this last possibility, it is interesting to note that the biphasic uptake rate is observed even during continuous incubation of the cells with the ligand. This suggests that the rapid receptor-mediated uptake mechanism is saturated very quickly and then is down-regulated or otherwise rendered incompetent for days. The slow phase could then be due to a completely separate uptake mechanism, as just mentioned. Alternatively, the slow phase may represent the rate of reutilization or insertion of new functional receptors into the membrane.

The presence of high-affinity heparin binding sites on the SMC surface, combined with the rapid initial internalization and the pattern of FITC-heparin uptake, strongly suggests that this glycosaminoglycan can enter SMC via receptor-mediated endocytosis. Several other reports on the uptake of glycosaminoglycans by cultured cells exist.[37-39] However, in most cases heparin uptake was not studied, and quantitative measurements of both binding and uptake were not made. In addition, these studies were carried out before receptor-mediated endocytosis was recognized; thus the role of this important internalization mechanism was not examined.

In preliminary experiments, we have observed heparin degradation products in SMC at both early (1 hr) and late (18 hr) time points. However, the techniques for measurement of heparin degradation are not as straightforward as the methods for measuring protein degradation, and more work is needed to clarify this important point.

To our knowledge, these studies provide the first evidence for receptor-mediated endocytosis of a glycosaminoglycan. The radiolabeled and fluorescent heparin probes should prove very useful in answering a number of important questions, including the metabolic fate of the internalized heparin, degradation and recycling of the heparin receptors, and the relationship between the binding and uptake of heparin and its antiproliferative activity.

V. EFFECTS OF HEPARIN ON SMC METABOLISM

A. Heparin Blocks SMC in Late G_1 Phase or at the G_1/S Boundary

Flow microfluorimetric analysis of cell cycle distribution of heparin-treated SMC[20]

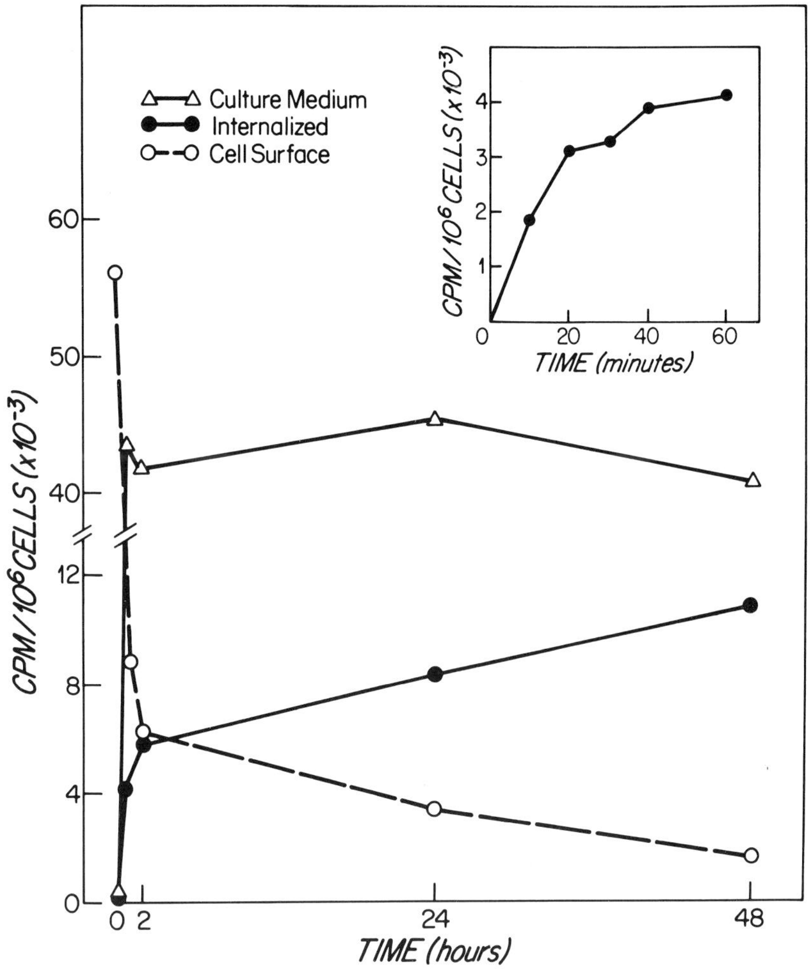

FIGURE 6. Uptake of radiolabeled heparin by SMC. Growth-arrested SMC were incubated in ^{3}H-heparin (13 μg/mℓ, 2×10^6 CPM per sample) for 60 min at 4°C. The cells were washed five times in ice-cold buffer and then warmed to 37°C. At the indicated times, the supernatant (Δ) was harvested and processed for scintillation counting as described. The cells were washed three times and then incubated in a 100-fold excess of unlabeled heparin for 60 min. This was followed by exposure to trypsin (50 μg/mℓ for 15 min). Heparin-displaceable and trypsin-releasable counts were pooled to give total surface counts (O). The cells (•) were solubilized in sodium hydroxide and processed for scintillation counting. The counts obtained from this sample were considered to be inside the cell.

revealed that heparin blocked either the $G_0 \rightarrow S$ transit or a very early S phase event in SMC (Figure 7). The $G_0 \rightarrow S$ transit can be functionally divided into two phases: (1) the competence phase, in which factors such as PDGF stimulate cells to leave the G_0 state and become "competent" to traverse the rest of G_1; (2) the progression phase, in which competent cells move through the rest of G_1 and enter S phase.[40] The progression phase requires a good supply of nutrients such as amino acids and appears to be mediated by factors such as somatomedins and steroids. In addition to the effect of heparin on the $G_0 \rightarrow S$ transition, a small but consistent increase in the G_2 compartment was observed in heparin-treated cells. Whether this represents true G_2 cells or tetraploid G_1 cells is not known.

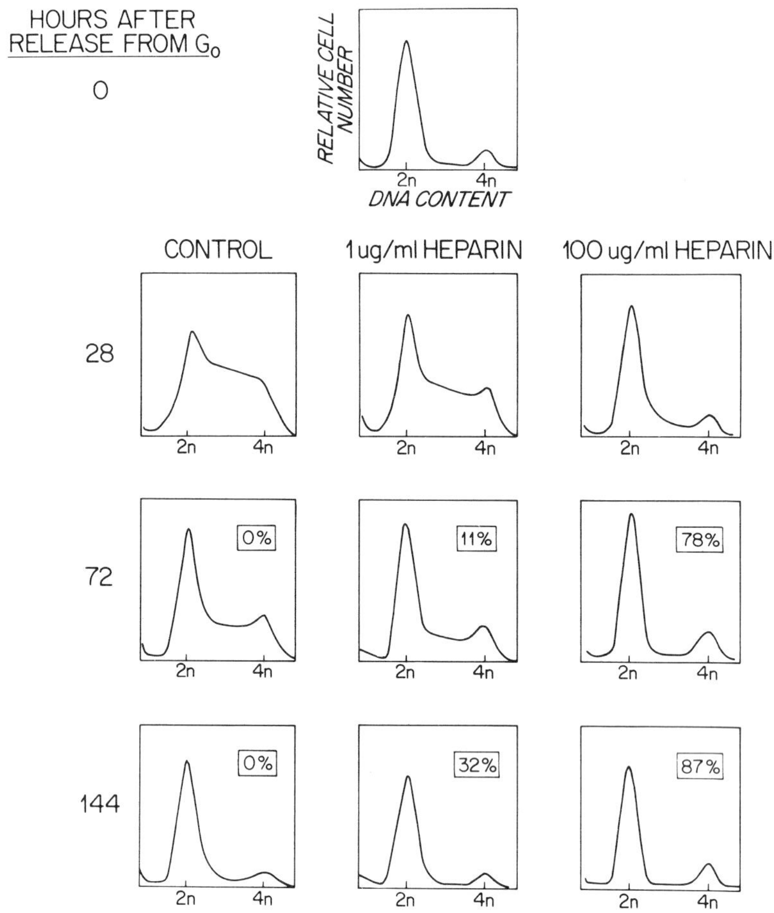

FIGURE 7. Flow microfluorimetric cell cycle analysis of heparin-treated SMC. Rat aortic SMC were growth-arrested and then exposed to normal growth medium with or without the indicated concentrations of heparin. At the indicated intervals, the cells were harvested and processed for flow microfluorimetry. Replicate cultures were harvested for cell counting, and the percent inhibition of growth was determined. DNA histograms are displayed for selected time points to demonstrate the relationship between the different cell cycle compartments and the antiproliferative effect of heparin. Note that at high concentrations of heparin, very few cells leave the growth-arrested state and reenter the cell cycle.

PDGF is a strongly cationic polypeptide that can bind avidly to anionic molecules like heparin. Because PDGF is a potent mitogen for SMC, it was important to determine whether heparin blocked the $G_0 \rightarrow S$ transition via an interaction with PDGF. We therefore determined how long after release from G_0 heparin could be added and still inhibit SMC growth (Figure 8). Heparin could be added up to 18 hr after serum stimulation with little or no loss of its antiproliferative effect. At 24 hr and later time points, however, heparin rapidly lost its ability to block SMC growth. The effectiveness of heparin, even when added 18 hr after serum stimulation, suggests strongly that it does not affect the competence phase. This makes the possibility that heparin inhibits growth via a direct interaction with PDGF highly unlikely, especially since this mitogen has been shown to exert its growth-promoting effect within 60 min after its addition to cells.[40] The loss of the antiproliferative effect after 18 hr of serum stimulation coincides

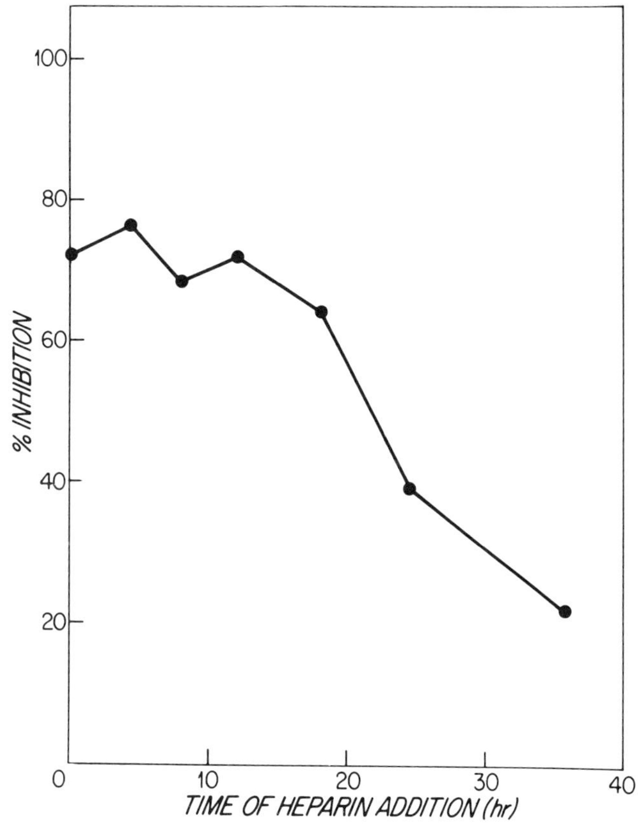

FIGURE 8. Kinetic analysis of heparin on the $G_0 \rightarrow S$ transit. Growth-arrested rat aortic SMC were released from the block by placing them in normal growth medium. At the indicated times after release from G_0, heparin was added to some cultures (final concentration, 100 μg/mℓ). Cell number was determined 7 days after heparin addition. Time points longer than 36 hr were not used because cell division occurs after this time, making interpretation of growth inhibition data difficult.

with the time that the cells are beginning to enter S-phase and provides additional evidence for the hypothesis that heparin is an antiprogression factor.

B. Heparin Inhibits DNA and RNA Synthesis, but not Protein Synthesis, Probably via Blocking Uptake of the Nucleoside Precursors

We determined the effect of heparin on DNA, RNA, and protein synthesis using standard metabolic labeling techniques.[20] SMC were growth-arrested and then released from the G_0 block by placing them in normal growth medium with or without heparin. At various intervals after release from G_0, cells were pulsed for 60 min with the appropriate radiolabeled precursor. The rates of macromolecular synthesis were determined by the incorporation of label into trichloroacetic acid-insoluble material. Immediate effects of heparin on DNA and RNA synthesis were observed, while protein synthesis was unaffected. Both DNA and RNA synthesis were inhibited by 60 to 80% within minutes after adding heparin.

Because of this rapid inhibition of nucleic acid synthesis, we considered the possibility that heparin could be blocking synthesis of these macromolecules by inhibiting

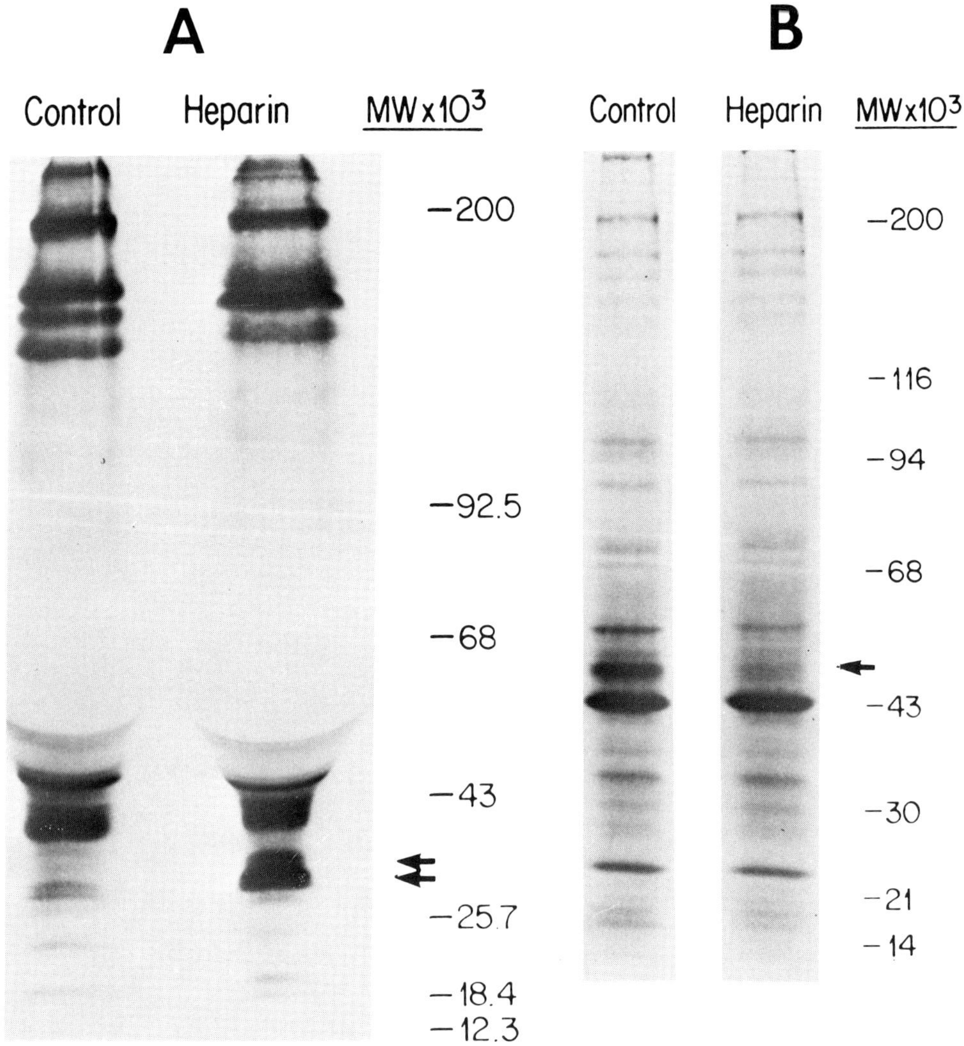

FIGURE 9. Alterations in specific protein synthesis by heparin. Proteins synthesized by serum-stimulated rat aortic SMC 4 hr after release from G_0 in the presence and absence of 100 μg/mℓ heparin were labeled with ^{35}S-methionine and examined by SDS polyacrylamide gel electrophoresis. Note the induction of a doublet in the 35-kdalton region in the culture medium of heparin-treated cells (A, heavy arrows). Also note the disappearance of a 48-kdalton protein in the substrate-attached material of heparin-treated SMC (B, heavy arrow).

uptake of the radiolabeled precursors. Using standard methods for measuring metabolite uptake into cells, we found that heparin inhibited thymidine and uridine uptake by 70 to 80% in SMC.[20] This degree of inhibition is sufficient to account entirely for the observed decrease in DNA and RNA synthesis. Aminoisobutyric acid (a leucine analog) and 3-*O*-methylglucose (a glucose analog) transport was unaffected by heparin. These metabolites were used because they are transported but not further metabolized by cells. In the case of thymidine and uridine, controls were performed to ensure that the radioactivity measured in the uptake assays was not due to incorporation of the metabolites into macromolecules by comparing trichloroacetic acid-soluble and trichloroacetic acid-insoluble counts. Less than 2% of the internalized metabolites were incorporated into macromolecules at the end of the assay period. Although a causal relationship, if any, between the inhibition of nucleoside uptake and the antiproliferative effect of heparin has not been established, this effect of heparin may provide valuable clues to the molecular mechanisms controlling the antiproliferative action of heparin. In addition, these two activities share many characteristics of biological and chemical specificity: (1) the effect is reversible, (2) the effect is specific for SMC, (3) AC and NAC heparin are equally effective, (4) the effect is lost with time in culture, (5) the effect is growth state specific, and (6) heparin is the most potent glycosaminoglycan in producing the effect.

C. Heparin Induces and Represses the Synthesis of Specific Proteins

Although the experiments described previously showed that overall rates of protein synthesis were not affected by heparin, we considered the possibility that heparin could selectively alter the synthesis of specific proteins.[41] SMC from rat aorta, rat mesenteric artery, and Cebus monkey aorta were first growth-arrested and then released from the G_0 block by placing them in normal growth medium with or without heparin. At intervals ranging from 0 to 144 hr after release, the cells were pulsed for 2 hr with ^{35}S-methionine. Incorporation of label into acid-insoluble pools was determined for the following pools: (1) *culture medium* was removed and added to a cocktail containing several protease inhibitors; protein was precipitated with 10% trichloroacetic acid, and the insoluble proteins were dissolved in 4% sodium dodecyl sulfate (SDS) for 5 min at 37°C; (2) *cells* were washed three times with buffer containing protease inhibitors and then removed from the dish by the addition of 1.0 m*M* EGTA with gentle rocking for 30 to 45 min at 37°C; and (3) *substrate-attached material* was prepared by adding 4% SDS to the culture dishes after the cells had been removed; the dishes were incubated with gentle rocking for 1 hr at 37°C and scraped with a rubber policeman.

We detected the induction into the culture medium of a pair of acidic (pI 5.0 to 5.5) proteins of approximately 35 kdaltons in heparin-treated SMC[41] (Figure 9). The induction of the 35-kdalton proteins was inhibited by actinomycin D, and was not affected by treatment with collagenase. Many characteristics of this protein alteration parallel the growth inhibitory property of heparin, including the reversibility, target cell specificity, glycosaminoglycan specificity, effectiveness of NAC heparin, growth state specificity, and loss of effect with time in culture. Furthermore, heparin caused a transient suppression of a 48-kdalton substrate-attached protein. We have not characterized this protein as extensively as the 35-kdalton proteins, but the 48-kdalton protein also appears to be noncollagenous and is most effectively suppressed by heparin compared to other glycosaminoglycans. Recently, Majack and Bornstein[42] have observed the induction of a novel 60-kdalton collagen in the cell fraction of heparin-treated SMC. They have also detected a pair of 37-kdalton proteins in the culture medium of heparin-treated SMC.[43] While it is quite likely that the 35- and 37-kdalton culture medium proteins are the same, to date this has not been directly established. It must be noted that, as is the case for the inhibition of nucleoside uptake, a direct relationship between these specific protein changes and the antiproliferative activity of heparin has not been proven.

The above findings demonstrate that heparin can both induce and suppress the synthesis of specific proteins. The fact that an inhibitor of cell growth can alter the synthesis of selected excreted and intracellular proteins may provide an important communications mechanism for coordinating growth within the vascular wall.

D. Heparin Inhibits Growth of Glomerular Mesangial Cells In Vivo and In Vitro

The glomerular mesangial cell is closely related to the vascular SMC by several criteria, including contractility,[44] ultrastructure,[45] and the presence of SMC-specific myosin.[46] Because this cell proliferates abnormally in certain kidney diseases, we tested the ability of heparin to inhibit the growth of this cell type in vivo and in vitro.

Using Habu snake venom to induce glomerular injury and subsequent mesangial hyperplasia,[47,48] we found that the administration of AC heparin beginning 18 hr after Habu venom resulted in a dramatic decrease in the percentage of injured glomeruli with mesangial cell proliferation. NAC heparin was only partially effective; the reasons for this are not yet known, but could be due to inherent differences in antiproliferative mechanism, inherent differences between mesangial and SMC, or to altered metabolism and clearance of AC and NAC heparins. Olson, using a renal ablation model for kidney injury, also found that heparin protected against such injury,[49] although a direct effect on mesangial cells was not determined.

Cultured mesangial cells were also inhibited by heparin.[50] The antiproliferative effect on these cells was similar to SMC in that the effect was reversible and it was also specific for heparin. Unlike the in vivo situation, cultured mesangial were inhibited by NAC heparin. Interestingly, glomerular epithelial cells were found to secrete a heparin-like inhibitor of mesangial cell growth.[50] In addition, a peptide inhibitor was also excreted by these cells. To make the analogy to the vascular wall more complete, the epithelial cells also secreted a mitogen for mesangial cells. Depending on the precise culture and postcollection treatment conditions, either the inhibitory or the growth-promoting effect can predominate. Much more work is needed to fully understand the precise interrelationships between the growth effectors operating in this system.

VI. A MODEL FOR GROWTH REGULATION IN THE VASCULAR WALL

Based on the results described above, we have postulated that heparin or heparin-like molecules may function as physiological growth regulators in the vascular wall (see also Chapter 4). In the normal, healthy vessel heparin is secreted by EC, SMC, or both into the extracellular matrix, where it functions to help maintain SMC in a quiescent growth state. When the endothelium is damaged, this growth control mechanism is lost, and the medial SMC react to the presence of mitogens by migrating into the intima and proliferating. A key point in this hypothesis is that SMC will not respond to PDGF, macrophage, or other mitogens in the presence of heparin. Indeed, we have recently shown[51] that macrophages from hypercholesterolemic rats strongly stimulate the proliferation of SMC. This effect is abolished by heparin. Therefore, heparin present in the arterial wall must be degraded or otherwise inactivated before SMC can undergo the hyperplastic response. There are at least four possible mechanisms for overcoming the antiproliferative effect of heparin, none of them mutually exclusive: (1) damage to or loss of endothelium may remove one source of heparin; (2) endoglycosidases released from platelets adhering to the injured site or from SMC might cleave cell-bound or matrix-bound heparin into soluble fragments that would be diluted or washed away because endothelial damage has removed a physical barrier to increased hydraulic flux; support for this mechanism comes from studies in our laboratory[52] showing that an endoglycosidase isolated from platelets[53] is capable of cleaving heparin from the EC surface in vitro; (3) the local concentration of mitogens may be so high that SMC can proliferate despite the presence of heparin-like species; and (4) other molecules which have a high affinity for heparin, such as Platelet Factor IV, could inactivate heparin in situ; the observations that Platelet Factor IV penetrates into an injured region in vivo[54] and that this substance blocks the antiproliferative effect of heparin in vitro[72] lend credence to this possibility. When the injured area is re-endothelialized, SMC proliferation appears to cease. This might be due to the elaboration of heparin by EC.

Until now, most of the results discussed were obtained in our laboratory. However, many other investigators have provided experimental support for the above model. For example, Benitz et al.[55] have recently demonstrated that heparin is a potent inhibitor of vascular SMC isolated from fetal pulmonary artery. The characteristics of the inhibition of this SMC type is similar to the inhibition of other types of vascular SMC. These findings may have important implications for the treatment of primary fetal hypertension.

Several laboratories[56-58] have shown that EC secrete heparan sulfates (the class of glycosaminoglycan to which heparin belongs). About half of all the glycosaminoglycans synthesized by EC are heparin sulfates secreted into the culture medium. In addition, the heparan sulfates made by EC were more heparin-like (i.e., more highly sulfated) than the heparan sulfates made by SMC. In contrast to EC, SMC and fibroblasts secrete only about 10% of their complex carbohydrates as heparan sulfates.[59,60]

Other observations implicate heparin-like species and EC as growth regulators in the arterial wall. Eisenstein et al.[61] prepared fractions of bovine aorta extracts and tested their ability to alter the growth of cultured SMC. Both positive and negative growth effects were observed. One of the fractions that inhibited SMC growth contained a heparin-like molecule. It has not been shown that this inhibitory activity was actually mediated by heparin, but in light of our previous results, it is possible that the active material in this fraction of the aortic extract was indeed heparin.

Changes in the glycosaminoglycans of arteries after experimentally induced injury have been reported by several groups,[62-65] and these observations are generally supportive of our hypothesis. Wight et al.[65] carried out careful biochemical analyses of the glycosaminoglycan profile in rabbit aortic intimas after endothelial denudation. Areas that had been reendothelialized accumulated much more glycosaminoglycan than nonendothelialized regions. Most of this accumulation consisted of heparan and chondroitin sulfates. Although the source of the heparan sulfate could not be determined, their results implicate EC in influencing both the amount and class of complex carbohydrate present in the arterial intima.

Ausprunk and her collaborators[66,67] have reported on the ultrastructural localization of glycosaminoglycans in both actively proliferating and quiescent microvascular beds in the rabbit eye. These investigators used ruthenium red to stain complex carbohydrates combined with selective degradation by glycosaminoglycan-degrading enzymes. They found that in actively developing vascular beds the predominant species was hyaluronic acid. In contrast, in quiescent vascular beds the predominant species were heparan sulfates that were found surrounding the SMC, as well as on the abluminal side of the EC. These observations in small vessels are consistent with the putative role of heparin-like molecules in regulating SMC growth in large vessels because the heparan sulfates were found under the quiescent EC and around the SMC; they also suggest that the growth state of EC — proliferative vs. quiescent — plays a crucial role in determining the amount of heparan sulfate present. Conceptually, this agrees with our own data, in which we have shown that confluent, but not proliferating, EC produce a heparin-like inhibitor of SMC.

Another example of the potential relationship between heparin-like compounds and the cessation of growth comes from the work of Bernfield and colleagues on the development of embryonic mouse salivary and mammary tissue.[68,69] In these systems, the predominant glycosaminoglycan in proliferating regions of the tissue is hyaluronic acid, whereas in terminally differentiated regions the major species are heparan sulfates. It is possible that the accumulation of heparin-like species is a control mechanism in development.

VII. POTENTIAL CLINICAL USES OF NAC HEPARIN

The development of NAC, antiproliferative heparin analogs may have clinical significance. A substantial number (perhaps 15%) of vascular surgical procedures such as grafts, shunts, bypasses, angioplasties, and endarterectomies fail within a year, apparently due to SMC proliferation.[70] These surgical failures might be preventable by treating patients with NAC, antiproliferative heparin compounds, thus avoiding hemorrhagic complications. In addition, such heparin derivatives might be useful in the treatment of primary fetal hypertension, the most common cardiovascular defect in newborns, and in the treatment of certain kidney diseases which are characterized by the proliferation of mesangial cells.

REFERENCES

1. Schwartz, S. M., Gajdusek, C. M., and Owens, G. K., Vessel growth control, in *Pathobiology of the Endothelial Cell,* Nossel, H. L. and Vogel, H. T., Eds., Academic Press, New York, 1982, 63.
2. Ross, R., Glomset, J., Kariya, B., and Harker, L., A platelet-dependent serum factor that stimulates the proliferation of arterial smooth muscle cells in vitro, *Proc. Natl. Acad. Sci. U.S.A.,* 71, 1207, 1974.
3. Grotendorst, G. R., Seppa, H. E. J., Kleinman, H. K., and Martin, G. R., Attachment of smooth muscle cells to collagen and their migration toward platelet-derived growth factor, *Proc. Natl. Acad. Sci. U.S.A.,* 78, 3669, 1981.
4. Greenberg, G. B. and Hunt, T. K., The proliferative response in vitro of vascular endothelial and smooth muscle cells exposed to wound fluids and macrophages, *J. Cell. Physiol.,* 97, 353, 1978.
5. Martin, B. M., Gimbrone, M. A., Unanue, F. R., and Cotran, R. S., Stimulation of nonlymphoid mesenchymal cell proliferation by a macrophage-derived growth factor, *J. Immunol.,* 126, 1510, 1981.
6. Gajdusek, C. M., DiCorleto, P., Ross, R., and Schwartz, S. M., An endothelial cell-derived growth factor, *J. Cell Biol.,* 85, 467, 1980.
7. Fishman, J. A., Ryan, G. B., and Karnovsky, M. J., Endothelial regeneration in the rat carotid artery and the significance of endothelial denudation in the pathogenesis of myointimal thickening, *Lab. Invest.,* 32, 339, 1975.
8. Moore, S., Thromboatherosclerosis in normolipemic rabbits. A result of continued endothelial damage, *Lab. Invest.,* 29, 478, 1973.
9. Poole, J. C. F., Cromwell, S. B., and Benditt, E. P., Behavior of smooth muscle cells and formation of extracellular structures in the reaction of arterial walls to injury, *Am. J. Pathol.,* 62, 391, 1970.
10. Ross, R. and Glomset, J. A., Atherosclerosis and the arterial smooth muscle cell, *Science,* 180, 1332, 1973.
11. Spaet, T. H., Stemerman, M. B., Veith, F. J., and Lejnieks, I., Intimal injury and regrowth in the rabbit aorta: medial smooth muscles as a source of neointima, *Circ. Res.,* 36, 58, 1975.
12. Schwartz, S. M., Haudenschild, C. C., and Eddy, E. M., Endothelial regerneration. I. Quantitative analysis of initial stages of endothelial regeneration in rat aortic intima, *Lab. Invest.,* 38, 568, 1978.
13. Chen, L. B. and Buchanan, J. M., Mitogenic activity of blood components. I. Thrombin and prothrombin, *Proc. Natl. Acad. Sci. U.S.A.,* 72, 131, 1975.
14. Clowes, A. W. and Karnovsky, M. J., Suppression by heparin of smooth muscle cell proliferation in injured arteries, *Nature (London),* 265, 625, 1977.
15. Lam, L. H., Silbert, J. E., and Rosenberg, R. D., The separation of active and inactive forms of heparin, *Biochem. Biophys. Res. Commun.,* 69, 570, 1976.
16. Hook, M., Bjork, I., Hopwood, J., and Lindahl, U., Anticoagulant activity of heparin: separation of high activity and low activity species by affinity chromatography on immobilized antithrombin, *FEBS Lett.,* 69, 51, 1976.
17. Guyton, J. R., Rosenberg, R. D., Clowes, A. W., and Karnovsky, M. J., Inhibition of rat arterial smooth muscle cell proliferation by heparin. In vivo studies with anticoagulant and non-anticoagulant heparin, *Circ. Res.,* 46, 625, 1980.
18. Hoover, R. L., Rosenberg, R. D., Haering, W., and Karnovsky, M. J., Inhibition of rat arterial smooth muscle cell proliferation by heparin. II. In vitro studies, *Circ. Res.,* 47, 578, 1980.

19. Castellot, J. J., Addonizio, M. L., Rosenberg, R. D., and Karnovsky, M. J., Cultured endothelial cells produce a heparin-like inhibitor of smooth muscle cell growth, *J. Cell Biol.*, 90, 372, 1981.
20. Castellot, J. J., Cochran, D. L., and Karnovsky, M. J., Effect of heparin on vascular smooth muscle cells. I. Cell metabolism, *J. Cell. Physiol.*, 124, 21, 1985.
21. Lippman, M. and Mathews, M. B., Heparins: varying effects on cell proliferation in vitro and lack of correlation with anticoagulant activity, *Fed. Proc.*, 36, 55, 1977.
22. Fritze, I. M. S., Reilly, C. F., and Rosenberg, R. D., An antiproliferative heparan sulfate species produced by post-confluent smooth muscle cells, *J. Cell Biol.*, 100, 1041, 1985.
23. Oosta, G. M., Gardner, W. T., Beeler, D. L., and Rosenberg, R. D., Multiple functional domains of the heparin molecule, *Proc. Natl. Acad. Sci. U.S.A.*, 78, 829, 1981.
24. Choay, J., Petitou, M., Lormeau, J. C., Sinay, P., Casu, B., and Gatti, G., Structure-function relationships in heparin: a synthetic pentasaccharide with high affinity for antithrombin III and eliciting high anti-factor Xa activity, *Biochem. Biophys. Res. Commun.*, 116, 492, 1983.
25. Kazatchkine, M. D., Fearon, D. T., Metcalfe, D. D., Rosenberg, R. D., and Austen, K. F., Structural determinants of the capacity of heparin to inhibit formation of the human amplification C3 convertase, *J. Clin. Invest.*, 67, 223, 1981.
26. Castellot, J. J., Beeler, D. L., Rosenberg, R. D., and Karnovsky, M. J., Structural determinants of the capacity of heparin to inhibit the proliferation of vascular smooth muscle cells, *J. Cell. Physiol.*, 120, 315, 1984.
27. Castellot, J. J., Wong, K., Herman, B., Hoover, R. L., Albertini, D. F., Wright, T. C., Caleb, B. L., and Karnovsky, M. J., Binding and internalization of heparin by vascular smooth muscle cells, *J. Cell. Physiol.*, 124, 13, 1985.
28. Yamada, K. M., Cell surface interactions with extracellular materials, *Annu. Rev. Biochem.*, 52, 761, 1983.
29. Pastan, I. H. and Willingham, M. C., Journey to the center of the cell: role of the receptosome, *Science*, 214, 504, 1981.
30. Brown, M. S. and Goldstein, J. L., Receptor-mediated endocytosis: insights from the lipoprotein receptor system, *Proc. Natl. Acad. Sci. U.S.A.*, 76, 3330, 1979.
31. Carpenter, G. and Cohen, S., ^{125}I-labeled human epidermal growth factor: binding, internalization and degradation in human fibroblasts, *J. Cell Biol.*, 71, 159, 1976.
32. Karin, M. and Mintz, B., Receptor-mediated endocytosis of transferrin in developmentally totipotent mouse teratocarcinoma stem cells, *J. Biol. Chem.*, 256, 3245, 1981.
33. Helenius, A., Kartenbeck, J., Simons, K., and Fries, E., On the entry of Semliki Forest virus into BHK-21 cells, *J. Cell Biol.*, 84, 404, 1980.
34. Salisbury, J. L., Condeelis, J. S., and Satir, P., Role of coated vesicles, microfilaments, and calmodulin in receptor-mediated endocytosis of cultured B lymphoblastoid cells, *J. Cell Biol.*, 87, 132, 1980.
35. Dunn, W. A. and Hubbard, A. L., Receptor-mediated endocytosis of epidermal growth factor by hepatocytes in the perfused rat liver: ligand and receptor dynamics, *J. Cell Biol.*, 98, 2148, 1984.
36. Robinson, M. S., Rhodes, J. A., and Albertini, D. F., Slow internalization of human chorionic gonadotropin by cultured granulosa cells, *J. Cell. Physiol.*, 117, 43, 1984.
37. Saito, H. and Uzman, B. G., Uptake of chondroitin sulfate by mammalian cells in culture, *Exp. Cell Res.*, 66, 97, 1971.
38. Kresse, H., Tekolf, W., von Figura, K., and Buddecke, E., Metabolism of sulfated glycosaminoglycans in cultivated bovine arterial cells. II. Quantitative studies on the uptake of $^{35}SO_4$-labeled proteoglycans, *Hoppe-Seyler's Z. Physiol. Chem.*, 356, 943, 1975.
39. Wasteson, A., Lindahl, U., and Hallen, A., Mode of degradation of the chondroitin sulfate proteoglycan in rat costal cartilage, *Biochem. J.*, 130, 729, 1972.
40. Pledger, W. J., Stiles, C., Antoniades, H., and Scher, C., Induction of DNA synthesis in Balb/c3T3 cells by serum components: reevaluation of the commitment process, *Proc. Natl. Acad. Sci. U.S.A.*, 74, 4481, 1977.
41. Cochran, D. L., Castellot, J. J., and Karnovsky, M. J., Effect of heparin on vascular smooth muscle cells. II. Specific protein synthesis, *J. Cell. Physiol.*, 124, 29, 1985.
42. Majack, R. A. and Bornstein, P., Heparin-like glycosaminoglycans regulate the phenotype of cultured vascular smooth muscle cells. Induced synthesis of a novel short chain collagen, *J. Cell Biol.*, 97, 2a, 1983.
43. Majack, R. A. and Bornstein, P., Heparin and related glycosaminoglycans modulate the secretory phenotype of vascular smooth muscle cells, *J. Cell Biol.*, 99, 1688, 1984.

44. Ausiello, D. A., Kreisberg, J. I., Roy, C., and Karnovsky, M. J., Contraction of cultured rat glomerular mesangial cells after stimulation with angiotensin II and arginine vasopressin, *J. Clin. Invest.*, 65, 754, 1980.
45. Latta, H. and Maunsbach, A. B., Relations of the centrolobular region of the glomerulus to the juxtaglomerular apparatus, *J. Ultrastruct. Res.*, 6, 563, 1962.
46. Harper, P. A., Robinson, J. M., Hoover, R. L., Wright, T. C., and Karnovsky, M. J., Improved methods for culturing rat glomerular cells, *Kidney Int.*, 26, 91, 1984.
47. Bradfield, J. W. B. and Cattell, V., The mesangial cell in glomerulonephritis. I. Mechanisms of hypercellularity in experimental immune complex disease, *Lab. Invest.*, 36, 481, 1977.
48. Coffey, A. K. and Karnovsky, M. J., Heparin inhibits mesangial cell proliferation in Habu venom induced glomerular injury, *Am. J. Pathol.*, 120, 248, 1985.
49. Olson, J. L., Role of heparin as a protective agent following reduction of renal mass, *Kidney Int.*, 25, 376, 1984.
50. Castellot, J. J., Harper, P. A., Hoover, R. L., and Karnovsky, M. J., Glomerular epithelial cells secrete a heparin-like inhibitor of mesangial cell proliferation, *Am. J. Pathol.*, 120, 427, 1985.
51. Karnovsky, M. J., Castellot, J. J., Robinson, J. M., and Hoover, R. L., Properties of macrophages from hypercholesterolemic rats, *J. Cell Biol.*, 99, 327a, 1984.
52. Castellot, J. J., Favreau, L., Rosenberg, R. D., and Karnovsky, M. J., Inhibition of vascular smooth muscle cell growth by endothelial cell-derived heparin: possible role of platelet endoglycosidase, *J. Biol. Chem.*, 257, 11256, 1982.
53. Oosta, G. M., Favreau, L., and Rosenberg, R. D., Purification and properties of a platelet endoglycosidase, *J. Biol. Chem.*, 257, 11249, 1982.
54. Goldberg, I. D., Stemerman, M. B., and Handin, R. I., Vascular permeation of platelet factor 4 after endothelial injury, *Science*, 209, 611, 1980.
55. Benitz, W. E., Coulson, J. D., Lessler, D. S., Kasnowski, C., and Bernfield, M., Smooth muscle cells from fetal bovine pulmonary arteries in vitro: growth inhibition by heparin, *J. Clin. Invest.*, in press, 1985.
56. Buonassisi, V., Sulfated mucopolysaccharide synthesis and secretion in endothelial cell cultures, *Exp. Cell Res.*, 76, 363, 1973.
57. Busch, C., Ljungman, C., Heldin, C. M., Waskson, E., and Obrink, B., Surface properties of cultured endothelial cells, *Haemostasis*, 8, 142, 1979.
58. Gamse, G., Fromme, H. G., and Kresse, H., Metabolism of sulfated glycosaminoglycans in cultured endothelial cells and smooth muscle cells from bovine aorta, *Biochem. Biophys. Acta*, 544, 514, 1978.
59. Kraemer, P. M., Heparan sulfate of cultured cells. II. Acid-soluble and -precipitable species of different cell lines, *Biochemistry*, 10, 1445, 1971.
60. Wight, T. N. and Ross, R., Proteoglycans in primate arteries. II. Synthesis and secretion of glycosaminoglycans by arterial smooth muscle cells in culture, *J. Cell Biol.*, 67, 675, 1975.
61. Eisenstein, R., Schumacher, B., and Matijevitch, B., Intrinsic regulators of arterial cell growth, *Fed. Proc.*, 38, 1075a, 1979.
62. Minick, C. R., Litrenta, M. M., Alonso, B. R., Silane, M. F., and Stemerman, M. B., Further studies on the effect of regenerated endothelium on intimal lipid accumulation, *Prog. Biochem. Pharmacol.*, 13, 115, 1977.
63. Richardson, M., Ihnatowycz, I., and Moore, S., Glycosaminoglycan distribution in rabbit aortic wall following balloon catheter deendothelialization: an ultrastructural study, *Lab. Invest.*, 43, 509, 1980.
64. Stevens, R. L., Colombo, M., Gonzales, J. J., Hollander, W., and Schmid, K., The glycosaminoglycans of the human artery and their changes in atherosclerosis, *J. Clin. Invest.*, 58, 470, 1976.
65. Wight, T. N., Curwen, K. D., Holman, W., and Minick, C. R., Effect of regenerated endothelium on glycosaminoglycan accumulation in the arterial wall, *Fed. Proc.*, 38, 1075a, 1979.
66. Ausprunk, D. H., Boudreau, C. L., and Nelson, D. A., Proteoglycans in the microvasculature. I. Histochemical localization in microvessels of the rabbit eye, *Am. J. Pathol.*, 103, 353, 1981.
67. Ausprunk, D. H., Boudreau, C. L., and Nelson, D. A., Proteoglycans in the microvasculature. II. Histochemical localization in proliferating capillaries of the rabbit cornea, *Am. J. Pathol.*, 103, 367, 1981.
68. Bernfield, M. R., Banerjee, S. D., and Cohn, R. H., Dependence of salivary epithelial morphology and branching morphogenesis upon acid mucopolysacharide-protein (proteoglycan) at the epithelial cell surface, *J. Cell Biol.*, 52, 674, 1972.
69. David, G. and Bernfield, M. R., Type I collagen reduces the degradation of basal lamina proteoglycan by mammary epithelial cells, *J. Cell Biol.*, 91, 281, 1981.
70. Whittemore, A. D., Clowes, A. W., Couch, N. P., and Mannick, J. A., Secondary femoropopliteal reconstruction, *Ann. Surg.*, 193, 35, 1981.

71. Castellot, J. J., Jr., Choay, J., Lormeau, J.-C., Petitou, M., Sache, E., and Karnovsky, M. J., Structural determinants of the capacity of heparin to inhibit the proliferation of vascular smooth muscle cells. II. Evidence for a pentasaccaride sequence that contains a 3-0-sulfate, *J. Cell Biol.*, 102, 1979, 1986.
72. Castellot, J. J., Jr. and Karnovsky, M. J., unpublished observation.

Chapter 8

BIOSYNTHESIS AND MODULATION OF EXTRACELLULAR MATRIX COMPONENTS BY CULTURED VASCULAR SMOOTH MUSCLE CELLS

Richard A. Majack and Paul Bornstein

TABLE OF CONTENTS

I. INTRODUCTION

Vascular smooth muscle cells (SMC) are the predominant cell type in the media of the blood vessel wall and serve both a major contractile function and an important synthetic function. SMC produce a spectrum of products which regulate vascular tone and platelet aggregation.[1-7] In addition, SMC produce a variety of molecules which, in the aggregate, comprise the extracellular matrix (ECM). This highly developed ECM is composed of proteoglycans, glycoproteins (such as thrombospondin and fibronectin), elastin, and at least five genetically distinct types of collagen. SMC also produce enzymes capable of degrading elastin[8] and presumably other matrix components. SMC-derived proteases (such as collagenases and elastases) undoubtedly play important roles in cellular movement, tissue remodeling and development, and in the regulation of production of ECM molecules.

In this review we focus on recent in vitro studies of the production and modulation of ECM components by vascular SMC and the reciprocal modulation of SMC functions by the ECM. The SMC connective tissue matrix, in vivo, forms the structural framework of the vessel wall and determines, in part, its mechanical properties. Matrix components can act as a thrombogenic surface,[9] can sequester biologically active molecules such as growth factors,[10] and may serve as important determinants of SMC function (e.g., growth, migration, and differentiation). The production of matrix molecules by vascular SMC is undoubtedly altered both quantitatively and qualitatively during hypertension, atherosclerosis, angiogenesis, and early development. Modulation of ECM components in vitro, as discussed here, presumably reflects similar mechanisms which operate in vivo and which may alter the structural and/or functional properties of the vessel wall and the cells therein.

II. MATRIX COMPONENTS SYNTHESIZED BY CULTURED VASCULAR SMOOTH MUSCLE CELLS

Vascular SMC from a variety of species produce an extensive ECM in culture.[11] The primary components of the SMC matrix include fibronectin, thrombospondin, elastin, and collagen; these macromolecules will be discussed below. The production and modulation of proteoglycans by vascular SMC will not be covered in this chapter.

A. Fibronectin

Fibronectins are high molecular weight, dimeric modular glycoproteins (subunit M_r 200,000 to 250,000) found in body fluids and in connective tissue matrices. The structure, distribution, and biological functions of the fibronectins have been the subject of several recent reviews.[12-15] Fibronectins contain structurally distinct domains which interact with collagen, fibrin, cell surfaces, and heparan sulfate[12-14] and play important roles in cell adhesion, spreading, proliferation, cytoskeletal organization, migration, chemoattraction, phagocytosis, and differentiation.[12,13,15] The synthesis of fibronectin by SMC in vitro has been established by metabolic labeling of monkey[16] and porcine[17] aortic SMC and by detection with antibodies in cultures of monkey aortic SMC.[18] We have determined, using immunoisolation techniques, that rat aortic SMC also produce fibronectin in culture (see Figures 1 and 2). The function of fibronectin in SMC cultures may encompass the wide range of functions ascribed to the fibronectins in general. Fibronectin is known to act as an attachment factor for guinea pig and monkey SMC in vitro.[19] In addition, fetal sheep SMC use fibronectin to attach to collagen types I and III.[20] Fibronectin may also play a role in the control of "nodulation" in porcine aortic SMC cultures.[17,21]

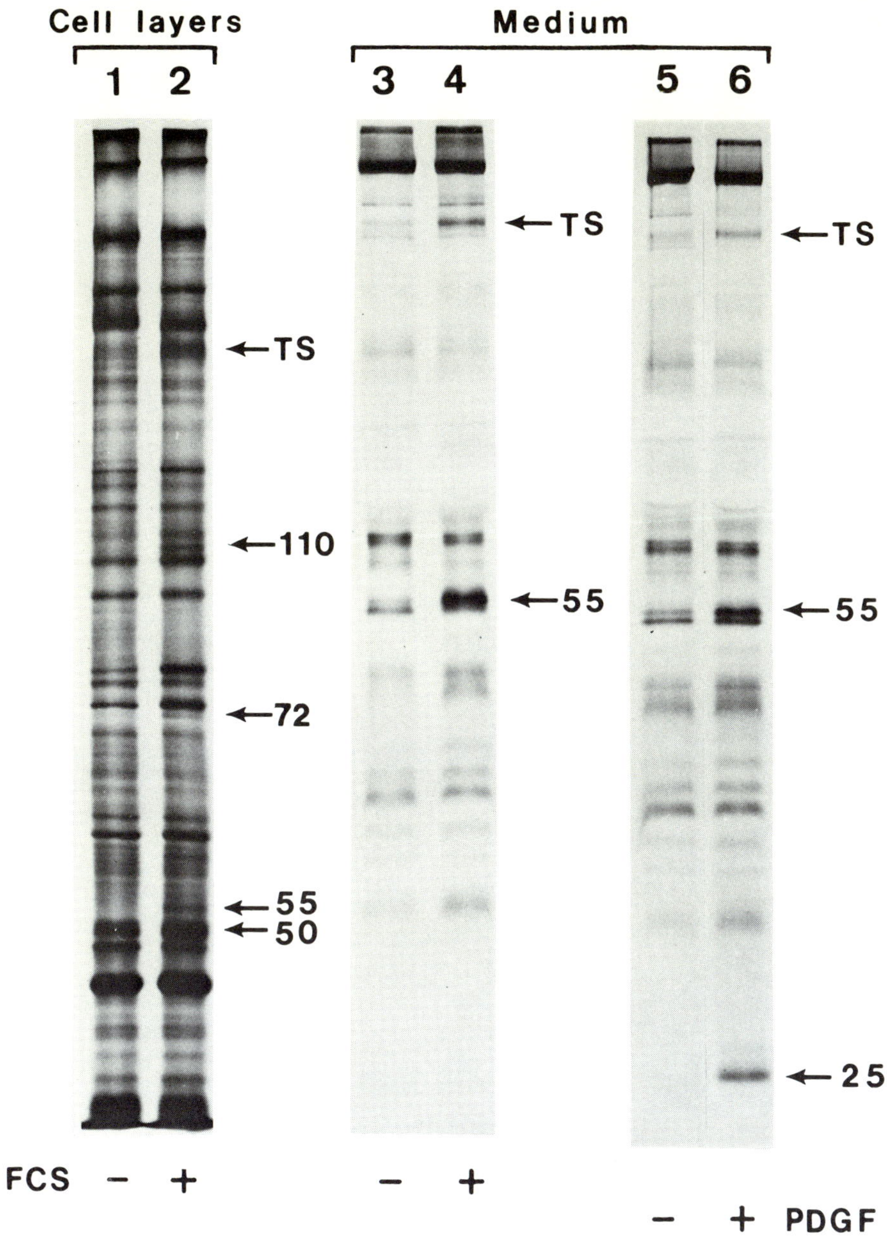

FIGURE 1. Modulation of SMC biosynthetic phenotype by serum and PDGF. Rat aortic SMC were maintained in a growth factor-deficient state by culture in 10% plasma-derived serum (PDS). PDS-SMC were metabolically labeled with [^{35}S]methionine in methionine-free Waymouth's medium for 1 hr at 37°C or following a 1 hr treatment with 10% fetal calf serum (FCS) or 5 ng/mℓ platelet-derived growth factor (PDGF). Cell layer and medium proteins were harvested into protease inhibitors and resolved by SDS-PAGE under reducing conditions using 8 (lanes 1 and 2) or 10% (lanes 3 to 6) separating gels. Proteins were visualized by autoradiography. In the cell layer, FCS consistently stimulated the production of thrombospondin (TS) and protein chains with approximate M_r 50,000, 55,000, 72,000, and 110,000 (lanes 1 and 2). TS and the M_r 55,000 protein were secreted into the culture medium (lanes 3 and 4). The effect of FCS on SMC secreted proteins could be completely mimicked by treatment of PDS-SMC with highly purified PDGF (kindly provided by E. Raines and Dr. R. Ross). Exposure of PDS-SMC to PDGF also induced the production of an M_r 25,000 secreted protein not observed in FCS-stimulated SMC (lane 6). Molecular weights (10^{-3}) of the induced proteins are indicated at arrows.

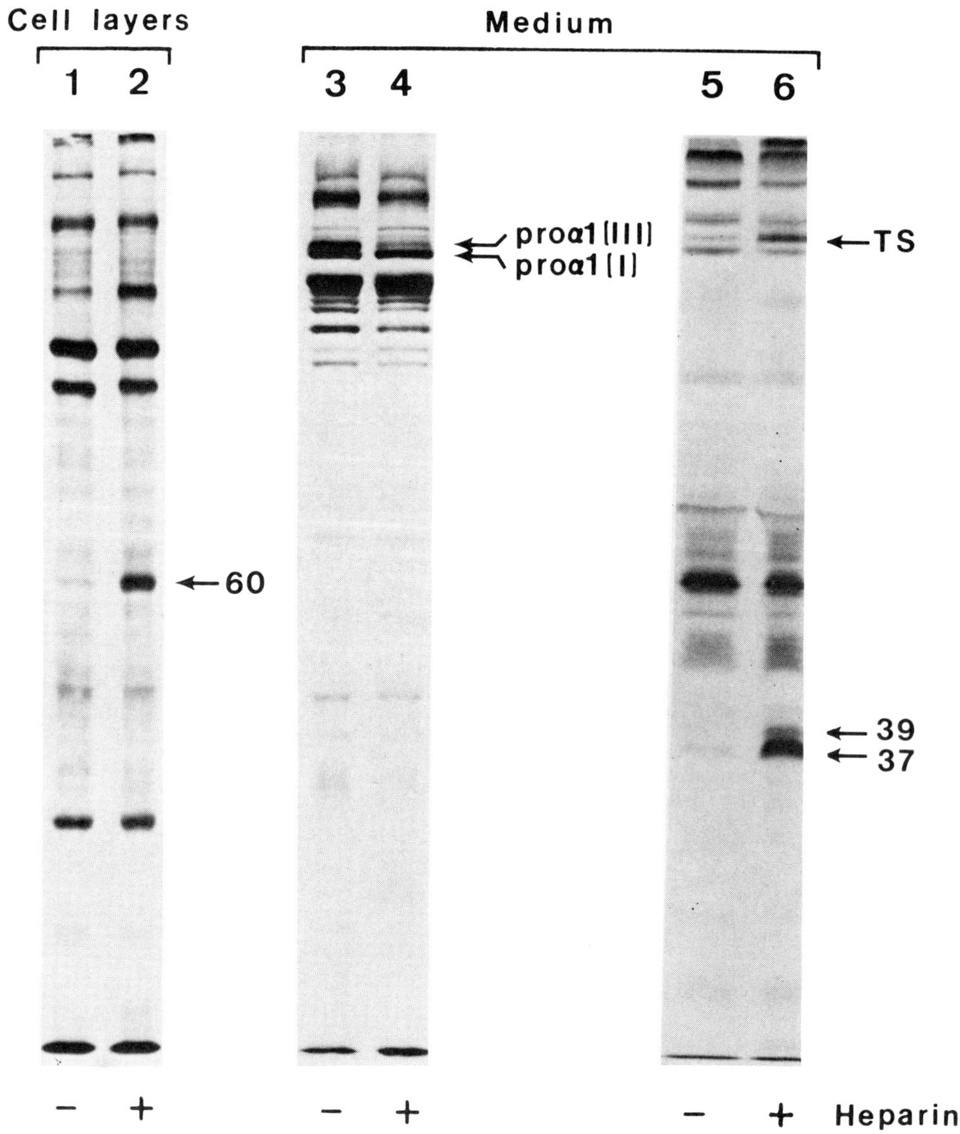

FIGURE 2. Modulation of SMC biosynthetic phenotype by heparin. Rat aortic SMC were grown to overconfluence and maintained in medium containing 10% FSC. Following exposure of SMC to 100 μg/mℓ heparin, cell proteins were metabolically labeled with [^{3}H]proline or [^{35}S]methionine and visualized by SDS-PAGE on 8 (lanes 1 to 4) or 10% (lanes 5 and 6) separating gels as described in the legend for Figure 1. SMC were exposed to heparin for 72 hr, then labeled with [^{3}H]proline for 24 hr in the continued presence of heparin (lanes 1 to 4). Heparin-treated SMC synthesized increased amounts of a cell-layer-associated short chain (M_r 60,000) collagenous protein and reduced the production of secreted type III procollagen (proα1(III)). In other experiments, SMC were exposed to heparin during a short (2 hr) labeling period with [^{35}S]methionine (lanes 5 and 6). In the presence of heparin, SMC synthesized and secreted increased amounts of two noncollagenous proteins (M_r 37,000 and 39,000) and augmented the release of thrombospondin (TS) into the culture medium. Details are given in the text. Molecular weights ($\times 10^{-3}$) are given for the proteins indicated at arrows; the position of migration of the proα1 chain of type I procollagen (proα1(I)) is also shown.

B. Thrombospondin

Thrombospondin (TS) is an M_r 450,000 glycoprotein first described as a component of platelet α granules[22,23] but now known to be synthesized by fibroblasts, bovine aortic SMC, and endothelial cells in culture.[24-27] The TS molecule consists of three probably identical disulfide-bonded chains of M_r 145,000,[23,28,29] with a heparin-binding region located in an NH_2-terminal domain.[30-32] Incorporation of TS into the ECM of cultured fibroblasts,[26,27] endothelial cells,[26] and SMC[26] has been demonstrated immunologically. The incorporation of TS into extracellular matrices undoubtedly reflects its ability to interact with heparan sulfate proteoglycan and other matrix components.[33-35] While platelet-derived TS is thought to act as an endogenous platelet lectin,[36] mediating platelet:platelet[36,37] or platelet:connective tissue[34] interactions, the function of cell-derived TS and its role in the ECM has not been elucidated.

TS production by cultured bovine SMC has been documented by metabolic labeling[24,26] and by indirect immunofluorescence.[26] The production of TS by cultured human SMC was found to be dependent on cell density; SMC at sparse density secreted more TS into the culture medium than did confluent cultures.[38] We have recently shown that TS is produced in vitro by rat aortic SMC and that its production is regulated by platelet-derived growth factor (see later).[39] While the function of matrix TS is not known for any cell type, our data suggest that TS participates in some manner in the SMC growth response.

C. Elastin

Elastin is a major structural component of the vessel wall and is synthesized by cultured arterial SMC as an M_r 72,000 to 76,000 protein.[40-42] The newly synthesized elastin (tropoelastin) is soluble but can be converted into insoluble elastin by the formation of unique lysine-derived desmosine and isodesmosine crosslinks.[43] Synthesis of both soluble and insoluble forms of elastin has been demonstrated in cultures of arterial SMC derived from rabbit,[44-47] pig,[48] and monkey.[49] Another component of elastic fibers, the microfibrillar protein,[50] has been identified morphologically in cultures of monkey, rabbit, pig, guinea pig, and rat SMC.[42,50-53] Biochemical characterization of the microfibrillar protein is incomplete[54] and will not be discussed here. Morphological data suggest that the fibrillar component of elastic fibers may appear first in the ECM and may act as a framework upon which insoluble elastin is deposited.[42,50,51]

D. Collagens

Vascular SMC are now known to produce at least five distinct types of collagen in culture, including types I, III, V, and VI, CP45 (a pepsin-resistant fragment of unknown origin), an M_r-60,000-short-chain collagen, and possibly type IV.[40,55] Collagen production by cultured SMC has been studied quantitatively, by assessing the relative amount of total collagen produced as a fraction of total protein synthesis and qualitatively, by determining the relative amounts of specific collagen types, primarily by SDS-PAGE. The production of collagens by cultured SMC has been shown to be selectively and quantitatively increased (as a percent of total protein synthesis) by cyclic stretching[56] and heparin treatment[57,58] and decreased by treatment of SMC with 17β-estradiol.[59] Cells cultured from atherosclerotic aortas[60] or treated with growth factors[40,61] also produced more collagen per cell, but collagen production relative to total protein synthesis was unchanged.

1. Type I Collagen

The type I collagen molecule consists of three chains with subunit composition

$[\alpha 1(I)]_2\alpha 2(I)$. Each α chain has a molecular weight of 95,000 (see Bornstein and Sage[62] for a recent review of the biosynthesis, processing, and structures of collagen types I to V). Production of type I collagen by SMC in vitro has been extensively documented (see References 40 and 63 to 66 and references therein). Type I is an interstitial collagen which is believed to be essential for normal development of the vessel wall[67] and can serve in culture as a substrate for SMC adhesion.[19,20] The production of type I collagen by bovine SMC was found to be decreased in confluent cultures.[63] This decrease occurred to a greater extent than a concomitant decrease in type III collagen production, thus leading to an increase in the ratio of types III:I in confluent SMC cultures. In contrast, Beldekas et al.[68] described an increase in type I production by bovine SMC with increasing cell density.

2. Type III Collagen

Type III collagen is a trimer with chain composition $[\alpha 1(III)]_3$. The α chains also have individual molecular weights of 95,000 and are products of a single gene. The pathway of processing of type III collagen in cultured bovine SMC appears to be the same as that described for type I; however, the rate of processing of type III procollagen is markedly slower.[69] The production of type III collagen by SMC and a discussion of the inter- and intraspecies discrepancies in the type I:III ratio reported by various workers have been reviewed previously;[40] additional reports of type III synthesis by cultured SMC have subsequently appeared.[59,63-66,68]

The function of type III collagen appears to be related to its distribution as an interstitial collagen. Patients with type IV Ehlers-Danlos syndrome, in which there is a defect in type III collagen synthesis or secretion, show a number of tissue defects, including a tendency to rupture large blood vessels.[70] Production of type III collagen was found to be reduced in heparin-treated SMC,[71] in bovine SMC treated with 17β-estradiol,[59] in confluent as compared with sparse cultures of rabbit SMC,[63] and in guinea pig and monkey aortic SMC after repeated passage in culture.[72] Beldekas et al.,[68] in studies of cultured bovine SMC, have reported an increased production of type III (and type I) procollagen with increasing cell number. Additionally, the relative amount of type III collagen (compared with type I) was increased twofold in dense cultures.

A number of reports have suggested that the relative content of types I and III collagens differs in atherosclerotic plaques, compared with normal aortic media.[73,74] While several reports have indicated a greater proportion of type III collagen in vivo in diseased or proliferative tissues,[73] other studies have indicated the opposite[74] or no change in the type I:III ratio.[75] Attempts to study this question by culturing aortic SMC from control or proliferative tissues have not clarified the issue. Pietila and Nikkari[60] analyzed collagen production by rabbit SMC cultured from control and atherosclerotic aortas and found no specific alterations in collagen production in cells from diseased tissues (see Chapter 13).

3. Type IV Collagen

Type IV collagen is synthesized as two genetically distinct chains of M_r 185,000 and 170,000 and occurs as a heterotrimer of chain composition $[\alpha 1(IV)]_2\alpha 2(IV)$.[76] Type IV is a normal constituent of most basal laminae;[77] its synthesis by SMC is therefore expected in view of the extensive external lamina elaborated by these cells in vivo and in vitro.[11] Sankey and Barnes[78] have presented preliminary evidence that cultured porcine aortic SMC may produce type IV collagen. In their study, a pepsin-resistant, collagenase-sensitive polypeptide (reduced M_r 140,000) was thought to be derived from type IV collagen on the basis of its molecular weight and solubility characteristics.

4. Type V Collagen

The biosynthesis of type V procollagen chains and processing of the molecules to functional extracellular forms are complex processes whose details remain to be established.[79] Several forms of the protein exist including a heterotrimer of three different chains α1(V), α2(V), and α3(V).[80] Mayne et al.[81] demonstrated the presence of the α1 and α2 chains of type V collagen following pepsin digestion of metabolically labeled cultures of rhesus monkey aortic SMC. Type V collagen has also been identified by immunoprecipitation techniques in the medium of cultured rat SMC.[134]

Grotendorst et al.[20] have shown that sheep aortic SMC attach to type V collagen matrices in a fibronectin-independent manner, in contrast to the attachment of SMC to types I and III collagens.[19,20] SMC preferentially attached to matrices composed of the α2(V) chain (compared to α1(V)), suggesting the presence of an SMC binding site on the α2(V) collagen chain. The SMC type V "receptor" was found to be trypsin-resistant, neuraminidase-sensitive, and blocked by treatment with concanavalin A. These data, together with immunofluorescence studies indicating a pericellular distribution of type V around SMC *in situ*,[82] suggest an important role for type V collagen in the interaction of SMC with their extracellular environment.

5. Type VI Collagen

Type VI collagen has been characterized primarily as a pepsin-resistant fragment containing three distinct chains,[83-85] but the primary biosynthetic product and tissue forms are substantially larger.[86-88] The production of type VI collagen by cultured human SMC has been detected, using both immunoblotting and immunofluorescence techniques.[89] The presence of type VI collagen in the aortic media was also demonstrated immunologically,[89] suggesting the synthesis of type VI by SMC in vivo.

6. CP45 and the M_r 60,000 SMC Collagen

Mayne et al.[72,81] and Majack and Bornstein[57,58] have reported the production of other collagenous proteins by cultured SMC. Mayne et al.[72,81] prepared pepsin extracts of guinea pig and monkey aortic SMC and found a short-chain (M_r 45,000) pepsin-resistant collagen, which they termed CP45. Production of CP45 was found to be greatest in early-passage SMC. The molecular weight of CP45 was not affected by reducing agents, suggesting an absence of inter- or intramolecular disulfide bonds. Cyanogen bromide peptides of CP45 were not comparable to those of collagen types I, III, or V. Little else is known concerning the size, structure, or nature of the precursor to CP45. We have recently reported that rat SMC produce an M_r 60,000 collagenous protein which is cell-layer associated, heparin-inducible, and digested by pepsin to an M_r 45,000 to 50,000 fragment.[57,58] The relationship of the M_r 60,000 heparin-induced SMC collagen to other known collagen types is not known.

In recent years the number of recognized collagen types has increased dramatically; at least 18 separate gene products have now been described. Among these new collagens are several "short-chain" collagens that are considerably smaller than the well-known interstitial collagens such as types I and III. The M_r 60,000 SMC collagen, based on its molecular weight, may be related to the pepsin-resistant collagenous protein referred to as CP45. The M_r 60,000 SMC collagen may also be related to an M_r 59,000 chondrocyte collagen (type X collagen) extensively described from in vitro sources.[90,91] The M_r 60,000 SMC protein is similar to type X collagen in several respects: (1) both have M_r of approximately 60,000, (2) both contain pepsin-resistant fragments of M_r approximately 45,000,[58,90] (3) neither contains disulfide bonds,[90] (4) both are inducible by matrix components,[91] and (5) both contain similar amounts of hydroxyproline.[91] Schmid and Linsenmayer, in a recent abstract,[92] have described the distribution of type X collagen using monoclonal antibodies and immunofluorescence.

Type X collagen was localized to hypertrophied chondrocytes in developing bone, but not to tissues which remain permanently cartilagenous. The collagen was also present in endochondral and membrane bone, but not in any other tissue, suggesting it may not be an SMC protein. The exact relationship, if any, between the M_r 60,000 SMC collagen and type X is therefore unclear and must await future studies.

III. SECRETORY PHENOTYPES OF VASCULAR SMC IN CULTURE: MODULATION BY GROWTH FACTORS AND HEPARIN-LIKE GLYCOSAMINOGLYCANS

SMC migration and proliferation are believed to be essential steps in the early vascular response to injury and consequently may play an important role in atherogenesis. The platelet-derived growth factor (PDGF) is mitogenic,[93] chemokinetic,[94,95] and chemotactic[20,96] for vascular SMC and is now recognized as a major determinant of SMC function, at least in vitro. Recent studies have indicated that other regulatory molecules, such as heparin-like glycosaminoglycans (GAG), may also control certain SMC functions. In contrast to PDGF, these molecules may be continually present in the normal vascular wall[97,98] and are inhibitory to SMC growth and movement. It is likely that PDGF and regulatory GAG play important roles in angiogenesis, normal development, and tissue repair as well.

We are interested in defining the molecular basis for SMC growth regulation. Accordingly, we have analyzed the biosynthetic phenotype of growth factor-deprived, growth factor-stimulated, and heparin-treated rat aortic SMC in culture.

A. Modulation of SMC Phenotype by Factors in Serum

PDGF has been identified as the principal mitogen responsible for SMC growth in vitro.[99] Addition of nanogram quantities of PDGF to fibroblastic cells in culture elicits a pleiotropic response, resulting in many cellular changes.[100,101] These alterations include an overall increase in protein synthesis,[102,103] stimulation of polysome formation,[102] induction of specific mRNAs,[104,105] and the induction of synthesis of specific "competence" proteins.[106] Data on growth factor-induced protein synthesis have been derived, almost exclusively, from studies on fibroblasts. In 3T3 cells, PDGF induces the rapid transcription of several known oncogenes including c-fos[107] and c-myc.[108] PDGF also stimulates the rapid (within 1.5 hr) production of cytoplasmic proteins, detectable by SDS-PAGE after metabolic labeling, with M_r 29,000, 35,000, 45,000, 60,000, and 70,000.[106] Growth factor-inducible secreted proteins of M_r 12,000, 24,000, 29,000, 34,000, 48,000, and 62,000 have also been described from 3T3 cells.[109,110]

We have recently defined the effects of serum and purified growth factors on the synthesis of specific proteins by vascular SMC.[39] The results, as described in part below, suggest that specific cell types may differ qualitatively in their response to growth stimuli. The data also support previous suggestions[111,112] that the character of the ECM may be an important determinant of cellular growth.

Rat aortic SMC were maintained in growth factor-deficient medium by culturing the cells for 4 to 7 days in Waymouth's medium supplemented with 10% plasma-derived fetal bovine serum (PDS), for 4 days in Waymouth's plus 0.5% fetal bovine serum (FCS), or for 4 days in a defined medium as described by Libby and O'Brien.[113] Cells were stimulated for 1 hr with 10% FCS in Waymouth's medium, then metabolically labeled for 1 hr with [^{35}S]methionine (see Reference 39 for protocols). Control cultures were not stimulated with FCS prior to labeling. Cell layer and medium proteins were resolved by SDS-PAGE under reducing conditions and visualized by autoradiography. As shown in Figure 1, the pattern of proteins synthesized by growth-arrested SMC differed qualitatively from that of serum-stimulated cells; the results were qualitatively similar regardless of the method of growth arrest used. In the cell layer (Figure 1, lanes 1 and 2), serum specifically and reproducibly induced the production of proteins with approximate M_r 50,000, 55,000, 72,000, 110,000, and 150,000. Other cell layer proteins were inconsistently increased or decreased following serum stimulation. Serum also altered the pattern of SMC secreted proteins (Figure 1, lanes 3 and 4). Cultures stimulated with FCS secreted increased amounts of proteins with reduced M_r 55,000 and 150,000.

We have identified the protein present in the cell layer and medium compartments with a chain M_r 150,000 as cellular thrombospondin.[39] The M_r 150,000 chain comigrated on SDS-PAGE with human platelet thrombospondin and was immunoprecipitated by antibodies prepared against human platelet or bovine endothelial cell thrombospondin. The induction of synthesis of thrombospondin and the M_r 55,000 protein can be elicited by treating SMC with purified PDGF (Figure 1, lanes 5 and 6) but not with other growth factors (fibroblast growth factor, epidermal growth factor, multiplication stimulating activity, or insulin). PDGF also stimulated the synthesis of an M_r 25,000 secreted protein not detected in the medium of serum-stimulated cells. It should be noted that these experiments were designed to study only the earliest events following growth factor stimulation and that our gel system was optimized for the resolution of higher molecular weight abundant proteins. It is likely that other specific protein synthetic events occur transiently and/or at later times following stimulation of SMC.

Our data suggest that PDGF treatment of vascular SMC may result in the induction of a unique set of "competence" proteins (compare with the PDGF-regulated 3T3 proteins listed above). While it is likely that many factor-regulated proteins may be common to all cells, other inducible proteins (especially matrix components) may be specific for each cell type. The most interesting results of our studies, in terms of the biology of connective tissue molecules, is the observation that PDGF selectively stimulated SMC thrombospondin production. To date the function of cell-derived or matrix-bound thrombospondin has been unclear. Our data suggest that thrombospondin may play some as-yet-unidentified role in the SMC growth response.

The role of ECM in the growth of cells has been the subject of extensive investigation in recent years.[111,112,114,115] It is clear that cells require an appropriate ECM for optimal growth,[116] and that growth factors may regulate the production of specific matrix molecules. Epidermal growth factor and fibroblast growth factor both appear to selectively inhibit the synthesis of type I collagen in several cell types.[117-119] Fibronectin, another component of the ECM of most cells, has been shown to act as a competence factor for HFL-1 fibroblasts.[115] These studies emphasize the hypothesis[114] that one function of growth factors may be to direct the synthesis of a growth-supportive ECM. For vascular SMC, the ECM optimal for cell proliferation and movement may contain thrombospondin.

B. Modulation of SMC Phenotype by Heparin-Like Glycosaminoglycans

In 1977 Clowes and Karnovsky[120] demonstrated that heparin treatment of animals significantly reduced the proliferative response of neointimal SMC following experimental vascular injury in vivo. A follow-up study[121] established that the growth-inhibitory effect of heparin was not related to the anticoagulant properties of heparin or to an inhibitory effect of heparin on platelet adherence or endothelial cell regeneration. Subsequent studies, using cultured rat SMC, verified that heparin was a cell-specific inhibitor of SMC proliferation.[122-124]

The importance of these observations was emphasized by data suggesting that heparin-like molecules may be normally present within the vascular wall. Gamse et al.[125] studied GAG synthesized by cultured vascular endothelial and SMC and found that endothelial heparan sulfate molecules were very similar to heparin in charge density and N-sulfate content. Conditioned medium from cultured quiescent aortic endothelium was found to be growth-inhibitory for vascular SMC.[126-128] The inhibitory activity required low concentrations of serum for release and was destroyed specifically by heparinase.[126] The enzyme present in serum that was responsible for release of the inhibitor has been shown to be a platelet-derived heparitinase.[129] This enzyme, which releases heparin-like GAG fragments from proteoglycans, is believed to be present in endothelium and in smooth muscle as well.[130]

SMC also produce heparan sulfate proteoglycans.[125,131] SMC heparan sulfate may also be growth inhibitory for SMC in culture, especially when derived from quiescent confluent SMC cultures rather than from cells in log-phase growth.[130] The above data collectively indicate that (1) vascular wall cells produce heparan sulfate proteoglycans, (2) a heparitinase may be present in normal and injured vessel walls which is capable of cleaving proteoheparan sulfates and generating heparin-like GAG fragments, and (3) these GAG are growth inhibitory to SMC. Thus SMC growth may be controlled, in an unknown fashion, by heparin-like GAG derived from endothelium or SMC (see Chapters 4 and 7).

Recently, Majack and Clowes[132] reported that heparin-like molecules inhibit the migration of rat vascular SMC in vitro, suggesting that other SMC functions may also be regulated by GAG. The mechanism(s) underlying this phenomenon and its potential role in SMC growth regulation remain unclear.

We have recently demonstrated that heparin and related molecules dramatically alter the synthetic phenotype of cultured rat vascular SMC[57,58,71] (Figure 2). Addition of heparin to the culture medium of early passage rat SMC resulted in a marked (3- to 15-fold) increase of a cell-layer associated M_r 60,000 protein which was sensitive to digestion by purified bacterial collagenase and contained significant amounts of hydroxyproline (Figure 2, lanes 1 and 2). Pulse-chase analysis of heparin-treated SMC revealed that the M_r 60,000 collagen was a primary and abundant product of these cells and was not processed extracellularly to a smaller form. The inductive effect of heparin could be mimicked by iota carrageenan or dextran sulfates but not by hyaluronic acid, dermatan sulfate, or chondroitin sulfates. The induction was concentration-dependent with a maximal effect observed at a heparin concentration of 10 μg/mℓ. Synthesis of the M_r 60,000 collagen increased 18 to 24 hr following addition of heparin to the cultures. Following induction and subsequent removal of heparin, synthesis of the protein remained maximal for at least 12 hr and required 72 hr to return to a basal level.

Heparin-treated SMC also produce decreased amounts of type III procollagen relative to type I procollagen[71] (Figure 2, lanes 3 and 4), and synthesize increased amounts of two noncollagenous proteins (M_r 37,000 and 39,000) (Figure 2, lanes 5 and 6). This effect could be mimicked by heparan and dermatan sulfates and iota carrageenan but not by hyaluronic acid, chondroitin-4-sulfate, or chondroitin-6-sulfate. The inductive effect of heparin was dose-dependent and occurred rapidly (within 1 hr) with maximal induction (three- to fivefold over controls) occurring after 10 to 12 hr of treatment. The effect was rapidly reversible (within 1 hr) and was not altered in the presence of actinomycin D, suggesting regulation at a posttranscriptional level. The relationship between the M_r 37,000 and 39,000 heparin-inducible proteins and an M_r 38,000 heparin-binding protein secreted from "nodular" cultures of bovine SMC[133] is not presently known.

We have recently characterized one additional change in the secretory phenotype of heparin-treated SMC.[39] Following heparin treatment, rat SMC released increased amounts of an M_r 150,000 (reduced) protein which we have identified (using specific immunoprecipitation) as cellular thrombospondin. The increased amount of thrombospondin secreted into the culture medium was directly correlated with a concomitant decrease in cell layer-associated thrombospondin. Analysis of Triton-X-100-insoluble

SMC matrices prepared from control and heparin-treated cells revealed that this effect resulted from the inhibition of incorporation of newly synthesized thrombospondin into the SMC extracellular matrix. The release of thrombospondin from cell layers was concentration-dependent, with a half-maximal effect observed at 0.1 μg/mℓ heparin and a maximal effect at heparin concentrations greater than 1.0 μg/mℓ. Dermatan sulfate, several heparan sulfate preparations, and a variety of heparins with a range of anticoagulant activities were effective in altering the distribution of thrombospondin in culture; other GAG tested were not active. Time-course studies indicated that maximal release of newly synthesized thrombospondin from SMC was achieved with 4 hr of heparin addition; the effect was completely reversible within 8 hr of removal of heparin from the cultures. These data suggest that heparin-like molecules may alter the composition and/or structure of the SMC extracellular matrix without direct cellular (i.e., biosynthetic) involvement. The data are especially significant in view of our recent observation (discussed above) that thrombospondin may be involved in the SMC growth response. We have proposed[39] that heparin-mediated inhibition of SMC:thrombospondin interactions may be involved in the inhibition of SMC migration and growth by heparin-like molecules.

IV. CONCLUSION

Vascular SMC maintained in culture produce many known components of the extracellular matrix. Expression of specific ECM molecules in vitro undoubtedly reflects expression of these matrix components at some point during SMC development. Similarly, modulation of production of ECM components in culture may reflect similar processes in vivo and may provide valuable insight into the functional role of these molecules.

In this paper we have described the primary collagen and glycoprotein matrix products of vascular SMC in culture and have noted, where applicable, the conditions under which synthesis of these molecules is modulated. Production of interstitial collagens (types I and III) can be altered by estrogens,[59] cell density,[63] or glycosaminoglycan treatment.[58,71] Synthesis of SMC thrombospondin varies according to cell density,[38] a finding which may be explained by our recent observation that SMC thrombospondin production is regulated by PDGF.[39] Heparin-like molecules induce the production of a novel SMC matrix protein, an M_r 60,000 short-chain collagen.[57,58] In addition, PDGF and heparin-like glycosaminoglycans, which regulate the growth and migration of vascular SMC in an antagonistic fashion, induce the production of a number of uncharacterized SMC proteins which may or may not be associated with the extracellular matrix.[39,71] Finally, heparin-like growth inhibitors alter the secretory phenotype of cultured SMC by regulating the interaction between thrombospondin and the SMC surface or matrix.[39] These observations, taken together, suggest an important role for thrombospondin and other matrix molecules in the control of SMC growth, migration, and differentiation. Future studies of the regulation, structure, molecular interactions, and function of each of these molecules should advance our understanding of the processes underlying atherogenesis, angiogenesis, and the normal development of the vessel wall.

ACKNOWLEDGMENT

Original contributions from this laboratory were supported in part by NIH Grants AM 11248, HL 18645, and DE 02600 and by a grant from R. J. Reynolds, Inc. R. A. Majack was the recipient of a postdoctoral fellowship from training grant NIH HL 67312.

REFERENCES

1. Dejana, E., Balconi, G., de Castellarnau, C., Barbieri, B., Veragara-Dauden, M., and de Gaetano, G., Prostacyclin production by human endothelial and bovine smooth muscle cells in culture, *Biochim. Biophys. Acta,* 750, 261, 1983.
2. Booyse, F. M., Scheinbuks, J., Radek, J., Osikowicz, G., Feder, S., and Quarfoot, A. J., Immunological identification and comparison of plasminogen activator forms in cultured normal human endothelial cells and smooth muscle cells, *Thromb. Res.,* 24, 495, 1981.
3. Tansik, R. L., Namm, D. H., and White, H. L., Synthesis of prostaglandin 6-keto $F_{1\alpha}$ by cultured aortic smooth muscle cells and stimulation of its formation in a coupled system with platelet lysates, *Prostaglandins,* 15, 399, 1978.
4. Baenziger, N. L., Dillender, M. J., and Majerus, P. W., Cultured human skin fibroblasts and arterial cells produce a labile platelet inhibitory prostaglandin, *Biochem. Biophys. Res. Commun.,* 78, 294, 1977.
5. Larrue, J., Rigaud, M., Daret, D., Demond, J., Durand, and Bricand, H., Prostaglandin production by cultured smooth muscle cells from atherosclerotic rabbit aorta, *Nature (London),* 285, 480, 1980.
6. Re, R., Fallon, J. T., Dzau, J., Quay, S. C., and Haber, E., Renin synthesis by canine aortic smooth muscle cells in culture, *Life Sci.,* 30, 99, 1982.
7. Ager, A., Gordon, J. L., Moncada, S., Pearson, J. D., Salmon, J. A., and Trevethick, M. A., Effects of isolation and culture on prostaglandin synthesis by porcine aortic endothelial and smooth muscle cells, *J. Cell. Physiol.,* 110, 9, 1982.
8. Hornebeck, W., Brechemier, D., Bourdillon, M. C., and Robert, L., Isolation and partial characterization of an elastase-like protease from rat aorta smooth muscle cells. Possible role in the regulation of elastin biosynthesis, *Connect. Tissue Res.,* 8, 245, 1981.
9. Sakariassen, K. S., Bolhuis, P. A., and Sixma, J. J., Human platelet adhesion to artery subendothelium is mediated by Factor VIII:VWF bound to subendothelium, *Nature (London),* 279, 636, 1979.
10. Smith, J. C., Singh, J. P., Lillquist, J. S., Goon, D. S., and Stiles, C. D., Growth factors adherent to cell substrate are mitogenically active *in situ, Nature (London),* 296, 154, 1982.
11. Oakes, B. W., Batty, A. C., Handley, C. J., and Sandberg, L. B., The synthesis of elastin, collagen, and glycosaminoglycans by high density primary cultures of neonatal rat aortic smooth muscle cells. An ultrastructural and biochemical study, *Eur. J. Cell Biol.,* 27, 34, 1982.
12. Hynes, R. O. and Yamada, K. M., Fibronectins: multifunctional modular glycoproteins, *J. Cell Biol.,* 95, 369, 1982.
13. Hynes, R. O., Fibronectin and its relation to cellular structure and behavior, in *Cell Biology of the Extracellular Matrix,* Hay, E. D., Ed., Plenum Press, New York, 1982, 295.
14. Mosher, D. F., Fibronectin, *Prog. Hemostasis Thromb.,* 5, 111, 1980.
15. Yamada, K. M., Cell surface interactions with extracellular materials, *Annu. Rev. Biochem.,* 52, 761, 1983.
16. Burke, J. M., Balian, G., Ross, R., and Bornstein, P., Synthesis of types I and III procollagen and collagen by monkey aortic smooth muscle cells *in vitro, Biochemistry,* 16, 3243, 1977.
17. Brennan, M. J., Millis, A. J. T., and Fritz, K. E., Fibronectin inhibits morphological changes in cultures of vascular smooth muscle cells, *J. Cell. Physiol.,* 112, 284, 1982.
18. Bornstein, P. and Ash, J. F., Cell surface-associated structural proteins in connective tissue cells, *Proc. Natl. Acad. Sci. U.S.A.,* 74, 2480, 1977.
19. Gold, L. I. and Pearlstein, E., Fibronectin-collagen binding and requirement during cellular adhesion, *Biochem. J.,* 186, 551, 1980.
20. Grotendorst, G. R., Seppa, H. E. J., Kleinman, H. K., and Martin, G. R., Attachment of smooth muscle cells to collagen and their migration towards platelet-derived growth factor, *Proc. Natl. Acad. Sci. U.S.A.,* 78, 3669, 1981.
21. Brennan, M. J., Millis, A. J. T., Mann, D., and Fritz, K. E., Structural alterations in fibronectin correlated with morphological changes in smooth muscle cells, *Dev. Biol.,* 97, 391, 1983.
22. Baenziger, N. L., Brodie, G. N., and Majerus, P. W., A thrombin-sensitive protein of human platelet membranes, *Proc. Natl. Acad. Sci. U.S.A.,* 68, 240, 1971.
23. Baenziger, N. L., Brodie, G. N., and Majerus, P. W., Isolation and properties of a thrombin-sensitive protein of human platelets, *J. Biol. Chem.,* 248, 2723, 1972.
24. McPherson, J., Sage, H., and Bornstein, P., Isolation and characterization of a glycoprotein secreted by aortic endothelial cells in culture: apparent identity with platelet thrombospondin, *J. Biol. Chem.,* 256, 11330, 1981.
25. Mosher, D. F., Doyle, M. F., and Jaffe, E. A., Synthesis and secretion of thrombospondin by cultured endothelial cells, *J. Cell Biol.,* 93, 343, 1982.
26. Raugi, G. J., Mumby, S. M., Abbott-Brown, D., and Bornstein, P., Thrombospondin: synthesis and secretion by cells in culture, *J. Cell Biol.,* 95, 351, 1982.

27. Jaffe, E. A., Ruggiero, J. T., Leung, L. L. K., Doyle, M. J., McKeown-Longo, P. J., and Mosher, D. F., Cultured human fibroblasts synthesize and secrete thrombospondin and incorporate it into extracellular matrix, *Proc. Natl. Acad. Sci. U.S.A.*, 80, 998, 1983.
28. Lawler, J. W., Slayter, H. S., and Coligan, J. E., Isolation and characterization of a high molecular weight glycoprotein from human blood platelets, *J. Biol. Chem.*, 253, 8609, 1978.
29. Margossian, S. S., Lawler, J. W., and Slayter, H. S., Physical characteristics of platelet thrombospondin, *J. Biol. Chem.*, 256, 7495, 1981.
30. Dixit, V. M., Grant, G. A., Santoro, S. A., and Frazier, W. A., Isolation and characterization of a heparin-binding domain from the amino terminus of platelet thrombospondin, *J. Biol. Chem.*, 259, 10100, 1984.
31. Raugi, G. J., Mumby, S. M., Ready, C. A., and Bornstein, P., Location and partial characterization of the heparin-binding fragment of platelet thrombospondin, *Thromb. Res.*, 36, 165, 1984.
32. Coligan, J. E. and Slayter, H. S., Structure of thrombospondin, *J. Biol. Chem.*, 259, 3944, 1984.
33. Mumby, S. M., Raugi, G. J., and Bornstein, P., Interactions of thrombospondin with extracellular matrix proteins: selective binding to type V collagen, *J. Cell Biol.*, 98, 646, 1984.
34. Lahav, J., Schwartz, M. A., and Hynes, R. O., Analysis of platelet adhesion with a radioactive chemical crosslinking reagent: interaction of thrombospondin with fibronectin and collagen, *Cell*, 31, 253, 1982.
35. Lahav, J., Lawler, J., and Gimbrone, M. A., Thrombospondin interactions with fibronectin and fibrinogen. Mutual inhibition in binding, *Eur. J. Biochem.*, 145, 151, 1984.
36. Jaffe, E. A., Leung, L. L. K., Nachman, R. L., Levin, R. I., and Mosher, D. F., Thrombospondin is the endogenous lectin of human platelets, *Nature (London)*, 295, 246, 1982.
37. Leung, L. L. K., Role of thrombospondin in platelet aggregation, *J. Clin. Invest.*, 74, 1764, 1984.
38. Mumby, S. M., Abbott-Brown, D., Raugi, G. J., and Bornstein, P., Regulation of thrombospondin secretion by cells in culture, *J. Cell. Physiol.*, 120, 280, 1984.
39. Majack, R. A., Cook, S. C., and Bornstein, P., Platelet-derived growth factor and heparin-like glycosaminoglycans regulate thrombospondin synthesis and deposition in the matrix by smooth muscle cells, *J. Cell Biol.*, 101, 1059, 1985.
40. Burke, J. M. and Ross, R., Synthesis of connective tissue molecules by smooth muscle, *Int. Rev. Connect. Tissue Res.*, 8, 119, 1979.
41. Foster, J. A., Elastin structure and biosynthesis: an overview, *Methods Enzymol.*, 82, 559, 1982.
42. Franzblau, C. and Faris, B., Biosynthesis of insoluble elastin in cell and organ cultures, *Methods Enzymol.*, 82, 615, 1982.
43. Eyre, D. W., Paz, M. A., and Gallop, P. M., Crosslinking in collagen and elastin, *Annu. Rev. Biochem.*, 53, 717, 1984.
44. Dunn, D. M. and Franzblau, C., Effects of ascorbate on insoluble elastin accumulation and cross-link formation in rabbit pulmonary artery smooth muscle cell cultures, *Biochemistry*, 21, 4195, 1982.
45. Faris, B., Salcedo, L. L., Cook, V., Johnson, L., Foster, J. A., and Franzblau, C., The synthesis of connective tissue protein in smooth muscle cells, *Biochim. Biophys. Acta*, 418, 93, 1976.
46. Snider, R., Faris, B., Verbitzski, V., Moscaritolo, R., Salcedo, L., and Franzblau, C., Elastin biosynthesis and cross-link formation in rabbit aortic smooth muscle cell cultures, *Biochemistry*, 20, 2614, 1981.
47. Foster, J. A., Mecham, R. P., Rich, C. B., Cronin, M. F., Levine, A., Imberman, M., and Salcedo, L. L., Proelastin. Synthesis in cultured smooth muscle cells, *J. Biol. Chem.*, 253, 2797, 1978.
48. Abraham, P. A., Hart, M. L., Winge, A. R., and Carnes, W. H., The biosynthesis of elastin by an aortic medial cell culture, *Adv. Exp. Med. Biol.*, 79, 397, 1977.
49. Narayanan, A. S., Sandberg, L. B., Ross, R., and Layman, D. L., The smooth muscle cell. VI. Elastin synthesis in arterial smooth muscle cell culture, *J. Cell Biol.*, 68, 411, 1976.
50. Ross, R., The smooth muscle cell. II. Growth of smooth muscle in culture and formation of elastic fibers, *J. Cell Biol.*, 50, 172, 1971.
51. Hinek, A. and Thyberg, J., Electron microscopic observations on the formation of elastic fibers in primary cultures of aortic smooth muscle cells, *J. Ultrastruct. Res.*, 60, 12, 1977.
52. Muir, L. W., Bornstein, P., and Ross, R., A presumptive subunit of elastic fiber microfibrils secreted by arterial smooth muscle cells in culture, *Eur. J. Biochem.*, 64, 105, 1976.
53. Rucker, R. B. and Tinker, D., Structure and metabolism of arterial elastin, *Int. Rev. Exp. Pathol.*, 17, 1, 1977.
54. Cleary, E. G. and Gibson, M. A., Elastin-associated microfibrils and microfibrillar proteins, *Int. Rev. Connect. Tissue Res.*, 10, 97, 1983.
55. Mayne, R., Vascular connective tissue: normal biology and derangement in human diseases, in *Diseases of Connective Tissue: The Molecular Pathology of the Extracellular Matrix*, Uitto, J. and Perejda, Z., Eds., Marcel Dekker, New York, 1984.

56. Leung, D. Y. M., Glagov, S., and Mathews, M. B., A new *in vitro* system for studying cell response to mechanical stimulation, *Exp. Cell Res.*, 109, 285, 1977.
57. Majack, R. A. and Bornstein, P., Heparin regulates the collagen phenotype of vascular smooth muscle cells: induced synthesis of an M_r 60,000 collagen, *J. Cell Biol.*, 100, 613, 1985.
58. Majack, R. A. and Bornstein, P., Regulation of collagen biosynthesis: heparin alters the biosynthetic phenotype of vascular smooth muscle cells in culture, *Ann. N.Y. Acad. Sci.*, 460, 172, 1985.
59. Beldekas, J. C., Smith, B., Gerstenfeld, L. C., Sonenshein, G. E., and Franzblau, C., Effects of 17β-estradiol on the biosynthesis of collagen in cultured bovine aortic smooth muscle cells, *Biochemistry*, 20, 2162, 1981.
60. Pietila, K. and Nikkari, T., Enhanced synthesis of collagen and total protein by smooth muscle cells from atherosclerotic rabbit aortas in culture, *Atherosclerosis*, 37, 11, 1980.
61. Stavenow, L., Kjellstrom, T., and Malmquist, J., Stimulation of collagen production in growth-arrested myocytes and fibroblasts in culture by growth factors from platelets, *Exp. Cell Res.*, 136, 321, 1981.
62. Bornstein, P. and Sage, H., Structurally distinct collagen types, *Annu. Rev. Biochem.*, 49, 957, 1980.
63. Holderbaum, D. and Ehrhart, L. A., Modulation of types I and III procollagen synthesis at various stages of arterial smooth muscle cell growth *in vitro*, *Exp. Cell Res.*, 153, 16, 1984.
64. Scott, D. M., Harwood, R., Grant, M. E., and Jackson, D. S., Characterization of the major collagen species present in porcine aortae and the synthesis of their precursors by smooth muscle cells in culture, *Connect. Tissue Res.*, 5, 7, 1977.
65. Rauterberg, J., Allam, S., Brehmer, U., Wirth, W., and Hauss, W. H., Characterization of the collagen synthesized by cultured human smooth muscle cells from fetal and adult aorta, *Hoppe Seyler's Z. Physiol. Chem.*, 358, 401, 1977.
66. Layman, D. L., Epstein, E. H., Dodson, R. F., and Titus, J. L., Biosynthesis of type I and III collagens by cultured smooth muscle cells from human aorta, *Proc. Natl. Acad. Sci. U.S.A.*, 74, 671, 1977.
67. Lohler, J., Timpl, R., and Jaenisch, R., Embryonic lethal mutation in mouse collagen I gene causes rupture of blood vessels and is associated with erythropoietic and mesenchymal cell death, *Cell*, 38, 597, 1984.
68. Beldekas, J. C., Gerstenfeld, L., Sonenshein, G. E., and Franzblau, C., Cell denstiy and estradiol modulation of procollagen type III in cultured calf smooth muscle cells, *J. Biol. Chem.*, 251, 12252, 1982.
69. Gerstenfeld, L., Beldekas, J. C., Sonenshein, G. E., and Franzblau, C., Processing of procollagen types III and I in cultured bovine smooth muscle cells, *J. Biol. Chem.*, 259, 9158, 1984.
70. Byers, P. H., Holbrook, K. A., McGillivray, B., MacLeod, P. M., and Lowry, R. B., Clinical and structural heterogeneity of type IV Ehlers-Danlos syndrome, *Hum. Genet.*, 47, 141, 1979.
71. Majack, R. A. and Bornstein, P., Heparin and related glycosaminoglycans regulate the secretory phenotype of vascular smooth muscle cells, *J. Cell Biol.*, 99, 1688, 1984.
72. Mayne, R., Vail, M. S., Miller, E. J., Blose, S. H., and Chacko, S., Collagen polymorphism in cell cultures derived from guinea pig aortic smooth muscle: comparison with three populations of fibroblasts, *Arch. Biochem. Biophys.*, 181, 462, 1977.
73. Aumailley, M. and Bricaud, H., Collagen synthesis in organ culture of normal and atherosclerotic aortas, *Atherosclerosis*, 39, 1, 1981.
74. MacCallaugh, K. A. and Balian, G., Collagen characterization and cell transformation in human atherosclerosis, *Nature (London)*, 258, 73, 1975.
75. Morton, L. F. and Barnes, M. J., Collagen polymorphism in the normal and diseased blood vessel wall, *Atherosclerosis*, 42, 41, 1982.
76. Odermatt, B. F., Lang, A. B., Ruttner, J. R., Winterhalter, K. H., and Trueb, B., Monoclonal antibodies to human type IV collagen: useful reagents to demonstrate the heterotrimeric nature of the molecule, *Proc. Natl. Acad. Sci. U.S.A.*, 81, 7343, 1984.
77. Timpl, R. and Martin, G. R., Components of basement membranes, in *Immunochemistry of the Extracellular Matrix*, Vol. 2, Furthmayr, H., Ed., CRC Press, Boca Raton, Fla., 1982, 119.
78. Sankey, E. A. and Barnes, M. J., Comparison of the collagenous products synthesized in culture by pig aortic endothelial and smooth muscle cells, *Biochem. J.*, 218, 11, 1984.
79. Fessler, J. H. Shigaki, N., and Fessler, L. I., Biosynthesis and properties of type V procollagens, *Ann. N. Y. Acad. Sci.*, 460, 181, 1985.
80. Niyibizi, C., Fietzek, P. P., and van der Rest, M., Human placenta type V collagens. Evidence for the existence of an $\alpha 1(V)\alpha 2(V)\alpha 3(V)$ collagen molecule, *J. Biol. Chem.*, 259, 14170, 1984.
81. Mayne, R., Vail, M. S., and Miller, E. J., Characterization of the collagen chains synthesized by cultured smooth muscle cells derived from rhesus monkey thoracic aorta, *Biochemistry*, 17, 446, 1978.

82. Gay, S., Martinez-Hernandez, A., Rhodes, R. K., and Miller, E. J., The collagenous exocytoskeleton of smooth muscle cells, *Collagen Rel. Res.*, 1, 377, 1981.
83. Chung, E., Rhodes, R. K., and Miller, E. J., Isolation of three collagenous components of probable basement membrane origin from several tissues, *Biochem. Biophys. Res. Commun.*, 71, 1167, 1976.
84. Odermatt, E., Risteli, J., Van Delden, V., and Timpl, R., Structural diversity and domain composition of a unique collagenous fragment (intima collagen) obtained from human placenta, *Biochem. J.*, 211, 295, 1983.
85. Jander, R., Rauterberg, J., and Glanville, R. W., Further characterization of the three polypeptide chains of bovine and human short-chain collagen (intima collagen), *Eur. J. Biochem.*, 133, 39, 1983.
86. Jander, R., Troyer, D., and Rauterberg, J., A collagen-like glycoprotein of the extracellular matrix is the undegraded form of type VI collagen, *Biochemistry*, 23, 3675, 1984.
87. Trueb, B. and Bornstein, P., Characterization of the precursor form of type VI collagen, *J. Biol. Chem.*, 259, 8597, 1984.
88. Hessle, H. and Engvall, E., Type VI collagen. Studies of its localization, structure and biosynthetic form with monoclonal antibodies, *J. Biol. Chem.*, 259, 3955, 1984.
89. von der Mark, H., Aumailley, M., Wick, G., Fleischmajer, R., and Timpl, R., Immunochemistry, genuine size and tissue localization of collagen VI, *Eur. J. Biochem.*, 142, 493, 1984.
90. Schmid, T. M. and Conrad, H. E., A unique low molecular weight collagen secreted by cultured chick embryo chondrocytes, *J. Biol. Chem.*, 257, 12444, 1982.
91. Gibson, G. J., Schor, S. L., and Grant, M. E., Effects of matrix molecules on chondrocyte gene expression: synthesis of a low molecular weight collagen species by cells cultured within collagen gels, *J. Cell Biol.*, 93, 767, 1982.
92. Schmid, T. M. and Linsenmayer, T. F., Localization of short chain skeletal collagen, *Fed. Proc.*, 43, 1588, 1984.
93. Ross, R. and Vogel, A., The platelet-derived growth factor, *Cell*, 14, 203, 1978.
94. Bernstein, L. R., Antoniades, H., and Zetter, B. R., Migration of cultured vascular cells in response to plasma and platelet-derived factors, *J. Cell Sci.*, 56, 1, 1982.
95. Nakao, J., Ooyama, T., Chang, W. C., Murota, S., and Orimo, H., Platelets stimulate aortic smooth muscle cell migration, *in vitro, Atherosclerosis*, 43, 143, 1982.
96. Grotendorst, G. R., Chang, T., Seppa, H. E. J., Kleinman, H. K., and Martin, G. R., Platelet-derived growth factor is a chemoattractant for vascular smooth muscle cells, *J. Cell. Physiol.*, 113, 261, 1983.
97. Clowes, A. W., Clowes, M. M., Gown, A. M., and Wight, T. N., Localization of proteoheparan sulfate in rat aorta, *Histochemistry*, 80, 379, 1984.
98. Marcum, J. A. and Rosenberg, R. D., Anticoagulantly active heparin-like molecules from vascular tissue, *Biochemistry*, 23, 1730, 1984.
99. Ross, R., Vogel, A., Davies, P., Raines, E., Kariya, B., Rivest, M. J., Gustafson, C., and Glomset, J., The platelet-derived growth factor and plasma control cell proliferation, in *Hormones and Cell Culture*, Book A, Sato, G. and Ross, R., Eds., Cold Spring Harbor Press, Cold Spring Harbor, N.Y., 1979, 3.
100. Stiles, C. D., Pledger, W. J., Tucker, R. W., Martin, R. G., and Scher, C. D., Regulation of the Balb/c-3T3 cell cycle — effects of growth factors, *J. Supramol. Struct.*, 13, 489, 1980.
101. Scher, C. D., Shepard, R. C., Antoniades, H. N., and Stiles, C. D., Platelet-derived growth factor and the regulation of the mammalian fibroblast cell cycle, *Biochim. Biophys. Acta*, 560, 217, 1979.
102. Cochran, B. H., Lillquist, J. S., and Stiles, C. D., Post-transcriptional control of protein synthesis in Balb/c-3T3 cells by platelet-derived growth factor and platelet-poor plasma, *J. Cell. Physiol.*, 109, 429, 1981.
103. Burke, J. M. and Ross, R., Collagen synthesis by monkey arterial smooth muscle cells during proliferation and quiescence in culture, *Exp. Cell Res.*, 107, 387, 1977.
104. Cochran, B. H., Reffel, A. C., and Stiles, C. D., Molecular cloning of gene sequences regulated by platelet-derived growth factor, *Cell*, 33, 939, 1983.
105. Hendrickson, S. L. and Scher, C. D., Platelet-derived growth factor-modulated translatable mRNAs, *Mol. Cell. Biol.*, 3, 1478, 1983.
106. Pledger, W. J., Hart, C. A., Locatell, K. L., and Scher, C. D., Platelet-derived growth factor-modulated proteins: constitutive synthesis by a transformed cell line, *Proc. Natl. Acad. Sci. U.S.A.*, 79, 4358, 1981.
107. Greenburg, M. E. and Ziff, E. B., Stimulation of 3T3 cells induces transcription of the c-fos proto-oncogene, *Nature (London)*, 311, 433, 1983.
108. Kelly, K., Cochran, B. H., Stiles, C. D., and Leder, P., Cell-specific regulation of the c-myc gene by lymphocyte mitogens and platelet-derived growth factor, *Cell*, 35, 603, 1983.

109. Nilsen-Hamilton, M., Shapiro, J. M., Massoglia, S. L., and Hamilton, R. T., Selective stimulation by mitogens of incorporation of [^{35}S]-methionine into a family of proteins released into the medium by 3T3 cells, *Cell,* 20, 19, 1980.
110. Nilsen-Hamilton, M., Hamilton, R. T., and Adams, G. A., Rapid selective stimulation by growth factors of the incorporation by Balb/c-3T3 cells of (^{35}S)-methionine into a glycoprotein and 5 superinducible proteins, *Biochem. Biophys. Res. Commun.,* 108, 158, 1982.
111. Gospodarowicz, D. and Ill, C. R., Do plasma and serum have different abilities to promote cell growth? *Proc. Natl. Acad, Sci. U.S.A.,* 77, 2726, 1980.
112. Gospodarowicz, D., Vlodavsky, I., and Savion, N., The extracellular matrix and the control of proliferation of vascular endothelial and vascular smooth muscle cells, *J. Supramol. Struct.,* 13, 339, 1980.
113. Libby, P. and O'Brien, K. V., Culture of quiescent arterial smooth muscle cells in a defined serum-free medium, *J. Cell. Physiol.,* 115, 217, 1983.
114. Salomon, D. S., Liotta, L. A., and Kidwell, W. R., Differential response to growth factor by rat mammary epithelium plated on different collagen substrata in serum-free medium, *Proc. Natl. Acad. Sci. U.S.A.,* 78, 382, 1981.
115. Bitterman, P. B., Rennard, S. I., Adelberg, S., and Crystal, R. G., Role of fibronectin as a growth factor for fibroblasts, *J. Cell Biol.,* 97, 1925, 1983.
116. Wicha, M. S., Liotta, L. A., Garbisa, S., and Kidwell, W. R., Basement membrane collagen requirements for attachment and growth of mammary epithelium, *Exp. Cell Res.,* 124, 181, 1979.
117. Tseng, S. C. G., Savion, N., Stern, R., and Gospodarowicz, D., Fibroblast growth factor modulates synthesis of collagen in cultured vascular endothelial cells, *Eur. J. Biochem.,* 122, 355, 1982.
118. Hata, R., Hori, H., Nagai, Y., Tanaka, S., Kondo, M., Hiramatsu, M., Utsum, N., and Kumegawa, M., Selective inhibition of type I collagen synthesis in osteoblastic cells by epidermal growth factor, *Endocrinology,* 115, 867, 1984.
119. Steinmann, B. U., Abe, S., and Martin, G. R., Modulation of type I and III collagen production in normal and mutant human skin fibroblasts by cell density, prostaglandin E_2 and epidermal growth factor, *Collagen Rel. Res.,* 2, 185, 1982.
120. Clowes, A. W. and Karnovsky, M. J., Suppression by heparin of smooth muscle cell proliferation in injured arteries, *Nature (London),* 265, 625, 1977.
121. Guyton, J. R., Rosenberg, R. D., Clowes, A. W., and Karnovsky, M. J., Inhibition of rat arterial smooth muscle cell proliferation by heparin. I. *In vivo* studies with anticoagulant and non-anticoagulant heparin, *Circ. Res.,* 46, 625, 1980.
122. Hatcher, V. B., Tsien, G., Oberman, M. S., and Burk, P. G., Inhibition of cell proliferation and protease activity by cartilage factors and heparin, *J. Supramol. Struct.,* 14, 33, 1980.
123. Nilsson, J., Ksiazek, T., Thyberg, J., and Wasteson, A., Cell surface components and growth regulation in cultivated arterial smooth muscle cells, *J. Cell Sci.,* 64, 107, 1983.
124. Hoover, R. L., Rosenberg, R. D., Haering, W., and Karnovsky, M. J., Inhibition of rat arterial smooth muscle cell proliferation by heparin. II. *In vitro* studies, *Circ. Res.,* 47, 578, 1980.
125. Gamse, G., Fromme, H. G., and Kresse, H., Metabolism of sulfated glycosaminoglycans in cultured endothelial cells and smooth muscle cells from bovine aorta, *Biochim. Biophys. Acta,* 544, 514, 1978.
126. Castellot, J. J., Addonizio, M. L., Rosenberg, R. D., and Karnovsky, M. J., Cultured endothelial cells produce a heparinlike inhibitor of smooth muscle cell growth, *J. Cell Biol.,* 90, 372, 1981.
127. Castellot, J. J., Favreau, L. V., Karnovsky, M. J., and Rosenberg, R. D., Inhibition of vascular smooth muscle cell growth by endothelial cell-derived heparin, *J. Biol. Chem.,* 257, 11256, 1982.
128. Willems, C., Astaldi, G. C. B., de Groot, P. G., Janssen, M. C., Gonsalvez, M. D., Zeijlemaker, W. P., van Mourik, J. A., and van Aken, W. G., Media conditioned by cultured human vascular endothelial cells inhibit the growth of vascular smooth muscle cells, *Exp. Cell Res.,* 139, 191, 1981.
129. Oosta, G. M., Favreau, L. V., Beeler, D. L., and Rosenberg, R. D., Purification and properties of human platelet heparitinase, *J. Biol. Chem.,* 257, 11249, 1982.
130. Fritze, L. M. S. and Rosenberg, R. D., Bovine aortic smooth muscle cells produce an inhibitor of smooth muscle cell growth *in vitro, J. Cell Biol.,* 97, 90a, 1983.
131. Wight, T. N. and Hascall, V. C., Proteoglycans in primate arteries. III. Characterization of the proteoglycans synthesized by arterial smooth muscle cells in culture, *J. Cell Biol.,* 96, 167, 1983.
132. Majack, R. A. and Clowes, A. W., Inhibition of vascular smooth muscle cell migration by heparin-like glycosaminoglycans, *J. Cell. Physiol.,* 118, 253, 1984.
133. Millis, A. J. T., Hoyle, M., and Reich, E., Nodular smooth muscle cells secrete a unique heparin-binding protein, *J. Cell Biol.,* 99, 29a, 1984.
134. Majack, R. A., unpublished observations.

Chapter 9

SYNTHESIS OF GLYCOSAMINOGLYCANS AND PROTEOGLYCANS

M. J. Merrilees

TABLE OF CONTENTS

I. INTRODUCTION

Vascular smooth muscle cells (SMC) synthesize and secrete proteoglycans (PG) and constituent glycosaminoglycans (GAG), matrix components which together with collagen and elastin play a vital role in maintaining the structural integrity of vessel walls. Interest in factors and mechanisms controlling the production of PG and GAG by SMC stems in large part from observations that the amounts and proportions of the various types of GAG are changed at sites of atherosclerotic lesion formation[1,2] and from findings that sulphated GAG (SGAG) have the ability to form complexes with low- and very low-density lipoproteins.[3-7] These two features have provided the impetus in recent years for a large number of investigations on the effects of atherosclerotic risk factors on GAG synthesis, and many of these studies have been conducted in vitro, using cell and organ culture techniques.

Like other connective tissue cells in culture SMC synthesize a spectrum of GAG including hyaluronic acid (HA), heparan sulfate (HS), dermatan sulfate (DS), and chondroitin sulfates A (CSA or CS_4) and C (CSC or CS_6). These GAG, except for HA, do not exist as free chains but are covalently bound to protein to form PG macromolecules, which may further link with HA to form very large PG aggregates.[8] These PG and PG aggregates are the functional components of the matrix, but, interestingly, there have been comparatively few studies on PG synthesis by SMC in culture. Most investigators have preferred to analyze the constituent GAG. While PG production is currently receiving increased attention,[9,10,98] analyses of GAG are nevertheless of considerable value since the amounts and proportions of GAG are very good indicators to the mechanical properties of tissues.[11] The amounts and proportions of GAG produced by SMC under conditions of cell and organ culture, however, are highly variable, and the interpretation of results from in vitro studies and their extrapolation to in vivo requires considerable caution. This chapter will review the effects of those factors which contribute to this variability in GAG synthetic patterns in culture and, further, will review the effects on GAG production of a number of factors considered to play a role in atherogenesis.

II. FACTORS AFFECTING GLYCOSAMINOGLYCAN LEVELS IN CULTURE

A. Culture Conditions

1. Cell Density and Phase of Growth

Changes in the amounts and proportions of GAG with changes in cell density probably best illustrate the importance of carefully monitoring culture conditions during experimental work. The relationship is complex and, surprisingly, only a few papers have reported in detail on the effects of cell density and phase of growth on SMC GAG synthesis.

Immediately after seeding at a low density, SMC are particularly active in the synthesis of GAG,[12] and HA is usually the predominate component.[12,13] This high level of activity is not solely due to increased synthesis associated with initial attachment and cell migration. Wight and Ross[14] found that cultures of primate SMC, maintained at a low density for an extended period by culturing initially in 1% serum for 7 days followed by serum-free medium for 12 days, also displayed a high level of GAG synthesis compared with more dense cultures.

The exponential or proliferative phase of growth, whether occurring in the first few days after seeding[12] or initiated at a later stage by increasing the serum level,[14] is associated with a marked reduction in GAG synthesis compared to low-density cultures

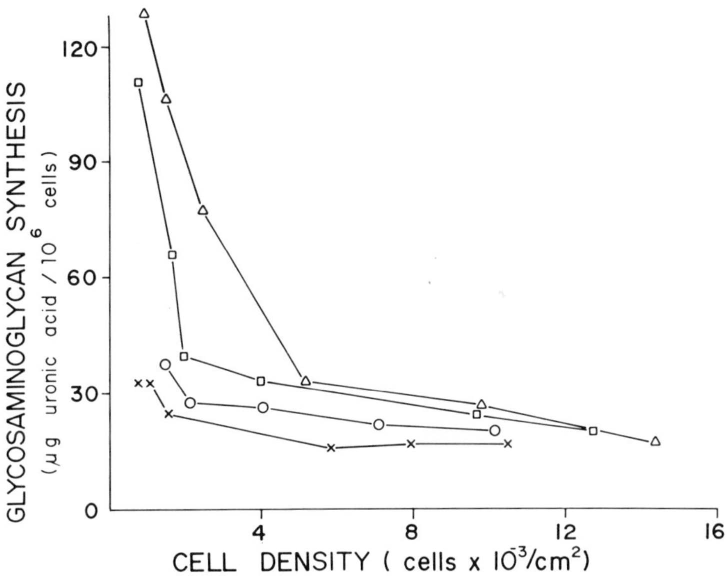

FIGURE 1. Effect of serum concentration and cell density on GAG production by SMC in culture. Cells were plated out at six different densities from 9 to 100 × 10^2 cells per cm^2 and when established given a serum-free medium for 24 hr. Subgroups were then given medium containing 0% (×), 1% (○), 5% (□), or 10% (△) serum. After a further 24 hr, cell counts were made and medium assayed for total GAG. (From Wosu, L., Parisella, R., and Kalant, N., *Atherosclerosis*, 48, 205, 1983. With permission.)

(Figure 1). Furthermore, during the proliferation phase and as cultures approach the stationary phase, the proportion of HA decreases while that of the SGAG increases.[12,13,15,16]

Few studies, however, have distinguished between the effect of cell density per se and the effect of proliferation rate. Wosu et al.[17] recently examined this feature and concluded that the fall in the rate of GAG synthesis which occurs with increasing cell density was a direct effect of density and not related to proliferation rate which was biphasic.

The reduced rate of synthesis in high-density stable cultures is not necessarily a constant feature. Pietilä[12] measured GAG synthesis in cultures of rabbit SMC maintained from 5 to 16 days in a stationary phase at high density and found an increase in GAG synthesis, including an increase in HA, compared to the proliferative and early stationary phases. The rates of synthesis, however, were not as high as that found for the low-density cultures immediately after seeding. Others have found that while SMC maintained at high densities for prolonged periods are still active in GAG synthesis, only very small amounts of HA are detectable,[14,18] and the proportions of GAG in these cultures more closely resemble the proportions in vivo.

2. Serum

Serum concentration is positively correlated with cell density, and the effects of serum on GAG synthesis can in part be explained on the basis of changes in cell densities. Serum does, however, affect GAG synthesis independently of cell density. Wosu et al.[17] showed that total GAG synthesis by human SMC increased with increasing serum concentration (0 to 10%), although at higher densities (where GAG synthesis was reduced) the effect was much less marked (Figure 1). Both SGAG and HA are stimulated by serum. The response of SGAG to changed serum levels, however, is more complicated than that for HA. Pietila[12] found that reduction in the serum level of cultures maintained in 10% serum resulted initially (24 to 48 hr) in an increase in SGAG synthesis, but after 7 days in the appropriate serum concentration, SGAG synthesis was positively correlated with serum levels. In contrast, HA was immediately responsive and positively correlated with serum concentration irrespective of the length of time of preincubation with serum. HA also shows a greater response to serum than SGAG,[16] which may relate to the finding that serum contains a factor capable of stimulating hyaluronic acid synthetase activity in fibroblasts.[19]

3. pH

Pietilä[12] examined the effect of pH, ranging from 6.8 to 7.9, on rabbit SMC cultured both in the presence of 10% serum and in serum-free medium. Synthesis of both SGAG and HA was shown to be positively correlated with pH and over the range tested there was a seven- to tenfold difference in incorporation irrespective of serum levels.

Other factors such as hypoxia and additives such as ascorbic acid also affect GAG synthesis, but these will be considered under other headings later. Cell density, serum, and pH are variables encountered under standard culture conditions, and it is evident that alterations in any one of these factors results in marked changes to both the amounts and proportions of GAG.

B. Source of SMC

1. Vessels

Almost all SMC cultures for the study of GAG metabolism have been derived from thoracic aortas, and most cultures have been established from medial or intimal-medial explants. Where SMC derived from intima have been compared to SMC from the media of the same animal, the patterns of GAG synthesis have been found to be very similar, apart from some minor differences in the pericellular pools.[20] Interestingly, muscular arteries, such as the coronary arteries where atherosclerotic plaques of primary significance occur, have rarely been used. Wosu et al.[17] used SMC from adult human tibial arteries (muscular) and from fetal human aortas in their study on the effect of lipoprotein on GAG secretion, but a direct comparison between the two types of SMC was not made. Thus it remains to be determined whether or not SMC cultured from different types of vessels have similar or different GAG synthetic patterns.

SMC from the same vessel of the same species, however, can display quite marked differences in the amounts and proportions of GAG, and these differences relate to the state of the vessel wall from which the SMC cultures were derived. Pietila et al.[21] examined GAG synthesis by rabbit SMC, established from intimal-medial explants, from normal vessels, and from vessels made atherosclerotic by 6 months of cholesterol feeding. They found that SMC derived from the thickened atherosclerotic vessels had a significantly higher rate of GAG synthesis than normal cells and that most of the increase was due to an increase in SGAG, predominately DS. This finding, however, was a feature only of proliferative lesions. In more advanced stable fibrous lesions, formed by 6 months of cholesterol feeding followed by 6 months on a normal diet, the synthesis of sulfated GAG was slightly but significantly reduced compared to control SMC, while the synthesis of HA was increased.[22]

The synthesis of SGAG by SMC derived from atherosclerotic-susceptible White Carneau (WC) pigeons is also greater than for SMC from the atherosclerotic-resistant Show Racer (SR) breed. SMC from WC pigeons synthesized three to four times as much SGAG as SR pigeons, although the relative proportions of the individual SGAG remained the same.[23] Another example of intraspecific variation in GAG synthesis is from SMC cultured from hypertensive rats. Their SMC synthesize more SGAG than SMC from normotensive rats, although this difference can be related directly to the higher average protein content of SMC from hypertensive rats.[24]

2. Species

The percentage distribution of the individual GAG varies considerably between species (Table 1). Not all of this variation, however, is attributable to true differences between species. Some of the variation is clearly due to culture conditions while differences in methods of GAG analysis may also be a factor.

Differences in methodology probably contribute only a small amount to the variation. In the majority of studies the separation of individual GAG has been by similar methods: protease digestion, ethanol or quarternary ammonium salt precipitation, followed by electrophoresis. Methods for the isolation and analysis of GAG were recently reviewed by Taniguchi,[25] and electrophoretic techniques were considered to give good separation of most GAG, recognizing that GAG display appreciable heterogeneity including differences in degree of sulfation, polydispersity of molecular weight, and variable amounts of attached residual peptides. Problems with methodology are partly resolved where comparative studies have been undertaken in the same laboratory using a standardized method. Under these circumstances, it would appear that at least some of the apparent species variability can be explained by variations in culture conditions, particularly cell density.

The major apparent variation between species relates to the amount of HA. Confluent cultures of nonhuman primates are characterized generally by a low percentage (0 to 10%) of HA, while confluent SMC from adult and fetal humans, pigs, and rabbits have, in general, a high proportion of HA, frequently more than 50% of the total GAG. Unfortunately, in most studies cell densities are not specified but only reported as being confluent, subconfluent, or in the growth phase. Where cell densities have been specified, or where stationary and growth phase cultures have been compared directly, it is apparent that low-density cultures are usually characterized by a high proportion of HA. Thus rat SMC, for example, produce mostly HA (70%) at low densities (0.6×10^6 cells per 25 cm^2) but only a small proportion (10%) at a high densities (3×10^6 cells per 25 cm^2).[16] If cultured for an extended period of up to 4 weeks, during which time cells are allowed to accumulate and form multilayers, only a trace of HA is detectable.[18] A similar reduction in the proportion of HA with increasing density has been found for porcine SMC,[13] but it would appear that human SMC, even when confluent, still produce mostly HA (see Table 1).

The proportions of the SGAG are also variable but unlike HA not so clearly correlated with changes in cell density. Dense cultures generally show an increased proportion of DS compared to low-density cultures, but there is no consistent pattern of dominance by either DS or CS with respect to density. Rather there seems to be a species-specific pattern for the SGAG, and this pattern correlates in most instances with the pattern occurring in vivo. For example, in some nonhuman primates and in rats, DS is dominant both in vivo and in vitro while in pigs, bovines, pigeons, and humans, CS is dominant in both situations. There are, however, a number of inconsistencies with this correlation. Very dense long-term cultures of rat SMC[18] have a predominance of CS (43%), although DS still constitutes a significant proportion (32%). A similar distribution has been found in some low-density cultures of rat SMC.[26] Chondroitin sulfate is dominant in rabbit aorta,[27,28] but in culture, rabbit SMC usually synthesize as much or more DS.[29,30]

Heparan sulfate constitutes on average about 20 to 25% of the total GAG in the intima and media, and, as for the other SGAG, there is species variability. Rat aorta for example is especially rich in HS (40 to 50%),[27,28,31] while the proportion in pigeon

Table 1
PERCENTAGE DISTRIBUTION OF GLYCOSAMINOGLYCANS PRODUCED BY SMC

Species[a]	Cell density	Serum level (%)	Distribution of GAG HA	HS	DS	CS A/C	Compartment	Ref.
Human (fetal)	Confluent	15	71	7	3	19	Medium	60
Human (fetal)	Confluent	15	50	(	50	)	Total GAG	48
Human (fetal)	Confluent	10	60	(	40	)	Total GAG	61
Human (fetal)	Confluent	15	71	(	29	)	Medium	50
			45	(	55	)	Cell layer[b]	
			67	(	33	)	Total GAG	
Human (fetal)	Confluent	LPF[c]						
		5	65	(	35	)	Total GAG	17
		2	70	(	30	)	Total GAG	
		LDL[d]						
		5	56	(	44	)	Total GAG	
		2	61	(	39	)	Total GAG	
Pigtail monkey	Confluent	5	0—5	ND[e]	80	15	Medium	14
Cynomolgus monkey	Organ culture	0	9	12	27	53	Whole vessel wall	42
Bovine	Subconfluent	0	5	2	2	91	Medium	98
			14	10	10	66	Cell Layer	
Bovine (fetal)		10	0	60	8	32	Pericellular coat	95
Bovine	Confluent	10	ND[e]	22	20	58	Medium	20
Bovine	Organ culture		30	11	10	49	Whole vessel wall	100
Porcine	Subconfluent	2	49	13	18	20	Medium	13
	Confluent for 10 days	2	18	17	31	34	Medium	
Porcine	Confluent	10	20	10	15	55	Medium	43
			17	40	(43	)	Pericellular coat	
Porcine	Confluent	2	24	9	20	47	Total GAG	26
Porcine	Confluent	10	23	10	(67	)	Medium	9
Porcine	Confluent	1	25	10	30	35	Total GAG	78
Rabbit (weanlings)	Confluent	10	64	2	23	11	Medium	30
	$1—1.5 \times 10^{6}$[f]	10	13	31	40	16	Cell Layer	
Rabbit	Confluent	10	62	(	38	)	Total GAG	21
Rabbit	Subconfluent	0	57	(	43	)	Total GAG	12
	Confluent	10	89	(	11	)	Total GAG	
Rabbit	Confluent	10	63	(	37	)	Total GAG	22
Rat (Neonatal)	Confluent multilayers	20	Trace	30	30	40	Medium	18
Rat	Subconfluent	2	24	8	21	47	Total GAG	26
	Confluent	2	9	11	50	30	Total GAG	
Rat	Subconfluent (lag phase)	10	70	13	12	5	Intracellular 1° cultures	15
	Confluent (stationary phase)	10	9	34	55	2	Intracellular 1° cultures	
	Confluent	10	10	59	24	7	Pericellular coat 1° culture	
	Confluent	10	3	7	88	2	Intracellular S10	
	Confluent	10	19	37	42	2	Pericellular coat S10	
Rat	3.0×10^{6}	1	10	10	43	37	Medium	16
	2.0×10^{6}	1	18	9	61	12	Medium	
	1.5×10^{6}	1	28	5	41	26	Medium	
	0.6×10^{6}	1	72	5	13	10	Medium	
	2.0×10^{6}	1	56	23	15	6	Cell layer	
	1.5×10^{6}	1	45	26	11	18	Cell layer	

Table 1 (continued)
PERCENTAGE DISTRIBUTION OF GLYCOSAMINOGLYCANS PRODUCED BY SMC

Species[a]	Cell density	Serum level (%)	Distribution of GAG HA	HS	DS	CS A/C	Compartment	Ref.
Pigeon								
White Carneau	Confluent	15	ND	5	35	60	Medium	23
Show Racer	Confluent	15	ND	5	35	60	Medium	

[a] All SMC for all species are from aortas.
[b] Cells plus pericellular coat.
[c] Lipoprotein-free serum.
[d] Low-density lipoprotein-containing serum.
[e] Not determined.
[f] Cell density per 25 cm² flask.

aorta may be as low as 11%.[32] Electron microscopical[33] and immunohistochemical[34] analyses suggest that HS is located primarily in the basement membrane-like material which surrounds individual SMC in the arterial walls (see Chapters 4 and 7). This basement membrane-like material has been isolated from rabbit SMC in culture and shown to contain predominantly HS (55%) and chondroitin sulfate with a small amount of HA and a trace of DS.[35] HS and CS also predominate in the pericellular coat immediately adjacent to the plasma membrane of cultured SMC.[36] In other culture studies, where the cell layer and growth medium have been analyzed separately, the proportion of HS is markedly increased in the pericellular pool (Table 1), a feature characteristic of other cell types in culture.[37-39]

C. SMC Phenotype

Variability in the amounts and proportions of GAG synthesized by SMC in culture may also be due partly to variability in SMC phenotype. The vast majority of studies, however, have not taken into account the degree of modulation of SMC which may occur in culture (see Chapter 4). Recently, Yamamoto et al.[15] did address this point directly by measuring GAG synthesis by rat SMC as the cells changed from a contractile phenotype in primary culture to a synthetic phenotype during successive subcultures. The change in phenotype was monitored by immunofluorescent staining of actin and myosin; by the third passage, myosin was absent. The pattern of GAG synthesis at this stage, however, was still similar to the primary culture with the pericellular GAG characterized by a large amount of HS (58%) and moderate amounts of DS (26%). By the seventh and subsequent subcultures, by which stage actin exhibited a decreased staining intensity, HS was replaced by DS as the dominant pericellular GAG. Superimposed on these changes were other changes, of the type discussed earlier, associated with alterations in cell density.

Yamamoto et al.[15] also compared primary cultures to medial explants of the rat aortic wall and found that over a 48-hr incubation period the explants synthesized much less HS and more HA. Although no comment was made on the state of the SMC in the explants, presumably they would have retained the contractile phenotype since SMC of rat carotid arteries maintained under organ culture conditions retain the morphological features of the contractile phenotype for more than a week.[40] Like the aortic explants, the rat carotid in organ culture also displayed a change in GAG synthesis. Although the percentage distribution of the individual GAG was not determined, the pattern of [^{3}H] glucosamine incorporation across the vessel wall, while initially very similar to carotids labeled in vivo, changed progressively with time in culture.[41] The carotids in culture, however, still had their endothelium intact, and it is likely that these cells were responsible for some of the changes in GAG synthesis by the SMC in the vessel wall.

Mozzicato et al.[42] investigated GAG synthesis in intimal-medial explants from the aorta of Cynomolgus monkey. Although it is not clear if endothelial cells were present, over the first 5 hr in culture the percentage distribution of newly synthesized GAG was the same as for that for GAG present in the wall at the start of culturing. The relative percentages were CS 53%, DS 27%, HS 12% and HA 9%. With increasing time in culture, however, the percentage distribution pattern for the newly synthesized GAG gradually changed, and by 22 hr the amount of labeled DS (30%) was almost equal to CS (32%) with HS (22%) and HA (16%) still contributing the least to total labeled GAG.

Thus even short-term maintenance of artery wall in organ culture, where the cell/matrix relationship more closely resembles normal wall and where the SMC still display the morphological features of a contractile phenotype, leads to changes in GAG synthetic patterns. But it remains to be determined whether or not these changes occurring in whole vessel wall in organ culture are truly dependent or independent of SMC phenotype.

D. Degradation

A potential source of the variation in the amounts of individual GAG produced by SMC in culture is a difference in the rate of degradation rather than a difference in the rate of synthesis. In most studies, while it is acknowledged that labeling levels or actual amounts of GAG are the net result of synthesis and degradation, it is usually assumed that any differences in GAG levels between control and test samples are due to altered rates of synthesis. The evidence from those studies which have investigated turnover would support, in general, this premise.

First, studies with both SMC[43] and fibroblasts[44] have shown that most newly synthesized GAG passes rapidly from the intracellular pool to the pericellular pool and into the medium. Addition of exogenous GAG has shown that there is virtually no degradation of GAG in the medium. Pulse chase experiments have shown, however, that 30 to 50% of the total labeled SGAG is degraded by between 1 and 5 days and that this loss exceeds amounts initially present in the intracellular pool. Thus some degradation is occurring in the pericellular pool, and this GAG probably contributes most to the degradative pool. Diehl et al.[45] showed that inhibitors of lysosomal function had no effect on the rate of loss of material from the intracellular pool and in view of the absence of degradation in the medium, they also concluded that degradation occurs from the pericellular compartment. More recently, Volker et al.[46] have shown conclusively that cell surface proteoglycans, visualized by attached gold particles, are endocytosed via coated and noncoated cell surface pits and degraded in lysosomes.

Studies on fibroblasts[44] have further shown that the turnover of individual GAG in the pericellular layer varies. Heparan sulfate is retained for a longer period than DS and accumulates. With increasing time in culture, the proportion of HS in the medium also increases as it is released from the pericellular pool. Thus the proportions of the individual GAG in the medium will be dependent in part upon the length of time in culture and the labeling times, whereas the proportions in the pericellular layer will be additionally influenced by rates of degradation.

Although turnover studies have been made of cells maintained under constant conditions, there have been few studies attempting to determine if changed levels of GAG under experimental conditions are the result of changes in rates of synthesis or rates of degradation. Merrilees and Scott[41] have shown that the pattern of incorporation of [^{3}H] glucosamine across the wall of the rat carotid artery maintained in organ culture is markedly different in the presence and absence of endothelium. Both pulse and continuous labeling, however, showed that net rates of degradation were the same under both conditions. Rates of degradation for some of the individual GAG may have varied, but if that did occur they were offset by changed rates for others. Overall it was concluded that changed labeling levels were due to changes in rates of synthesis.

III. EFFECT OF FACTORS RELATED TO ATHEROGENESIS

The primary purpose of many of the studies on GAG production by SMC in culture has been to investigate the effect of factors related to atherogenesis in isolation from the complexity of the in vivo environment. Although some of the results are contradictory, after elimination of effects due to methodology and to culture conditions, it would appear that in general there is a good correlation between factors associated with atherogenesis in vivo and their effects on GAG production in vitro (Table 2). In vivo, developing atherosclerotic lesions are characterized by increased amounts of GAG compared with unaffected parts of vessel walls and especially an increase in SGAG relative to HA. The increase in total GAG may not be particularly large, but the change in the HA to SGAG ratio can be a valuable indicator to changed vessel structure. Thus a decrease in the HA to SGAG ratio is associated with factors that increase the risk of atherosclerosis, while the converse is generally true for factors which decrease the risk.[61]

A. Lipoproteins

The effect of lipoproteins on GAG metabolism has been the most controversial of all factor studies, probably due in large part to the fact that there have been more studies on lipoproteins than any other factor and thus more scope for variability in methodology and culture conditions. For example, the recovery of GAG by methods using cetylpyridinium chloride is reduced in the presence of hyperlipidemic serum.[47] Also, lipoproteins may effect cell growth, thus making interpretation of changes in GAG more difficult. Where cell growth has been carefully monitored, however, it is evident that lipoproteins can have a direct effect of GAG synthesis.

The most significant finding is that the atherogenic low-density lipoproteins (LDL) have an opposite effect from the antiatherogenic high-density lipoproteins (HDL). The most consistent finding is that LDL produces a decrease in the HA to SGAG ratio, while HDL produces an increase.

In the presence of LDL or in the presence of hyperlipidemic serum, the decrease in the ratio may be achieved either by a decrease in HA with little change to the amount of SGAG[48-50] or by an increase, usually small, in the amount of SGAG.[51,52] It should be noted, however, that while it is possible to generalize in this way, the effect of LDL on SMC is complex.

Wosu et al.[17] have shown that the LDL-stimulated increase in GAG is more marked when the cells are proliferating but that high levels of LDL have a cytotoxic effect, a feature noted previously for SMC[53] and for other cell types.[54,55] Similar results were obtained for both SMC and fibroblasts from adults, but fetal SMC responded differently. With fetal SMC, low levels of LDL in the presence of a low serum concentration had a stimulatory effect on SMC growth, as well as on GAG secretion; however, with

Table 2
EFFECT OF ATHEROSCLEROTIC RISK FACTORS ON GLYCOSAMINOGLYCAN PRODUCTION BY SMC IN CULTURE

		Effect on GAG levels[a]						
Risk factor	Source of SMC	HA	HS	DS	CS A/C	Total	HA/SGAG[a]	Ref.
LDL[b]	Human	—	↔	↔	↔	↔	—	56
LDL	Human							
	Adult	—	—	—	—	↑	↓	17
	Fetal	—	—	—	—	↔	—	
LDL	Bovine	—	↑	(↑)		↑	—	51
LDL-Sera	Human (fetal)	↔	(	↔	)	—	↔	59
LDL-Sera	Human (fetal)	↓	(	↔	)	—	↓	48
LDL-Sera (Type IIA hyperlipidemia)	Human (fetal)	↓	(	↔	)	—	↓	49
LDL-Sera (Type IIA hyperlipidemia)	Human (fetal)	↓	(	↔	)	—	↓	50
LDL-Sera (long-term culture, 28 days)	Rabbit	↓	(	↑	)	—	↓	52
HDL[c]	Bovine	—	↓	(↓)		↓	—	51
HDL-Sera	Human (fetal)	↓	(	↓	)	—	↑	59
HDL-Sera	Human (fetal)	↓	↓	↓	↓	↓	↑	60
HDL-Sera	Human (fetal)	↔	(	↓	)	—	↑	48
HDL-Sera	Human (fetal)							
Lumberjacks		↓	(	↓	)	—	↑	49
Runners		↔	(	↓	)	—	↑	
Hormones	Human (fetal)							
Cortisol		↓	(	↔		—	↓	48, 61
Estradiol		↔	(	↔		—	↔	
Testosterone		↔	(	↔		—	↔	
Insulin		↔	(	↔		—	↔	
Prostaglandins (E_1, E_2, $F_1\alpha$, $F_2\alpha$)	Rabbit	↑E_2	(	↑	)	—	—	70
Hypoxia	Rabbit	↑	(	↑	)		↓	72
Mechanical forces								
Cyclic stretching	Rabbit	↑	—	↔	↑	—	—	29
Centrifugation	Porcine	↑	↑	↑	↑	↑	↓	13
Endothelial cells	Porcine	↑	↑	↑	↑	↑	↑	26
Low density		↑	↑	↑	↑	↑	↑	26
High density		↔	↑	↑	↑	↑	↓	102
Ascorbic acid	Rat	—	↓	↑	↑	—	—	95
(50 μg/mℓ)	Bovine	—	↓	↑	↑	—	—	

[a] ↑ increase; ↓ decrease; ↔ no change; — not determined.
[b] Low-density lipoprotein.
[c] High-density lipoprotein.

increasing concentration of LDL, both cell number and GAG secretion were significantly reduced. Interestingly, confluent cultures of SMC did not respond to LDL with an increase in GAG secretion. Sudhakaran et al.[56] also found that LDL had no effect on confluent cultures of SMC, but Ehrlich and Murray[57] found that confluent primary cultures of SMC from rabbit and rhesus monkey did respond to LDL by increasing very significantly SGAG synthesis.

This variability in the response of SMC to LDL and to hyperlipidemic serum illustrates very clearly the complexity of the system and the necessity for further detailed studies. For example, the effect of LDL on the individual SGAG species has not been fully investigated, although Pillai et al.[51] did note that increases in HS and the other SGAG were of a similar magnitude. The effects of the various subspecies of LDL are a further avenue for future studies since it has been shown that whereas the small LDL subspecies exhibit no mitogenic action on SMC growth in culture, the large subspecies can have a marked proliferative action.[58]

The effect of HDL[51] or high-density lipoproteinemic sera[48,49,59,60] on SMC is more marked and less variable than LDL. HDL decreases the synthesis of SGAG[48,49,51,59] and may[59,60] or may not[48,49] decrease the synthesis of HA. Where HA is decreased, however, the ratio of HA to SGAG still favors HA. The effects on GAG synthesis can also be more clearly separated from cell density effects than for LDL. Tammi et al.[60] found that HDL-rich sera, collected from lumberjacks, had no effect on [^{3}H] thymidine incorporation by human SMC up to a concentration of 10%, although at 15% there was significant inhibition compared with control sera. Within the range of serum concentration where [^{3}H] thymidine incorporation was not affected, the synthesis of SGAG decreased significantly, and the individual SGAG were decreased by the same extent. HA was also decreased although at serum concentrations up to 5% the synthesis of HA was increased compared to the absence of serum. The mechanism by which HDL-sera affects GAG synthesis is not known, but there is some evidence that the effect may be dependent on the platelet-derived growth factor (PDGF).[48]

B. Hormones

Little is known about the effects of hormones on GAG synthesis. Rönnemaa et al.[49] in their studies on the effects of lipoproteins also included results on the effects of a number of hormones, including cortisol, estradiol, testosterone, and insulin. The only hormone to affect GAG synthesis was cortisol, which, at concentrations slightly above physiological level, decreased the synthesis of HA by 50% but had no effect on SGAG. Further studies showed that the decrease in HA was not due to a direct effect on the HA synthesizing system.[61] Rather, cortisol may act by changing the properties of the cell membrane,[62] the site where hyaluronate is synthesized.[63] Elevated levels of cortisol and other glucorticoids are considered to be risk factors for atherosclerosis.[64]

The role of estrogens in atherosclerosis is not clear. While epidemiological studies indicate that premenopausal women have less coronary artery disease than men, there are no data to support such a protective function. To the contrary, elevated levels seem to be associated with increased risk.[65] Interestingly, administration of estrogen or estrogen-progesterone increases the GAG content of rabbit thoracic aorta and with a marked decrease in the HA to CS ratio[66] — which implies an increased risk. The percentage distribution of the individual GAG after treatment, however, resembled that for canine thoracic aorta, which is resistant to atherosclerosis. Thus interpretation of the significance of the results is difficult. The response of vessel wall to estrogen may also be different from other tissues. It has been shown (in mice) that estradiol administration markedly increases HA content of dermal tissues while not affecting DS.[67] From the limited data available, however, it would seem that GAG production by SMC in culture is not affected by estradiol.[49]

C. Prostaglandins

The synthesis of prostaglandin E_2 is elevated in atherosclerotic rabbit aortas[68] and also in the aortas of atherosclerotic-susceptible White Carneau pigeons when compared to the resistant Show Racer breed,[69] but it is not clear if prostaglandins play a direct role in lesion development. The effects of prostaglandins E_1, E_2, $F_1\alpha$, and $F_2\alpha$ on SMC in culture have been investigated by Pietila et al.[70] Although all of these prostaglandins enhanced the incorporation of [^{3}H] glucosamine into SGAG by about 50%, they also inhibited [^{3}H] thymidine uptake; thus some of the increase may be accounted for by a lower cell density. The effect of prostaglandins on HA, however, indicates that density effects were not solely responsible since for all prostaglandins except E_2 there was less change in HA than SGAG, whereas at lower densities relatively more HA would be expected. Prostaglandin E_2 did stimulate HA, but SGAG also increased by a similar amount again indicating that the effect was probably independent of cell density.

D. Hypoxia

In experimental animals, systemic hypoxia can induce atherosclerosis with an associated increase in the synthesis and accumulation of GAG.[71] In culture the synthesis of GAG by rabbit SMC incubated in medium with oxygen saturation lowered from 20% to 2 to 3% is increased, especially SGAG (twofold increase), although HA is also increased significantly.[72] The amount of cell protein changed little with hypoxia; thus the effect on GAG levels was probably independent of cell density and may even have bee underestimated since the hypoxic cultures had a lower pH than controls. As previously discussed, pH is positively correlated with GAG synthesis.

E. Mechanical Forces

An association has been demonstrated between hypertension and increased SGAG.[73-76] While this association may not be the result of a direct effect of mechanical stress acting on the SMC in the vessel wall, connective tissues in general are very responsive to their mechanical environment.[11] In cell culture there is evidence that SMC can respond to changes in physical forces acting on the cells. Leung et al.[29] have shown that rabbit SMC grown on purified elastin membranes and subjected to repeated elongation and relaxation increase their synthesis of HA and CS6 threefold — and without any change in cell number, compared to stationary cultures. DS and CS4, however, did not increase. SMC also respond to increased pressure generated by centrifuging cultures at low speeds (45 × g).[13] Confluent cultures, centrifuged for 16 hr/day for a total spin time of 48 hr over a 72-hr period, increased their GAG by 50%. All GAG increased, but there was a greater proportional increase for SGAG (60 to 90%) than for HA (-35%).

Thus, SMC are capable of responding to the mechanical environment, but interpretation of these results must be made with considerable caution. Apart from the fact that the experimental designs used in the above experiments may be quite inappropriate models for SMC subjected to stress in vivo, changes in GAG levels observed with hypertension may be mediated not through a direct effect but through, for example, the endothelium. Endothelial cells are known to respond to acute hypertension by increasing their turnover,[77] and the increase in GAG (which is primarily intimal) may be mediated by factors released by active endothelium.

F. Endothelium

Endothelial cells in culture produce a factor or factors able to stimulate GAG synthesis by SMC.[26,78] This stimulation occurs both with endothelial cells grown in coculture with SMC and with growth medium conditioned on endothelial cells and then placed on SMC. Generally the increase in HA is greater than that for SGAG; HA usually shows at least a two- to threefold increase, although the increase may be as much as seven- to eightfold over controls, while SGAG usually doubles in amount. This stimulation by endothelial cells also occurs across species[26] and also with other cells such as fibroblasts.[78] More recent evidence indicates that conditioned media from low-density cultures of endothelial cells is more effective than media from confluent cultures, although the latter media still stimulates SGAG synthesis.[102]

These results suggest that in vivo endothelium could play a role in modulating GAG synthesis by SMC in the intima or inner media and that the modulation may be dependent upon the state of the endothelium. Similar ideas have been advanced for the control of SMC growth by endothelium. In culture, endothelial cells produce both stimulatory[79] and inhibitory[80] factors for SMC growth depending upon culture conditions. There is also some support for the idea of endothelial control of SMC GAG from studies of rat carotid artery maintained in organ culture with endothelium present, absent, and regenerating.[41] In the presence of mitotically active endothelium, the synthesis of GAG in the inner layer of the media is increased compared with the rest of the media. In the absence of endothelium, removed by air-drying, there is a marked drop in the rate of synthesis in the inner layer, but this returns to normal following regeneration of endothelium. Throughout these changed levels of GAG the rates of degradation, as measured by pulse and continuous labeling, remained the same as for controls. Furthermore, throughout the various experimental conditions, there was no significant growth of SMC. Similar changes in intimal medial GAG levels in the absence and presence of regenerating endothelium have been observed in experimental animal models,[81,82] but the changes observed in organ culture occurred in serum-free medium and thus independently of factors such as PDGF. Endothelium in an active state may thus play a direct role in modulating GAG levels and independently from SMC growth.

G. Platelets and Monocytes

Platelets are thought to play a pivotal role in the initiation of SMC growth and lesion development through the release of PDGF. Platelets also produce connective tissue activating peptides (CTAP III and CTAP-P2)[83,84] that stimulate GAG synthesis, especially HA, in fibroblasts. The effect on SMC is not known, but it is possible that they would respond in a similar manner.

The role of monocytes in atherogenesis, especially the early stages, is currently receiving increased attention.[85-87] While their primary role appears to be one of lipid uptake, in culture they have been shown to release a growth factor for SMC;[88] therefore, in addition to forming foam cells they may contribute to lesion development by stimulating SMC growth. Their effect on GAG synthesis, however, is not known although it is possible that they could play a role in degradation since peripheral blood mononuclear cells can release distinct latent enzymes capable of degrading both collagen and proteoglycans.[89]

H. Ascorbic Acid

Ascorbic acid (AA) deficiency is considered to be a risk factor for atherosclerosis.[90,91] It must be noted, however, that overt AA deficiency, or scurvy, is a rare occurrence, which implies that if AA does play a role in the pathogenesis of atherosclerosis, then either there are local deficiencies in vessel walls or AA affects vessel wall structure in prescorbutic states. With true AA deficiency it is clearly apparent that connective tissue structure and organization is affected, and it is well known that AA is required for hydroxylation of collagen, without which proper fibril formation will not take place.[92]

AA also affects GAG levels in vessel walls. For example Verlangieri and Stevens[93] showed that aortic GAG levels (and especially CS4) in rabbits fed an atherogenic diet supplemented with AA were increased compared with animals on the same diet but without AA. The increased GAG levels here were interpreted as evidence in support of the idea that AA is necessary to maintain adequate levels of GAG in vessels to maintain the structural integrity and resist atherosclerotic changes. The lower levels of GAG found in animals on the atherogenic diet without AA were thus considered to contribute to the process of atherogenesis.

Evidence from cell culture studies supports the idea that AA plays a role in maintaining the production of extracellular materials by SMC. Like fibroblasts, SMC in culture require adequate levels of AA for the formation of insoluble collagen.[94] Furthermore, addition of AA to SMC cultures also enhances both the synthesis and degree of sulfation of SGAG, except for HS, and independently of increased collagen synthesis.[95] In these studies morphology and rates of proliferation were not affected by the addition of AA, although others[96] have found that AA affects both parameters of bovine SMC in culture, with cell doubling time being decreased from 62 to 47 hr in the presence of AA and cells changing from an elongated to a polygonal shape. Further, in this latter study there was evidence that HS increased.

In the above studies, AA was added to a level of 50 μg/mℓ. In some unpublished studies using porcine and rat SMC, increasing concentrations of AA ranging from 25 to 300 μg/mℓ were found to have a biphasic effect on GAG synthesis.[16] At concentrations of 25 μg/mℓ and 50 μg/mℓ all GAG, including HA, were stimulated to a small degree (25 to 30%), but above 50 μg/mℓ GAG synthesis was decreased markedly. Cell density was also reduced but only at 200 μg/mℓ and 300 μg/mℓ, whereas the reduction in GAG was apparent at 100 μg/mℓ where cell densities and morphologies were the same as for lower concentrations of AA. A concentration of 50 μg/mℓ, however, is above the normal physiological level of 0.7 to 1.2 mg/100 mℓ of plasma. It would appear, therefore, that GAG synthesis may be increased by AA supplementation even if only to a small degree.

These studies on AA also illustrate the importance of being able to compare changes in GAG levels in culture with changes in GAG levels in vivo. Otherwise the increased GAG levels in culture could be interpreted as increasing the risk of atherosclerosis by increasing available GAG for binding to lipoproteins rather than bringing GAG levels up to a level adequate to maintain normal vessel structure. Interestingly, while studies on changes in collagen synthesis have been invariably conducted with AA-supplemented media, few studies on GAG metabolism have included AA in the media. Stimulation of SMC GAG synthesis by endothelial cells, however, still occurs in media supplemented with AA.[78]

IV. PROTEOGLYCAN SYNTHESIS

Only recently have attempts been made to characterize in detail the types of PG synthesized by SMC in culture. Studies on SMC from bovine,[97] porcine,[9] and primate[10] aortas have shown that at least two distinct size classes of proteoglycans are produced with physicochemical properties similar to PG isolated from intact vessel walls. More recently, Arumugham and Anderson[98] have established for bovine SMC in culture that although both the medium and cell layer contain predominately CS proteoglycans, the cell layer contains a higher proportion of HS and DS proteoglycans. As yet, however, there is virtually no information on the effects of either culture conditions or atherogenic risk factors on PG production. Nevertheless, the demonstration that SMC in culture secrete PG with characteristics similar to those present in vivo is important since investigations on factors suspected of modulating PG synthesis can now be carried out using the advantages of cell culture and with some confidence that the cells will retain their differentiated function.

V. CONCLUDING REMARKS

It is apparent from the results of these cell culture studies that many of the changes to the amounts and proportions of GAG seen in intact vessel walls can be explained by the direct effects of stimulatory or inhibitory factors on GAG synthesis by the SMC. It is also clear that the synthesis of GAG by SMC in culture is highly variable and that before concluding that any particular factor has a direct effect, care must be taken to ensure that differences between control and test cultures are not due to changes in culture conditions, especially changes in cell density, serum concentration, and pH.

This review also highlights a number of apparent gaps in our knowledge of SMC synthesis by SMC in culture. Perhaps foremost is that virtually all studies have been carried out using SMC from a single vessel, the aorta, and while it is likely that SMC from other vessels are no different from aortic SMC, it would seem worthwhile to examine SMC from other sources such as coronary arteries.

It is also notable that while SMC from fetal human aortas have been used fairly extensively for the investigation of factors associated with atherosclerosis, there is little information available on GAG production by adult human SMC. Furthermore, in only one study on human SMC[60] have the individual SGAG been analyzed separately. Of further interest is the finding that human SMC in culture produce a large amount of HA, much more than would be expected from amounts present in the whole aorta.[31,99] SMC from nonhuman primates and from many other animals are characterized by a low proportion of HA; thus it would be of interest to know if HA production by human SMC in culture is a specific trait or relates to cell density. Although many of the cultures with a high HA production were apparently confluent, the effect of cell density on HA production for these SMC is not known.

Although it has been shown that SMC of a contractile phenotype produce a slightly different profile of SMC compared to synthetic SMC,[15] further studies are required to confirm and extend these findings. In particular, a strong argument can be advanced for investigating the effect of atherosclerotic risk factors on contractile SMC. In the vast majority of cell culture studies, the SMC have been of the synthetic phenotype, but Chamley-Campbell et al.[101] have shown that contractile SMC do not respond to PDGF, hyperlipidemic LDL, and other serum-derived mitogens. Once they have modulated to a synthetic phenotype, however, they are immediately responsive and undergo proliferation. It would be of interest to determine if changes in GAG production by SMC are similarly dependent on phenotype.

Further studies are also warranted on the effects of other factors such as hormones and ascorbic acid, and it may also be appropriate with these and other studies to make more extensive use of vessels in organ culture where the cell/matrix relationship more closely resembles the condition in vivo. Finally, it is important to reiterate that a change in the HA to SGAG ratio is just as important as a change in GAG amounts and that whenever possible the effect of factors on both HA and SGAG should be determined.

REFERENCES

1. Kramsch, D. M., Biochemical changes in the arterial wall in atherosclerosis with special reference to connective tissue: promising experimental avenues for their prevention, in *Connective Tissues in Arterial and Pulmonary Disease,* McDonald, T. F. and Chandler, A. B., Eds., Springer-Verlag, New York, 1981, 95.
2. Pietilä, K. and Nikkari, T., Role of the arterial smooth muscle cell in the pathogenesis of atherosclerosis, *Med. Biol.,* 61, 31, 1983.
3. Amenta, J. S. and Waters, L. L., The precipitation of serum lipoproteins by mucopolysaccharides extracted from aortic tissue, *Yale J. Biol. Med.,* 33, 112, 1960.
4. Gerö, S., Gergely, J., Devenyi, T., Jakob, L., Szekely, J., and Virag, S., Role of intimal mucoid substances in the pathogenesis of atherosclerosis. I. Complex formation in vitro between mucopolysaccharides from atherosclerotic aortic intimas and plasma β-lipoprotein and fibrinogen, *J. Atheroscler. Res.,* 1, 67, 1961.
5. Srinivasan, S. R., Lopez, S. A., Radhakrishnamurthy, B., and Berenson, G. S., complexing of serum pre-β- and β-lipoproteins and acid mucopolysaccharides, *Atherosclerosis,* 12, 321, 1970.
6. Iverius, P. H., The interaction between human plasma lipoproteins and connective tissue glycosaminoglycans, *J. Biol. Chem.,* 247, 2607, 1972.
7. Iverius, P. H., Possible role of glycosaminoglycans in the genesis of atherosclerosis, in *Atherogenesis: Initiating Factors,* Ciba Symposium No. 12, Elsevier, Amsterdam, 1973, 185.
8. McMurtrey, J., Radhakrishnamurthy, B., Dalferes, E. R., Berenson, G. S., and Gregory, J. D., Isolation of proteoglycan-hyaluronate complexes from bovine aorta, *J. Biol. Chem.,* 254, 1621, 1979.
9. Horn, M. C., Breton, M., Deudon, E., Berrou, E., and Picard, J., The structural characterisation of proteoglycans of cultured aortic smooth muscle cells and arterial wall of the pig, *Biochim. Biophys. Acta,* 755, 95, 1983.
10. Wight, T. N. and Hascall, V. C., Proteoglycans in primate arteries. III. Characterization of the proteoglycans synthesized by arterial smooth muscle cells in culture, *J. Cell Biol.,* 96, 167, 1983.
11. Flint, M. H., Gillard, G. C., and Merrilees, M. J., The effect of local physical environmental factors on connective tissue organization and glycosaminoglycan synthesis, in *Fibrous Proteins: Scientific, Industrial and Medical Aspects,* Vol. 2, Parry, D. A. D. and Creamer, L. K., Eds., Academic Press, London, 1980, 107.
12. Pietilä, K., Incorporation of [^{3}H] glucosamine into glycosaminoglycans in different cell culture conditions by rabbit aortic smooth muscle cells, *Biochim. Biophys. Acta,* 677, 318, 1981.
13. Merrilees, M. J., Merrilees, M. A., Birnbaum, P. S., Scott, P. J., and Flint, M. H., The effect of centrifugal force on glycosaminoglycan production by aortic smooth muscle cells in culture, *Atherosclerosis,* 27, 259, 1977.
14. Wight, T. N. and Ross, R., Proteoglycans in primate arteries. II. Synthesis and secretion of glycosaminoglycans by arterial smooth muscle cells in culture, *J. Cell Biol.,* 67, 675, 1975.
15. Yamamoto, H., Kanaide, H., and Nakamura, M., Metabolism of glycosaminoglycans of cultured rat aortic smooth muscle cells altered during subculture, *Br. J. Exp. Pathol.,* 64, 156, 1983.
16. Merrilees, M. J. and Scott, L., unpublished data, 1984.
17. Wosu, L., Parisella, R., and Kalant, N., Effect of low density lipoprotein on glycosaminoglycan secretion by cultured human smooth muscle cells and fibroblasts, *Atherosclerosis,* 48, 205, 1983.
18. Oakes, B. W., Batty, A. C., Handley, C. J., and Sandberg, L. B., The synthesis of elastin, collagen, and glycosaminoglycans by high density primary cultures of neonatal rat aortic smooth muscle. An ultrastructural and biochemical study, *Eur. J. Cell Biol.,* 27, 34, 1982.
19. Tomida, M., Koyama, H., and Ono, T., A serum factor capable of stimulating hyaluronic acid synthesis in cultured rat fibroblasts, *J. Cell. Physiol.,* 91, 323, 1977.
20. Gamse, G., Fromme, H. G., and Kresse, H., Metabolism of sulphated glycosaminoglycans in cultured endothelial cells and smooth muscle cells from bovine aorta, *Biochim. Biophys. Acta,* 544, 514, 1978.
21. Pietilä, K., Ylä-Herttuala, S., Jaakkola, O., and Nikkari, T., Metabolism of glycosaminoglycans and lipids in smooth muscle cells from atherosclerotic rabbit aortas in culture, *Atherosclerosis,* 37, 449, 1980.
22. Pietilä, K., Ylä-Herttuala, S., Rantala, I., and Nikkari, T., Characterisation of cells cultured from advanced atherosclerotic lesions of the rabbit, *Med. Biol.,* 60, 221, 1982.
23. Wight, T. N., Differences in the synthesis and secretion of sulphated glycosaminoglycans by aorta explant monolayers cultured from atherosclerotic-susceptible and resistant pigeons, *Am. J. Pathol.,* 101, 127, 1980.
24. Schmidt, A., Grünwald, J., and Buddecke, E., [^{35}S] Proteoglycan metabolism of arterial smooth muscle cells cultured from normotensive and hypertensive rats, *Atherosclerosis,* 45, 299, 1982.

25. Taniguchi, N., Isolation and analysis of glycosaminoglycans, in *Glycosaminoglycans and Proteoglycans in Physiological Processes of Body Systems,* Varma, R. S. and Varma, R., Eds., S. Karger, Basel, 1982.
26. Merrilees, M. J. and Scott, L., Interaction of aortic endothelial and smooth muscle cells in culture, *Atherosclerosis,* 39, 147, 1981.
27. Engel, U. R., Glycosaminoglycans in the aorta of six animal species, *Atherosclerosis,* 13, 45, 1971.
28. Stefanovich, V. and Akiyama, K., Comparative studies of aortic acid mucopolysaccharides in fifteen species, *Comp. Biochem. Physiol.,* 34, 125, 1970.
29. Leung, D. Y. M., Glagov, S., and Mathews, M. B., Cyclic stretching stimulates synthesis of matrix components by arterial smooth muscle cells in vitro, *Science,* 191, 475, 1976.
30. Namiki, O., Faris, B., Tschopp, F., Fuglistaller, P., Hollander, W., Franzblau, C., and Schmid, K., Synthesis of glycosaminoglycans by cultured rabbit smooth muscle, *Biochemistry,* 19, 1900, 1980.
31. Gardais, A., Picard, J., and Hermelin, B., Glycosaminoglycan (GAG) distribution in aortic wall from five species, *Comp. Biochem. Physiol. B,* 44, 507, 1973.
32. Curwen, K. D. and Smith, S. S., Aortic glycosaminoglycans in atherosclerosis-susceptible and resistant pigeons, *Exp. Mol. Pathol.,* 27, 121, 1977.
33. Wight, T. N. and Ross, R., Proteoglycans in primate arteries. I. Ultra-structural localization and distribution in the intima, *J. Cell Biol.,* 67, 660, 1975.
34. Hassell, J. R., Robey, P. G., Barrach, H.-J., Wilczek, J., Rennard, S. I., and Martin, G. R., Isolation of a heparan sulphate-containing proteoglycan from basement membrane, *Proc. Natl. Acad. Sci. U.S.A.,* 77, 4494, 1980.
35. Heickendorff, L. and Ledet, T., Glycosaminoglycans of arterial basement membrane-like material from cultured rabbit aortic myomedial cells, *Biochim. Biophys. Acta,* 798, 276, 1984.
36. Nilsson, J., Ksiazek, T., Thyberg, J., and Wasteson, A., Cell surface components and growth regulation in cultivated arterial smooth muscle cells, *J. Cell Sci.,* 64, 107, 1983.
37. Kraemer, P. M., Heparan sulphates of cultured cells. I. Membrane-associated and cell-sap species in Chinese hampster cells, *Biochemistry,* 10, 1437, 1971.
38. Kraemer, P. M., Heparan sulphates of cultured cells. II. Acid-soluble and precipitable species of different cell lines, *Biochemistry,* 10, 1445, 1971.
39. Kraemer, P. M., Mucopolysaccharides: cell biology and malignancy, in *Surfaces of Normal and Malignant Cells,* Hynes, R. O., Ed., John Wiley & Sons, New York, 1979, 149.
40. Merrilees, M. J. and Scott, L., Organ culture of rat carotid artery: maintenance of morphological characteristics and of pattern of matrix synthesis, *In Vitro,* 18, 900, 1982.
41. Merrilees, M. J. and Scott, L., Effects of endothelial removal and regeneration on smooth muscle glycosaminoglycan synthesis and growth in rat carotid artery in organ culture, *Lab. Invest.,* 52, 409, 1985.
42. Mozzicato, P., Faris, B., Hollander, W., Franzblau, C., and Schmid, K., A method to evaluate the biosynthesis of glycosaminoglycans by the aorta of Cynomolgus Monkey, *Atherosclerosis,* 45, 359, 1982.
43. Deudon, E., Breton, M., Berrou, E., and Picard, J., Metabolism of glycosaminoglycans in cultured smooth muscle cells from pig aorta, *Biochimie,* 62, 811, 1980.
44. Vogel, K. G. and Kendall, V. F., Cell-surface glycosaminoglycans: turnover in cultured human embryo fibroblasts (IMR-90), *J. Cell. Physiol.,* 103, 475, 1980.
45. Diehl, T., Scott-Burden, T., and Gevers, W., Sulphate turnover of surface proteoglycans in cultured rat smooth muscle cells, *Biochim. Int.,* 6, 29, 1983.
46. Volker, W., Schmidt, A., Robenek, H., and Buddecke, E., Binding and degradation of proteoglycans by cultured arterial smooth muscle cells. I. Endocytosis and intracellular translocation of proteoglycan-gold conjugates, *Eur. J. Cell Biol.,* 34, 110, 1984.
47. Pietilä, K. and Nikkari, T., Hyperlipidemic rabbit serum reduces recovery of acidic glycosaminoglycans from tissue culture medium, *Anal. Biochem.,* 116, 317, 1981.
48. Rönnemaa, T., Serum lipoprotein composition, platelet factor and arterial smooth muscle cells, *Acta Med. Scand. Suppl.,* 642, 55, 1980.
49. Rönnemaa, T., Jarvelainen, H., Lehtonen, A., Tammi, M., Larjava, H., Saarni, H., Vihersaari, T., and Viikari, J., Serum lipoprotein composition, hormones, and the synthesis of glycosaminoglycans by human aortic smooth muscle cells, *Artery,* 8, 323, 1980.
50. Järveläinen, H., Rönnemaa, T., Tammi, M., Vihersaari, T., Lehtonen, A., and Viikari, J., Type IIA Hyperlipoproteinemic sera decreases the synthesis of hyaluronic acid by cultured human aortic smooth muscle cells, *Atherosclerosis,* 39, 61, 1981.
51. Pillai, S., Donnelly, P. V., Mourao, P. A. S., Di Ferrante, N., and Eskin, S. G., Effect of high density lipoproteins and low density lipoproteins on the glycosaminoglycans metabolism of cultured bovine smooth muscle cells, *Biochem. Int.,* 1, 55, 1980.

52. Pietilä, K., Long-term effect of hyperlipidemic serum on the synthesis of glycosaminoglycans and on the rate of growth of rabbit aortic smooth muscle cells in culture, *Atherosclerosis,* 42, 67, 1982.
53. Hessler, J. R., Robertson, A. L., and Chisolm, G. M., LDL induced cytotoxicity and its inhibition by HDL in human vascular smooth muscle and endothelial cells in culture, *Atherosclerosis,* 32, 213, 1979.
54. Curtiss, L. K. and Edginton, T. S., Regulatory serum lipoproteins — regulation of lymphocyte stimulation by a species of low density lipoprotein, *J. Immunol.,* 116, 1452, 1976.
55. Henricksen, T., Evensen, S. H., and Carlander, B., Injury to human endothelial cells in culture induced by low density lipoprotein, *Scand. J. Clin. Lab. Invest.,* 39, 361, 1979.
56. Sudhakaran, P. R., Prinz, R., Filipovic, I., von Figura, K., and Buddecke, E., Homologous low density lipoprotein does not affect proteoglycan metabolism of cultured skin fibroblasts and arterial smooth muscle cells, *Hoppe Seyler's Z. Physiol. Chem.,* 361, 129, 1980.
57. Ehrlich, K. and Murray, M., Effect of low density lipoprotein on proteoglycan synthesis by aorta cells in culture, *Experientia,* 34, 179, 1978.
58. Fless, G. M., Kirchhausen, T., Fischer-Dzoga, K., Wissler, W., and Scanu, A. M., Serum low density lipoproteins with mitogenic effect on cultured aortic smooth muscle cells, *Atherosclerosis,* 41, 171, 1982.
59. Tammi, M., Rönnemaa, T., Vihersaari, T., Saarni, H., Lehtonen, A., and Viikari, J., Effect of sera from hyperlipidemic subjects and high-density-lipoproteinemic runners on the synthesis of DNA and glycosaminoglycans by cultured human aortic smooth muscle cells, *Med. Biol.,* 57, 118, 1979.
60. Tammi, M., Rönnemaa, T., Vihersaari, T., Lehtonen, A., and Viikari, J., High density lipoproteinemia due to vigorous physical work inhibits the incorporation of [^{3}H] thymidine and the synthesis of glycosaminoglycans by human aortic smooth muscle in culture, *Atherosclerosis,* 32, 23, 1979.
61. Larjava, H., Saarni, H., Tammi, M., Penttinen, R., and Ronnemaa, T., Cortisol decreases the synthesis of hyaluronic acid by human aortic smooth muscle cells in culture, *Atherosclerosis,* 35, 135, 1980.
62. De Duwe, C., Walleaux, R., and Wibo, M., Effect of fat-soluble compounds on lysosomes in vitro, *Biochem. Pharmacol.,* 9, 97, 1972.
63. Prehm, P., Hyaluronate is synthesized at plasma membranes, *Biochem. J.,* 220, 597, 1984.
64. Troxler, R., Sprague, E. A., Albanese, R. A., Fuchs, R., and Thompson, A. J., The association of elevated plasma cortisol and early atherosclerosis as demonstrated by coronary angiography, *Atherosclerosis,* 26, 151, 1977.
65. Phillips, G. B., Sex hormones, risk factors and cardiovascular disease, *Am. J. Med.,* 65, 7, 1978.
66. Aikawa, J., Munakata, H., Isemura, M., Ototani, N., and Yosizawa, Z., Hormonal effects on glycosaminoglycans in thoracic aortas of rabbits, *Tohoku J. Exp. Med.,* 143, 113, 1984.
67. Uzuka, M., Nakajima, K., Ohta, S., and Mori, Y., The mechanism of estrogen-induced increase in hyaluronic acid biosynthesis with special reference to estrogen receptor in the mouse skin, *Biochim. Biophys. Acta,* 627, 199, 1980.
68. Berberian, P. A., Ziboh, V. A., and Hsia, S. L., Prostaglandin E_2 biosynthesis: changes in rabbit aorta and skin during experimental atherogenesis, *J. Lipid Res.,* 17, 46, 1976.
69. Subbiah, M. T. R., Prostaglandin E biosynthesis and effect in pigeon aorta — possible role in atherogenesis, *Atherosclerosis,* 29, 487, 1978.
70. Pietilä, K., Moilanen, T., and Nikkari, T., Prostaglandins enhance the synthesis of glycosaminoglycans and inhibit the growth of rabbit aortic smooth muscle cells in culture, *Artery,* 7, 509, 1980.
71. Helin, G., Helin, P., and Lorenzen, I., The aortic glycosaminoglycans in arteriosclerosis induced by systemic hypoxia, *Atherosclerosis,* 12, 235, 1970.
72. Pietilä, K. and Jaakkola, O., Effect of hypoxia on the synthesis of glycosaminoglycans and collagen by rabbit aortic smooth muscle cells in culture, *Atherosclerosis,* 50, 183, 1984.
73. Crane, W. A. J., Sites of mucopolysaccharide synthesis in the lesions of experimental hypertension in rats, *J. Pathol. Bacteriol.,* 83, 183, 1962.
74. Hollander, W., Kramsch, D. M., Farmelant, N., and Madoff, I. M., Arterial wall metabolism in experimental hypertension of coarctation of the aorta of short duration, *J. Clin. Invest.,* 47, 1221, 1968.
75. Sharpe, D. N., Scott, P. J., and Flint, M. H., Connective tissue changes in artery walls in experimental hypertension, *Aust. N. Z. J. Surg.,* 44, 427, 1974.
76. Hauss, W. H., Tissue alterations due to experimental arteriosclerosis, in *Connective Tissue and Ageing,* Vol. 1, Vogel, H. G., Ed., Excerpta Medica, Amsterdam, 1973, 23.
77. Chobanian, A. V., The influence of hypertension and other hemodynamic factors in atherogenesis, *Prog. Cardiovasc. Dis.,* 26, 177, 1983.
78. Merrilees, M. J., Sodek, J., and Aubin, J. E., Effect of cells of epithelial rests of Malassez and endothelial cells on synthesis of glycosaminoglycans by periodontal ligament fibroblasts in vitro, *Dev. Biol.,* 97, 146, 1983.

79. Gajdusek, C., DiCorleto, P., Ross, R., and Schwartz, S. M., An endothelial cell-derived growth factor, *J. Cell Biol.*, 85, 467, 1980.
80. Castellot, J. J., Addonizio, M. L., Rosenberg, R., and Karnovsky, M. J., Cultured endothelial cells produce a heparinlike inhibitor of smooth muscle cell growth, *J. Cell Biol.*, 90, 372, 1981.
81. Richardson, M., Ihnatowycz, I., and Moore, S., Glycosaminoglycan distribution in rabbit aortic wall following balloon catheter deendothelialization. An ultrastructural study, *Lab Invest.*, 43, 509, 1980.
82. Wight, T. N., Curwen, K. D., Litrenta, M. M., Alonso, D. R., and Minick, C. R., Effect of endothelium on glycosaminoglycan accumulation in injured rabbit aorta, *Am. J. Pathol.*, 113, 156, 1983.
83. Myers, S. L. and Castor, C. W., Connective tissue activation. XV. Stimulation of glycosaminoglycan and DNA synthesis by a polymorphonuclear leukocyte factor, *Arthritis Rheum.*, 23, 556, 1980.
84. Castor, C. W. and Cobel-Geard, S. R., Connective tissue activation: evidence for a second human platelet growth factor, *Clin. Res.*, 28, 139a, 1980.
85. Gerrity, R. G., The role of the monocyte in atherogenesis. I. Transition of blood-borne monocytes into foam cells in fatty lesions, *Am. J. Pathol.*, 103, 181, 1981.
86. Gerrity, R. G., The role of the monocyte in atherogenesis. II. Migration of foam cells from atherosclerotic lesions, *Am. J. Pathol.*, 103, 191, 1981.
87. Joris, I., Zand, T., Nunnari, J. J., Krolikowski, F. J., and Majno, G., Studies on the pathogenesis of atherosclerosis. I. Adhesion of mononuclear cells in the aorta of hypercholesterolemic rats, *Am. J. Pathol.*, 113, 341, 1983.
88. Ziats, N. P. and Robertson, A. L., Effects of peripheral blood monocytes on human vascular cell proliferation, *Atherosclerosis*, 38, 401, 1981.
89. Golds, E. E., Santer, V., Killackey, J., and Roughley, P. J., Mononuclear cell factors stimulate the concomitant secretion of distinct latent proteoglycan, gelatin and collagen degrading enzymes from human skin fibroblasts and synovial cells, *J. Rheumatol.*, 10, 861, 1983.
90. Shaffer, C. F., Ascorbic acid and atherosclerosis, *Am. J. Clin. Nutr.*, 23, 27, 1970.
91. Krumdieck, C. and Butterworth, C. E., Ascorbate-cholesterol-lecithin interactions: factors of potential importance in the pathogenesis of atherosclerosis, *Am. J. Clin. Nutr.*, 27, 866, 1974.
92. Prockop, J. J., Kivirikko, K. I., Tuderman, L., and Guzman, N. A., The biosynthesis of collagen and its disorders, *N. Engl. J. Med.*, 301, 13, 1979.
93. Verlangieri, A. J. and Stevens, J. W., L-ascorbic acids: effects on aortic glycosaminoglycan ^{35}S incorporation in rabbit-induced atherosclerosis, *Blood Vessels*, 16, 177, 1979.
94. De Clerck, Y. A. and Jones, P. A., The effect of ascorbic acid on the nature and production of collagen and elastin by rat smooth-muscle cells, *Biochem. J.*, 186, 217, 1980.
95. Scott-Burden, T., Murray, E., Diehl, T., and Gevers, W., Glycosaminoglycan synthesis by smooth muscle cells cultured in the absence and presence of ascorbic acid, *Hoppe Seyler's Z. Physiol. Chem.*, 364, 61, 1983.
96. Schwartz, E., Bienkowski, R. S., Coltoff-Schiller, B., Goldfisher, S., and Blumenfeld, O. O., Changes in the components of extracellular matrix and in growth properties of cultured aortic smooth muscle cells upon ascorbate feeding, *J. Cell Biol.*, 92, 462, 1982.
97. Kresse, H., von Figura, K., Buddecke, E., and Fromme, H. G., Metabolism of sulphated glycosaminoglycans in cultivated bovine arterial cells. I. Characterization of different pools of sulphated glycosaminoglycans, *Hoppe Seyler's Z. Physiol. Chem.*, 356, 929, 1975.
98. Arumugham, R. and Anderson, J. C., Distribution in caesium chloride gradients of proteoglycans secreted by bovine aorta smooth muscle cells and study of their aggregation with hyaluronate and cartilage proteoglycan, *Biochim. Biophys. Acta*, 797, 128, 1984.
99. Aikawa, J., Munakata, H., Isemura, M., Ototani, N. and Yosizawa, Z., Comparison of glycosaminoglycans from thoracic aortas of several mammals, *Tohoku J. Exp. Med.*, 143, 107, 1984.
100. Kresse, H. and Buddecke, E., Stoffwechselheterogenität ^{14}C- und ^{35}s-markieter glycosaminoglykane (saurer mucopolysaccharide) bei in-vitro-inkubation, *Hoppe Seyler's Z. Physiol. Chem.*, 351, 151, 1970.
101. Chamley-Campbell, J. H., Campbell, G. R., and Ross, R., Phenotype-dependent response of cultured aortic smooth muscle to serum mitogens, *J. Cell Biol.*, 89, 378, 1981.
102. Scott, L. J. and Merrilees, M. J., Stimulation of smooth muscle cell glycosaminoglycan synthesis by cultured endothelial cells is dependent on endothelial cell density, *Atherosclerosis*, 1986, in press.

Chapter 10

GLYCOPROTEINS ASSOCIATED WITH BOVINE AORTIC SMOOTH MUSCLE CELLS IN CULTURE — SELECTED ASPECTS

James R.A. Leushner and M. Daria Haust

TABLE OF CONTENTS

I. INTRODUCTION

The significance of smooth muscle cells (SMC) in atherosclerosis has been well documented.[1,2] Many of the advances in our understanding of their role, both in the normal and diseased arteries, have been obtained from the in vitro tissue culture system. Central to their involvement in the disease are the components they secrete into the extracellular compartment. These consist primarily of the fibrous elements of the interstitial collagens and the elastic tissue, all of which have been characterized in detail both morphologically[3-5] and biochemically.[6-11]

Other components such as glycoproteins, glycosaminoglycans, and other substances that do not form definable fibrous elements are also constituents of the extracellular matrix produced by SMC.[6,12] Generally, SMC are "wrapped" by a morphologically definable basement membrane (BM) whose major structural constituent is type IV collagen.[13,14] Closely associated with this BM are a number of high-molecular-weight structural glycoproteins such as fibronectin[15,16] and laminin.[17,18] Several other structural glycoproteins[19] have been demonstrated in the extracellular matrix. For the purpose of this presentation, these macromolecules are defined as oligosaccharide-containing matrix proteins. Therefore, this class would include the above structural glycoproteins as well as the procollagens[20] and some nonfibrous collagens such as type IV collagen.[21]

Recent studies suggest that in addition to the interstitial and BM collagens a separate class, termed "intermediate collagens",[22] also is present in the extracellular compartment. The major member of this intermediate class is the type V collagen,[7,23] which is distributed in an "intermediate zone" between the BM-cell interface (i.e., the pericellular matrix) and the interstitial matrix. Some other glycoproteins such as fibronectin[15,16] were shown to have a similar pericellular distribution. Macromolecules with this type of distribution have been implicated in the structural organization of both the BM and the intercellular matrix, serving as an organizational lattice upon which the other components of the matrix are deposited.[19] Many of these glycoproteins are intimately associated with the cytoskeletal elements and thus may provide a structural and functional link between the cell and the extracellular matrix. In this capacity the macromolecules are important in cell migration, spreading, and differentiation.[24]

In this presentation some of our studies using bovine aortic SMC in culture will be summarized in the following areas: (1) the synthesis of oligosaccharide (oligo)-containing glycoproteins in general and the interstitial and type V procollagens in particular, (2) the binding of type V collagen to the SMC surface and the role of this collagen in the transference of forces in SMC function, and (3) biochemical and morphological comparison of the features of a polypeptide complex synthesized by SMC, which has characteristics similar to both, the type VI collagen, and the microfibrils.

II. GLYCOPROTEINS IN THE SMC MATRIX

The cellular functions of SMC in culture have been shown to be dependent on the extracellular matrix adjacent to the cell (also termed the "pericellular matrix"[25]). Regulatory roles have been proposed for the matrix produced by the SMC themselves in culture[26] and that derived from other sources.[27] Studies such as these underscore the fact that rather than playing just a simple structural role, the components of the matrix are directly involved in modifying the behavior of cells.

The oligo groups of the glycoproteins in the matrix are thought to mediate the cell-matrix interconnections,[28,29] as well as cell to cell interactions.[30] Changes in the oligos at the surface of fibroblasts have been observed during cell transformation[31] and cell growth in culture.[32-34] Modifications of the oligos on the cell surface have been shown to alter the way the cell adheres to the intercellular matrix[35] and binds certain substances.[36]

Whereas the effects of various components within the matrix on SMC growth have been documented, no information on the oligo composition of the matrix had been available. Therefore, efforts in our laboratories have been directed towards testing whether the changes of the oligos associated with glycoproteins of the matrix of SMC occur in different phases of growth in culture.[37]

A. Methodology

SMC were obtained from medial explants of bovine aorta. They were grown in M199 media supplemented with 20% fetal calf serum and an antimycotic-antibiotic mixture. The proliferative stage of SMC growth was characterized by rapidly dividing cells, as shown in Figure 1A. This phase was followed by a confluent phase with multilayered growth of "hill and valley" appearance, characteristic of SMC (Figure 1B). The latter phase of growth was characterized by uptake of [^{3}H] thymidine, as shown in Table 1, column A; the labeling of these cultures was similar to the quiescent or confluent phase observed in fibroblast cultures. During the same time interval, proliferating cells incorporated more thymidine label than those in confluent cultures.

B. Glycoproteins and Oligosaccharides

The results of a 24-hr labeling of SMC in both phases of growth with either [^{3}H] Pro or [^{3}H] Man are summarized in Table 1. The cell cultures were divided into three compartments: the medium, the detergent soluble cell layer, and the insoluble matrix remaining attached to the culture flask. As indicated in column B, the level of [^{3}H] Pro incorporation was similar in all three compartments from both types of cultures. The amount of [^{3}H] Man (Table 1, column C) was consistently higher in all three compartments from proliferating than those of confluent cultures; the largest difference was present in the soluble cell fractions.

The nature of the oligos attached to the matrix secreted by both phases of cell growth were determined by several biochemical techniques.[37] The addition of the antibiotic tunicamycin, which specifically interferes with oligosynthesis,[38] resulted in a marked decrease in Man incorporation, and the level of inhibition was greater in proliferating cultures. Glycoprotein preparations were analyzed by affinity chromatography on concanavalin A-Sepharose columns which "recognize" oligos with Man residues on the nonreducing termini or substituted in their carbon 2 positions.[39,40] The results indicated that greater amounts of label from proliferating cultures were retained by the columns than from confluent cells.

Endoglycosidases (endo) were also used to characterize the mannose-labeled oligos in matrix glycoproteins. Endo H and endo D remove simple and complex oligos, respectively.[41-43] The oligomannosyl cores generated by endo treatment of glycopeptides were analyzed by molecular seiving, and the size differences are summarized in Table 2. The oligomannosyl cores derived from endo H digestion of glycopeptides from proliferating cultures consisted of eight to ten carbohydrates; those from confluent cultures were smaller and averaged four to six carbohydrates. The endo D-derived oligomannosyl cores from preparations obtained from proliferating cultures contained primarily small-core, four to six carbohydrates and small amounts of large-core subunits. On the other hand, endo D-derived preparations from confluent cultures contained larger amounts of large core subunits (15%) than the smaller cores (10%). Similar amounts of glycopeptides remained in the high-molecular-weight region after both endo treatments. In general, therefore, the matrix from proliferating cultures contains

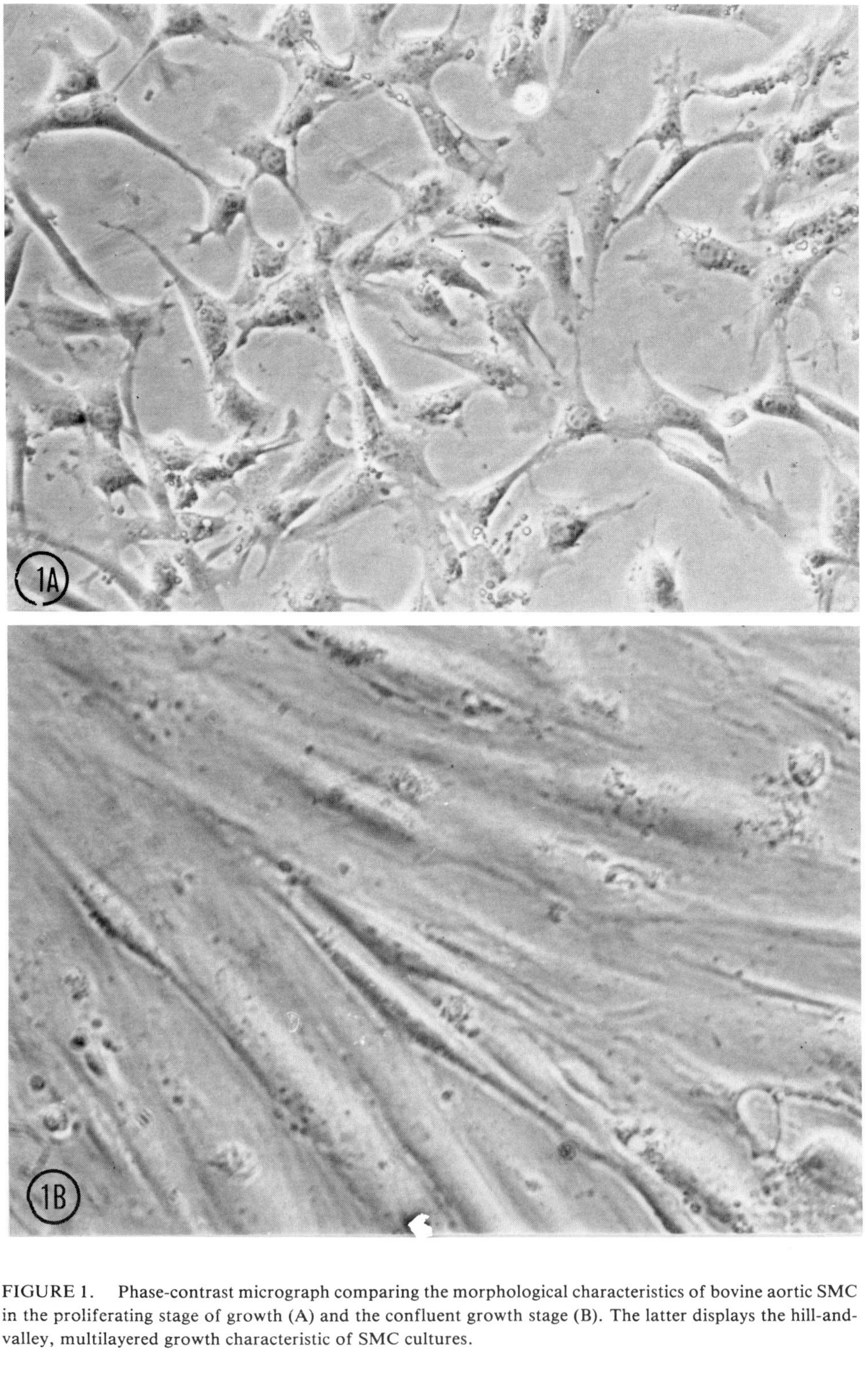

FIGURE 1. Phase-contrast micrograph comparing the morphological characteristics of bovine aortic SMC in the proliferating stage of growth (A) and the confluent growth stage (B). The latter displays the hill-and-valley, multilayered growth characteristic of SMC cultures.

Table 1
THE INCORPORATION OF [^{3}H] THYMIDINE, [^{3}H] PROLINE, AND [^{3}H] MANNOSE INTO COMPONENTS SYNTHESIZED BY PROLIFERATING AND CONFLUENT SMC IN CULTURE

	A Thymidine (dpm × 10/ mg protein)	B Proline (dpm × 10/ mg protein)	C Mannose (dpm × 10/ mg protein)
Proliferating SMC			
Medium		5.0	1.89
Cell layer	1.6	0.75	5.4
Insoluble matrix		0.58	2.08
Confluent SMC			
Medium		4.5	1.4
Cell layer	0.4	0.68	2.2
Insoluble matrix		0.41	0.86

Note: Mean values based on the level of incorporation in three identical flasks.

Table 2
SIZE DIFFERENCES[a] IN THE OLIGOMANNOSYL CORES DERIVED FROM ENDOGLYCOSIDASE TREATMENT OF CLYCOPEPTIDES FROM THE EXTRACELLULAR MATRIX OF SMC IN DIFFERENT PHASES OF GROWTH

	Endo H-sensitive (carbohydrate size)			Endo D-sensitive (carbohydrate size)		
Glycopeptide preparation	8—10	4—6	>10[b]	8—10	4—6	>10
Proliferating cells	24%	10%	66%	5%	30%	65%
Confluent cells	11%	19%	70%	15%	10%	75%

[a] Based on chromatographic analyses on Bio Gel P 4.[37]

[b] The oligosaccharides resistant to the endo cleavage were grouped in the fraction designated 10 carbohydrates.

higher amounts of large-core, endo H-sensitive oligos, and confluent cells have higher amounts of large-core, endo D-sensitive oligos.

The glycoproteins of the matrix from both phases of cell growth were radiolabeled with Man and separated on the basis of molecular weight. The overall pattern of glycoproteins synthesized by both phases of growth was similar. Profiles representative of either culture type are presented in Figure 2. Matrix components separated by polyacrylamide gel electrophoresis are presented in panel A (Figure 2), and similar preparations analyzed on gel permeation columns are shown in panel B (Figure 2). Several glycoproteins were observed by both methods ranging in molecular weight from under 20 kdaltons (band 10, panel A: peak at fraction 42, panel B) to over 500 kdaltons (band 1, panel A: peak at fraction 15, panel B). Whereas qualitatively the pattern of glycoproteins were similar in both phases of growth, the individual components differed with respect to their endo sensitivity.[37] The interstitial procollagens (Figure 2, panel A,

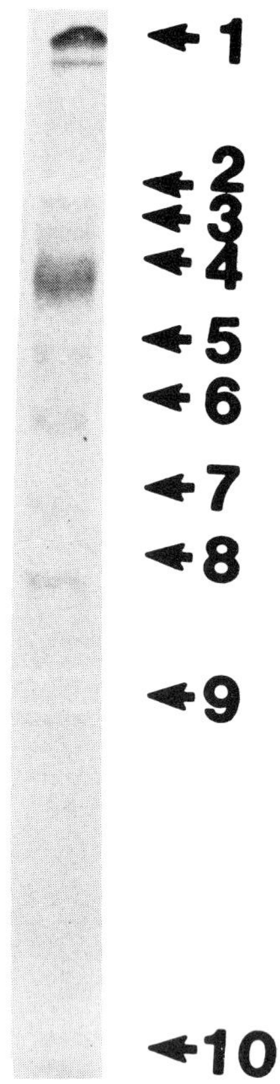

A

FIGURE 2. Slab gel electrophoresis of the Man-labeled glycoproteins associated with the insoluble matrix of SMC cultures. After deoxycholate treatment (0.5%) to remove soluble, cell-related components, the matrix was solubilized and analyzed on a 7.5% polyacrylamide slab gel. Glycoproteins were visualized by fluorography. At least ten bands of incorporation were evident and ranged in size from under 20 kdaltons (band 10) to over 500 kdaltons (band 1). The position of fibronectin (band 4) and the interstitial procollagens (band 5) were determined from the migration of standard glycoproteins under similar conditions. (B) Gel permeation chromatography of [^{3}H]-Man-labeled (open circles) and [^{35}S]-Met-labeled (closed circles) glycoproteins associated with the extracellular matrix of SMC. Components were analyzed on a 1.5 × 150-cm-column in a buffer containing 5 *M* urea. Molecular weight estimates were determined on the basis of elution volumes of glycoproteins with known molecular weights.

band 5) and fibronectin (Figure 2, panel A, band 4) were the Man-labeled components in these preparations. The other macromolecules corresponded to a class of components termed "structural glycoproteins".[12] Whereas the existence of Man-containing glycoproteins in the SMC matrix has been questioned by some,[44] our data support the concept of a distinct structural glycoprotein class in this context. Moreover, the results suggest that the transition from rapid growth to confluency (i.e., slow growth) in SMC cultures generally does not involve major qualitative changes in the extracellular glycoprotein. However, in accordance with previous studies employing other cell types,[33,34] our data support the contention that differences in the synthesis and/or processing of the oligos attached to components in the pericellular matrix are correlated with the state of growth of the SMC.[37]

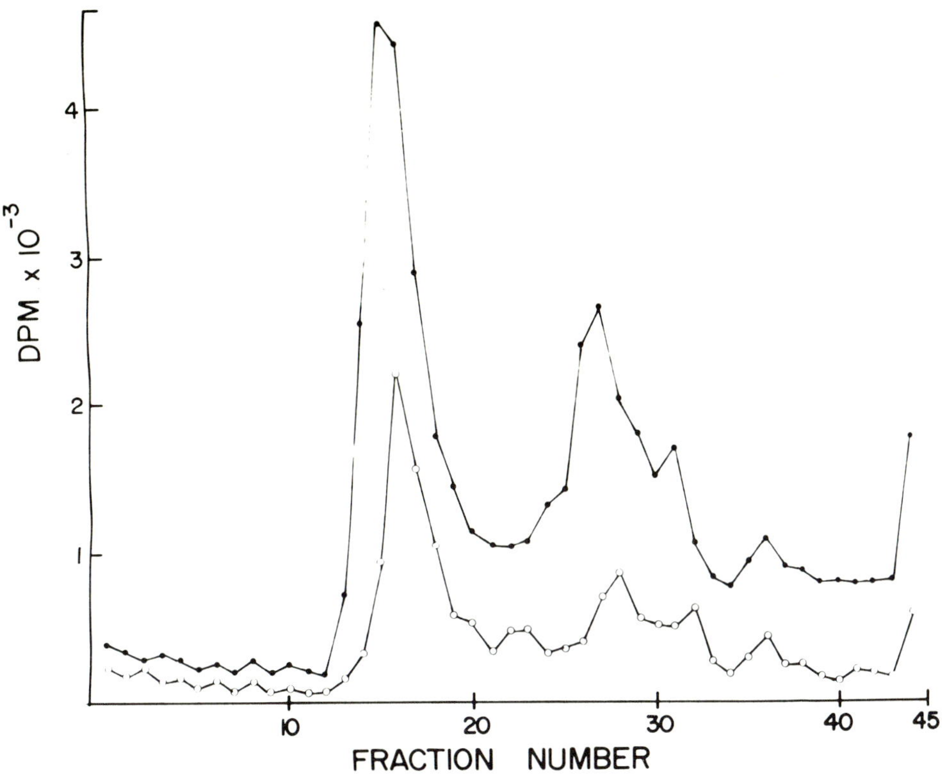

FIGURE 2B.

C. Intermediate and Interstitial Collagen Synthesis

Collagens associated with detergent extracts of the cellular layer or from the medium were routinely purified on DEAE cellulose to obtain interstitial and type V procollagen fractions using routine procedures.[23,45,46]

The simple oligos of many glycoproteins such as fibronectin[48] are converted to the complex type by the elimination of glucose and mannose residues. Subsequently, elongation takes place in the Golgi apparatus (with the addition of *N*-acetylglucosamine, galactose, sialic acid, and fucose) prior to the transportation to the cell membrane.[38,43] However, the data presented in Table 3 suggest that the oligos associated with the interstitial collagens (types I and III) are endo H-sensitive (simple or high mannose type) also after secretion from the cell, in analogy to observations made with other cell types.[20,47] In contrast to the interstitial procollagens the oligos attached to the type V procollagens were both endo H- and endo D-sensitive, suggesting that some processing had occurred already. Gel filtration (Figure 3) confirmed that endo D was primarily releasing oligos from these preparations, and all the products eluted as two major peaks in the region as expected for these carbohydrates.

Type V collagen may be deposited in the matrix as a procollagen without cleavage of the terminal extensions in a manner analogous to type IV.[49,50] Therefore, the oligos may play a role in determining the fate of the noncollagenous propeptides. The presence of endo D-sensitive oligos may prevent cleavage of the type V propeptides, while the simple oligos on the interstitial propeptides may "signal" their removal by the specific peptidases. Alternatively, the differences between the oligo content of the propeptides of the interstitial and type V collagens may be due to the presence of the unique P peptide that has been observed to be attached to type V procollagen during

Table 3
ENDOGLYCOSIDASE TREATMENT OF PROCOLLAGENS SECRETED BY SMC IN CULTURE

	Percent label released by Endo H		Percent label released by Endo D	
	Proliferating	Confluent	Proliferating	Confluent
Pro type V	48.9	40.2	25.6	31.2
Pro type I and III	59.0	45.6	4.6	5.2

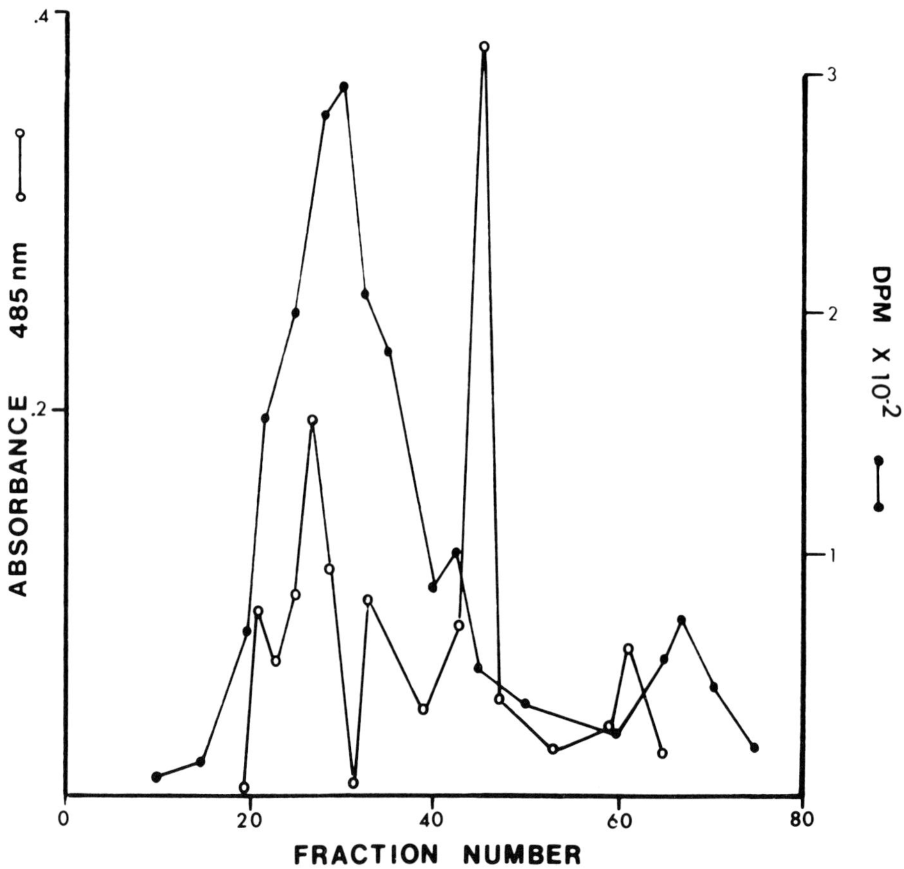

FIGURE 3. Gel filtration of endo D-cleaved oligos from type V procollagen. Solid circles represent label released, while the open circles depict the elution profile of pronase-derived carbohydrates from standard aortic type IV collagen. The peak at fraction 27 represents the oligo-sized components.

secretion.[50] Since differences were also observed in the levels of endo H- and endo D-sensitive oligos attached to type V between proliferating and confluent cultures (see Table 3), these components may be involved in determining the fate of this collagen during changes in the growth and interactions of cells. This collagen has been shown to play a role in cell proliferation and movement, and it is possible that its oligo composition is variable, pending the status of the cells.[51]

III. INTERACTION BETWEEN TYPE V COLLAGEN AND THE SMC SURFACE

A. Surface Glycoconjugates

At the ultrastructural level SMC in culture may be shown to be associated with a fairly well-defined BM (Figure 4). It was shown that the BM consists of a relatively lucent inner zone adjacent to the cell membrane, a poorly defined midzonal fibrillar network, and an outermost dense or compact zone. Fine discrete fibrils often are present within and account for the filamentous nature of the BM when it is cut tangentially.[52] Immunohistochemical observations suggest that these fibrils may be primarily type V collagen, which forms an extensive pericellular coat over the outer surface of the BM adjacent to the interstitial matrix.[53-55] It was also shown by immunohistochemical methods that this collagen was distributed on the surface of the SMC in such a way as to form a three-dimensional lattice anchoring the cell to the interstitial collagen matrix. Therefore, type V collagen seems to serve as a binding or connecting collagen linking the interstitial collagen fibers to the structures of the BM.[22,25]

Type V collagen covers the cell surface penetrating the BM at sites where it attaches to the plasma membrane at specific glycoconjugate receptors.[56] This form of direct-membrane interaction appears to be a unique property of the type V collagen since other classes of collagen interact with the cell surface by means of glycoprotein intermediaries, i.e., fibronectin for the interstitial and laminin for the BM collagens.[16,25] In addition to these two well characterized glycoprotein classes, several other polypeptides are thought to be involved in cell-collagen interactions, but the exact nature of these substances is not known.[57-61] The direct binding of type V collagen to the plasma membrane suggests that the biological function of this collagen differs, at least in some aspects, from that of the other collagens.

Deducing from the above, it was reasonable to assume that several independent systems were involved in SMC interaction with any one collagen. Therefore, several components at the surface of SMC involved in attachment to type V collagen have been investigated in our laboratories.[62] Our studies suggest that at least two surface glycoproteins on the SMC are either involved in binding type V directly or in a "cooperative" fashion in conjunction with a glycolipid. These studies were carried out according to procedures published by other workers.[56] Table 4 shows that the primary type V collagen-attachment system at the surface of SMC is probably a glycolipid since it was neuraminidase-sensitive and occurred even when protein synthesis was inhibited. However, in our system slightly elevated concentrations of cycloheximide (20 $\mu g/m\ell$ compared to 10 $\mu g/m\ell$)[56] caused a significant decrease in the final numbers of cells attached to type V collagen (approximately 25%). Moreover, the treatment with endo H resulted in a 20% decrease in binding, whereas that with endo D had no effect.

The nature of this cycloheximide-dependent system was determined by electrophoretic analyses of preparations of crude plasma membranes from radiolabeled cultures [^{35}S] methionine of [^{3}H] Man). Characteristic densitometric profiles are presented in Figure 5. Glycoprotein synthesis was compared in cells which were labeled in the process of attaching to a type V substrate and those grown on plastic (Figure 5, panels A and D, respectively). In general, the patterns of the major methionine (panels A and D) and Man-labeled (panels B and E) glycoproteins from the two culture types were comparable both in terms of numbers and positions (compare peaks 1 to 10 in panels A and D and peaks 1′ to 12′ in panels B and E). The components within the Man-labeled preparations that selectively bound to affinity columns composed of type V collagen attached to Sepharose were analyzed under similar conditions (Figure 5, panels C and E). Four peaks corresponding to glycoproteins were isolated from both culture types and corresponded to molecular weights of 50, 80, 180, and 200 kdaltons.

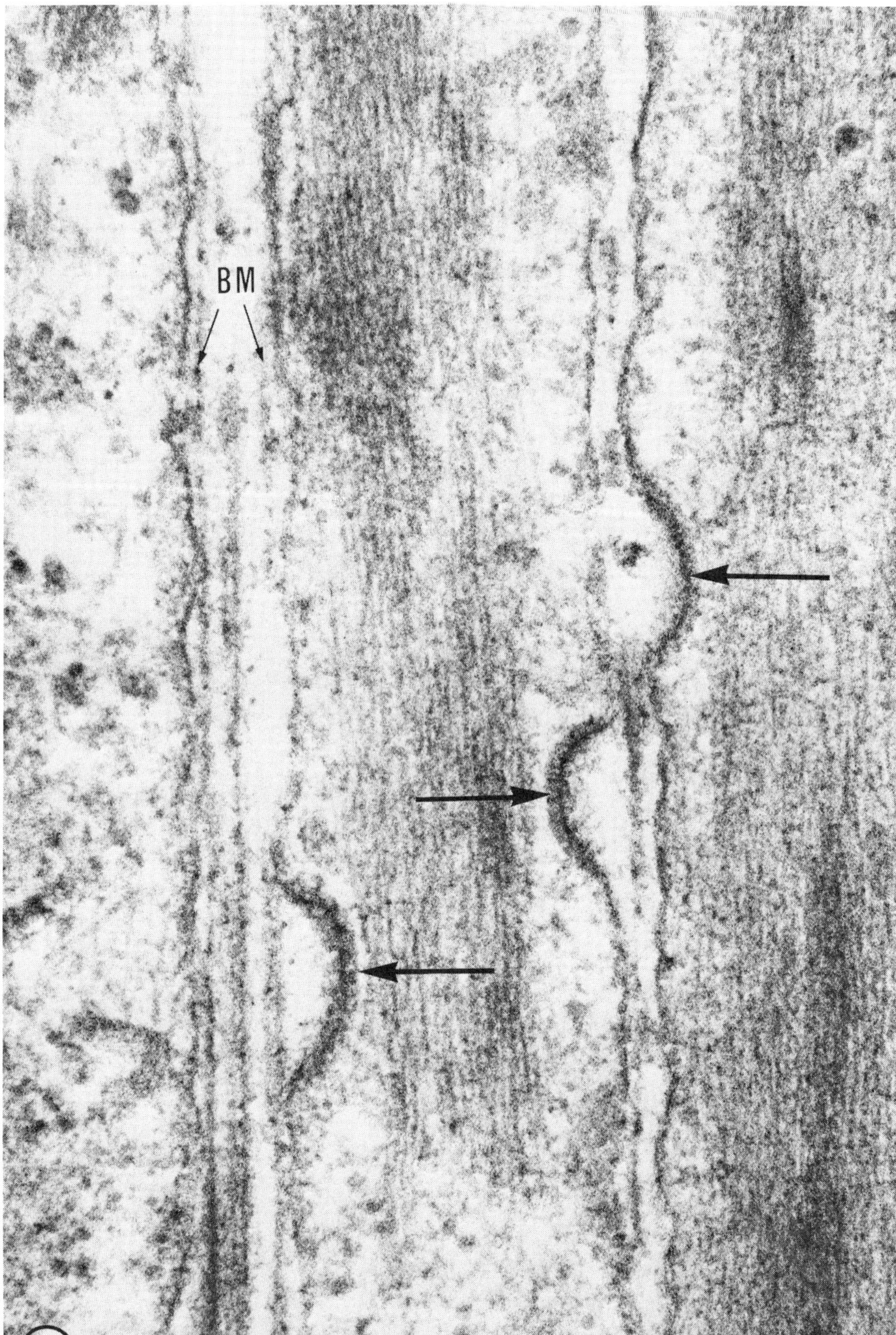

FIGURE 4A. Electron micrograph of a section through the "hill" of an early confluent (stationary) phase of bovine SMC in culture (ascorbate untreated). Complete or incomplete basement membranes (BM, small arrows) are adjacent to each of the three cells. Prominent Porter pits (large arrows) "open" in two of three instances, opposite a segment of a basement membrane. (Magnification × 100,000.)

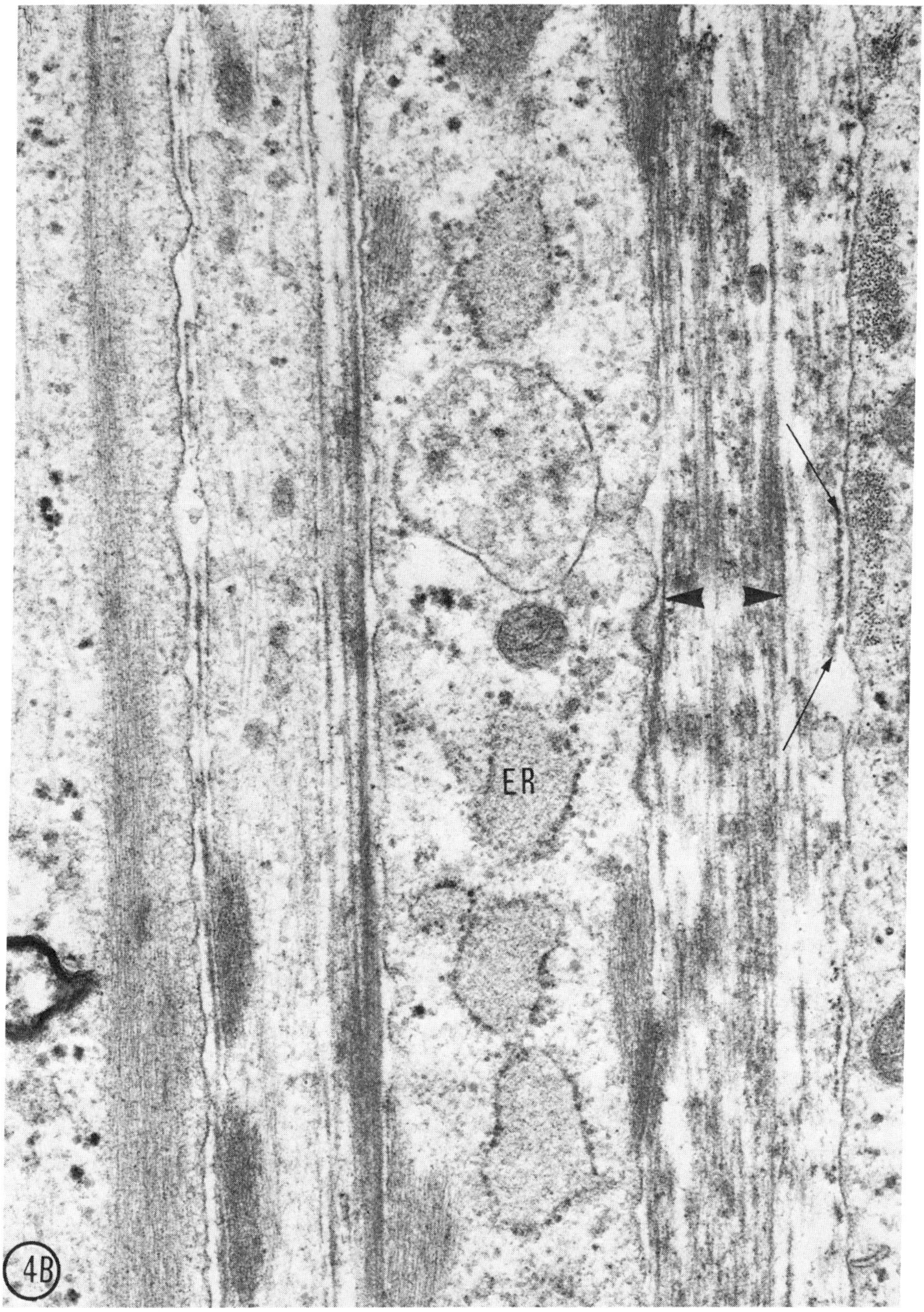

FIGURE 4B. Tissues as in Figure 4A but at a later stage in culture. The parallel-arranged SMC are in various stages of development, some containing longitudinal tracts (extreme left) or peripheral densities (=aggregates) (second cell from left) of myofilaments, whereas others are largely secretory with dilated profiles of rough surface endoplasmic reticulum (ER). Note that the intercellular space contains now more abundant basement membrane-like substance than that depicted in Figure 4A, but it is uncertain whether the ''fibrils'' in the space indicated (between two arrowheads) represent extracellular fibrils or remnants of (?tangential section through) a cell. Note that some segments of basement membranes appear ''beaded'' as if reflecting a cross-section through its constituent fibrils (between two arrows). (Magnification × 38,000.)

Table 4
THE EFFECT OF VARIOUS PRETREATMENTS ON BOVINE AORTIC SMC BINDING TO TYPE V COLLAGEN SUBSTRATES

Pretreatment[a]	Percentage[b] cells attached
None	76 ± 3.0
PBS	72 ± 4.0
Endo H	53 ± 2.6
Neuraminidase	31 ± 5.1
Endo H + neuraminidase	12 ± 3.8
Endo D	68 ± 4.8
Endo D + neuraminidase	33 ± 3.5
Cycloheximide[c] (20 μg/mℓ)	51 ± 4.4

[a] All enzymatic treatments were carried out immediately before attachment assay, as outlined.[62].

[b] The means ± SEM were computed from four independent determinations.

[c] Cycloheximide was present after trypsin/EDTA treatment and during attachment testing. This value is significantly smaller than that for nontreated cells with a *p*-value of 0.001 as determined by student's *t*-test.

The level of label associated with the 50- and 80-kdalton glycoproteins isolated from attaching cultures was consistently greater than that observed in cells grown independent of a type V collagen substrate. These type V collagen-binding components were also analyzed by gel permeation high-performance liquid chromatography (HPLC) (Figure 6). The 50- and 80-kdalton peaks both contained methionine and mannose label, had an affinity for concanavalin A, and were endo H-sensitive.

One of the type V collagen-binding glycoprotein fractions was similar in size (Figure 6, fraction 12, 200 kdaltons) to fibronectin, reacted to antibody against this protein, and had an ability to bind to several different collagens. Fibronectin has been shown to have this affinity for collagens, including the type V.[63] It could be expected to be present in the extracts reported herein primarily because it serves as the element of attachment for the SMC interaction with the interstitial collagens.[56] Some of the material in the 180 kdaltons (Figure 6, fraction 15) reacted to fibronectin antibody, but most of it was thought to be related to thrombospondin, which also has an affinity for type V collagen and is produced by SMC in culture.[64]

The 50-kdalton component had several features in common with another group of plasma membrane-associated glycoproteins which have been implicated in endodermal cell binding to collagen.[61] This class of molecules contained a 47-kdalton glycoprotein which not only shared a similarity to the 50-kdalton species because of its size, but also contained endo H-sensitive carbohydrates and selectively attached to a native undenatured type IV collagen substrate.[61] This 47-kdalton component was termed "colligin,"[61] and our studies suggest that molecules of this size may be common mediators of cell-collagen interactions. Support for this contention is provided by the findings that platelets attach themselves to type I collagen by means of a 65-kdalton species.[60] Moreover, a 47-kdalton, gelatin-binding component has been isolated from serum,[65] and a polypeptide of this size has been observed attached to fibronectin in hamster

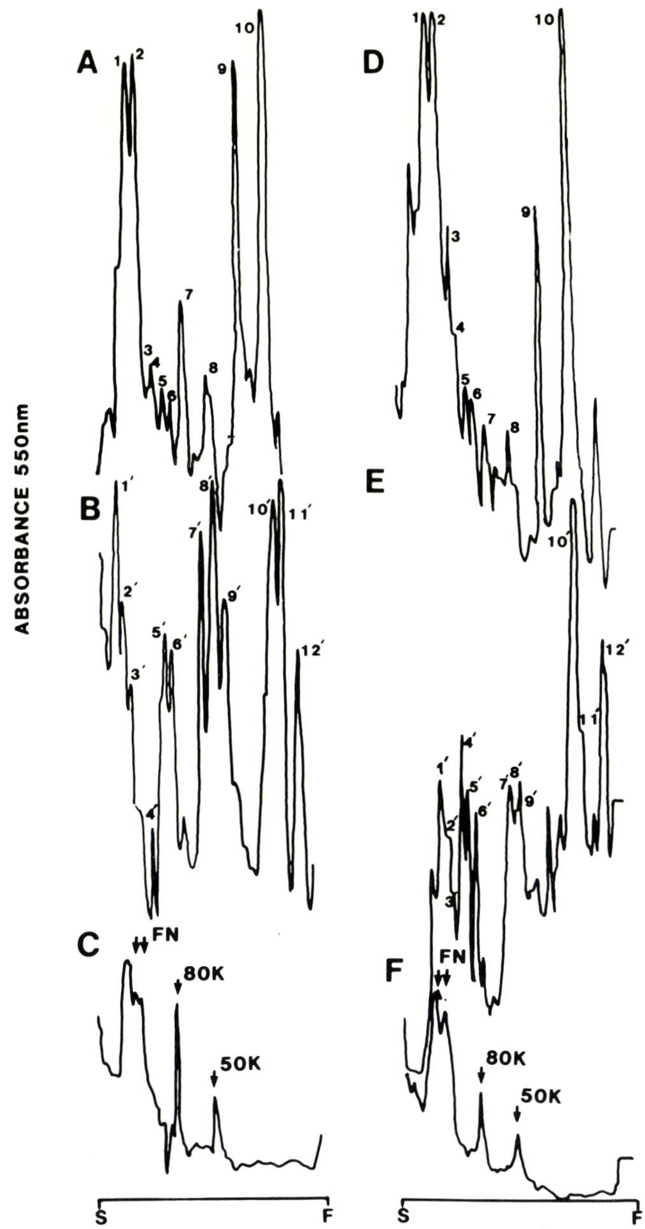

FIGURE 5. Slab gel electrophoresis of putative plasma membrane proteins from SMC labeled with [^{35}S] Met or [^{3}H] Man. After electrophoresis, the proteins were visualized by fluorography and subsequently scanned using an EC densitometer at 550 nm. Representative profiles obtained from cells attached to type V collagen are presented in panels A (Met-labeled, peaks 1 to 10) and B (Man-labeled, peaks 1′ to 12′). For comparison, similar preparations from SMC that had grown independent of type V substrates are presented in panels D (Met-labeled, peaks 1 to 10) and E (Man-labeled, peaks 1′ to 12′). Panels C and F represent the electrophoretic profiles of components contained in the preparations shown in panels A and D which were selectively retained by type V-Sepharose. The positions of fibronectin in panels C and F (arrows, FN), 80- and 50-kdalton glycoproteins, are indicated. The start (S) and dye front (F) of the gels are also indicated. Reproduced with permission of the National Research Council of Canada (re: Ref. 62).

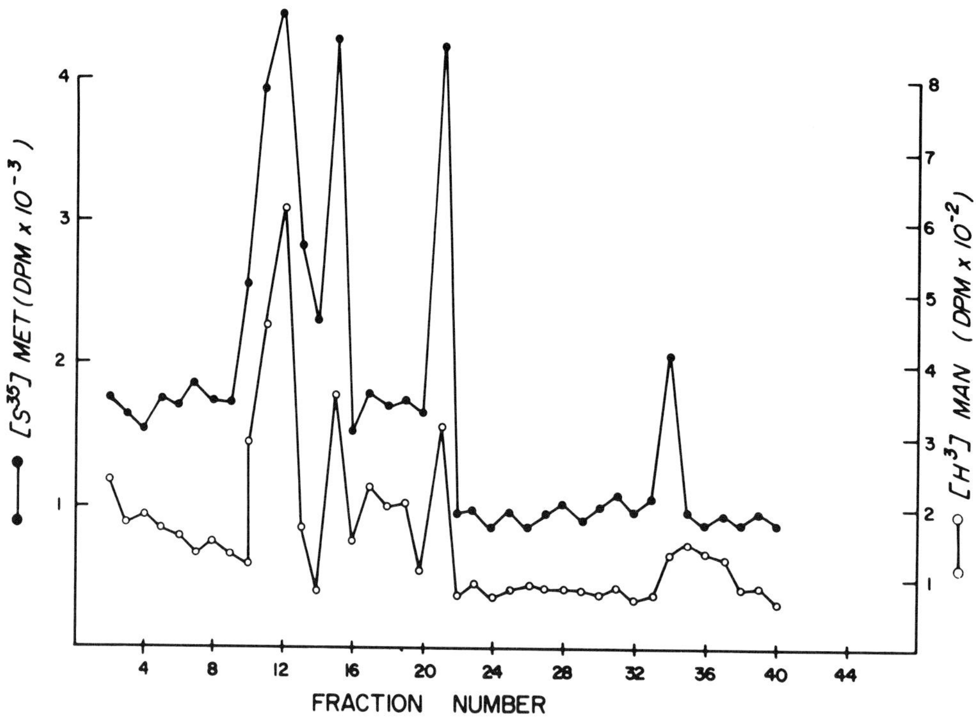

FIGURE 6. HPLC-elution profile of SMC-membrane glycoproteins selectively retained by affinity chromatography on type V collagen Sepharose shows that Met-labeled (closed circles) and Man-labeled (open circles) substances are both present in a given fraction. Molecular weight estimates based on the elution volumes of standard proteins indicated that the peaks at fractions 12, 15, and 21 correspond to molecular weights of 200, 180, and 50 kdaltons, respectively. The material eluting between fractions 16 and 20 had a mean molecular weight of 80 kdaltons (fraction 18). Reproduced with permission of the National Research Council of Canada (re: Ref. 62).

BHK cells.[66] Components similar in size to the 80-kdalton species have also been implicated in the binding of other cell types to collagen.[58,59]

Type V collagen consists of a helix composed of two dissimilar chains: (1) two $\alpha 1(V)$ chains and (2) one $\alpha 2(V)$ chain.[23] Previously, the type Vα2 chain was shown to contain the attachment region for SMC.[56] In our studies, cyanogen bromide peptides from radiolabeled type V chains were tested for their ability to bind to and promote SMC adhesion (Figure 7). They showed that the binding region is probably within the cyanogen bromide fragment 6 of this chain.[67,68] This fragment has a nonspecific amino acid composition which is a feature of these cell-attaching fragments such as the αCB 7 peptide of the $\alpha 1(I)$ chain.[69] Direct comparison between these fragments is difficult because the latter is almost three times the size of type V, α2, CB 6.

B. Function Significance of Type V Collagen — A Role in Force Transference?

As outlined above, type V collagen has a unique distribution in the extracellular matrix,[22,53] especially at the surface of SMC and interacts with the cell with two distinct attachment systems.[62] These data suggest that its function in the matrix may be more than strictly of a structural nature.[70] A "collagenous net" has been suggested to play a role in the force transference of SMC,[71] and its existence was confirmed by ultrastructural studies.[72,73] According to this hypothesis, an SMC, after stimulation, actively increases in diameter, placing tension on the surrounding interstitial collagen fibers (in the same manner that the Chinese finger trap works). The stressed connective tissue

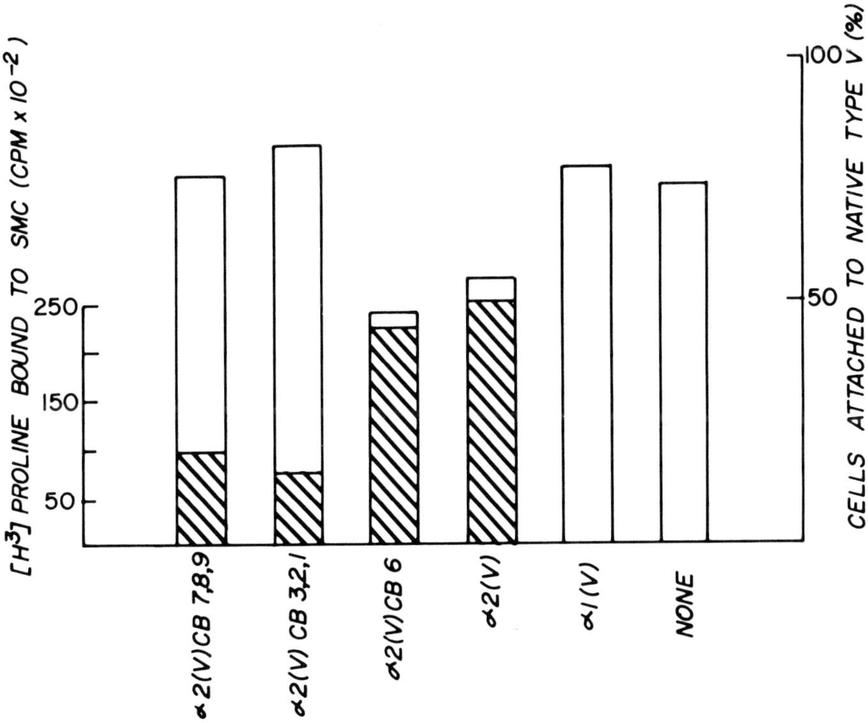

FIGURE 7. Histogram showing the percentage cells attached to type V collagen in the presence of collagen α chains and peptides from the same collagen (open bars). When these test components were radiolabeled, the amount of radioactivity associated with the cells was determined, as indicated by the cross-hatched bars. (From Leushner, J. R. A. and Haust, M. D., *Can. J. Biochem. Cell. Biol.*, in press, 1985. Reproduced with permission of the National Research Council of Canada.)

transmits force to the load. It is unlikely that the interstitial collagen fibers of types I and III[74,75] play an active role in this system. These latter fibers possess the characteristic properties generally ascribed to collagen; namely, high tensile strength, lack of extensibility, and structural stability. Therefore, the interstitial collagens probably play a relatively passive structural role in the process. On the other hand, data suggest that type V collagen is a major structural component of this "collagenous net". Since the arrangement of type V collagen may be envisaged as a latticework of pliable filaments, the original designation of this collagen as an exoskeleton[52] does not seem appropriate. This term may be better applied to the encompassing fibers of the interstitial collagens.

IV. TYPE VI COLLAGEN? A COMMON DENOMINATOR FOR COLLAGEN AND ELASTIC TISSUE

It was demonstrated that focal, tight, and relatively inflexible binding sites exist between SMC and the elastic laminae.[72,73] These appear to assure overall coordination of configurational changes between cell groups and elastic systems and to prevent slippage of cell layers. The material involved at these binding sites is probably a BM collagen. This was deduced from ultrastructural studies,[76,77] which have shown a spatial relation between the developing connective tissues and the BM of the SMC. In the original study,[76] elastic units were often observed to be attached to the BM of the SMC, and this appeared to be similar to that of the BM. Type III collagen has been shown to

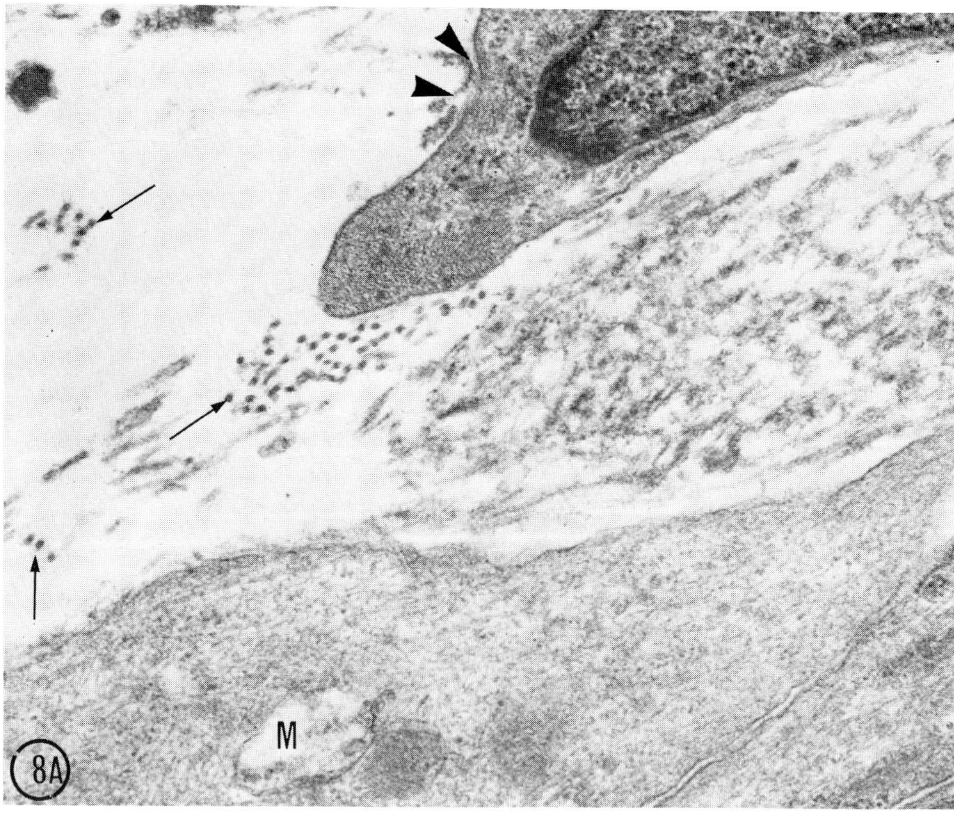

A

FIGURE 8(A). Electron micrograph of proliferative phase of SMC in culture with added ascorbate. Collagen fibrils (arrows) intermingled with fine and short fibrils are present in the intercellular space. Note the "beaded" short segment (between arrowheads) of the basement membrane of uppermost SMC. (M) poorly preserved mitochondrion. (Magnification × 30,000.) (B) Tissues as in Figure 8A. The collagen "bundle", indicated by an arrow, developed in close vicinity to an invagination of plasma membrane (of the SMC). Note that plasma membrane and the immediately adjacent cytoplasm opposite the developing collagen "bundle" is electron-opaque. The collagen fibrils are of varying and small diameter. The basement membrane "trailing" the cell (upper right corner, between the two arrowheads) has a "beaded" appearance. Much of this cell is otherwise not surrounded by a basement membrane. (Magnification × 90,000.)

be condensed at these attachment sites.[78] It is conceivable that type V filaments also terminate at these locations. The exact nature of the interaction of the cell with the elastin complexes remains unknown, but recent evidence has implicated a member of the intermediate class of collagens, particularly the type VI collagen, in this interaction.[79,80] Our observations suggest that in culture, type VI collagen is secreted in a form that shares characteristics with both type VI collagen and those of the aortic microfibrils.[24a,81]

A. Ultrastructural Analysis

In the absence of ascorbic acid, SMC secrete decreased amounts of the interstitial procollagens, while the production of glycoproteins (such as the microfibrillar component) increases.[26,81] At the ultrastructural level, ascorbate-treated (Figure 8) and untreated (Figure 9) cultures displayed marked differences. In the presence of ascorbate,

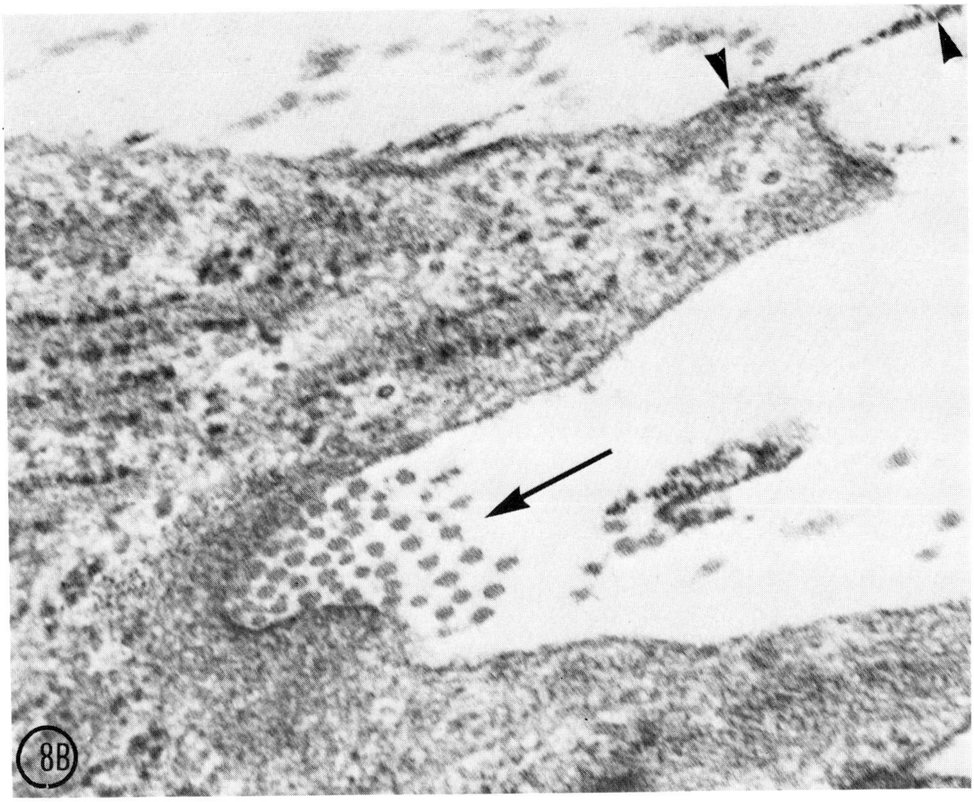

FIGURE 8B.

the extracellular spaces contained a considerable number of collagen fibrils (Figure 8), whereas, in its absence, microfibrillar (Figure 9) components dominated the field, and only a few collagen fibrils were observed on occasion.

B. Biochemical Analysis

Biochemical studies revealed that the secretion of the interstitial collagens decreased from 30 to 11% when ascorbate was omitted from the labeling media.[81] On the other hand, there was a concomitant increase in the more soluble collagenase-sensitive components in the 50% ammonium sulfate fraction in the absence of ascorbate. Several high-molecular-weight components could be demonstrated in this 50% fraction. Whereas the biochemical characteristics of type VI collagen have not been determined with certainty,[82-84] this collagen has several unique distinguishing features that are shared by the substance precipitating in the 50% ammonium sulfate fractions. These include:

1. It has a higher solubility than that of the other collagen types.[82,83]
2. In nonreduced form, it consists of high-molecular-weight aggregates, which, upon reduction, give rise to several low-molecular-weight polypeptides (from 30 to 70 kdaltons).[83]
3. Recent studies on a soluble form of this collagen suggest that these commonly found smaller chains may be derived from a 140-kdalton precursor.[85]

Our studies confirm that a 140-kdalton chain is associated with type VI collagen. They also indicate that it is very susceptible to proteolytic cleavage, being rapidly con-

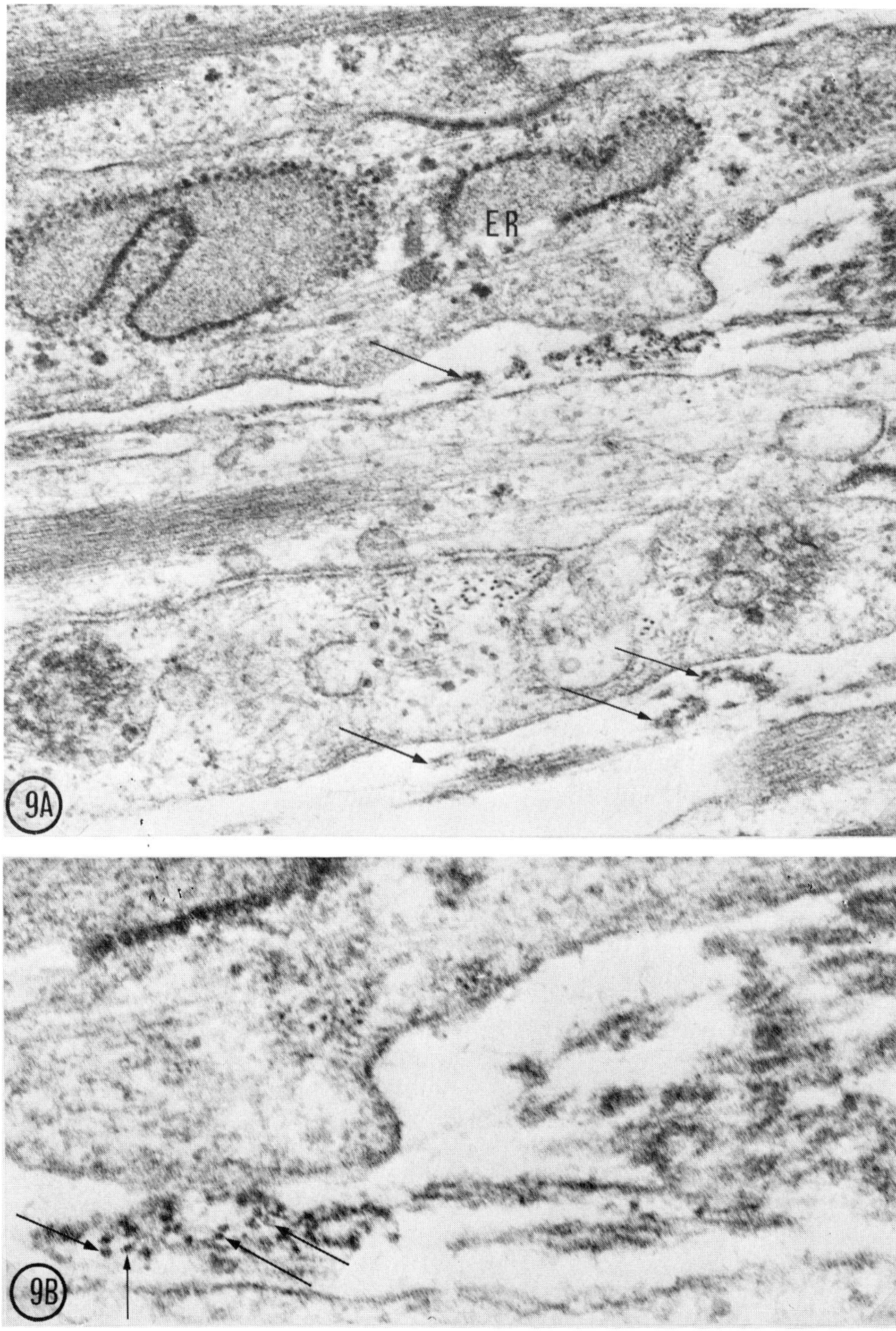

FIGURE 9(A). Electron micrograph of a "hill" of the confluent stationary phase of SMC in culture "untreated" with ascorbate. The cells are in various stages of differentiation and maturation, and some are in a distinctly secretory phase, with dilated profiles of endoplasmic reticulum (ER). No collagen fibrils are present. At this early stage, the intercellular space contains a modest number of microfibrils that appear to have a spatial relation to the cellular basement membrane (arrows). (Magnification × 40,000.) (B) Higher magnification of the area of and to the right indicated by the uppermost arrow in Figure 9B shows the microfibrils in cross- (arrows) and oblique (right half of photograph) cut. (Magnification × 80,000.)

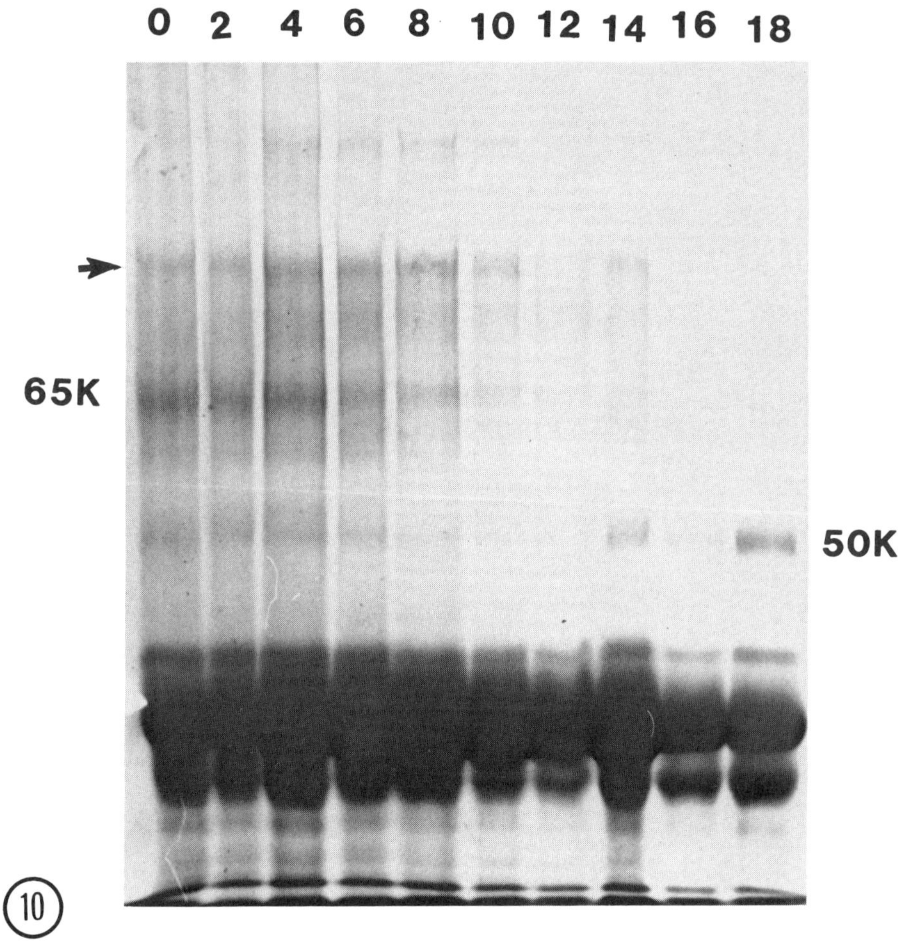

FIGURE 10. Slab gel electrophoresis of the 50% ammonium sulfate precipitate which had been incubated over an 18-hr interval in the absence of protease inhibitors. Aliquots of the sample were analyzed every 2 hr. The gradual disappearance of the 65- and 140-kdalton (arrow) chains with a concomitant increase in the 50-kdalton chain was apparent.

verted to smaller polypeptides in cultures. This is demonstrated by the experiment represented in Figure 10. The 50% ammonium sulfate precipitate (see previously) was incubated at room temperature in the absence of protease inhibitors for 16 hr, and aliquots were analyzed by electrophoresis at various times. A gradual decrease in the 140- (arrow) and 65-kdalton components and a concomitant increase in the smaller chains was evident with time. This protease sensitivity has been observed in previous studies on type VI collagen.[80]

It has been suggested once previously that low-molecular-weight collagens were produced by SMC in culture.[7] These polypeptides, designated CP 45, were assumed to be derived from BM and were present in equal proportions both in the medium and the cell layer. Whereas it is not possible to compare the components isolated in our own studies with the CP 45 because of limited information on the latter, it is tempting to postulate that they are the same or similar.

Other features of the collagen observed in our studies also indicate that it is type VI-like, e.g., the amino acid composition (see Table 5, column A). The high levels of hydroxyproline and hydroxylysine suggest that it is collagenous in nature, but features

Table 5
AMINO ACID COMPOSITION OF HIGH-MOLECULAR-WEIGHT COLLAGEN FROM SMC CULTURES[80,86]

Amino acid	A HMW-collagen	B Type VI	C Microfibril
4-HYP	37	39	26
ASP	92	102	102
THR	25	28	37
SER	38	47	45
GLU	102	93	117
PRO	93	76	64
GLY	227	243	179
ALA	80	51	69
CYS	30	23	57
VAL	36	37	18
MET	15	5	9
ILE	39	29	35
LEU	33	43	61
TYR	20	15	19
PHE	33	22	30
HYL	36	37	25
HIS	4	6	14
LYS	11	28	38
ARG	48	63	56

such as the low glycine levels and elevated amounts of half-cystine indicate noncollagenous sequences. These latter features are comparable to both: the published characteristics of type VI collagen (Table 5, column B) and the aortic microfibrillar component (Table 5, column C).

Recent electron microscopic examination of placental type VI collagen revealed its fibrillar nature,[79] which was similar to that of microfibrillar components of elastic tissue. These findings suggest that the type VI collagen and microfibrils of the extracellular space[24a] may be related. Moreover, the soluble form of microfibrils has been shown to be similar in size to the 140-kdalton type VI chain,[86,87] and our observations support this contention.

V. CLOSING COMMENTS

This report concerned recent work carried out in our laboratories on the isolation and characterization of glycoproteins and oligosaccharides associated with the extracellular matrix of bovine aortic SMC in culture. Two types of cell growth were distinguished during our studies: (1) a proliferative constantly growing phase and (2) a quiescent or confluent phase. Differences in composition and/or processing of oligosaccharides attached to the extracellular macromolecules were found depending upon the state of growth of the cell, including variation in size and sensitivity to endoglycosidases (endo). The endo H-sensitive oligomannosyl cores from the matrix of proliferating cells were larger than those associated with confluent cultures. On the other hand, the latter cells contained endo D-sensitive oligomannosyl residues which were larger than those from the matrix of proliferating cells. In the presence of ascorbic acid, procollagens and fibronectin were the major glycoproteins, while up to 11 other minor mannose-containing components were observed in the matrix secreted by both phases of the cell growth. Variation in the endo sensitivity was observed in several of the glycoproteins when the different cells were compared, especially with respect to the procollagens and fibronectin. Some of the variability in thc procollagen fraction was ascribed to procollagen type I, which, unlike the interstitial types, contained endo D-sensitive components.

Data indicate that SMC interaction with type V collagen may involve both glycolipid and glycoprotein components. The latter are 50,000 and 80,000 daltons in size, contain simple oligosaccharides, and bind preferentially to the cyanogen bromide number 6 of the $\alpha 2(V)$ chain. The observations on type V collagen were interpreted in terms of a hypothetical "collagenous net" theory. Evidence suggested that type V collagen was the major structural component of this net, and therefore type V collagen may be involved in force transference in the SMC function.

In the absence of added ascorbic acid, the SMC cultures secreted reduced amounts of interstitial collagens but produced a collagenous high-molecular-weight polypeptide complex into the media. Reduction of disulfide cross-links within this complex gave rise to a series of low-molecular-weight subunits comparable in size and composition to type VI collagen and sharing some features with the aortic microfibrils. These data were confirmed and correlated with the ultrastructural features of the extracellular components of SMC cultures.

SMC in culture synthesize a heterogeneous group of carbohydrate-containing proteins. The exact role of these components remains uncertain, primarily because of their diversity. It is by complex associations, possibly involving their carbohydrate side chains, that these macromolecules form diverse but integrated matrices. These vary in composition from the plasma membrane to the cell surface and finally to the intercellular space. Compositional differences in these substances are believed to be associated with functional changes that occur in the cell during adhesion, proliferation, and migration. Therefore, changes in the amounts and types of both the polypeptide and carbohydrate components of these macromolecules may play an important role in the physiological and pathological changes that occur in aorta. This complex interplay is exemplified by our observations on the interaction of the cell with type V collagen, as well as the possible shared identity of type VI collagen and microfibrillar components associated with elastic elements. Moreover, the unique characteristics of these macromolecules have necessitated a complete reevaluation of our concepts that collagens serve strictly as structural elements of either an interstitial or BM distribution. On the contrary, as more data accumulate on such components, e.g., the intermediate collagens, their functional roles will prove as diverse as their biochemical characteristics.

ACKNOWLEDGMENTS

This work was supported by a grant-in-aid T.3-11 from the Ontario Heart and Stroke Foundation, Toronto, Canada. The authors wish to thank Mrs. M. John and Mr. R. Dewar for their skillful technical assistance and Mrs. B. Gardiner and Ms. J. Balint for their efficient typing of the manuscript.

REFERENCES

1. Haust, M. D. and More, R. H., Significance of the smooth muscle cell in atherogenesis, in *Evolution of the Atherosclerotic Plaque,* Jones, R. J., Ed., University of Chicago Press, Chicago, 1963.
2. Haust, M. D., Atherosclerosis and smooth muscle cells, in *Biochemistry of Smooth Muscles,* Vol. 2, Stephens, N. L., Ed., CRC Press, Boca Raton, Fla., 1983, 189.

3. Boissel, J. P., Bourdillon, M. C., Loire, R., and Grouzet, B., Histological arguments for collagen and elastin synthesis by primary cultures of rat aortic media cells, *Atherosclerosis*, 25, 107, 1976.
4. Daoud, A. S., Fritz, K. E., Singh, J., Augustyn, J. M., and Jarmolych, J., Arterial mesenchyme and arteriosclerosis. Production of monosaccharides, collagen and elastic tissue by aortic medial explants, *Adv. Exp. Med. Biol.*, 43, 281, 1974.
5. Jarmolych, J., Daoud, A. S., Landau, J., Fritz, K. E., and McElvene, E., Aortic media explants. Cell proliferation and production of mucopolysaccarides, collagen and elastic tissue, *Exp. Mol. Pathol.*, 9, 171, 1968.
6. Schwatrz, E., Adamany, A. M., and Blumenfeld, O. O., Extracellular proteins of the calf aortic media smooth muscle cells in culture, *Biochim. Biophys. Acta*, 624, 531, 1980.
7. Mayne, R., Vail, M. S., and Miller, E. J., Characterization of the collagen chains synthesized by cultured smooth muscle cells derived from rhesus monkey thoracic aorta, *Biochemistry*, 17, 446, 1978.
8. Rauterberg, J., Allam, S., Brehmer, U., Wirth, W., and Hauss, W. H., Characterization of the collagen synthesized by cultured human smooth muscle cells from fetal and adult aorta, *Hoppe Seyler's Z. Physiol. Chem.*, 358, 401, 1977.
9. Scott, D. M., Harwood, R., Grant, M. E., and Jackson, D. S., Characterization of the major collagen species present in porcine aortae and the synthesis of their precursors by smooth muscle cells in culture, *Connect. Tissue Res.*, 5, 7, 1977.
10. Layman, D. L. and Titus, J. L., Synthesis of type I collagen by human smooth muscle cells in vitro, *Lab. Invest.*, 33, 103, 1975.
11. De Clerck, Y. A. and Jones, P. A., The effect of ascorbic acid on the nature of production of collagen and elastin by rat smooth muscle cells, *Biochem. J.*, 186, 217, 1980.
12. Jones, P. A., Scott-Burden, T., and Gevers, W., Glycoprotein, elastin and collagen secretion by rat smooth muscle cells, *Proc. Natl. Acad. Sci. U.S.A.*, 76, 353, 1979.
13. Kefalides, N. A., Basement membranes: structural and biosynthetic considerations, *J. Invest. Dermatol.*, 65, 85, 1975.
14. Bornstein, P. and Sage, H., Structurally distinct collagen types, *Annu. Rev. Biochem.*, 49, 957, 1980.
15. Ruoslahti, E., Engvall, E., and Hayman, E. G., Fibronectin: current concepts of its structure and function, *Collagen Rel. Res.*, 1, 95, 1981.
16. Kleinman, H. K., Klebe, R. J., and Martin, G. R., Role of collagenous matrices in the adhesion and growth of cells, *J. Cell Biol.*, 88, 473, 1981.
17. Timpl, R., Rohde, H., Gehron-Robey, P., Rennard, S. I., Foidart, J-M., and Martin, G. R., Laminin — a glycoprotein from basement membranes, *J. Biol. Chem.*, 254, 9933, 1979.
18. Foidart, J-M., Bere, E. W., Yaar, M., Rennard, S. I., Gullino, M., Martin, G. R., and Katz, S. I., Distribution and immunoelectron microscopic localization of laminin, a noncollagenous basement membrane glycoprotein, *Lab. Invest.*, 42, 336, 1980.
19. Robert, A. M., Robert, B., and Robert, L., Chemical and physical properties of structural glycoproteins, in *The Chemistry and Molecular Biology of the Intercellular Matrix*, Balazs, I., Ed., Academic Press, New York, 1970.
20. Clark, C. C., The distribution and initial characterization of oligosaccharide units on the COOH-terminal propeptide extensions of the Pro- 1 and Pro- 2 chains of type I procollagen, *J. Biol. Chem.*, 254, 10798, 1979.
21. Levine, M. J. and Spiro, R. G., Isolation from glomerular basement membrane of a glycopeptide containing both asparagine-linked and hydroxylysine-linked carbohydrate units, *J. Biol. Chem.*, 254, 8121, 1979.
22. Konomi, H., Hayashi, T., Nakayasu, K., and Arima, M., Localization of type V collagen and type IV collagen in human cornea, lung, and skin, *Am. J. Pathol.*, 116, 417, 1984.
23. Leushner, J. R. A. and Haust, M. D., Characterization of basement membrane collagens of bovine aorta, *Atherosclerosis*, 50, 11, 1984.
24. Poste, G. and Nicolson, G. L., Eds., *Cytoskeletal Elements and Plasma Membrane Organization*, North-Holland, Amsterdam, 1981.
24a. Haust, M. D., Fine fibrils of extracellular space (microfibrils). Their structure and role in connective tissue organization, *Am. J. Pathol.*, 47, 1113, 1965.
25. Hedman, K., Kurkinen, M., Alitalo, K., Vaheri, A., Johansson, S., and Hook, M., Isolation of the pericellular matrix of human fibroblast cultures, *J. Cell Biol.*, 81, 83, 1979.
26. Schwartz, E., Bienkowski, R. S., Coltoff-Schiller, B., Goldfischer, S., and Blumenfeld, O. O., Changes in the components of extracellular matrix and in growth properties of cultured aortic smooth muscle cells upon ascorbate feeding, *J. Cell Biol.*, 92, 462, 1982.
27. Gospodarowicz, D., Hirabayashi, K., Giguere, L., and Tauber, J. P., Factors controlling the proliferative rate, final cell density, and final life span of bovine vascular smooth muscle cells in culture, *J. Cell Biol.*, 89, 568, 1981.

28. Poste, G. and Nicolson, G. L., *Cell Surface Reviews*, Vol. 5, Elsevier, Amsterdam, 1978.
29. Alpin, J. D. and Hughes, R. C., Complex carbohydrates of the extracellular matrix structures, interactions and biological roles, *Biochim. Biophys. Acta*, 694, 375, 1982.
30. Subtelny, S. and Wessels, N. K., *The Cell Surface: Mediator of Developmental Processes*, Academic Press, New York, 1980.
31. Buck, C. A., Glick, M. C., and Warren, L., Effect of growth on the glycoproteins from the surface of control and Rous sarcoma-virus transformed hamster cells, *Biochemistry*, 10, 2176, 1971.
32. Ceccarini, C., Muramatsu, T., Tsang, J., and Atkinson, P. H., Growth-dependent alterations in oligomannosyl cores of glycopeptides, *Proc. Natl. Acad. Sci. U.S.A.*, 72, 3139, 1975.
33. Muramatsu, T., Koide, N., Ceccarini, C., and Atkinson, P. H., Characterization of mannose-labelled glycopeptides from human diploid cells and their growth-dependent alterations, *J. Biol. Chem.*, 251, 4673, 1976.
34. Sasak, W., Herscovics, A., and Quaroni, A., Cell-density-dependent changes in cell-surface glycopeptides and in adhesion of cultured intestinal epithelial cells, *Biochem. J.*, 201, 359, 1982.
35. Dennis, J., Waller, C., Timpl, R., and Schirrmacher, V., Surface sialic acid reduces attachment of metastatic tumour cells to collagen type IV and fibronectin, *Nature (London)*, 300, 274, 1982.
36. Görög, P. and Born, G. V. R., Increased uptake of circulating low-density lipoproteins and fibrinogen in arterial walls after removal of sialic acids from their endothelial surface, *Br. J. Exp. Pathol.*, 63, 447, 1982.
37. Leushner, J. R. A. and Haust, M. D., Oligosaccharides of matrix glycoproteins synthesized by cultured bovine aortic smooth muscle cells during various phases of growth, submitted for publication, 1985.
38. Staneloni, R. J. and Leloir, L. F., The biosynthetic pathway of the asparagine-linked oligosaccharides of glycoproteins, *CRC Crit. Rev. Biochem.*, 12(4), 289, 1982.
39. Baenziger, J. U. and Fiete, D., Structural determinants of concanavalin A specificity for oligosaccharides, *J. Biol. Chem.*, 254, 2400, 1979.
40. Narasimhan, S., Wilson, J. R., Martin, E., and Schachter, H., A structural basis for four distinct elution profiles on Concanavalin-A-Sepharose affinity chromatography of glycopeptides, *Can. J. Biochem.*, 57, 83, 1979.
41. Arakawa, M. and Muramatsu, T., Endo-*N*-acetylglucosaminidases acting on the carbohydrate moieties of glycoproteins. The differential specificities of the enzymes from Streptomyces griseus and Diplococcus pneumoniae, *J. Biochem. (Tokyo)*, 76, 307, 1974.
42. Varki, A. and Kornfeld, S., The spectrum of anionic oligosaccharides release by endo-*N*-acetylglucosaminidase H from glycoproteins, *J. Biol. Chem.*, 258, 2808, 1983.
43. Kornfeld, S., Li, E., and Tabas, I., The synthesis of complex-type oligosaccharides, *J. Biol. Chem.*, 253, 7771, 1978.
44. Bach, P. R. and Bentley, J. P., Structural glycoprotein, fact or artefact, *Connect. Tissue Res.*, 7, 185, 1980.
45. Sodek, J. and Limeback, H. F., Comparison of the rates of synthesis, conversion, and maturation of type I and type III collagens in rat periodontal tissues, *J. Biol. Chem.*, 254, 10496, 1979.
46. Kumamoto, C. A. and Fessler, J. H., Biosynthesis of A,B procollagen, *Proc. Natl. Acad. Sci. U.S.A.*, 77, 6434, 1980.
47. Anttinen, H., Oikarinen, A., Ryhanen, L., and Kivirikko, K. I., Evidence for the transfer of mannose to the extension peptides of procollagen within the cisternae of the rough endoplasmic reticulum, *FEBS Lett.*, 87, 222, 1978.
48. Choi, M. G. and Hynes, R. O., Biosynthesis and processing of fibronectin in NIL.8 hamster cells, *J. Biol. Chem.*, 254, 12050, 1979.
49. Narayanan, A. S. and Page, R. C., Biosynthesis and regulation of type V collagen in diploid human fibroblasts, *J. Biol. Chem.*, 258, 11694, 1983.
50. Fessler, L. I., Kumamoto, C. A., Meis, M. E., and Fessler, J. H., Assembly and processing of procollagen V (AB) in chick blood vessels and other tissues, *J. Biol. Chem.*, 256, 9640, 1981.
51. Stenn, K. S., Madri, J. A., and Roll, F. J., Migrating epidermis produces AB_2 collagen and requires continual collagen synthesis for movement, *Nature (London)*, 277, 229, 1979.
52. Haust, M. D., Connective tissue in atherosclerosis, in *Atherosclerosis IV*, Schettler, G., Goto, Y., Hata, Y., and Kose, G., Eds., Springer-Verlag, New York, 1977.
53. Gay, S., Martinez-Hernandez, A., Rhodes, R. K., and Miller, E. J., The collagenous exocytoskeleton of smooth muscle cells, *Collagen Rel. Res.*, 1, 377, 1981.
54. Linsenmayer, T. F., Fitch, J. M., Schmid, T. M., Zak, N. B., Gibney, E., Sanderson, R. D., and Mayne, R., Monoclonal antibodies against chicken type V collagen: production, specificity, and use for immunocytochemical localization in embryonic cornea and other organs, *J. Cell Biol.*, 96, 124, 1983.
55. Martinez-Hernandez, A., Gay, S., and Miller, E. J., Ultrastructural localization of type V collagen in rat kidney, *J. Cell Biol.*, 92, 343, 1982.

56. Grotendorst, G. R., Seppa, H. E. J., Kleinman, H. K., and Martin, G. R., Attachment of smooth muscle cells to collagen and their migration toward platelet-derived growth factor, *Proc. Natl. Acad. Sci. U.S.A.*, 78, 3669, 1981.
57. Yamada, K. M., Cell surface interactions with extracellular materials, *Annu. Rev. Biochem.*, 52, 761, 1983.
58. Vartio, T. and Vaheri, A., A gelatin-binding 70,000-dalton glycoprotein synthesized distinctly from fibronectin by normal and malignant adherent cells, *J. Biol. Chem.*, 256, 13085, 1981.
59. Vartio, T., Hovi, T., and Vaheri, A., Human macrophages synthesize and secrete a major 95,000 dalton gelatin binding protein distinct from fibronectin, *J. Biol. Chem.*, 257, 8862, 1982.
60. Chiang, T. M. and Kang, A. H., Isolation and purification of collagen 1(I) receptor from human platelet membrane, *J. Biol. Chem.*, 257, 7581, 1982.
61. Kurkinen, M., Taylor, A., Garrels, J. I., and Hogan, B. L. M., Cell surface-associated proteins which bind native type IV collagen or gelatin, *J. Biol. Chem.*, 259, 5915, 1984.
62. Leushner, J. R. A. and Haust, M. D., Glycoproteins on the surface of smooth muscle cells involved with their interaction with type V collagen, *Can. J. Biochem. Cell Biol.*, in press, 1985.
63. Engvall, E., Ruoslahti, E., and Miller, E. J., Affinity of fibronectin to collagens of different genetic types and to fibrinogen, *J. Exp. Med.*, 147, 1584, 1978.
64. Mumby, S. M., Raugi, G. J., and Bornstein, P., Interactions of thrombospondin with extracellular matrix proteins: selective binding to type V collagen, *J. Cell Biol.*, 98, 646, 1984.
65. Isemura, M., Sato, N., and Yosizawa, Z., Isolation and characterization of glycine-rich gelatin binding protein; a plasma glycoprotein which interacts with gelatin, arginine, heparin and hyaluronic acid, *J. Biol. Chem.*, 257, 14854, 1982.
66. Hughes, R. C., Butters, T. D., and Aplin, J. D., Cell surface molecules involved in fibronectin-mediated adhesion. A study using specific antisera, *Eur. J. Cell Biol.*, 26, 198, 1981.
67. Rhodes, R. K., Gibson, K. D., and Miller, E. J., Isolation and characterization of the cyanogen bromide peptides derived from the human $\alpha 2(V)$ collagen chain, *Biochemistry*, 20, 3117, 1981.
68. Miller, E. J., Rhodes, R. K., and Furuto, D. K., Identification of collagen chains as a function of cyanogen bromide peptide patterns using gel permeation high-performance liquid chromatography, *Collagen Rel. Res. Clin. Exp.*, 3, 79, 1983.
69. Kleinman, H. K., McGoodwin, E. B., Martin, G. R., Klebe, R. J., Fietzek, P. P., and Woolley, D. E., Localization of the binding site for cell attachment in the $\alpha(I)$ chain of collagen, *J. Biol. Chem.*, 253, 5642, 1978.
70. Leushner, J. R. A., Type V collagen and the transmission of forces in smooth muscle cell function: Dupuytren's disease as a model system, *J. Inferential Deductive Biol.*, in press, 1985.
71. Mullins, G. L. and Guntheroth, W. G., A collagen net hypothesis for force transference of smooth muscle, *Nature (London)*, 206, 592, 1965.
72. Wolinsky, H. and Glagov, S., Structural basis for the static mechanical properties of the aortic media, *Circ. Res.*, 14, 400, 1964.
73. Clark, J. M. and Glagov, S., Structural integration of the arterial wall. I. Relationships and attachments of the medial smooth muscle cells in normally distended and hyperdistended aortas, *Lab. Invest.*, 40, 587, 1979.
74. Trelstad, R. L., Human aorta collagens: evidence for three distinct species, *Biochem. Biophys. Res. Commun.*, 57, 717, 1974.
75. Chung, E. and Miller, E. J., Collagen polymorphism: characterization of molecules with the chain composition $[\alpha 1(III)]_3$ in human tissues, *Science*, 183, 1200, 1974.
76. Haust, M. D., More, R. H., Benscome, S. A., and Balis, J. U., Elastogenesis in human aorta: an electron microscopic study, *Exp. Mol. Pathol.*, 4, 508, 1965.
77. Leung, D. Y. M., Glagov, S., and Mathews, M. B., Elastin and collagen accumulation in rabbit ascending aorta and pulmonary trunk during postnatal growth. Correlation of cellular synthetic response with medial tension, *Circ. Res.*, 41, 316, 1977.
78. Gay, S., Balleisen, L., Remberger, K., Fietzek, P. P., Adelmann, B. C., and Kuhn, K., Immunohistochemical evidence for the presence of collagen type III in human arterial walls, arterial thrombi, and in leucocytes incubated with collagen in vitro, *Klin. Wochenschr.*, 53, 899, 1975.
79. Furthmayr, H., Widemann, H., Timpl, R., Odermatt, E., and Engel, J., Electron-microscopical approach to a structural model of intima collagen, *Biochem. J.*, 211, 303, 1983.
80. Odermatt, E., Risteli, J., VanDeldin, V., and Timpl, R., Structural diversity and domain composition of a unique collagenous fragment (intima collagen) obtained from human placenta, *Biochem. J.*, 211, 295, 1983.
81. Leushner, J. R. A. and Haust, M. D., The effect of ascorbate on the synthesis of the minor (non-interstitial) collagens by cultured bovine aortic smooth muscle cells, *Biochim. Biophys. Acta.*, in press, 1986.
82. Chung, E., Rhodes, R. K., and Miller, E. J., Isolation of three collagenous components of probable basement membrane origin from several tissues, *Biochem. Biophys. Res. Commun.*, 71, 1167, 1976.

83. Furuto, D. K. and Miller, E. J., Isolation of a unique collagenous fraction from limited pepsin digests of human placental tissue, *J. Biol. Chem.*, 255, 290, 1980.
84. Jander, R., Rauterberg, J., Voss, B., and vonBassewitz, D. B., A cysteine-rich collagenous protein from bovine placenta, *Eur. J. Biochem.*, 114, 17, 1981.
85. Jander, R., Troyer, D., and Rauterberg, J., A collagen-like glycoprotein of the extracellular matrix is the undegraded form of type VI collagen, *Biochemistry*, 23, 3675, 1984.
86. Gibson, M. A. and Cleary, E. G., A collagen-like glycoprotein from elastin-rich tissues, *Biochem. Biophys. Res. Commun.*, 105, 1288, 1982.
87. Sear, C. H. J., Grant, M. E., and Jackson, D. S., The nature of the microfibrillar glycoprotein of elastic fibers, *Biochem. J.*, 194, 587, 1981.

INDEX

A

B

C

F

G

H

I

K

L

M

R

S

T

U

V

W